Nephrology

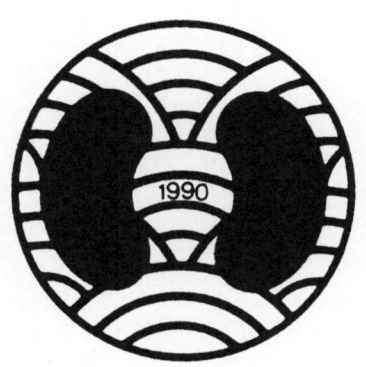

Nephrology VOLUME I

PROCEEDINGS OF THE
XIth INTERNATIONAL CONGRESS OF NEPHROLOGY

Editor
Michinobu Hatano

Associate Editors
Nishio Honda · Hyoe Ishikawa · Kenkichi Koiso
Kiyoshi Kurokawa · Tadao Niijima
Nobuhiro Sugino · Susumu Takahashi

With 253 Figures

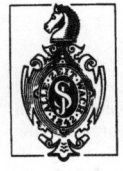

Springer Japan KK

Editor

MICHINOBU HATANO, M.D., Professor of Medicine, Director, Department of Internal Medicine, Nihon University School of Medicine, Tokyo, Japan

Associate Editors

NISHIO HONDA, Tokyo Senbai Hospital, Tokyo
HYOE ISHIKAWA, Nara Medical University, Nara
KENKICHI KOISO, The University of Tsukuba, Ibaraki
KIYOSHI KUROKAWA, University of Tokyo, Tokyo
TADAO NIIJIMA, Tokyo Seamen's Medical College, Tokyo
NOBUHIRO SUGINO, Tokyo Women's Medical College, Tokyo
SUSUMU TAKAHASHI, Nihon University, Tokyo

ISBN 978-3-540-70074-6

Library of Congress Cataloging-in-Publication Data
International Congress on Nephrology (11th: 1990: Tokyo, Japan); Nephrology: proceedings of the XIth International Congress of Nephrology/editors, Michinobu Hatano: associate editors, Nishio Honda...[et al.].
p. cm. Congress held in Tokyo, Japan, July 15-20, 1990. Includes bibliographical references. Includes index.
ISBN 978-3-540-70074-6   ISBN 978-3-662-35158-1 (eBook)
DOI 10.1007/978-3-662-35158-1
1. Kidneys – Diseases – Congresses.
2. Nephrology – Congresses. 3. Kidney Diseases – congresses. 4. Nephrology – congresses. I. Hatano, Michinobu, 1926- . II. Honda, Nishio. III. Title. [DNLM: WJ 300 I59n 1990]. RC902.A2I56 1990. 616.6'1 –dc20. DNLM/DLC. for Library of Congress 91-4651

© Springer Japan 1991
Originally published by Springer-Verlag Tokyo Berlin Heidelberg New York in 1991
Softcover reprint of the hardcover 1st edition 1991

Typesetting: Publishers Service of Montana, Bozeman, Montana

Foreword

The proceedings of the XIth International Congress of Nephrology held in Tokyo in 1990, form the most international and complete document of the present state of basic and clinical science in nephrology. In addition, they document the progress made in this field during the 3 years since the London Congress. The result is nothing short of impressive. The material presented by the invited lecturers and the participants of the symposia all show a remarkable pattern; not only the "height" of the science, but also the depth of the specialized knowledge, both prerequisites of excellency in science, which do not necessarily imply narrowness of outlook. On the contrary, this written document of the Tokyo Congress is a witness to the enormous progress made over the last few years in communication between basic scientists and clinical scientists.

The International Society of Nephrology is a fine example of how fruitful and productive this interaction can be, if it is conducted with the desire to understand each other. The members of the Scientific Program Committee of the Tokyo Congress are to be congratulated, not only for a thoughtful and well designed program, but also for carefully selecting those speakers who, besides their own contribution to nephrological science, also have the talent of being able to communicate with a large, international audience. In particular, I would like to express my deep appreciation to the editors of the Proceedings for their commitment and industriousness which made it possible for this publication to appear so soon after the Congress.

Since the first Congress of the International Society of Nephrology in Evian in 1960, nephrologists have witnessed a phenomenal increase in knowledge, a progress which still continues and will do so in the future. The present proceedings are a snapshot of this process. The counterpoint to the intellectual challenge of acquiring deeper understanding is the duty and promise to utilize that understanding for the benefit of our patients.

KLAUS THURAU, M.D.
President,
International Society of Nephrology
(1987–1990)

v

Preface

The XIth International Congress of Nephrology was held in Tokyo, Japan from July 15–20, 1990.

Since the first congress in Evian, France in 1960, this is the first time that this prestigious congress has been held in Asia. Therefore, enthusiastic expectations were held by nephrologists not only in Japan but also throughout the world.

In organizing the congress under the estimable guidance of Prof. Klaus Thurau, President of the International Society of Nephrology, the ISN Executive Committee and the International Advisory Committee, Prof. Michinobu Hatano, Chairman of the local organizing committee as well as the organizing committee made every effort to make the congress a success.

Over three thousand participants from 71 countries attended the congress. These included 1,470 participants from Japan, 472 from the United States, 150 from France, and 128 from Italy. We were particularly pleased to welcome eight representatives from Czechoslovakia as well as an increased participation from other eastern European countries, the Soviet Union, and China. Forty-nine delegates from Taiwan were also in attendance.

The opening ceremony was held at the New Takanawa Prince Hotel in the presence of the Crown Prince, whose address noted that progress in nephrology would contribute greatly to the welfare of patients worldwide.

The scientific program consisted of 15 state-of-the-art lectures, 36 symposia, 11 workshops, 256 oral and 1,778 poster presentations. Following the advice of the ISN Executive Committee, the Scientific Program Committee encouraged the presentation of clinical and research papers at the same time in each session. This ensured that throughout the scientific program, discussions were constructive, and this helped to make the congress both stimulating and fruitful.

A total of 12 ISN satellite symposia, 4 overseas and 8 in Japan, were also held. The specific topics discussed at each symposium, combined with sightseeing tours at each site, contributed greatly to exchanges of both friendship and information.

Finally, we would like to express our sincere thanks and appreciation to the ISN Committee and all the participants of the congress.

KENZO OSHIMA, M.D.
President

YAWARA YOSHITOSHI, M.D.
Vice-President

YASUSHI UEDA, M.D.
Vice-President

HIROSHI ABE, M.D.
Vice-President

XIth International Congress of Nephrology

ORGANIZED BY: The Organizing Committee of the XIth International
Congress of Nephrology

UNDER THE AUSPICES OF: International Society of Nephrology

SPONSORED BY: Japanese Society of Nephrology
The Kidney Foundation, Japan

IN COOPERATION WITH: The Japanese Association of Medical Science
Japan Medical Association
The Japanese Urological Association
The Japan Society for Transplantation
Japanese Society for Artificial Organs
Japanese Society for Dialysis Therapy
The Japanese Society of Pediatric Nephrology
Japan Incorporated Medical Association for Dialysis

SUPPORTED BY: Ministry of Education, Science and Culture
Ministry of Health and Welfare
Science Council of Japan
Tokyo Metropolitan Government

The International Society of Nephrology

EXECUTIVE COMMITTEE 1987–1990

Klaus Thurau	FRG	President
Donald W. Seldin	USA	Past President
Roscoe R. Robinson	USA	President Elect
John Stewart Cameron	UK	Vice-President
Claude Amiel	France	Secretary-General
Robert W. Schrier	USA	Treasurer
Thomas E. Andreoli	USA	Editor, Kidney International

ADVISORY COMMITTEE FOR THE 1990 CONGRESS

Klaus Thurau	FRG	Chairman
Robert C. Atkins	Australia	
Claude Amiel	France	
John Stewart Cameron	UK	
Jared James Grantham	USA	
Roscoe R. Robinson	USA	

NOMINATING COMMITTEE

Paul Michielsen	Belgium	President
Franklin H. Epstein	USA	
Gerhard Giebisch	USA	
Richard J. Glassock	USA	
Colin I. Johnston	Australia	
Norman F. Jones	UK	
Franciszek Kokot	Poland	
Jean-Philippe Mery	France	
Jose C. Pena	Mexico	
Mordecai M. Popovtzer	Israel	
Yawara Yoshitoshi	Japan	

MANAGEMENT COMMITTEE

Klaus Thurau	FRG	President
Roscoe R. Robinson	USA	President Elect
Claude Amiel	France	Secretary-General
Robert W. Schrier	USA	Treasurer
Thomas E. Andreoli	USA	Editor, Kidney International
Saulo Klahr	USA	Councillor
D. Keith Peters	UK	Councillor

COUNCIL

Stephen Angielski	Poland
Robert C. Atkins	Australia
Knut Auklund	Norway
Vittorio Bonomini	Italy
Barry M. Brenner	USA
Giuseppe D'Amico	Italy
Vincent W. Dennis	USA
John H. Dirks	Canada
Evert J. Dorhout Mees	The Netherlands
Carl W. Gottschalk	USA
Jean-Pierre Grünfeld	France
Jean Hamburger	France
Klaus Hierholzer	FRG
David N.S. Kerr	UK
Saulo Klahr	USA
Robert T. McCluskey	USA
Gerhard Malnic	Brazil
D. Keith Peters	UK
Hidekazu Shigematsu	Japan
Jay Stein	USA
Nobuhiro Sugino	Japan
Guillermo Whittembury	Venezuela

XIth International Congress Officers

President	Kenzo Oshima
Vice Presidents	Yawara Yoshitoshi
	Yasushi Ueda
	Hiroshi Abe

ORGANIZING COMMITTEE

Chairman	Michinobu Hatano
Secretary-General	Susumu Takahashi

Members

Yoshio Aso	Tadashi Miyahara
Toshiyuki Furukawa	Toshihiko Nagasawa
Kohei Hara	Mitsuharu Narita
Nishio Honda	Hiromi Nihira
Takeshi Hoshi	Tadao Niijima
Kazunari Iidaka	Teruo Omae
Hyoe Ishikawa	Zensuke Ota
Chuichi Kawai	Fuminori Sakai
Teruo Kitagawa	Takao Sonoda
Kenkichi Koiso	Nobuhiro Sugino
Kiyoshi Kurokawa	Shizuo Tojo
Sunao Maki	

SCIENTIFIC PROGRAM COMMITTEE

Chairmen

Nobuhiro Sugino
Nishio Honda

Executive Secretary

Kiyoshi Kurokawa

Members
Akitoshi Ando
Kikuo Arakawa
Masaaki Arakawa
Hitoshi Endou
Mamoru Fujimoto
Gerhard Giebisch
Takashi Harada
Eiji Higashihara
Kazunari Iidaka
Masashi Imai
Hiroshi Kida
Hikaru Koide
Kenkichi Koiso
Shozo Koshikawa
Akio Koyama
Kenji Maeda
Sunao Maki

Koichi Matsumoto
Toshihiko Nagasawa
Mitsumasa Nagase
Yasushi Nakamoto
Hiroshi Nihei
Michio Odaka
Hiroyuki Ohi
Yoshimasa Orita
Kazuo Ota
Hideto Sakai
Osamu Sakai
Tadasu Sakai
Takao Saruta
Hidekazu Shigematsu
Kenjiro Yamamoto
Nobuyuki Yoshizawa

FUND RAISING COMMITTEE

Chairmen

Tadao Niijima
Hyoe Ishikawa

Members
Keishi Abe
Yoshio Aso
Tohru Azuma
Kohei Hara
Yoshihei Hirasawa
Hiroshi Kida

Joichi Kumazawa
Yuji Nagura
Zensuke Ota
Tsutomu Sanaka
Takao Sonoda
Naohiko Ueda

FINANCE COMMITTEE

Chairman

Kenkichi Koiso

Members
Hiroshi Kawamura

Gengo Osawa

Contents of Volume I

State of the Art Lectures

Symposia

Systemic Dysfunctions in Renal Failure and Their Management

ATPases of the Kidney

Vitamin D and Uremic Bone Disease

AIDS/AIDS — Nephropathy

Cyclosporine Nephrotoxicity: From Experimental Animal to Clinical Practice

Cell Volume Regulation in Health and Disease

Mechanisms of Renal Cell Injury of Acute Renal Failure

Cellular and Integrative Regulation of Renal Circulation

Dietary Factors and Progression of Chronic Renal Failure

Renal Diseases in Asia

Pathobiology of Glomerular and Tubular Basement Membranes

Index *see Volume II*

Contents of Volume II

Symposia

Cytokines, Mitogens and Their Receptors on Glomerular Cells

Frontiers of Research on Natriuretic Peptides

List of Contributors

For contributors' addresses see chapter opening pages

List of Contributors

State-of-the-Art Lectures

Pathogenesis of Glomerulonephritis – 1990

ROBERT C. ATKINS

Chair: Yasushi Ueda

Pathogenesis of Glomerulonephritis – 1990

ROBERT C. ATKINS[1]

SUMMARY. Recent advances in our understanding of the pathogenesis of glomerulonephritis are reviewed, focusing on evidence for the importance of the role of sensitized T cells and/or activated macrophages in causing glomerular injury, either directly, or via production of cytokines capable of modulating the normal biosynthetic and proliferative activities of intrinsic glomerular cells. In addition, recent data on the hitherto unrecognized importance of interstitial mononuclear cell infiltration to the progression of renal injury and declining function in glomerulonephritis is discussed. Insights gained from these developing areas of nephrologic research suggest important new approaches to the understanding and improved therapy of glomerulonephritis.

Introduction

Glomerulonephritis has long been considered to result from activation of immune mechanisms. This was first recognized at the turn of the century, and the concept of induction of glomerular injury by immune mechanisms leading to glomerulonephritis still pertains today. The evidence for human glomerular disease being immunologically induced stems, in part, from the localization of immune reactants within glomeruli. The understanding of its immune pathogenesis, as originally proposed by Dixon [1,2] has served us well over the ensuing years, although the linear staining of anti-GBM antibody and the classic deposits of circulating immune complexes within glomeruli may well represent opposite poles of a spectrum of antibody localization, rather than discrete disease entities [3].

Probably most glomerulonephritides, apart from those initiated by an exogenous antigen, such as in post-infectious glomerulonephritis, result from an auto-immune

[1]Department of Nephrology, Prince Henry's Hospital, Monash Medical Centre, Melbourne, Victoria 3004, Australia

reaction to self antigen. Autoimmune mechanisms and their relationship to the kidney have been recently reviewed [4]. Renal damage in glomerulonephritis is caused by immune products which are derived from B or T lymphocytes activated by the nominal antigen [5]. Details of humoral immunity and glomerulonephritis, a field which has historically been the subject of intense study, were recently reviewed [6,7]. The role of sensitized T-cells has not been completely assessed, but we now know that these cells do contribute to the inflammatory process [8–10]. Over the past few years there has been an increasing awareness of the contribution to the glomerular nephritic process by both intrinsic glomerular cells and infiltrating glomerular leucocytes. The cytokine interrelationships of these cells and the balance of their effects are just beginning to be unravelled. Such studies, using approaches made possible by the recent technical advances in cell and molecular biology, have considerably changed research direction in glomerulonephritis over the past few years. This chapter will review three areas where recent work has resulted in conceptual advances in the understanding of the pathogenesis of glomerulonephritis:

1. The role of T-cells and monocytes in glomerular injury.
2. The contribution of intrinsic glomerular cells to the glomerulonephritis process.
3. Involvement of the interstitium in the initiation and evolution of glomerulonephritis.

The Role of T Lymphocytes and Monocytes in Glomerular Injury

T Lymphocytes

Over the past 10 years, evidence for the initiation of glomerular injury by sensitized T cells has been convincingly demonstrated in several models. Initial experiments by Bhan and co-workers demonstrated, both in anti-GBM and in immune complex models of glomerulonephritis, that adoptive transfer of sensitized T lymphocytes produced mild proliferative glomerulonephritis [11]. Further evidence of the capacity of sensitized T cells to induce glomerular injury was provided by Bolton et al. Chickens were depleted of B cells by bursectomy, and an auto-immune glomerulonephritis of varying histologic severity, including, in some cases, glomerulonephritis with crescent formation was induced by injection of heterologous glomeruli in Freund's adjuvant [12,13]. Injury was associated with the presence of intraglomerular T cells, and was also induced in naive chickens by transfer of T cells from affected, but not control, hosts. The fact that T cell depleted nude mice cannot be induced to produce a crescentic glomerulonephritis due to anti·GBM disease also supports the concept that T cells are involved in the genesis of this type of experimental glomerulonephritis [14].

Studies using monoclonal antibodies as specific markers of lymphocyte subsets have demonstrated that in experimental anti-GBM disease, glomerular accumulation of T cells precedes monocyte infiltration and glomerular injury [15]. Such T cells produce the lymphokine, migration inhibition factor [16], and express receptors for interleukin-2 (IL-2 (IL-2R)) [17], indicating their functional activation.

Two recent studies have demonstrated that a proliferative glomerulonephritis can also be induced, in the absence of antibody, by cellular immune responses to exogenous antigens which lodge in the glomeruli. Otie et al. [18] immunized rats with the hapten TNP; this produced sensitized T cells as demonstrated by a local delayed-type hypersensitivity (DTH) reaction to injected antigen, 7 days after immunization. When the hapten was coupled to cationized albumin and injected into the renal arteries of sensitized rats, a proliferative glomerulonephritis with proteinuria developed, without evidence of antibody involvement. Rennke et al. [19] also reported induction of a crescentic glomerulonephritis with marked interstitial involvement in a similar model, using a different antigen. In addition to producing crescentic nephritis after renal artery infusion, transfer of sensitized T cells to naive recipients, followed by antigen injection into the renal artery, produced a focal crescentic glomerulonephritis. Together with the work of Bhan et al. and Bolton et al., these studies provide impressive evidence that T cells alone can induce proliferative crescentic glomerulonephritis in a variety of experimental models of glomerulonephritis.

The evidence for T cell directed glomerulonephritis in human disease is understandably more circumstantial. It has been known for many years that there are no glomerular immune humoral reactants detected in 20% of patients with glomerulonephritis, suggesting a possible cellular causation. Circulating T cells have been shown to be sensitized to renal antigens in some forms of human glomerulonephritis [20]. In addition, intraglomerular T cells have recently been demonstrated in crescentic glomeruli [21–24], and within glomeruli of patients with aggressive proliferative glomerulonephritides such as lupus nephritis and cryoglobulinemic glomerulonephritis [25]. Such T cells are almost certainly functionally active in proliferative and/or crescentic glomerulonephritis, as shown by their association with monocytes and fibrin, the other components of cell mediated immunity [26], and their expression of IL-2R [24].

Though the types of human glomerulonephritis and the extent to which cell mediated immunity is involved remain uncertain, the findings of activated T cells within damaged glomeruli, in conjunction with the mounting experimental evidence cited above, suggests that T cells probably participate in aggressive proliferative glomerular injury in human disease. However, it is likely that both antibody mediated and T cell directed cellular immune mechanisms are involved in many immune mediated glomerulonephritides, and future studies will have to delineate these initiator and effector mechanisms more clearly.

How T cells induce glomerular damage is, as yet, unknown. However, they could recruit and activate monocytes within glomeruli by cell mediated immune mechanisms, as in the classic delayed type hypersensitivity reaction. T cells may also cause damage by production and release of various cytokines, which can cause direct cell injury, or can stimulate intrinsic glomerular cells to proliferate and secrete inflammatory mediators. Direct damage to glomerular cells by cytotoxic T cells may also occur, although there is currently no evidence to support or refute this point [9,10].

Monocytes/Macrophages

Monocytes contribute to glomerular hypercellularity in both human and experimental glomerulonephritis [8,10]. Early workers used ultrastructural examination to demonstrate the presence of monocytes within glomeruli of rabbits with experimental anti-GBM disease [27]. Subsequently, using various identification techniques such as glomerular culture, enzyme histochemistry, and monoclonal antibody analysis, intraglomerular monocytes were demonstrated in experimental anti-GBM disease, immune complex disease, lupus nephritis, and focal glomerular sclerosis [10,28,29].

The presence of monocytes in diseased human glomeruli was first described by Jones in 1951 [30]. We initially used glomerular culture to quantitate macrophages within glomeruli from patients with crescentic glomerulonephritis [31], but with the use of specific monoclonal antibodies and sensitive immunohistochemical labelling techniques it became feasible to compare the degree of macrophage involvement among the various human glomerular nephritides [8,32,33]. Thus, from these and other studies, it is now apparent that macrophages are found within glomeruli in many forms of proliferative glomerulonephritis, but especially in crescentic disease (of all etiologies), and in post-infectious, cryoglobulinemic, and diffuse lupus nephritis [21–23,25,32–35].

Macrophages can be recruited to glomeruli in several ways [10]. Monocyte accumulation and activation can result from elaboration of cytokines by sensitized T cells, by Fc receptor binding to glomerular deposits of immunoglobulin [36], via surface receptors for activated complement components, or in response to chemotactic fragments of fibrin and its degradation products [37]. In addition, glomerular endothelial leucocyte adhesion molecules are transiently induced in response to stimulation by endotoxin or cytokines, such as IL-1 or TNF [38,39], and such a mechanism could be responsible for macrophage entrapment within inflamed glomeruli.

Once localized to glomeruli, macrophages produce inflammatory mediators such as reactive oxygen species [40], thromboxane A2 [41], and IL-1 [29,42]. Indeed, increased IL-1 production from glomeruli from patients with glomerulonephritis was recently reported, suggesting that this cytokine may be important in the pathogenesis of human disease as well [43]. Moreover, in addition to its well-known pro-inflammatory effects, IL-1 is now known to directly affect tubular transport mechanisms [44].

Macrophage induced fibrin deposition via activation of the extrinsic pathway of coagulation was shown in experimental disease [10,45]. The association of glomerular macrophages expressing the pro-coagulant tissue factor with fibrin deposition within glomeruli suggests that this may also be a mechanism of macrophage induced injury in patients with proliferative glomerulonephritis [26,46]. Macrophages are also involved in the generation of crescents, the presence of which usually signifies extensive renal damage and a poor prognosis [10,47].

Cytokines produced by macrophages can induce other complex alterations in the normal physiology of intrinsic glomerular cells [48]. Recently, additional evidence for this interaction of inflammatory and intrinsic glomerular cells was demonstrated in rats with accelerated anti-GBM nephritis by Matsumoto and Hatano [42]. Glomerular monocytes were eliminated by treatment with anti-macrophage serum, causing a reduction in mesangial cell numbers and IL-1 production from isolated glomeruli, and diminished proteinuria. One interpretation of these results is that macrophage-produced IL-1 stimulates mesangial cell proliferation. This explanation is further supported by experiments studying progressive glomerulosclerosis in rats, where the numbers of glomerular macrophages and mesangial cells were progressively reduced, in conjunction with decreasing production of glomerular IL-1, as the disease evolved [29].

Thus, there is ample evidence for T-cell directed mechanisms of injury, together with macrophage participation, in experimental and human glomerulonephritis, although the unravelling of the complex interplay of the initiation and mediation of glomerular injury, by cytokine cell to cell signalling, is just beginning.

Contribution of Intrinsic Glomerular Cells to the Glomerulonephritic Process

Though proliferation of intrinsic glomerular cells is one of the key histologic features for the diagnosis and classification of glomerulonephritis, just how and why these cells proliferate beyond the normal level is unknown. Few studies determining the actual increased cell numbers of the intrinsic glomerular types in the various forms of glomerulonephritis are available [49,50]. One of the major changes in recent thinking has been the realization that intrinsic glomerular cells respond to various stimuli, not as passive targets nor as innocent bystanders, but with specific structural and metabolic changes which can directly influence evolution of the glomerular inflammatory process. It is now realized that the three intrinsic glomerular cells — mesangial, endothelial, and epithelial cells — are potentially all capable of exhibiting an active role in the initiation and progression of glomerulonephritis. Studies of the complex interplay between glomerular cells, both in normal and in diseased states, has just begun.

The technical ability to obtain these cells as pure isolates in culture, thereby enabling controlled manipulation of their properties, has led to intensive study of their in vitro properties over the past few years [51,52]. There is now a considerable literature, especially relating to the properties of mesangial cells, reflecting the relative ease of their isolation and homogenous culture, compared to the other glomerular cell types. Mesangial cells are increasingly thought to play a significant pathophysiologic role, because of their pivotal position within the glomerulus, surrounded by matrix, yet directly accessible to the plasma, and with actions ranging from regulation of glomerular blood flow to modulation of matrix production.

Mesangial Cells

The mesangial cell is a pluripotential cell with many features of a smooth muscle cell. The properties of mesangial cells have been identified, largely using mesangial cells cultured in vitro. Such studies have shown that mesangial cells contract in response to vasoactive amines and peptides, proliferate in response to inflammatory agents such as cytokines and growth factors, complement, immune complexes, and endotoxin, and secrete many factors, including cytokines, matrix proteins, bioactive lipids, and enzymes [51,52]. However, since many of the characteristics demonstrated using cultured mesangial cells vary considerably depending upon the culture conditions, great care must be exercised when extrapolating from in vitro mesangial cell properties to an assumed function in vivo.

In vitro, the cytokines IL-1, IL-6, prostaglandin F (PGF), and epidermal growth factor (EGF) induce mesangial cell proliferation, whereas proliferation is inhibited by transforming growth factor (TGF) beta and gamma interferon (Kakazaki and Kraft, Atkins 1990, unpublished observations). Likewise, lipids produced by mesangial cells, such as platelet activating factor, induce mesangial cell proliferation, whereas the prostaglandins inhibit proliferation. Similarly, addition of some matrix proteins, such as fibronectin, stimulate proliferation of cultured mesangial cells, but others, like heparan sulfate, inhibit this effect. Clearly, this balance between proliferation and its inhibition could be easily perturbed during the inflammation process and, depending on the dominance of the various inflammatory mediators, could result in either mesangial proliferation and/or sclerosis.

Mesangial cells produce a host of secreted substances in culture. These products are produced under "normal" culture conditions and may be further increased by immune and other stimuli. These secretory products include cytokines: interleukin-1 (IL-1), interleukin-6 (IL-6), tumor necrosis factor (TNF), transforming growth factor beta (TGF-B), and epidermal growth factor (EGF); enzymes, such as neutral proteinase and collagenase; bioactive lipids, such as the prostaglandins and platelet activating factor; and matrix proteins including Collagen III, IV and V, fibrinectin, laminin, and heparan sulfate [51,52,59].

Since mesangial cells both make and respond to various cytokines, the concept of mesangial cell auto-regulation was introduced, by Sterzel and Lovett, particularly in regard to IL-1 production [48]. These workers suggested that the perpetuation of mesangial cell activity by the breakdown in this auto-regulation might be one reason for the progression of mesangial glomerular sclerosis following cessation of the initial glomerular insult, in some forms of glomerulonephritis.

Additional evidence for such a concept was the demonstration that IL-6 is an autocrine growth factor for mesangial cells. Horii et al. demonstrated that mesangial cells in culture produced IL-6, and IL-6 itself induces a dose-dependent proliferation of rat mesangial cells in culture [60]. This group further showed that IL-6 was present within glomeruli of patients with proliferative glomerulonephritis, but not in normal glomeruli or in glomeruli from patients with minimal change glomerulonephritis, and that IL-6 urinary excretion was raised only in patients with proliferative glomerulonephritis. By inference, these results suggest that unregulated production of IL-6, presumably by mesangial cells, is a factor in progressive mesangial dysfunction in proliferative types of glomerulonephritis. This would also support the findings that IL-6 transgenic mice develop mesangial proliferative glomerulonephritis [61].

Another cytokine, TGF beta, also promotes mesangial matrix accumulation in experimental glomerulonephritis [62]. In rat mesangial injury induced by anti-thymocyte serum, cultured nephritic glomeruli produced increased amounts of TGF beta and matrix proteins. Normal rat mesangial cells in culture increased proteoglycan production when stimulated by TGF-beta or conditioned media from these nephritic glomeruli. These changes were blocked by anti-TGF serum. The time-course of matrix accumulation in these animals paralleled TGF-beta mRNA expression in glomeruli. These results suggest that TGF beta has a central role in the accumulation of pathological extracellular matrix and raises the possibility that therapy to regulate TGF beta action might be salutary.

Endothelial Cells in Glomerulonephritis

Normal glomerular endothelial cells have complex functions, including growth, permeability, maintenance of an anti-coagulant state, and matrix production; these functions may be modified following interactions with circulating leucocytes. Most studies of endothelial cells in culture have relied on non-glomerular endothelial cells. However, recently, glomerular endothelial cells have been grown and sustained in culture [63,64], and hence the relevance of many of the properties of activated endothelial cells determined so far may soon be examined using glomerular endothelial cells.

With immune stimulation, cultured non-renal endothelial cells produce cytokines and vasoactive lipids, express leucocyte adhesion and HLA molecules, promote procoagulant activity, and undergo changes in their cell structure [39]. Proliferation of these cells is enhanced by the cytokines IL-1, TNF, PGF, and EGF, and inhibited by TGF beta and gamma interferon. Hence, as for mesangial cells, these cytokines appear to closely regulate proliferation, and this balance between competing agents may be disrupted in disease states.

No studies are, as yet, available concerning isolated glomerular endothelial cells. However, incubation of isolated human glomeruli with endotoxin or with cytokines such as IL-1 and tumor necrosis factor (TNF) induces leucocyte adhesion molecules [38]. Similarly, such cytokines induce glomerular endothelial expression of procoagulant molecules [38] and downregulation of endothelial thrombomodulin expression [53]. Moreover, infusion of TNF into rabbit causes glomerular endothelial damage [54], downregulation of thrombomodulin expression, and induction of fibrin deposition, features which are also found in experimental anti-GBM disease [53]. Hence, initial studies indicate that cytokines do have in vivo effects similar to those induced in culture, and which may be relevant to the glomerulonephritic inflammatory process. These observations raise the potential for therapy by specific blocking of cytokine actions.

Epithelial Cells and Glomerulonephritis

Role in Membranous Nephropathy

For many years idiopathic membranous nephropathy in humans was considered a classic immune complex nephropathy, caused by deposition of circulating immune complexes. However, evidence now suggests that membranous glomerulonephritis is the result of an autoimmune response to native renal epithelial cell antigens. Intensive study of Heymann's nephritis, induced by immunization of rats with brush border antigen FXIA, has changed our concept of the pathogenesis of membranous nephritis. Heymann nephritis, both passive and active, mimics human membranous nephropathy and was originally also thought to be due to deposition of circulating immune complexes. The antigen responsible for Heymann's nephritis, gp330 (recently sequenced and found to be homologous with the low density lipoprotein receptors [55], occurs both within cells of the proximal tubule and in the coated pits of glomerular epithelial cells [56]. Moreover, antibodies to epithelial cell antigens can redistribute antigens at the surface of human and monkey glomerular epithelial cells in vitro, in vivo, and ex vivo [57]. Furthermore, specific membrane proteins were detected in immune deposits of patients with membranous nephropathy [58]. Hence, these suggest that human membranous nephritis, like Heymann's nephritis in rats, is due to the formation of auto-antibodies to epithelial cell antigens, resulting in in-situ immune complex formation.

Modulation of Epithelial Cell Growth In Vitro

Both human and animal glomerular epithelial cells can now be reproducibly grown in culture, using special culture media, and their response to, and production of, inflammatory mediators are currently being assessed [63,65,66]. Glomerular epithelial cells in vitro proliferate in response to leukotrienes, thrombin, and EGF, and this proliferation is inhibited by heparan sulfate and transforming growth factor beta [66]. Based on these initial experiments, matrix proteins and inflammatory cytokines, such as EGF and TGF-b, may exert a regulatory influence on epithelial cell proliferation.

Epithelial Cells and Glomerular Crescent Formation

Crescent formation occurs in a heterogenous group of glomerulonephritides, but generally indicates an increased severity of disease and is frequently associated with a poorer outcome. Langhans originally proposed that proliferating glomerular epithelial cells formed the crescent, and this view became widely accepted [67]. However, numerous experimental and human studies [10,47] have now demonstrated that monocytes are also intimately involved in crescent formation. Thus, it is now generally accepted that both monocytes and epithelial cells contribute to crescent formation, and in fact the composition appears to depend upon the age of the crescent [68] and the integrity of Bowman's capsule [69]. Indeed, there is a prominent interstitial periglomerular infiltration of leucocytes associated with crescentic glomerulonephritis, and it may be that many of the leucocytes entering Bowman's space enter from the interstitium, as well as via the capillary tuft, perhaps in response to fibrin [10,47].

The mechanism leading to the migration of monocytes is only partially understood, and is almost certainly multifactorial, yet a recent study has again highlighted the importance of fibrin in this regard. Zoja et al. [70] showed that recombinant plasminogen activator, which causes lysis of fibrin clots by activating plasminogen to plasmin, markedly reduced glomerular fibrin deposition and crescent formation, and also prevented deterioration of renal function in rabbit nephrotic nephritis. Since fibrin is only one determinant of crescent formation, and can itself result from macrophage activation and initiation of the extrinsic pathway of coagulation, interpretation of these results may be complex [46]. Nevertheless, such studies emphasize the many complex interrelationships potentially active between inflammatory cells and mediators, intrinsic glomerular cells, particularly parietal and visceral epithelial cells, and the coagulation system.

With regard to further analysis of mononuclear cell involvement in crescentic glomerulonephritis, we have recently noted that with the advent of crescent formation in IgA nephropathy, there is increased T-cell and monocyte activation, particularly in the interstitium, and a decrease in renal function [24]. Indeed, our most recent studies of leucocyte composition of crescents, in 34 patients, have demonstrated that leucocytes make up some 80% of the cells in active cellular crescents; the majority of these leucocytes are monocytes, though a few T-cells and IL-2R+ mononuclear cells, as yet unidentified further, are present. In contrast, in inactive, sclerosed crescents, the proportion of leucocytes was reduced to about 20% of total cells, emphasizing the potential importance of cellular immune activation in crescent formation [71].

Involvement of the Interstitium in the Initiation and Evolution of Glomerulonephritis

In trying to understand the relationship between alteration of glomerular structure and decreased function in glomerulonephritis, the paradox arises that glomerular morphological changes do not correlate with renal functional impairment, whereas the interstitial changes do [72]. We demonstrated a relationship between a decreasing glomerular filtration rate and the intensity of interstitial leucocytic infiltration in 145 patients with glomerulonephritis [33]. This interstitial leucocytic infiltration was prominent in all forms of glomerulonephritis except minimal change glomerulo-nephritis, and its density reflected the severity of the underlying glomerular disease. The infiltrate was similar in composition to that seen in acute interstitial allograft rejection, as well as interstitial nephritis, consisting predominantly of T lymphocytes and macrophages, and with a notable absence of B cells. About 50% of T cells were of the CD4 + phenotype, and the ratio of CD4 + to CD8 + cells remained relatively constant within the varying disease types. The interstitial infiltrate increased in intensity with increasing degree of morphological evidence of glomerular injury, contained immune activated mononuclear cells expressing IL-2R, and activated macrophages producing the procoagulant tissue factor. A relationship between the glomerular crescentic activity and interstitial leucocyte infiltration was demon-strated in human IgA disease [24], whereby greater interstitial infiltration of leuco-cytes occurred in biopsies from patients with glomerular crescents. The number of T-cells and monocytes were greater in crescentic disease, and a higher proportion of mononuclear cells, approximately 20%, expressed IL-2R. Other recent studies have also examined the interstitial leucocytic infiltrate [73,74] and the degree of intersti-tial leucocytic infiltration has been shown to be a good predictor of clinical progres-sion, including cases of membranous nephritis [75], IgA disease [76,77], and lupus nephritis [25,78,79], providing additional credence to the importance of the intersti-tial events in progression of glomerulonephritis.

The relationship between glomerular and interstitial leucocyte involvement was studied experimentally, using both immune and non-immune models of glomerulo-nephritis. In accelerated anti-GBM disease, leucocytes appeared, within 15 minutes of disease induction, in the glomerulus and surrounding the afferent and efferent arterioles of the periglomerular stalk. These cells consisted of both T lymphocytes and monocytes, and over the ensuing days accumulated and encircled the glomerulus before spreading throughout the interstitium by day 7. However, the leucocyte profile differed between glomerulus and interstitium, the glomerular leucocytes consisting mainly of monocytes, whereas the periglomerular and interstitial cells consisted of approximately 50% monocytes and 50% T lymphocytes [17]. This rapid localization of leucocytes around hilar vessels, which occurred in the absence of local immunoglobulin deposition and concurrently with the glomerular leucocyte ingress, may provide a route for cytokine dispersal from the inflamed glomerulus and mesan-gium into the interstitial and other cortical areas.

An interstitial infiltrate was also present in a "non-immune" model of progressive focal glomerulosclerosis induced in rats by the concomitant injection of amino-nucleoside and protamine sulfate [80]. Prednisolone treatment begun 10 days after the instigation of the disease produced a significant improvement in renal function, corresponding to a decrease in severity of the interstitial changes, decrease in the relative interstitial volume, and reduction in leucocyte infiltration, yet without any glomerular alteration in sclerosis or leucocyte infiltration. This study further suggests that glomerular filtration rate and disease progression is more dependent on changes in the interstitium than in the glomerulus. Both studies are consistent with a hypothesis that infiltration of leucocytes into the interstitium in glomerulonephritis, of whatever etiology, determines evolution of the disease. Other recent studies have also evaluated the significance of the interstitial component in "non-immune" renal disease and the importance of interstitial macrophages and T cells in mediation of injury, including effects on tubular transport mechanisms [44,81].

Hence, though the pathogenesis of these interstitial changes and their relationship to the primary glomerular disease is currently uncertain, it could well be that the interstitial changes in glomerulonephritis may progress, regardless of the type of initial glomerular insult, perhaps due to cellular immune mechanisms. This interstitial leucocyte infiltration could result from classic T-cell directed cellular immunity to planted or unmasked tubular antigens. It might be the consequence of non-antigenic specific leucocyte accumulation following cytokine dispersal from injured glomeruli. Interstitial leucocytic accumulation could also follow increased expression of leucocyte adhesion molecules. Cytokine mediated upregulation of ICAM-1 in lupus nephritis in mice, which could well promote such leucocyte attraction to the interstitium, has recently been described [82]. Whatever the etiology, the interstitial component in glomerulonephritis has clinical implications for estimation of progression of disease and for therapy. Further understanding of the pathogenesis of the interstitial component of glomerulonephritis will perhaps lead to more specific therapy by targeting of the mediator systems involved. Such a therapeutic approach is vital for the current clinical situation, where the nephrologist is frequently faced with a disease which is ongoing, an initiating antigen which is unknown, and mediators which are obscure.

Concluding Remarks

Progress in our understanding of the pathogenesis of glomerulonephritis has occurred in recent years in incremental steps. Re-analysis of familiar animal models of glomerulonephritis, using monoclonal antibodies to markers of immune activation; widescale culture and passage of isolated glomerular cells (mesangial, epithelial, but still only with difficulty, endothelial cells) and their use in studies of proliferation, matrix production, and the effects of recombinant proteins, especially cytokines; and detailed clinicopathologic studies of biopsies from patients with glomerulonephritis have all contributed to this progress. However, the challenge remains to convert recent advances in basic cellular and molecular biology into clinically relevant, meaningful, and cost-effective applications. Meeting this challenge will require the clinician to become more conversant with the seemingly difficult, and increasingly complex, developments in biologic research, and the basic scientist to ask, and attempt answers to, clinically relevant questions. Nevertheless, the accelerating pace of development in nephrologic research, set against the ongoing revolution in biology brought about by the advent of monoclonal antibodies, and, more recently, molecular biology, is likely to yield quantum leaps in our understanding of the pathogenesis of glomerulonephritis.

References

1. Dixon FJ (1968) The pathogenesis of glomerulonephritis. Am J Med 44:493–494
2. Wilson CB, Dixon FJ (1986) The renal response to immunological injury. In: Brenner BJ, Rector FC (eds) The kidney, 3rd edn. WB Saunders, Philadelphia, pp 800–889
3. Bruijn JA, Hoedemaeker PJ, Fleuren GJ (1989) Pathogenesis of anti-basement membrane glomerulopathy and immune-complex glomerulonephritis: dichotomy dissolved. Lab Invest 61:480–488
4. Oliviera DBG, Peters DK (1989) Autoimmunity and the kidney. Kidney Int 35:923–928
5. Kelly CJ, Haverty T, Neilson EG (1988) Control of the nephritogenic immune response. In: Wilson CB (ed) Immunopathology of renal disease, vol 18. Churchill Livingstone, New York, pp 35–56
6. Wilson CB (1988) Antibody reactions with native or planted glomerular antigens producing nephritogenic immune deposits or selective glomerular cell injury. In: Wilson CB (ed) Immunopathology of renal disease, vol 18. Churchill Livingstone, New York, pp 1–34
7. Brentjens JR, Andres G (1989) Interaction of antibodies with renal cell surface antigens. Kidney Int 35:954–968
8. Atkins RC, Holdsworth SR, Hancock WW, Thomson NM, Glasgow EF (1982) Cellular immune mechanisms in human glomerulonephritis: The role of mononuclear leucocytes. Springer Semin Immunopathol 5:269–296
9. McCluskey RT, Bhan AK (1986) Cell mediated immunity in renal disease. Hum Pathol 17:146–153
10. Atkins RC, Holdsworth SR (1988) Cellular mechanisms of immune glomerular injury. In: Brenner and Stein (eds) Cellular mechanisms of injury in GN. Churchill Livingstone, New York, pp 111–135
11. Bhan AK, Schneeberger EE, Collins AB, McCluskey RT (1978) Evidence for a pathogenic role of a cell-mediated immune mechanism in experimental glomerulonephritis. J Exp Med 148:246–260
12. Bolton WK, Tucker FL, Sturgill BC (1984) New avian model of experimental GN consistent with mediation by cellular immunity. J Clin Invest 73:1263–1276
13. Bolton WK, Chandra M, Tyson TM, Kirkpatrick PR, Sadovnic MJ, Sturgill BC (1988) Transfer of experimental glomerulonephritis in chickens by mononuclear cells. Kidney Int 34(5):598–610
14. Okada K, Otie T, Kihara I, Morita T, Yamamoto T (1982) Masugi nephritis in the nude mice and their normal littermates. Acta Pathol Jpn 32:1
15. Tipping PG, Neale TJ, Holdsworth SR (1985) T lymphocyte participation in antibody-induced experimental glomerulonephritis. Kidney Int 27:530–537
16. Boyce NW, Tipping PG, Holdsworth SR (1986) Lymphokine (MIF) production by glomerular T-lymphocytes in experimental glomerulonephritis. Kidney Int 30:673
17. Lan HY, Paterson DJ, Atkins RC (1989) Evolving pattern of the interstitial leucocyte infiltrate in experimental anti-GBM glomerulonephritis (abstract). Kidney Int 36:1176
18. Otie T, Shimuzu F, Kagami S, Morioka T (1989) Hapten-specific cellular immune response producing glomerular injury. Clin Exp Immunol 76(3):463–468
19. Rennke HG, Klein PS, Mendrick DL (1990) Cell-mediated Immunity (CMI) in hapten-induced interstitial nephritis and glomerular crescent formation in the rat (abstract). Kidney Int 37:428
20. Rocklin R, Lewis E, David J (1970) In-vitro evidence for cellular hypersensitivity to glomerular-basement-membrane antigens in human glomerulonephritis. N Engl J Med 283:497–501
21. Nolasco FEB, Cameron JS, Hartley B, Coelho RA, Reuben R (1987) Intraglomerular T cells and monocytes in nephritis: study with monoclonal antibodies. Kidney Int 31:1160–1166

22. Bolton WK, Innes DJ, Sturgill BC, Kaiser DL (1987) T Cells and macrophages in rapidly progressive glomerulonephritis: clinicopathological correlations. Kidney Int 32:869–876
23. Muller GA, Muller CA, Markovic-Lipkovski J, Kilper RB, Risler T (1988) Renal major histocompatibility complex antigens and cellular components in rapidly progressive glomerulonephritis identified by monoclonal antibodies (with 1 color plate). Nephron 49:132–139
24. Li HL, Hancock WW, Hooke DH, Dowling JP, Atkins RC (1990) Mononuclear cell activation and decreased renal function in IgA nephropathy with crescents. Kidney Int 37: In Press
25. Castiglione A, Bucci A, Fellin G, D'Amico G, Atkins RC (1988) The relationship of infiltrating renal leucocytes to disease activity in lupus and cryoglobuilinaemic glomerulonephritis. Nephron 50:14–23
26. Neale TJ, Tipping PG, Carson SD, Holdsworth SR (1988) Participation of cell-mediated immunity in deposition of fibrin in glomerulonephritis. Lancet II(8608):421–424
27. Shigematsu H (1970) Glomerular events during the initial phase of rat Masugi nephritis. Virchows Arch [Cell Pathol] 5:187
28. Boyce NW, Holdsworth SR, Dijkstra CD, Atkins RC (1987) Quantitation of intraglomerular mononuclear phagocytes in experimental glomerulonephritis in the rat using specific monoclonal antibodies. Pathology 19:290–293
29. Matsumoto K, Atkins RC (1989) Glomerular cells and macrophages in the progression of experimental focal and segmental glomerulosclerosis. Am J Pathol 134(4):933–945
30. Jones DB (1951) Inflammation and repair of the glomerulus. Am J Pathol 27:991–1009
31. Atkins RC, Glasgow EF, Holdsworth SR, Matthews FE (1976) The macrophage in human rapidly progressive glomerulonephritis. Lancet I:830–832
32. Hooke DH, Hancock WW, Gee DC, Kraft N, Atkins RC (1984) Monoclonal antibody analysis of glomerular hypercellularity in human glomerulonephritis. Clin Nephrol 22(4):163–168
33. Hooke DH, Gee DC, Atkins RC (1987) Leukocyte analysis using monoclonal antibodies in human glomerulonephritis. Kidney Int 31:964–972
34. Magil AB, Wadsworth LD, Loewen M (1981) Monocytes and human renal glomerular disease. A quantitative evaluation. Lab Invest 44:23–33
35. D'Amico G, Colasanti G, Ferrario F, Sinico RA (1989) Renal involvement in essential mixed cryoglobulinemia. Kidney Int 35:1004–1014
36. Holdworth SR (1983) Fc dependence of macrophage accumulation and subsequent injury in experimental glomerulonephritis. J Immunol 130:735–739
37. Holdsworth SR, Thomson NM, Glasgow EF, Atkins RC (1979) The effect of defibrination on macrophage participation in rabbit nephrotoxic nephritis: Studies using glomerular culture and electromicroscopy. Clin Exp Immunol 37:38–43
38. Hancock WW, Cotran RS (1987) Induction of activation antigens on human glomerular endothelium by interleukin 1 (IL-1), interferon-gamma (IFN-g) and endotoxin (LPS) (abstract). Kidney Int 31:322
39. Cotran RS, Pober JS (1989) Effects of cytokines on vascular endothelium: their role in vascular and immune injury. Kidney Int 35:969–975
40. Boyce NW, Tipping PG, Holdsworth SR (1989) Glomerular macrophages produce reactive oxygen species in experimental glomerulonephritis. Kidney Int 35:778–782
41. Cook HT, Smith J, Salmon JA, Cattell V (1989) Functional characteristics of macrophages in glomerulonephritis in the rat: 02-generation, MHC class II expression, and eicosanoid synthesis. Am J Pathol 134:431–437
42. Matsumoto K, Hatano M (1989) Production of interleukin-1 in glomerular cell cultures from rats with nephrotoxic serum nephritis. Clin Exp Immunol 75:123–128
43. Matsumoto K, Dowling J, Atkins RC (1988) Production of Interleukin-1 in glomerular cell cultures from patients with rapidly progressive crescentic glomerulonephritis. Am J Nephrol 8:463–470

44. Schreiner GF, Kohan DE (1990) Regulation of renal transport processes and hemo-dynamics by macrophages and lymphocytes. Am J Physiol 258:F761–767
45. Tipping PG, Lowe MG, Holdsworth SR (1988) Glomerular macrophages express aug-mented procoagulant activity in experimental fibrin-related glomerulonephritis in rabbits. J Clin Invest 82(4):1253–1259
46. Hancock WW, Atkins RC (1985) Activation of coagulation pathways and fibrin deposition in human glomerulonephritis. Semin Nephrol 5:69–75
47. Atkins RC, Thomson NM (1988) Rapidly progressive glomerulonephritis. In: Schrier RW, Gooschalk CW (eds) Diseases of the kidney, vol 2. Little, Brown, Boston, pp 1903–1927
48. Sterzel RB, Lovett DH (1988) Interactions of inflammatory and glomerular cells in the response to glomerular injury. In: Wilson CB (ed) Immunopathology of renal disease, vol 18. Churchill Livingstone, New York, pp 137–173
49. Atkins RC, Glasgow EF, Holdsworth S, Thomson NM, Hancock WW (1980) Tissue culture of isolated glomeruli from patients with glomerulonephritis. Kidney Int 17(4):515–527
50. Sterzel RB, Pabst R, Kregeler M, Perfetto M (1982) The temporal relationship between glomerular cell proliferation and monocyte infiltration in experimental glomerulonephri-tis. Virchows Arch [Cell Pathol] 38:337–350
51. Mene P, Simonson MS, Dunn MJ (1989) Physiology of the mesangial cell. Physiol Rev 69:1347–1424
52. Hawkins NJ, Wakefield D, Charlesworth JA (1990) The role of mesangial cells in glomeru-lar pathology. Pathology 22
53. Hancock WW (to be published) IL-1 and TNF depress glomerular endothelial throm-bomodulin expressin in vitro and in vivo. Kidney Int
54. Bertani T, Abbate M, Zoja C, Corna D, Perico N, Ghezzi P, Remuzzi G (1989) Tumor necrosis factor induces glomerular damage in the rabbit. Am J Pathol 134:419–430
55. Raychowdhury R, Hiles JL, McCluskey RT, Smith JA (1989) Autoimmune target in Hey-mann nephritis is a glycoprotein with homology to the LDL receptor. Science 244(4909): 1163–1165
56. Kerjaschki D (1990) The pathogenesis of membranous glomerulonephritis: from morphol-ogy to molecules. Virchows Arch [Cell Pathol] 58:253–271
57. Fukatsu A, Yuzawa Y, Olson L, Miller J, Andres G (1989) Interaction of antibodies with human glomerular epithelial cells. Lab Invest 61:389–403
58. Kerjaschki D (1989) Kinetics of immune deposits in membranous nephropathy. Kidney Int 35:1423
59. Hancock WW, Kraft N, Clarke F, Atkins RC (1984) Production of monoclonal antibodies to fibronectin, type IV collagen and other antigens of the human glomerulus. Pathology 16:197–206
60. Horii Y, Muraguchi A, Iwano M, Matsuda T, Hirayama T, Yamada H, Fujii Y, Dohi K, Ishikawa H, Ohmoto Y, Yoshizaki K, Hirano T, Kishimoto T (1989) Involvement of IL-6 in mesangial proliferative glomerulonephritis. J Immunol 143(12):3949–3955
61. Suematsu S, Matsuda T, Aozasa K, Akira S, Nakano N, Ohno S, Miyazaki JI, Yamamura KI, Hirano, T, Kishimoto T (1989) IgG1 plasmacytosis in interleukin 6 transgenic mice. Proc Natl Acad Sci USA (Immunol) 86:7547–7551
62. Okuda S, Languino LR, Ruoslanti E, Border WA (to be published) Elevated expression of transforming growth factor-beta and proteoglycan production in experimental glomerulo-nephritis: possible role in expansion of the mesangial extracellular matrix. J Clin Invest
63. MacKay K, Striker LJ, Elliot S, Pinkert CA, Brinster RL, Striker GE (1988) Glomerular epi-thelial, mesangial and endothelial cell lines from transgenic mice. Kidney Int 33:677–684
64. Ballerman BJ (1989) Regulation of bovine glomerular endothelial cell growth in vitro. Am J Physiol 256(1 Pt 1):C182–C189
65. Quigg RJ, Abrahamson DR, Cybulsky AV, Badalamenti J, Minto AW, Salant DJ (1989) Studies of antibodies to cultured rat glomerular epithelial cells. Subepithelial immune deposit formation after in vivo injection. Am J Pathol 134(5):1125–1133

66. Adler S, Chen X, Eng B (1990) Control of rat glomerular epithelial cell growth in vitro. Kidney Int 37:1048–1054

67. Langhans T (1979) Über die Veränderungen der Glomeruli bei der Nephritis nebst einigen Bemerkungen über die Enstshung der Fibrinzylinder. Arch Pathol Physiol Klin Med 76:85

68. Hancock WW, Atkins RC (1984) Cellular composition of crescents in human rapidly progressive glomerulonephritis identified using monoclonal antibodies. Am J Nephrol 3:177–181

69. Boucher A, Droz D, Adafer E, Laure-Helene N (1987) Relationship between the integrity of Bowman's capsule and the composition of cellular crescents in human crescentic glomerulonephritis. Lab Invest 56(5):526–533

70. Zoja C, Corna D, Macconi D, Zilio P, Bertani T, Remuzzi G (1990) Tissue plasminogen activator therapy of rabbit nephrotoxic nephritis. Lab Invest 62(1):34–40

71. Li HL, Hancock WW, Dowling JP, Atkins RC (to be published) IL-2R mononuclear cell (MNC) composition of crescents in human crescentic glomerulonephritis (CGN) (abstract). Kidney Int

72. Risdon RA, Sloper JC, DeWardner HE (1968) Relationship between renal function and histological changes found in renal biopsy specimens from patients with persistent glomerulonephritis. Lancet II:363–366

73. D'Amico G (1988) Role of interstitial infiltration of leukocytes in glomerular diseases. Nephrol Dial Transplant 3(5):596–600

74. Markovic-Lipkovski J, Muller CA, Risler T, Bohle A, Muller GA (1990) Association of glomerular and interstitial mononuclear leukocytes with different forms of glomerulonephritis. Nephrol Dial Transplant 5:10–17

75. Alexopoulos E, Seron D, Hartley RB, Nolasco F, Cameron JS (1989) Immune mechanisms in idiopathic membranous nephropathy: the role of the interstitial infiltrates. Am J Kidney Dis 13(5):404–412

76. Sabadini E, Castiglione A, Colasanti G, Ferrario F, D'Amico G (1988) Characterisation of interstitial infiltrating cells in Berger's disease. Am J Kidney Dis 12:307–315

77. Alexopoulos E, Scron D, Hartley RB, Nolasco F, Cameron JS (1989) The role of interstitial infiltrates in IgA nephropathy: a study with monoclonal antibodies. Nephrol Dial Transplant 4:187–195

78. D'Agati UD, Appel GA, Estes D, Knowles DM, Pirani CL (1986) Monoclonal antibody identification of infiltrating mononuclear leucocytes in lupus nephritis. Kidney Int 30:573–581

79. Alexopoulos E, Seron D, Hartley RB, Cameron JS (1990) Lupus nephritis: correlation of interstitial cells with glomerular function. Kidney Int 37:100–109

80. Saito T, Atkins RC (1990) Contribution of mononuclear leucocytes to the progression of experimental focal glomerular sclerosis. Kidney Int 37:1076–1083

81. Schreiner GF, Harris KP, Purkerson ML, Klahr S (1988) Immunological aspects of acute ureteral obstruction: immune cell infiltrate in the kidney. Kidney Int 34(4):487–493

82. Wuthrich RP, Jeunikar AM, Takei F, Glimcher LH, Kelley VE (1990) Intercellular adhesion molecule-1 (ICAM-1) expression is unregulated in autoimmune murine lupus nephritis. Am J Pathol 136:441–450

Functional Morphology of the Nephron

C. CRAIG TISHER, KIRSTEN M. MADSEN, and
JILL W. VERLANDER

Chair: Wilhelm Kriz

Functional Morphology of the Nephron

C. Craig Tisher, Kirsten M. Madsen, and Jill W. Verlander[1]

Introduction

The mammalian nephron is composed of the renal corpuscle (commonly referred to as the "glomerulus") and the renal tubule. The tubular component of the nephron is traditionally divided into three functional regions: the proximal tubule, the thin limb, and the distal tubule. Strictly speaking, the collecting duct system is not part of the nephron since its embryonic derivation is from the ureteric bud rather than the metanephric mass. However, physiologists and anatomists now view the collecting duct as an integral portion of the nephron regardless of its embryonic origin.

During the past two decades a variety of investigative techniques have allowed scientists to more precisely define the structural and functional properties of the nephron. This effort received a major impetus with the development of the isolated perfused tubule technique, by Burg and his colleagues [1], which permitted examination of the functional properties of individual segments of the renal tubule under carefully controlled and defined experimental conditions. Concurrently, Morel [2] and Garg et al. [3] developed and adapted analytical biochemical techniques to measure enzyme activities in individually dissected segments of the renal tubule. Simultaneously, morphologists took advantage of improved methods of tissue preservation that made it possible to examine the renal tubule in greater detail, at both the cellular and subcellular level. The more recent availability of monoclonal and polyclonal antibodies directed against specific transport and structural proteins located in the kidney has allowed investigators to locate not only the segment of the renal tubule involved in a particular transport event, but also the exact cell(s) and often the precise subcellular location of a specific transport function. Currently under development are methods of in situ hybridization which permit scientists to examine gene expression and regulation in individual components of the nephron, at both the light microscopic and electron microscopic level.

[1]Laboratory of Experimental Morphology, Division of Nephrology, Hypertension and Transplantation, University of Florida College of Medicine, Gainesville, FL 32610, USA

The results of all of these technologies have underscored the fact that major structural and functional axial heterogeneity exists in the entire renal tubule. This review will focus on specific structural-functional relationships in the distal tubule and collecting duct, since it is in these regions of the renal tubule where the greatest progress has been made in the past few years in correlating structure with function.

Distal Tubule

Structure

Anatomically, the distal tubule consists of three distinct segments: the thick ascending limb (TAL) of Henle's loop, the macula densa, and the distal convoluted tubule (DCT). The macula densa actually represents a specialized segment of the TAL and will not receive further comment in this review. There is an abrupt transition from the TAL to the DCT, approximately 90–100 μm beyond the region of the macula densa. The DCT resembles the TAL by light microscopy, but major differences have been identified between these two segments ultrastructurally and functionally. Both the TAL and the DCT possess extensive invaginations of the basolateral membrane and lateral interdigitations between adjacent cells. Numerous elongate mitochondria in close apposition to the plasma membrane are present within the interdigitating processes, a feature that is common to epithelia involved in active solute transport. The cells of the DCT are generally taller and their nuclei are located in a more apical position than those of the TAL.

Thick Ascending Limb

Based on the location within the kidney, the TAL can be divided into two segments: the medullary and cortical TAL. Structural and functional differences exist between these two segments. Cells forming the inner stripe TAL measure 7–8 μm in height, but the height decreases progressively in the outer medullary and cortical TAL, finally reaching values of 2 μm in the rabbit and 5 μm in the rat [4]. The decrease in height is associated with a decrease both in the relative volume of mitochondria and in the surface area of the basolateral plasma membrane per millimeter of tubule length. However, because of an increase in lateral interdigitations in the apical region of the cells and an increase in the number of luminal surface microprojections, there is a significant increase in the surface area of the apical plasma membrane as the cortical TAL ascends toward its parent glomerulus [4]. The invaginations of the basolateral membrane, which are extensive throughout the TAL, form lateral cell processes that are oriented mainly parallel to the long axis of the cells and perpendicular to the long axis of the tubule. Some years ago we observed with scanning electron microscopy that cells of the medullary TAL had very few apical lateral interdigitations and a relatively smooth luminal surface, while in the cortical TAL apical lateral interdigitations were more prominent and the cells were covered by extensive luminal microprojections [5]. The functional significance of these two cell configurations, if any, remains to be established.

Immunocytochemical studies reveal the presence of Na,K-ATPase [6] and Tamm-Horsfall protein in this region of the nephron. Recent results from our own laboratory demonstrate the presence of a serotonin receptor, $5\text{-}HT_{1A}$, in the basolateral plasma membrane of the medullary and cortical TAL of both rat and human kidney (J.R. Raymond, C.C. Tisher 1990, unpublished observations).

Distal Convoluted Tubule

This region of the distal tubule corresponds to the "early distal tubule" described in the micropuncture literature. In both the rat and the rabbit the DCT measures 1 mm in length. The cells in this region are considerably taller than those of the TAL, especially the cortical TAL, and in contrast to the cortical TAL, there are no extensive apical lateral interdigitations. Surface microprojections are prominent, especially in the rabbit DCT. Basolateral invaginations of the plasma membrane extend two-thirds to three-fourths of the distance from the base to the apex of the cell and contain elongate mitochondria. Numerous small vesicles are located above the nucleus in the apical region of the cell. In the rat, intercalated cells begin to appear in the terminal portion of the DCT near the connecting segment, a transition region located between the DCT and the collecting duct.

Immunocytochemical studies have identified Na,K-ATPase in this segment of the distal tubule [6], and we have recently observed the presence of the $5\text{-}HT_{1A}$ serotonin receptor in the basolateral membrane of DCT cells (J.R. Raymond, C.C. Tisher 1990, unpublished observations). In contrast to its presence in the TAL, there is no evidence for the presence of Tamm-Horsfall protein in the DCT.

Structural-Functional Relationships

The distal tubule is involved in ion transport, including monovalent ions such as sodium, potassium, and chloride and divalent ions, including calcium and magnesium. There is also evidence for proton and ammonium ion transport in this region of the nephron. Na,K-ATPase provides most of the energy for these transport events and abundant levels of activity of this ATPase have been measured in both the TAL and the DCT.

Thick Ascending Limb

A major function of the TAL is the maintenance of a hypertonic medullary interstitium and the delivery of a dilute tubular fluid to the DCT. This is accomplished by the active reabsorption of NaCl, a process driven by the Na, K-ATPase pump that is located along the basolateral membrane of the cell [6]. Greger et al. [7] have demonstrated that throughout the TAL of the rabbit, NaCl reabsorption is mediated by a sodium-potassium-chloride ($Na^+\text{-}K^+\text{-}2\ Cl^-$) cotransport mechanism. Hebert et al. [8] have shown that the mouse medullary TAL possesses a similar transport mechanism.

Excellent correlations exist between the morphologic, biochemical, and physiologic characteristics of the TAL. For instance, the basolateral membrane area of the medullary TAL is greatest in the inner stripe [4], and it is in this segment of the TAL that Na,K-ATPase activity is the highest [9]. In addition, isolated perfused tubule studies have revealed a greater capacity for NaCl reabsorption in the medullary than the cortical TAL [10]. The cortical TAL is capable of maintaining a steeper concentration gradient for NaCl, which results in a lower concentration of this solute in the tubular fluid, and a lower fluid osmolality [11]. It is interesting to speculate that the more complicated apical lateral interdigitations between the cells of the cortical TAL, that result in an increase in the luminal surface area, may be responsible in some manner for this physiological characteristic.

Several hormones operating through activation of the adenylate cyclase system influence the function of the TAL. For instance, vasopressin stimulates NaCl reabsorption in the medullary TAL of the mouse [8] and rat [12], but not the rabbit [12], and biochemical studies have shown vasopressin stimulation of adenylate cyclase activity in the mouse and rat medullary TAL, but little in the rabbit. In contrast, there is no evidence for either vasopressin-stimulated NaCl transport or increased adenylate cyclase activity in the cortical TAL. Chronic administration of vasopressin to rats with hereditary hypothalamic diabetes insipidus leads to hypertrophy of the medullary TAL [13], presumably the result of enhanced NaCl transport, while acute vasopressin administration stimulates NaCl reabsorption in isolated perfused medullary TAL segments from the same animals [14]. These data suggest a role for vasopressin in the maintenance of a hypertonic medullary interstitium through regulation of NaCl transport by the medullary TAL.

We have demonstrated a decrease in cell height and an increase in surface area of the basolateral membrane in cells of the medullary TAL in drug-induced hypothyroidism in rats, which could be prevented by treatment with thyroid hormone [15,16]. Since hypothyroidism is associated with a decrease in adenylate cyclase activity, these morphological changes may be the result of impairment in vasopressin-stimulated ion transport.

Distal Convoluted Tubule

This segment of the distal tubule is actively involved in NaCl transport, although the exact transport mechanism, while incompletely understood, probably differs from the Na^+-K^+-$2Cl^-$ cotransport mechanism that is characteristic of the TAL. The morphology of the DCT is greatly affected by the delivery of NaCl to this segment. For instance, Kaissling et al. [17,18] have demonstrated that in rabbits fed a high sodium, low potassium diet there is an increase in the surface area of the basolateral plasma membrane of DCT cells and an increase in Na,K-ATPase activity. Furthermore, chronic administration of a loop diuretic is associated with a significant increase in cell height and basolateral membrane area in rat DCT cells [18]. In our own laboratory we have demonstrated that chronic bumetanide administration in the rat is associated with hypertrophy of the DCT only when animals receive augmented NaCl in their drinking water (K.M. Madsen, W.J. Welch, K. Jin 1990, unpublished observations), thus providing additional evidence that the morphologic and biochemical alterations described previously with a loop diuretic are quite likely due to enhanced NaCl delivery to the DCT.

Connecting Segment

Structure

This region of the renal tubule represents the transition from the DCT to the initial portion of the cortical collecting duct, commonly referred to as the initial collecting tubule (ICT). In superficial nephrons there is a direct one on one transition, whereas in mid-cortical and juxtamedullary nephrons connecting tubules join to form arcades that actually ascend in the cortex before joining an ICT. In most species, including humans and rats, the connecting segment is not well defined because of extensive intermingling of cells from the DCT and the ICT. This gives rise to a very gradual transition, which contrasts with the transition in the rabbit, where there is a well-defined connecting tubule (CNT) composed of two cell types, CNT cells and intercalated cells. In the rat kidney, the transition region is composed of four cell types — DCT cells, CNT cells, intercalated cells, and principal cells. The CNT cell which is characteristic of this region is intermediate in its ultrastructural appearance between the DCT cell and the principal cell and features a combination of basolateral interdigitations and true basal infoldings of the plasma membrane. Mitochondria, though prominent, are less numerous than in the cells of the DCT.

The intercalated cells vary greatly in their appearance in the same species and between species. For instance, in the rabbit CNT a black and a gray form have been described, both of which are rich in mitochondria [19]. The latter, however, possesses more tubulovesicular profiles in the apical cytoplasm. We have described two types of intercalated cells, type A and type B, in this region and throughout the cortical collecting duct of the rat (Fig. 1a, b) [20]. The type A cells in the rat resemble the gray intercalated cells of the rabbit.

Structural-Functional Relationships

High levels of parathyroid hormone — and isoproterenol-dependent adenylate cyclase activity — have been measured in the rabbit CNT [2], but there is no stimulation of this second messenger by vasopressin, nor is there any physiologic or morphologic evidence for increased water permeability in response to this hormone [21].

Both morphologic and physiologic data have identified a role in potassium secretion for the connecting segment [22,23] which, at least in part, is under the control of mineralocorticoids. Potassium secretion is decreased in the superficial distal nephron (which includes the DCT, the connecting segment, and the ICT) in adrenalectomized rats [24], and morphologic studies performed in the same segments reveal a decrease in the surface area of the basolateral membrane of principal cells of the ICT, which is a site of Na,K-ATPase activity [25]. The chronic administration of aldosterone can prevent the decrease in basolateral membrane area and larger doses will actually increase the surface area of the basolateral membrane of principal cells. Potassium loading, which stimulates aldosterone secretion, exerts a similar effect in both rats and rabbits. Potassium secretion in the late distal tubule (including the connecting segment and ICT) is increased and the surface area of the basolateral membrane is also increased in both principal cells and CNT cells [17,26].

Cortical Collecting Duct

Structure

Generally we divide the cortical collecting duct (CCD) into two major segments — the ICT and the medullary ray portion. Taken together, the connecting segment and the ICT of superficial nephrons constitute the so-called "late" distal tubule, which has

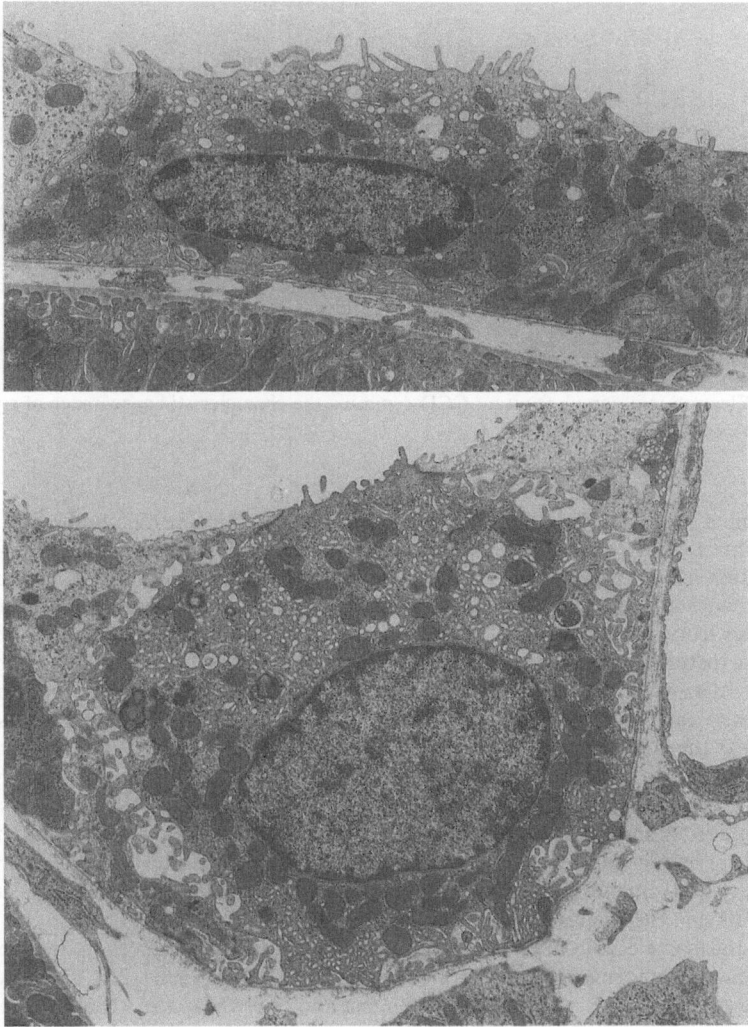

Fig. 1a,b. Electron micrographs from rat CCD illustrating the differences in structure of: **a** the type A intercalated cell, × 6370 and **b** the type B intercalated cell, × 5400

been studied extensively by renal micropuncturists. The medullary ray portion of the CCD is commonly used in isolated perfused tubule experiments. This region contains both intercalated cells, which in the rat and rabbit contribute from 37% to 39% of the total cell population, and principal cells. No major differences in the overall morphology of the principal cell have been reported to exist in the various regions of the CCD. However, it has become increasingly evident that structural as well as functional heterogeneity exists in the intercalated cells in the CCD.

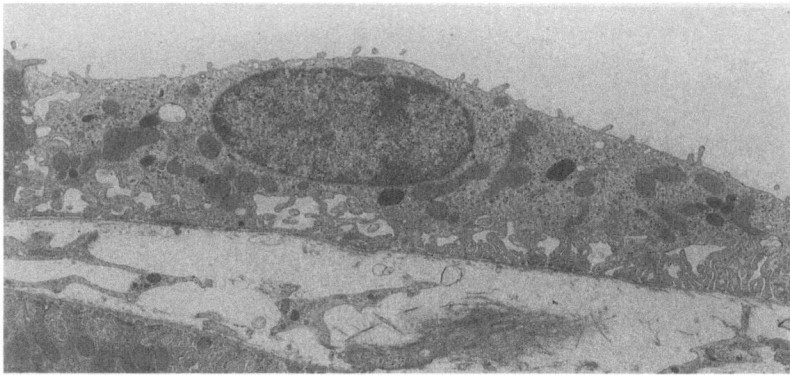

Fig. 2. Electron micrograph from rat CCD depicting the characteristic appearance of a principal cell, × 5200

Principal cells exhibit extensive infoldings of the basal plasma membrane, but lack lateral interdigitations (Fig. 2). The cells contain relatively few mitochondria, which are scattered randomly through a light staining cytoplasm. The luminal surface is covered with a few blunt microvilli and has a single centrally-positioned cilium.

Studies from our laboratory [20] and by other investigators [19] have identified at least two distinct populations of intercalated cells throughout the CCD. Type A intercalated cells, which are believed to be involved in proton secretion, are more common in the early portion of the ICT, whereas type B intercalated cells increase in number as the collecting duct approaches the medullary ray. With scanning electron microscopy it has been possible to identify distinct surface patterns for each cell type (Fig. 3). Type A cells are generally covered with microplicae, while type B cells exhibit microvilli. Microplicae are especially prominent in those cells located in the connecting segment and early ICT, but tend to be less extensive on type A cells in the medullary ray. In the rabbit, some intercalated cells have either microplicae or microvilli, but the majority exhibit both.

Transmission electron microscopy has revealed distinct differences in the appearance of these two forms of intercalated cells in the CCD (Fig. 1a, b) [20]. Type A cells have a cytoplasm that is rich in mitochondria and polyribosomes. Tubulovesicular membrane structures are extensive in the apical cytoplasm. Prominent studs are present on the cytoplasmic surface of many of the tubulovesicular structures and along the apical, but not the basolateral plasma membrane. The cytoplasm of the type B cells is generally more electron dense and, in addition to an extensive population of polyribosomes and mitochondria, contains numerous vesicular structures throughout the cell. In contrast to type A cells, the vesicles in these cells are generally smooth on the cytoplasmic surface and lack studs. Occasional studs have been observed on the cytoplasmic surface of the basolateral, but not the apical plasma, membrane of type B intercalated cells.

Immunocytochemical studies from our laboratory [27] and by other investigators have revealed striking differences between type A and type B intercalated cells in the CCD. For instance, we have demonstrated that antibodies against band 3 protein, an

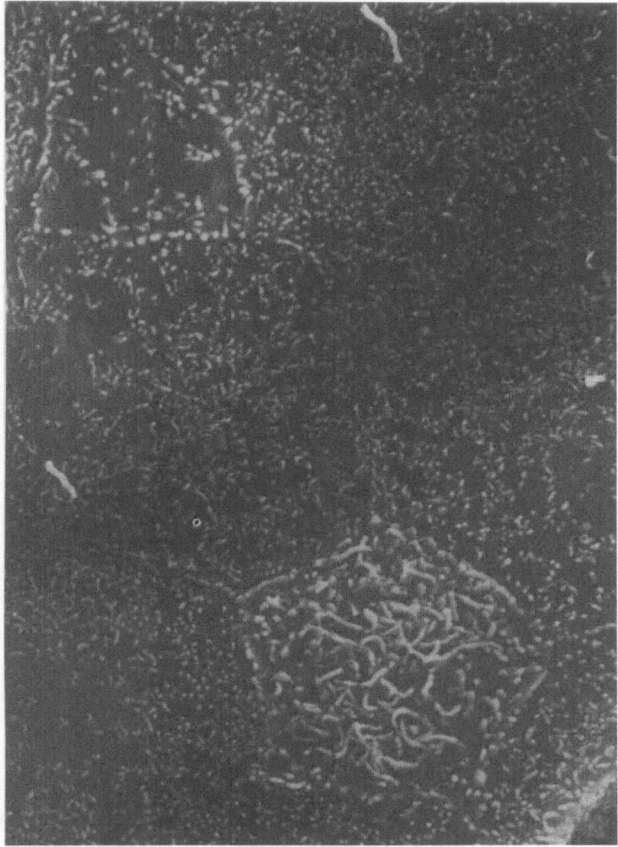

Fig. 3. Scanning electron micrograph from rat CCD illustrating the luminal surface of a type B intercalated cell (*upper left*) and a type A intercalated cell (*lower right*). Principal cells are covered with short, blunt microvilli and possess a single centrally-positioned cilium, × 9000

anion transporter involved in HCO_3-Cl exchange, bind to the basolateral membrane of type A cells (Fig. 4), but fail to label type B cells. Recently, it has been observed that antibodies against H-ATPase bind to tubulovesicular structures and the apical plasma membrane of type A cells (Fig. 5a) and to cytoplasmic vesicles and the basolateral plasma membrane of type B cells (Fig. 5b) [28].

Both types of intercalated cells in the rat and the rabbit have been found to possess high levels of carbonic anhydrase activity when subjected to the appropriate immunocytochemical procedures [29]. However, we have demonstrated recently that major differences do exist in the amount and distribution of carbonic anhydrase II immunoreactivity between these two populations of intercalated cells [30]. When we used a rabbit polyclonal antibody directed against mouse erythrocyte carbonic anhydrase II in combination with a horseradish peroxidase detection procedure, immuno-

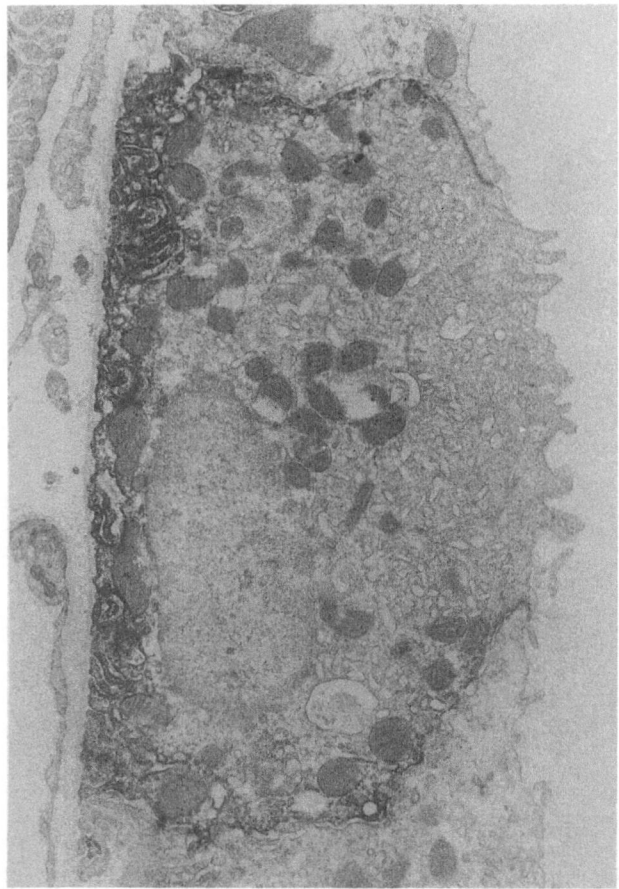

Fig. 4. Electron micrograph of type A intercalated cell from rat CCD, depicting localization of antibodies to band 3 protein along the basolateral plasma membrane of a type A intercalated cell, using an immunoperoxidase technique, × 12740

staining was strikingly more pronounced in type A than in type B cells (Fig. 6). In the former, the staining was especially prominent over the apical region, whereas type B cells had weak diffuse staining throughout the cytoplasm. In addition, the densely staining A cells had a spider-like cell configuration, while the type B cells were round or ovoid in appearance. Thus, this immunocytochemical reaction provides an excellent marker to separate type A from type B intercalated cells by both light and electron microscopy in the rat. The findings provide additional evidence that at least two distinct populations of intercalated cells exist in the CCD, populations that are morphologically, as well as functionally, distinct.

Wingo et al. [31], working in our laboratory, have recently published immunocytochemical evidence for the presence of H-K-ATPase activity in the intercalated

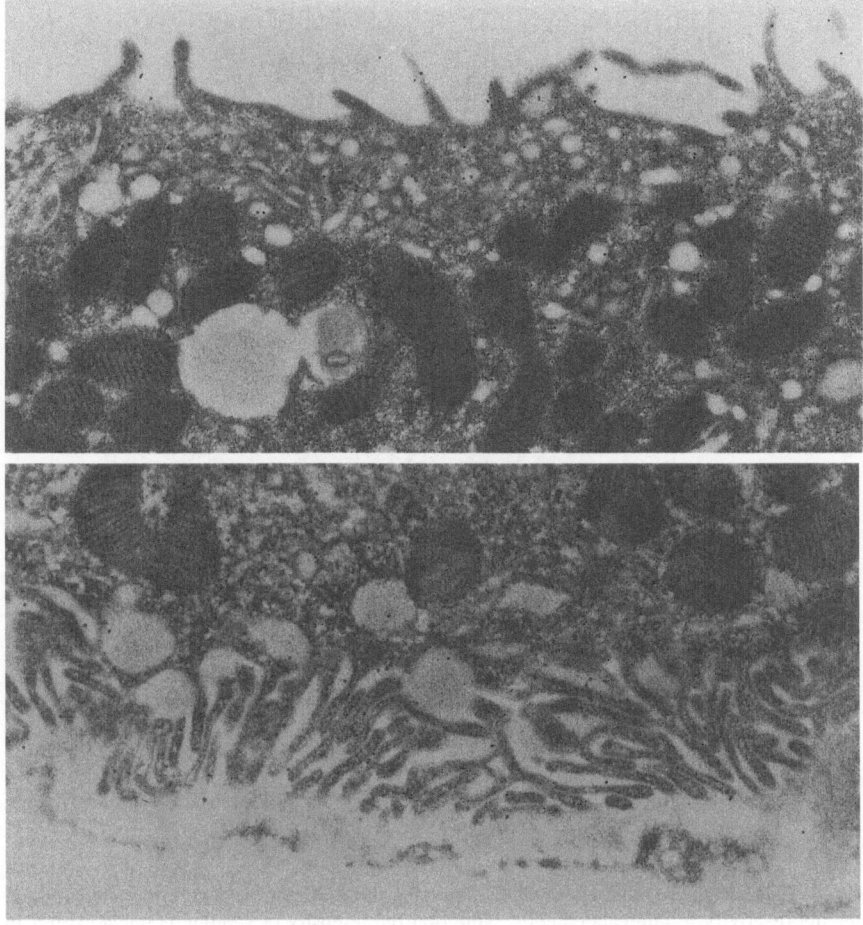

Fig. 5a,b. Electron micrographs from rat CCD depicting localization of antibodies against H⁺-ATPase: **a** along the luminal membrane and apical tubulovesicles in a type A intercalated cell, × 21060 and **b** along the basolateral membrane of a type B intercalated cell, × 19840

cells of the CCD and the outer medullary collecting duct (OMCD) of the rat and rabbit. Using a mouse monoclonal antibody against hog gastric H-K-ATPase that did not cross react with either Na,K-ATPase or H-ATPase, Wingo and coworkers found diffuse cytoplasmic staining, indicative of H-K-ATPase immunoreactivity, to be present in intercalated cells in the CCD and OMCD of rat and rabbit. In all segments except the rat CCD, the percentage of H-K-ATPase immunoreactive cells corresponded to the percentage of intercalated cells. However, in the rat, only 23% of the cells were reactive, which is less than the percentage of intercalated cells in this segment of the collecting duct. It is possible that, in the rat, only type A intercalated cells

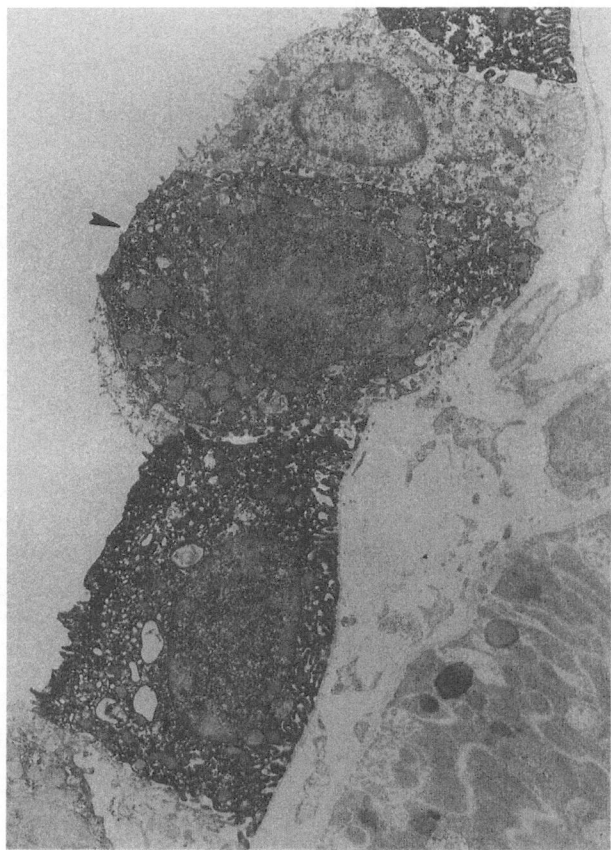

Fig. 6. Electron micrograph of rat CCD, depicting the localization of carbonic anhydrase II immunoreactivity in intercalated cells. Note that the intensity of staining is much greater in type A than in type B (*arrowhead*) cells. The principal cells have only faint staining for carbonic anhydrase II immunoreactivity, × 5250

possess H-K-ATPase activity, or that some intercalated cells did not have sufficient activity to be detected by the immunocytochemical method that was employed.

Structural-Functional Relationships

There is both structural and functional evidence that the ICT is involved in potassium secretion [23], hydrogen ion secretion, and vasopressin-induced water reabsorption. The ICT behaves in a manner similar to that of the connecting segment with respect to potassium secretion. Stanton and co-workers [26] have provided convincing evidence that chronic potassium loading, which stimulates aldosterone secretion, is associated with both an increase in potassium secretion in the so-called "late" distal tubule and with proliferation of the basolateral membrane of principal cells in the ICT. Moreover, in adrenalectomized rats these same cells exhibit a decrease in surface area of the basolateral membrane [25], and potassium secretion is impaired [24]. These defects can be either reversed or prevented with aldosterone administration [24,25]. Thus, the principal cells appear to be responsible for mineralocorticoid-dependent potassium secretion in the ICT.

Hydrogen ion secretion also appears to be a function of the ICT. Evidence from micropuncture studies has documented the presence of proton secretion in superficial distal tubules of acid-loaded rats [32]. We have observed a striking increase in the surface density of type A intercalated cells in both the ICT and the medullary ray portion of the CCD of the rat with acute respiratory acidosis [20].

The entire collecting duct, including the ICT, plays an important role in urine dilution and concentration. With vasopressin stimulation the apical membrane of the principal cells becomes permeable to water, due to the insertion of water channels [33]. Early morphologic studies from our laboratory [34] demonstrated that vasopressin-induced osmotic water reabsorption is associated with swelling of the principal cells and with intercellular space dilatation. In the absence of the hormone these morphologic features of transepithelial water flow are not observed.

Many of the structural-functional relationships described in the ICT are also present in the CCD. For instance, physiologic studies performed in the isolated perfused rabbit CCD have demonstrated that mineralocorticoids stimulate potassium secretion [35]. Biochemical studies have documented increased levels of Na,K-ATPase activity following mineralocorticoid administration in the CCD of both the rat [36] and the rabbit [3]. Morphologists have demonstrated a significant increase in the surface area of the basolateral plasma membrane of principal cells in the CCD of rabbits treated with deoxycorticosterone acetate [37] or fed a diet high in potassium and low in sodium [17]. In addition, optical and microelectrode studies have demonstrated that principal cells, but not intercalated cells, possess a barium-sensitive potassium conductance in the luminal membrane, thus providing further evidence that the principal cell is involved in potassium secretion [38,39]. These morphologic, physiologic, and biochemical data all suggest that the principal cells in the CCD are responsible for mineralocorticoid-stimulated potassium secretion in association with sodium reabsorption.

As described briefly in an earlier section, there is considerable structural and functional evidence that type A intercalated cells are involved in proton and bicarbonate transport. Depending on the physiologic condition of the animal, the CCD can either reabsorb or secrete bicarbonate. Using the isolated perfused tubule technique it has been found that the rabbit CCD dissected from normal and acid-loaded rabbits reabsorbs bicarbonate [40,41]. In contrast, CCD from bicarbonate-loaded rabbits [42] or rabbits treated with deoxycorticosterone [43] secretes bicarbonate. Furthermore, CCD from rats receiving an ammonium chloride load reabsorbs bicarbonate, while CCD dissected from rats receiving either deoxycorticosterone [44] or a bicarbonate load [45] secretes bicarbonate.

Morphologic studies performed in our laboratory by Verlander et al. [20] have demonstrated that, in the rat CCD, type A intercalated cells respond to acute respiratory acidosis with an increase in the apical or luminal membrane area, secondary to fusion of tubulovesicular structures, normally located in the apical cell cytoplasm, with the luminal plasma membrane. We and others [28], using immunocytochemical

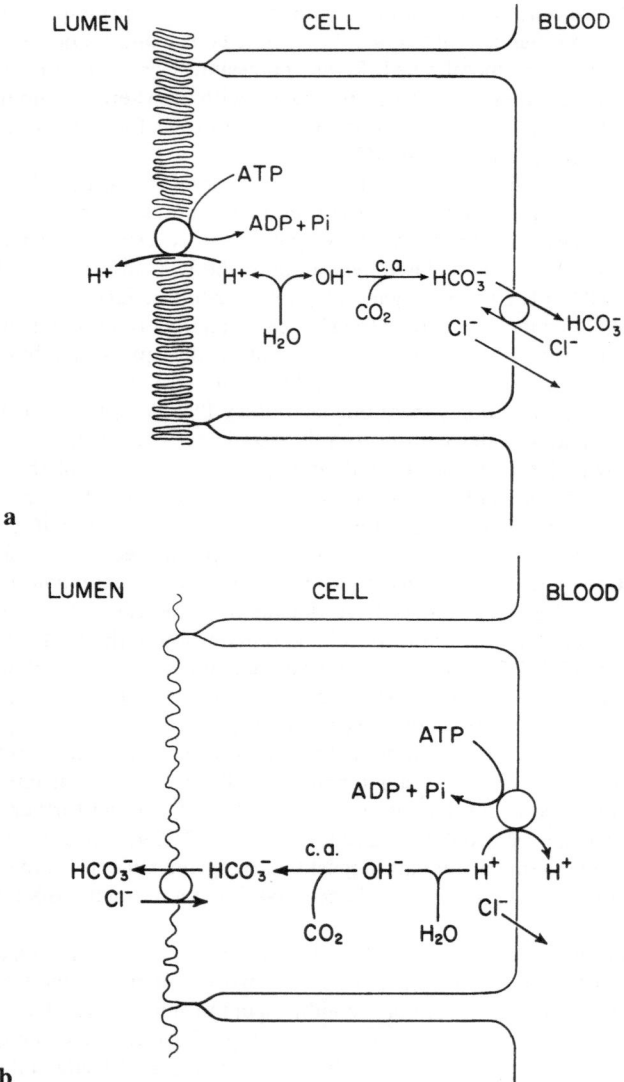

Fig. 7a,b. Functional characteristics of: **a** type A intercalated cell and **b** type B intercalated cell in the rat CCD. c.a., carbonic anhydrase

techniques, have demonstrated the presence of an H-ATPase in the tubulovesicular structures, and it is this transporter that is believed to be inserted into the luminal membrane of the type A intercalated cell in response to the need to secrete protons. There is also histochemical and immunocytochemical evidence for the presence of carbonic anhydrase II throughout the cytoplasm of both types of intercalated cells

[29,30,46]. We [27] and other investigators [47] have demonstrated that antibodies against erythrocyte band 3 protein, an anion transporter responsible for Cl-HCO_3 exchange, are located along the basolateral plasma membrane of type A intercalated cells. Thus, type A cells possess a Cl-HCO_3 exchanger to permit bicarbonate reabsorption, an H-ATPase to effect secretion of protons at the luminal surface, and carbonic anhydrase activity within the cytoplasm to catalyze the hydration of CO_2 to form hydroxyl ions and protons. This mechanism for proton secretion and bicarbonate reabsorption in the type A cells is illustrated in Fig. 7a.

Evidence is accumulating that type B intercalated cells are involved in bicarbonate secretion. As noted in an earlier section, CCD from both rats and rabbits secretes bicarbonate, following a bicarbonate load [42,45] or deoxycorticosterone treatment [43,44]. Functional studies employing fluorescent pH-sensitive probes have provided evidence for a Cl-HCO_3 exchange process across the luminal plasma membrane of peanut lectin-positive cells in the rabbit CCD, which correspond to type B intercalated cells in the rat. All intercalated cells in the rat and rabbit, including type B cells, are immunoreactive for carbonic anhydrase II [30]. There is additional immunocytochemical evidence for the presence of H-ATPase activity distributed diffusely in the cytoplasm or in the basal region of the type B cells. We have preliminary evidence from our laboratory suggesting that stimulation of bicarbonate secretion leads to an increase in both the volume of B cells and their basolateral plasma membrane area [48]. We have also observed that the type B intercalated cells decrease in size in chronic metabolic acidosis. Thus, type B cells appear to play a significant role in regulating bicarbonate secretion under the appropriate experimental conditions, as illustrated in Fig. 7b.

The presence of H-K-ATPase immunoreactivity in the rat and rabbit CCD [31] raises the distinct possibility that intercalated cells are also involved in the reabsorption of potassium in exchange for protons. This possibility will be explored in greater detail in the section on the OMCD that follows.

Outer Medullary Collecting Duct

Structure

The OMCD has two distinct segments, the $OMCD_o$, located in the outer stripe and the $OMCD_i$, located in the inner stripe of the outer medulla. In both segments in the rat, intercalated cells constitute approximately 36%–40% of the cells, with the percentage remaining representing principal cells [49]. In the rabbit, however, there is a gradual decrease in the number of intercalated cells along the entire OMCD, where they represent approximately 18% of the total cell population [50]. In the rat, the overwhelming majority of intercalated cells in the outer stripe, and essentially all intercalated cells in the inner stripe, resemble the type A cells in the CCD. Tubulovesicular membrane structures, often possessing studs on their cytoplasmic surface, are extensive throughout the apical cytoplasm, and micro-projections, so-called microplicae that are appreciated best with scanning electron microscopy, are extensive on the luminal membrane surface. The cytoplasmic surface of the luminal plasma membrane is, also, often studded. Rod-shaped particles have been described with freeze-fracture in the luminal membrane of these cells [51], but their relationship, if any, to the studs on the cytoplasmic side of the apical cell membrane remains unclear.

The principal cells in the OMCD resemble those located in the CCD, although some differences have been described. The basal infoldings of the former are less extensive and they have fewer organelles.

Immunocytochemical studies have documented that antibodies against band 3 protein, the anion transporter involved in Cl-HCO$_3$ exchange, bind along the basolateral membrane of all intercalated cells in the rat and rabbit OMCD. Antibodies against H-ATPase bind to tubulovesicular structures and to the apical membrane of these same intercalated cells [46], which are also positive for carbonic anhydrase II immunoreactivity. Finally, as noted in an earlier section, Wingo et al. [31] have demonstrated H-K-ATPase immunoreactivity in all intercalated cells in the OMCD of both the rat and the rabbit.

Structural-Functional Relationships

Physiologic, biochemical, and morphologic studies all provide evidence that the OMCD is a major site of proton secretion in the distal nephron. Proton secretion, measured as bicarbonate reabsorption, is well documented in the isolated perfused OMCD, dissected from the kidneys of both normal and acidotic rabbits [41]. This electrogenic sodium-independent process that is mineralocorticoid-sensitive [52] resembles the acidification process described in the turtle urinary bladder. Studies in both the turtle urinary bladder [53] and the bovine renal medulla [54] have led to isolation of an H-ATPase believed to be responsible for this electrogenic hydrogen-translocating process. Studies employing a fluorescent pH-sensitive dye, performed first in the turtle urinary bladder [55] and later in the rabbit OMCD, [56], demonstrated that an increase in the ambient carbon dioxide caused a simultaneous increase in hydrogen ion secretion and release of fluorescent vesicle contents from mitochondria-rich and intercalated cells, respectively. Based on the findings in the turtle, it was suggested that proton secretion is regulated by exocytotic insertion of H-ATPase into the luminal membrane of the mitochondria-rich cell [55]. Subsequent morphologic data supported this hypothesis by demonstrating that stimulation of proton secretion in the turtle urinary bladder caused an increase in surface area of the luminal membrane and a decrease in the volume density of apical vesicles in mitochondria-rich cells [57]. Studies from our own laboratory [58,59] demonstrated significant ultrastructural changes in OMCD intercalated cells of rats with either acute respiratory acidosis or chronic metabolic acidosis, suggesting that the intercalated cells are responsible for proton secretion in the OMCD. These morphologic changes with acidosis included an increase in the surface density and surface area of the luminal plasma membrane and a simultaneous decrease in the number of tubulovesicular membrane profiles in the apical cell region. The stud-like structures located on the cytoplasmic surface of the tubulovesicular profiles were transferred to the cytoplasmic surface of the luminal membranes. On the basis of these observations, we suggested that membrane containing a proton pump was inserted into the luminal membrane when hydrogen ion secretion was stimulated. Immunocytochemical studies by Brown et al. [28], using the immunogold technique, were reproduced later in our own laboratory and have demonstrated H-ATPase immunoreactivity within the tubulovesicular structures and along the luminal cell membrane of intercalated cells. Antibodies against band 3 protein, the Cl-HCO$_3$ exchanger, have been demonstrated along the basolateral membrane of these same cells [27]. As noted in an earlier section, the intercalated cells also possess a high level of immunoreactivity to carbonic anhydrase II [30]. Thus, intercalated cells in the OMCD resemble the type A cells in the CCD and appear capable of secreting protons.

Biochemical, physiologic, and morphologic studies have provided evidence for the presence of an H-K-ATPase in the CCD and OMCD, which is believed to be involved in the reabsorption of potassium in exchange for protons. K-ATPase activity that is ouabain-insensitive, but inhibited by omeprazole and SCH 28080 has been described in individual segments of the CCD and OMCD in both rat [60] and rabbit [60,61]. Wingo [62] has provided physiologic evidence for active potassium reabsorption and proton secretion that is also inhibited by omeprazole, a known inhibitor of gastric H-K-ATPase, in the isolated OMCD dissected from rabbits on a potassium restricted diet. Immunocytochemical studies by Wingo et al. [31] have identified H-K-ATPase immunoreactivity in all intercalated cells in the OMCD of both the rat and the rabbit. Taken together, these data provide strong support for an additional mechanism for acid secretion by the collecting duct, in which protons are exchanged for potassium in the intercalated cell, a process similar to that present in the parietal cell of the gastric mucosa.

Acknowledgments. The authors acknowledge the technical assistance of James K. Cannon, Frederick Kopp, and Wendy L. Wilber, and the secretarial support of Deborah S. Malis. The authors also thank Dr. W. Fischlschweiger, Director of the Electron Microscope Facility of the College of Dentistry at the University of Florida, where the electron microscope studies were performed.

This work was supported, in part, by National Institutes of Health Grant DK-28330.

References

1. Burg MB, Grantham J, Abramow M, Orloff J (1966) Preparation and study of fragments of single rabbit nephrons. Am J Physiol 210:1293–1298
2. Morel F (1981) Sites of hormone action in the mammalian nephron. Am J Physiol 240: F159–F164
3. Garg LC, Knepper MA, Burg MB (1981) Mineralocorticoid effects of Na-K-ATPase in individual nephron segments. Am J Physiol 240:F536–F544
4. Kone BC, Madsen KM, Tisher CC (1984) Ultrastructure of the thick ascending limb of Henle in the rat kidney. Am J Anat 171:217–226
5. Allen F, Tisher CC (1976) Morphology of the ascending thick limb of Henle. Kidney Int 9:8–22
6. Kashgarian M, Biemesderfer D, Caplan M, Forbus B (1985) Monoclonal antibody to Na,K-ATPase: immunocytochemical localization along nephron segments. Kidney Int 28:899–913
7. Greger R, Schlatter E, Lang F (1983) Evidence for electroneutral sodium chloride cotransport in the cortical thick ascending limb of Henle's loop of rabbit kidney. Pflugers Arch 396:308–314
8. Hebert SC, Culpepper RM, Andreoli TE (1981) NaCl transport in mouse medullary thick ascending limbs. I. Functional nephron heterogeneity and ADH-stimulated NaCl cotransport. Am J Physiol 241:F412–F431
9. Garg LC, Mackie S, Tisher CC (1982) Effect of low potassium diet on Na⁺-K⁺-ATPase in rat nephron segments. Pflugers Arch 394:113–117

10. Rocha AS, Kokko JP (1973) Sodium chloride and water transport in the medullary thick ascending limb of Henle. Evidence for active chloride transport. J Clin Invest 54:612–623
11. Burg MB, Green N (1973) Function of the thick ascending limb of Henle's loop. Am J Physiol 224:659–668
12. Sasaki S, Imai M (1980) Effects of vasopressin on water and NaCl transport across the in vitro perfused medullary thick ascending limb of Henle's loop of mouse, rat, and rabbit kidneys. Pflugers Arch 383:215–221
13. Bouby N, Bankir L, Thinh-Trang-Tan MM, Minuth WW, Kriz W (1985) Selective ADH-induced hypertrophy of the medullary thick ascending limb in Brattleboro rats. Kidney Int 28:456–466
14. Work J, Galla JH, Booker B, Schafer JA, Luke R (1985) Effect of ADH on chloride reabsorption in the loop of Henle of Brattleboro rats. Am J Physiol 249:F698–F703
15. Davis RG, Madsen KM, Fregly MJ, Tisher CC (1983) Kidney structure in hypothyroidism. Am J Pathol 113:41–49
16. Bentley AG, Madsen KM, Davis RG, Tisher CC (1985) Response of the medullary thick ascending limb to hypothyroidism in the rat. Am J Pathol 120:215–221
17. Kaissling B, LeHir M (1982) Distal tubular segments of the rabbit kidney after adaptation to altered Na- and K-intake. I. Structural changes. Cell Tissue Res 224:469–492
18. Kaissling B, Bachmann S, Kriz W (1985) Structural adaptation of the distal convoluted tubule to prolonged furosemide treatment. Am J Physiol 248:F374–F381
19. Kaissling B, Kriz W (1979) Structural analysis of the rabbit kidney. Adv Anat Embryol Cell Biol 56:1–123
20. Verlander JW, Madsen KM, Tisher CC (1987) Effect of acute respiratory acidosis on two populations of intercalated cells in the rat cortical collecting duct. Am J Physiol 253:F1142–F1156
21. Imai M (1979) The connecting tubule: a functional subdivision of the rabbit distal nephron segments. Kidney Int 15:346–356
22. Kaissling B (1982) Structural aspects of adaptive changes in renal electrolyte excretion. Am J Physiol 243:F211–F226
23. Wright FS, Giebisch G (1978) Renal potassium transport: contributions of individual nephron segments and populations. Am J Physiol 235:F515–F527
24. Field MJ, Stanton BA, Giebisch GH (1984) Differential acute effects of aldosterone, dexamethasone, and hyperkalemia on distal tubular potassium secretion in the rat kidney. J Clin Invest 74:1792–1802
25. Stanton B, Janzen A, Klein-Robbenhaar G, De Fronzo R, Giebisch G, Wade J (1985) Ultrastructure of rat initial collecting tubule. Effect of adrenal corticosteroid treatment. J Clin Invest 75:1327–1334
26. Stanton BA, Biemesderfer D, Wade JB, Giebisch G (1981) Structural and functional study of the rat distal nephron: effects of potassium adaptation and depletion. Kidney Int 19:36–48
27. Verlander JW, Madsen KM, Low PS, Allen DP, Tisher CC (1988) Immunocytochemical localization of band 3 protein in the rat collecting duct. Am J Physiol 255:F115–F125
28. Brown D, Hirsch S, Gluck S (1988) An H⁺-ATPase in opposite plasma membrane domains in kidney epithelial cell subpopulations. Nature 331:622–624
29. Brown D, Kumpulainen T, Roth J, Orci L (1983) Immunohistochemical localization of carbonic anhydrase in postnatal and adult rat kidney. Am J Physiol 245:F110–F118
30. Kim J, Tisher CC, Linser PJ, Madsen KM (1990) Ultrastructural localization of carbonic anhydrase II in subpopulations of intercalated cells of the rat kidney. J Am Soc Nephrol 1:245–256
31. Wingo CS, Madsen KM, Smolka A, Tisher CC (1990) H-K-ATPase immunoreactivity in cortical and outer medullary collecting duct. Kidney Int 38:985–990
32. Lucci MS, Pucacco LR, Carter NW, DuBose TD (1982) Evaluation of bicarbonate transport in rat distal tubule: effects of acid-base status. Am J Physiol 243:F335–F341

33. Strange K, Willingham MC, Handler JS, Harris HW, Jr (1988) Apical membrane endocytosis via coated pits is stimulated by removal of antidiuretic hormone from isolated, perfused rabbit cortical collecting tubule. J Membr Biol 103:17–28
34. Woodhall PB, Tisher CC (1973) Response of the distal tubule and cortical collecting duct to vasopressin in the rat. J Clin Invest 52:3095–3108
35. O'Neil RG, Helman SI (1977) Transport characteristics of renal collecting tubules: influences of DOCA and diet. Am J Physiol 233:F544–F558
36. Mujais SK, Chekal MA, Jones WJ, Hayslett JP, Katz AI (1984) Regulation of renal Na-K-ATPase in the rat: role of the natural mineralo- and glucocorticoid hormones. J Clin Invest 73:13–19
37. Wade JB, O'Neil RG, Pryor JL, Boulpaep EL (1979) Modulation of cell membrane area in renal collecting tubules by corticosteroid hormones. J Cell Biol 81:439–445
38. O'Neil RG, Hayhurst RA (1985) Functional differentiation of cell types of cortical collecting duct. Am J Physiol 248:F449–F453
39. Muto S, Giebisch G, Sansom S (1987) Effects of adrenalectomy on CCD: evidence for differential response of two cell types. Am J Physiol 253:F742–F752
40. McKinney TD, Burg MB (1978) Bicarbonate absorption by rabbit cortical collecting tubules in vitro. Am J Physiol 234:F141–F145
41. Lombard WE, Jacobson HR, Kokko JP (1983) Bicarbonate transport in cortical and outer medullary collecting tubules. Am J Physiol 244:F289–F296
42. McKinney TD, Burg MB (1978) Bicarbonate secretion by rabbit cortical collecting tubules in vitro. J Clin Invest 61:1421–1427
43. Star RA, Burg MB, Knepper MA (1985) Bicarbonate secretion by rabbit cortical collecting ducts. Role of chloride/bicarbonate exchange. J Clin Invest 76:1123–1130
44. Knepper MA, Good DW, Burg MB (1985) Ammonia and bicarbonate transport by rat cortical collecting ducts perfused in vitro. Am J Physiol 249:F870–F877
45. Atkins JL, Burg MB (1985) Bicarbonate transport by isolated perfused rat collecting ducts. Am J Physiol 249:F485–F489
46. Lonnerholm G, Ridderstrale Y (1980) Intracellular distribution of carbonic anhydrase in the rat kidney. Kidney Int 17:162–174
47. Schuster VL, Bonsib SM, Jennings ML (1986) Two types of collecting duct mitochondria-rich (intercalated) cells: lectin and band 3 cytochemistry. Am J Physiol 251:C347–C355
48. Tisher CC, Verlander JW, Madsen KM, Galla JH, Luke RG, Bonduris D (1989) Morphological findings in rat collecting duct during chloride-depletion metabolic alkalosis. Kidney Int 35:464A
49. Hansen GP, Tisher CC, Robinson RR (1980) Response of the collecting duct to disturbances of acid-base and potassium balance. Kidney Int 17:326–337
50. Le Furgey A, Tisher CC (1979) Morphology of rabbit collecting duct. Am J Anat 155:111–124
51. Stetson DL, Wade JB, Giebisch G (1980) Morphologic alterations in the rat medullary collecting duct following potassium depletion. Kidney Int 17:45–56
52. Stone DK, Seldin DW, Kokko JP, Jacobson HR (1983) Mineralocorticoid modulation of rabbit medullary collecting duct acidification. A sodium-independent effect. J Clin Invest 72:77–83
53. Gluck S, Kelly S, Al-Awqati Q (1982) The proton-translocating ATPase responsible for urinary acidification. J Biol Chem 257:9230–9233
54. Gluck S, Al Awqati Q (1984) An electrogenic proton-translocating adenosine triphosphatase from bovine kidney medulla. J Clin Invest 73:1704–1710
55. Gluck S, Cannon C, Al-Awqati Q (1982) Exocytosis regulates urinary acidification in turtle bladder by rapid insertion of H+ pumps into the luminal membrane. Proc Natl Acad Sci USA 79:4327–4331
56. Schwartz GJ, Al-Awqati Q (1985) Carbon dioxide causes exocytosis of vesicles containing H+ pumps in isolated perfused proximal and collecting tubules. J Clin Invest 75:1638–1644

57. Stetson DL, Steinmetz PR (1983) Role of membrane fusion in CO_2 stimulation of proton secretion by turtle bladder. Am J Physiol 245:C113–C120
58. Madsen KM, Tisher CC (1983) Cellular response to acute respiratory acidosis in rat medullary collecting ducts. Am J Physiol 245:F670–F679
59. Madsen KM, Tisher CC (1984) Response of intercalated cells of rat outer medullary collecting duct to chronic metabolic acidosis. Lab Invest 51:268–276
60. Doucet A, Marsy S (1987) Characterization of K-ATPase activity in distal nephron: stimulation by potassium depletion. Am J Physiol 253:F418–F423
61. Garg LC, Narang N (1988) Ouabain-insensitive K-adenosine triphosphatase in distal nephron segments of the rabbit. J Clin Invest 81:1204–1208
62. Wingo CS (1989) Active proton secretion and potassium absorption in the rabbit outer medullary collecting duct: functional evidence for H-K-ATPase. J Clin Invest 84:361–365

Function of Thin Segments of Henle's Loop

Masashi Imai, Koji Yoshitomi, Yoshiaki Kondo,
Junichi Taniguchi, Chizuko Koseki, Taisuke Isozaki,
Kaoru Tabei, and Shigeru Koyama

Chair: Donald W. Seldin

\

Function of Thin Segments of Henle's Loop

Masashi Imai[1], Koji Yoshitomi[1], Yoshiaki Kondo[2], Junichi Taniguchi[3],
Chizuko Koseki[3], Taisuke Isozaki[4], Kaoru Tabei[1],
and Shigeru Koyama[1]

Introduction

It is well known that the renal medulla plays an important role in the generation of concentrated urine, which is critical in the maintenance of body fluid osmolality. Since the proposal of the operation of countercurrent systems in the renal medulla by Kuhn and his associates [1–3], it has been widely accepted that the loop structures of the nephron in the renal medulla are essential for the generation and maintenance of a steep osmotic gradient along the axis of the renal medulla. However, the detailed mechanisms by which a steep osmotic gradient is generated by the countercurrent multiplication system remain to be established.

Micropuncture studies on exposed renal papilla of rodents have established essential characteristics of the loop of Henle [4]. The luminal fluid in the descending limb of Henle's loop is concentrated as it flows down toward the papillary tip, whereas the fluid in the ascending limb is diluted as it flows upward. The observations that the fluid in the ascending limb is relatively hypotonic as compared to that in the descending limb [5] are compatible with the view that the countercurrent multiplication system operates in the loop of Henle. Although the in vitro microperfusion studies of thin loop segments in renal papillary slices shed light on the membrane properties of the thin loop segments [6], detailed mechanisms of water and ion transport are unknown.

The in vitro microperfusion technique developed by Burg et al. [7] provides a useful tool with which to examine detailed transport properties across those nephron segments which are inaccessible by conventional micropuncture techniques. More

[1]Department of Pharmacology, Jichi Medical School, Minamikawachi, Kawachi, Tochigi, 329-04 Japan
[2]Department of Pediatrics, Tohoku University, Sendai 980, Japan
[3]Departments of Molecular Physiology and Cell Biology, National Cardiovascular Center, Osaka, 565 Japan
[4]Department of Internal Medicine, Hamamatsu University School of Medicine, Hamamatsu, 431-31 Japan

recently, technical advances have allowed us to apply intracellular impalement of microelectrodes or fluorescent dye technique on the in vitro microperfused thin loop segments, thereby providing information on the cell membrane properties of these segments.

In addition to operating the urine concentrating mechanism, the renal medulla also contributes to renal handling of potassium and regulation of acid-base balance. The purpose of the present communication is to review the works in which characteristics of water and ion transport across these segments have been studied by in vitro microperfusion and to discuss their functional significance, with respect to the three distinct but inter-related functions of the renal medulla; namely, the urine concentrating mechanism, K⁺ recycling, and regulation of acid-base balance.

Morphology of Henle's Loop

The thin loop segments belong to the intermediate segments [4]. They include descending thin limb for the short-looped nephron (short descending limb, SDL), and descending (long descending limb, LDL) and ascending thin limbs (ATL) for the long-looped nephron. Since comprehensive reviews on the morphological features of the thin loop segments have been reported [4,8,9], we will briefly mention only the essential features which are relevant for understanding the function of the thin loop segments (Fig. 1).

Architectural Organization

The descending limb and the ascending limb of Henle's loop do not necessarily make a simple countercurrent contact with each other. Rather, they a have complicated architectural organization, with vascular bundles and capillary networks supplied from the vasa rectae. The renal medullary vasculatures originate from efferent arterioles of the juxtamedullary glomeruli. A group consisting of arteriole and venous vasa recta constitutes a vascular bundle in the outer medulla. In some species, several vascular bundles are combined to make a giant bundle [4,8,9]. It should be emphasized that blood of the venous vasa recta of the vascular bundle is supplied mainly from the capillary network in the inner medulla. In contrast, blood supplied to the outer medulla returns directly to the interlobular vein. Such distinct separation of blood supply, between outer and inner medulla, must have some physiological significance.

In most animal species, the descending limbs of the long-looped nephron are distributed in the interbundle regions, and appear to be separated from the vascular bundles by interpositioned thick ascending limbs [4,8,9]. In marked contrast, the descending limbs of the short-looped nephron have much closer contact with the vascular bundles [4,8,9]. However, there are some species differences in the pattern of the contact of the SDL with the vascular bundle. The pattern can be classified into three types. In the first type, the SDL distributes within the vascular bundle. In this type, the SDL clearly constitutes a countercurrent system with the ascending vasa recta. The segments of SDL in *Psammomys* [10], *Meriones* [11], *Perognathus* [12], and mice [13] belong to this type. In the second type, the SDL distributes around the vascular bundle. The SDL of the rat belongs to this type [14]. In the third type, the SDL distributes in the interbundle region. The SDLs of rabbits and hamsters belong

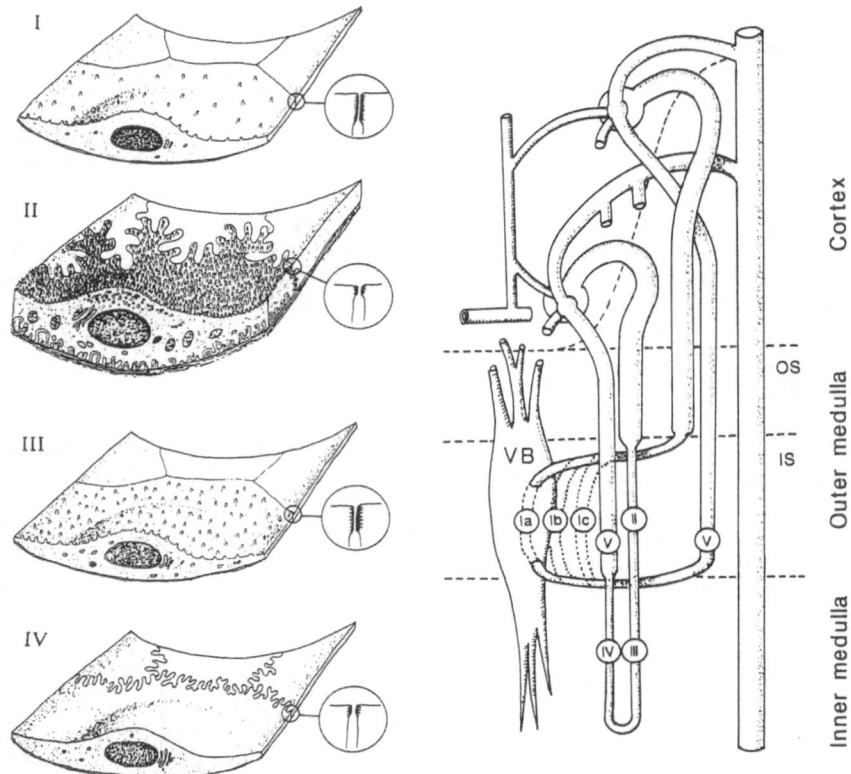

Fig. 1. Epithelial morphology and architectural organization of thin loop segments. I, Short looped descending limb (*SDL*); II, Upper portion of long-looped descending limb (*LDLu*); III, Lower portion of long-looped descending limb (*LDLl*); IV, Ascending thin limb (*ATL*). OS, outer stripe; IS, inner stripe; VB, vascular bundle. Figures in circles represent magnification of morphology of tight junctions

to this type [15,16]. Although it is not a general rule, there is a tendency that the species having closer contact of SDL with the vascular bundle have higher urine concentrating capacity.

Epithelial Morphology

With the exception of the rabbit, there are considerable heterogeneities in the morphology of the descending limb. Heterogeneity exists not only between short and long-looped nephrons (internephron heterogeneity), but also within the same long-looped nephron (intranephron or axial heterogeneity). These heterogeneities are prominent in rodent kidneys [4,8]. The short loop descending limb (SDL) consists of simple and flat epithelia (type I cells). The microvilli of the luminal membrane are not well developed. Only scarce organelles are present in cytoplasm. The apposition to the neighboring cells is simple and lacks interdigitation. The tight junctions are deep and contain several ramified junctional strands. These features are representative for tight epithelia.

In contrast, the morphology of the epithelia in the upper portion of the long-loop descending limb (LDLu) is more complicated [4]. The LDLu consists of the most elaborate cells, which have abundant microvilli in the apical membrane, are rich in cytoplasmic mitochondria, and have meticulously developed interdigitation with neighboring cells (Type II cells). The basal infolding of LDLu is also well developed. The tight junctions are very shallow, having only one or two junctional strands. These features are representative for leaky epithelia. Along the axis of the long-looped nephron, epithelial morphology changes gradually, with the height of epithelia becoming shorter. Qualitative changes in morphology occur somewhere near the border of the outer and inner medulla, but the position of the transition varies among nephrons. Sometimes the transition occurs in inner medulla.

The morphology of the lower portion of the long-loop descending limb (LDLl) is very similar to that of the SDL (Type III cell).

Functions of the Descending Limb

Water Permeability

Early micropuncture studies in exposed renal papilla of rats and hamsters have demonstrated that tubular fluid to plasma (TF/P) inulin concentration is about 11[17,18]. This value indicates that a considerable amount of water is absorbed along the descending limb, because TF/P inulin concentration in the latest part of the superficial proximal tubule is 5–6.

By perfusing the descending limb of tissue slices of rat renal papilla, Morgan and Berliner [6], demonstrated that the diffusional water permeability was high in the descending limb. Kokko [19] reported that the rabbit descending limb perfused in vitro exhibited high osmotic water permeability. This finding was later supported by several investigators [20,21].

In spite of the considerable heterogeneity of the epithelial morphology between SDL and LDLu, as mentioned above, both segments are highly permeable to water [22]. Although water permeability tended to be higher in the LDLu than in the SDL, because of the considerable scatter of the data, they were not significantly different.

Mechanism of Water Transport

Miwa and Imai [20] reported that in the rabbit descending thin limb, the osmotic water permeability was 56 times greater than the diffusional water permeability. This large difference in two parameters for water permeability could only be explained by the hypothesis that water is transported, at least in part, through a water channel having a single file mechanism, which has also been postulated to exist in two other water permeable nephron segments, namely vasopressin stimulated collecting duct [23] and proximal tubules [24].

More recently, Imai et al. [25] examined the mechanism of water transport across the hamster LDLu in more detail. Osmotic water permeability of the hamster LDLu

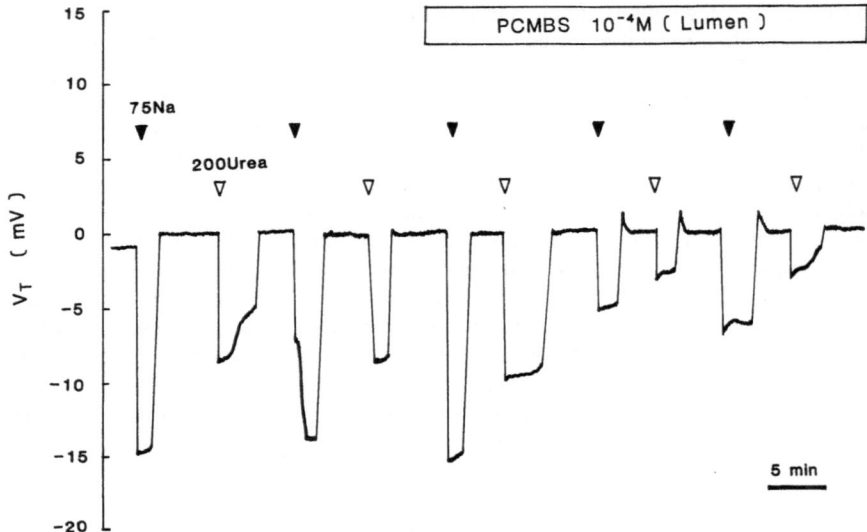

Fig. 2. A representative study showing that parachloromercuri-benzene sulfonate (*PCMBS*) inhibits both NaCl diffusion voltage and streaming voltage, induced by a urea osmotic gradient in hamster LDLu. (From [25])

was 26 times higher than diffusional water permeability. They showed that para-chloro-mercuribenzene sulfonate (PCMBS), which is known to be an inhibitor of the water channel, decreased both diffusional and osmotic water permeabilities of the hamster LDLu. Additional evidence which supports the existence of a water channel is the low activation energy for diffusion of water. Diffusional water permeability of the LDLu was measured at various temperatures, and apparent activation energy was calculated according to the following equation:

$$ln\,(P_{dw}) = -K_A/T + C$$

where P_{dw} is diffusional water permeability, K_A is activation energy, T is absolute temperature, and C is a constant value. Apparent activation energy thus calculated was 3.16 kCal/mol, a low value compatible with a channel mechanism for water transport.

The water channel of the LDLu has a unique characteristic in that it is also permeable to cations. As will be discussed in the next section, the LDLu is highly permeable to cations. Part of the cation selective permeability is mediated by the water channel. This view was supported by the observation that PCMBS reduced streaming potential, as well as NaCl diffusion potential, as shown in Fig. 2 [25]. To rule out the possibility that PCMBS also acts on the tight junction to inhibit paracellular cation conductance, we examined the effect of PCMBS on another nephron segment which is known to have a cation selective paracellular pathway, but is impermeable to water. The medullary thick ascending limbs of hamsters were chosen for this purpose. In the presence of 0.1 mM furosemide, reduction of NaCl concentration in the bath by a

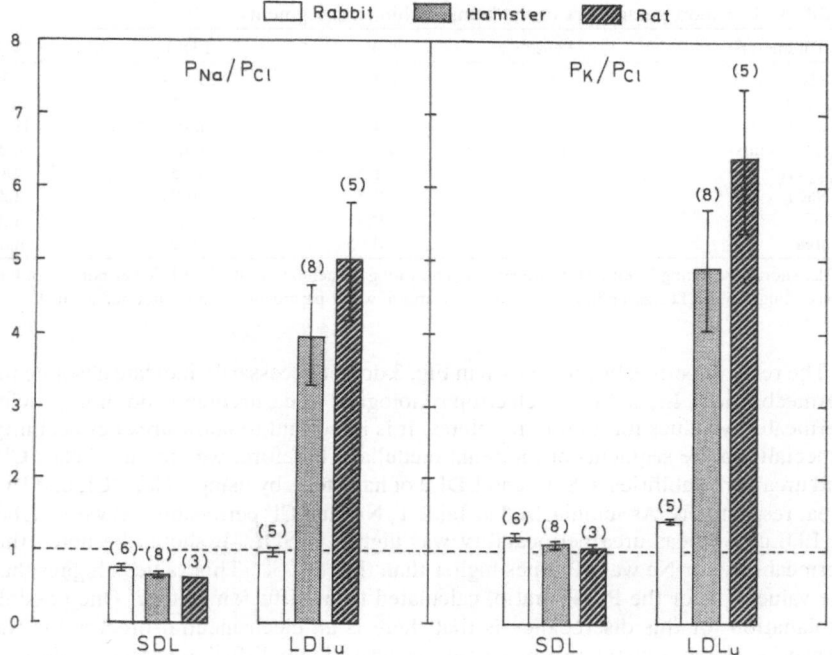

Fig. 3. Internephron heterogeneity and species differences of relative Na/Cl and K/Cl permeabilities, determined by diffusion voltage. (From [26])

half caused negative deflection of transepithelial voltage (V_T). However, addition of PCMBS to the lumen did not affect the diffusion voltage. This suggests that PCMBS does not affect paracellular cation selective conductance.

Solute Permeabilities

Heterogeneity of Ion and Urea Permeability

As suggested by the heterogeneity of epithelial morphology, it is possible that there is intranephron, as well as internephron, heterogeneity with respect to ion permeability properties. We have performed a series of studies, in which internephron heterogeneity and species differences were examined [22,26]. From the deflection of V_T when the composition of the bathing fluid was varied, we calculated the relative permeabilities of Na^+/Cl^- and of K^+/Cl^- in descending limbs of hamsters, rats, and rabbits.

The results are summarized in Fig. 3. In hamsters and rats, both P_{Na}/P_{Cl} and P_K/P_{Cl} are very much higher in the LDLu than in the SDL. This is definite evidence that there is internephron heterogeneity between the descending limbs of long-looped and short-looped nephrons. The data of this figure also show that there is species difference in the internephron heterogeneity: in contrast to the cases of hamsters and rats, no striking difference in relative ion permeability was observed in rabbits.

Table 1. Transport parameters of the hamster thin loop segments

Parameters	SDL	LDLu	LDLl	ATL
Pf (10^{-3} cm/s)	285	403	390	3
P_{Na} (10^{-5} cm/s)	4.2	5.0	3.5	87.6
P_{Cl} (10^{-5} cm/s)	1.3	4.2	n.d.	196.0
P_K (10^{-5} cm/s)	n.d.	85.4	n.d.	n.d.
P_{urea} (10^{-5} cm/s)	7.4	1.5	13.5	18.5
σ NaCl	n.d.	0.83	0.99	n.d.
σ KCl	n.d.	0.81	n.d.	n.d.
σ urea	n.d.	0.95	0.97	n.d.

SDL, short descending limb; LDLu, upper portion of long descending limb; LDLl, lower portion of long descending limb; ATL, ascending thin limb. Pf, osmotic water permeability; n.d., not determined

The relative permeabilities shown in Fig. 3 do not necessarily indicate absolute ion permeabilities. In addition, electrophysiological measurements do not provide permeability values for non-ionic solutes. It is important to know urea permeability, especially in the segments of the renal medulla. Therefore, we measured Na$^+$, Cl$^-$, and urea permeabilities in SDL and LDLu of hamsters, by using ^{22}Na, ^{36}Cl, and ^{14}C-urea, respectively. As summarized in Table 1, Na$^+$ and Cl$^-$ permeabilities were higher in LDLu, whereas urea permeability was higher in SDL. It should be noted that permeability for Na was 10 times higher than that for Cl$^-$. This value is higher than the value of 4 for the P_{Na}/P_{Cl} ratio, calculated from diffusion voltage. One possible explanation for this discrepancy is that there is an electroneutral process for Na$^+$ transport, which is distinct from a cation selective ionic diffusion process. However, no one has ever tested this possibility.

In addition to internephron heterogeneity, there is an axial heterogeneity in the permeability properties of the long-looped descending limb. As was expected from the morphological transition of epithelia along the axis of the long-loop descending limb [27], we demonstrated that the characteristic of preferential Na$^+$ permeability in LDLu diminished along the descending limb. Such transition occurred at various levels of the renal medulla. The transport parameters of the lower portion of long loop descending limb (LDLl) are essentially the same as those of SDL. In other words, the segment is less permeable to Na$^+$ and moderately permeable to urea.

Selectivity of Ion Permeability

As mentioned above, LDLu of hamster is more permeable to Na$^+$ than to Cl$^-$; it is of interest to know whether the permeability of this segment is specific for Na$^+$ or not. Tabei and Imai [28] examined relative ion permeabilities of hamster LDLu by observing V_T deflection upon ion substitution (biionic diffusion voltage). The sequence of relative permeabilities of cation to Cl$^-$ were: 8.89 for NH$_4^+$, 7.07 for K$^+$, 6.70 for Rb$^+$, 5.88 for Na$^+$, 5.76 for Cs, and 4.19 for Li$^+$. On the other hand, relative permeabilities of anions to Cl$^-$ were: 1.16 for NO$_3^-$, 0.80 for Br$^-$, and 0.58 for acetate. These findings indicate that this segment is permeable to cations in general.

Transepithelial Resistance and Paracellular Pathway

In accordance with species differences in ion permeability properties, the transepithelial resistance of the descending limb also differs between rabbits and hamsters.

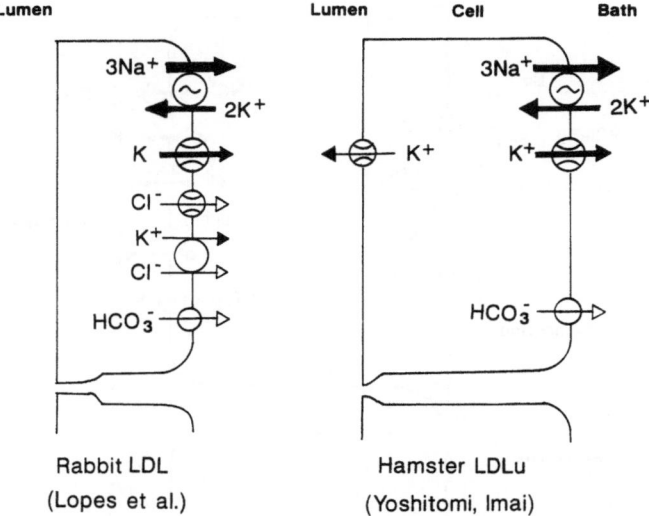

Fig. 4. Cell model for descending limb of rabbit, deduced from study of cell volume regulation and from electrophysiological study. (*left*, from [30], *right*, from [29])

Abramow and Orci [21] reported that in rabbit descending limb, transepithelial resistance (R_T) was 600 ohm cm². In contrast, Yoshitomi and Imai [29] found that R_T of hamster LDLu was 18 ohm cm².

Although, as discussed earlier, cation selective permeability is accounted for, in part, by the water channel associated with cation selective conductance, the contribution of the paracellular pathway should be also considered. This idea is supported by the observation that NaCl diffusion voltage was symmetrical when the direction of the concentration gradient was reversed [28]. A preliminary study by Koyama, Yoshitomi, and Imai further supported this view. They observed that protamine inhibited NaCl diffusion voltage, as well as transepithelial conductance. These effects were reversed by heparin. Along with other observations, they estimated that about 50% of the transepithelial resistance was accounted for by paracellular shunt resistance.

Transcellular Pathway

Lopez et al. [30] have conducted a very elegant study to clarify the mechanisms of ion transport across basolateral membrane of rabbit descending limb. They studied the ion transport mechanisms responsible for cell volume regulation of this segment. Based on ion substitution studies, they proposed a cell model, depicted in Fig. 4.

We have recently succeeded in impaling the epithelia of hamster LDLu [29]. Our current cell model, deduced from an electrophysiological mean, is also depicted in Fig. 4 for comparison. In steady state, basolateral membrane voltage (V_B) was -18 $\pm$ 2 mV ($n=55$). Because the basolateral membrane was depolarized by 40 mV by the action of ouabain, it is probable that the Na$^+$/K$^+$ pump may contribute to the generation of V_B.

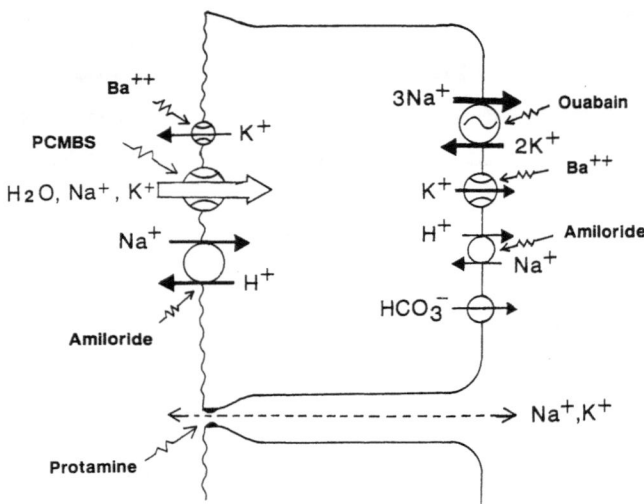

Fig. 5. Cell model of hamster LDLu based on pHi measurement and electrophysiological study

In addition to an ouabain sensitive pump, barium sensitive high K^+ conductance also exists in the basolateral membrane. This conclusion was based on the observations that the increase in K^+ concentration in the bath, from 5 to 50 mM, or application of 2 mM $BaCl_2$ to the bath, depolarized basolateral membrane by 36 mV or 46 mV, respectively. The electrophysiological method is insufficient for evaluating whether neutral carrier, such as K^+-Cl^- or Na^+-K^+-$2Cl^-$, cotransport exists in the basolateral membrane.

With regard to anion conductance, we could demonstrate a small, but significant, V_B deflection upon reduction of bath HCO_3^- from 25 to 2.5 mM, which became more prominent when K^+ conductance was suppressed by Ba^{2+}. On the other hand, we could not obtain definite evidence for the presence of Cl^- conductance. However, because of the technical difficulty in demonstrating a small Cl^- conductance, we cannot exclude such a possibility.

In the apical membrane, there is a small K^+ conductance. Increase in lumen K concentration, from 5 to 50 mM, or luminal addition of 2 mM $BaCl_2$, caused the apical membrane to depolarize by 10 mV or 8 mV, respectively. Thus, along with nonselective cation conductance associated with the water channel, there are significant ion conductances in the apical membrane. However, fractional apical membrane resistance was relatively high, at 0.92 [29].

H^+ Transport

Kurtz [31] reported for the first time that in rabbit descending limb, Na^+/H^+ antiporters exist in both apical and basolateral membranes. Independently, Koseki et al. [32] also reported that Na^+/H^+ antiporters exist in apical and basolateral membranes of hamster LDLu. They further showed that lumen pH, as determined by fluorescence of free BCECF, became acid when luminal flow was stopped by obstruction of tubular outflow. Under this condition, addition of ouabain to the bath

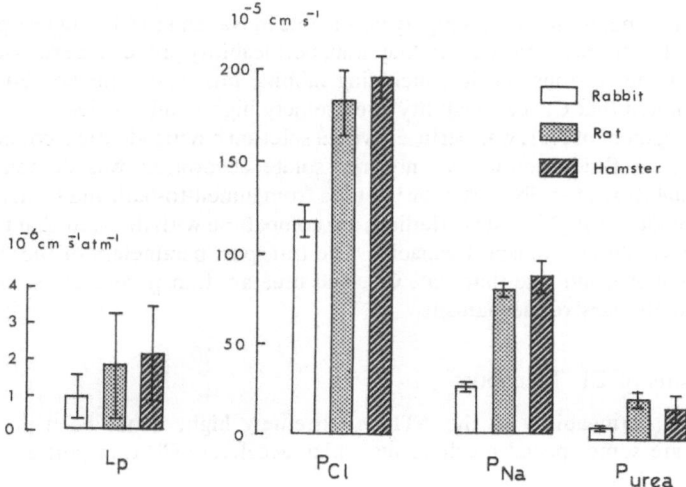

Fig. 6. Permeability properties of the ATL of rabbits, rats, and hamsters

dissipated the pH gradient, indicating that the generation of pH gradient is mediated by a process of luminal H^+ transport, secondarily driven by Na^+/K^+ pump in the basolateral membrane, possibly Na^+/H^+ antiporter.

Under the stopped flow condition, abrupt changes in bath pH caused rapid parallel changes in luminal pH, indicating that this segment is also highly permeable to proton. Therefore, it is suggested that the transepithelial pH gradient across this segment is maintained by a strong secondarily active H^+ secretory mechanism, which is associated with a leak of H^+, probably through the paracellular pathway.

Cell Model of LDLu

Based on our observations, which were the result of various approaches, we constructed a cell model, as in Fig. 5. The Na^+/K^+ pump in the basolateral membrane provides the driving force for Na^+/H^+ antiporters in both basolateral and apical membranes. Along with the presence of HCO_3^- conductance in the basolateral membrane, the LDLu may play a significant role in the acidification of tubular fluid. The existence of K^+ conductance in the apical membrane may, in part, account for K^+ recycling, which is known to occur along the descending limb [33].

Functions of the Ascending Thin Limb

Water and Solute Permeabilities

Water and solute permeabilities of the ascending thin limb (ATL) have been reported for rabbits, rats, and hamsters [34–40]. The data are summarized in Fig. 6. Osmotic water permeability of the ATL is very low. Diffusional water permeability was also shown to be low in the ATL of rabbits and hamsters.

On the other hand, the ATL is highly permeable to Na^+ and to Cl^-, but less permeable to urea. In contrast to the descending limb, permeability properties are essentially the same among various species, including rabbits, rats, and hamsters [34–36]. It should be noted that Cl^- permeability is extremely high in all species.

When a segment of ATL was perfused with a solution having identical composition to the bathing fluid, neither V_T nor net solute absorption was demonstrated. Bidirectional fluxes for ^{22}Na, ^{36}Cl, or ^{14}C urea from lumen-to-bath and from bath-to-lumen were identical [34]. These findings are compatible with the view that the ATL has no detectable net transport capacity. The transport parameters of the ATL, as mentioned above, indicate that Na^+, Cl^-, and urea are transported across this segment by purely passive mechanisms.

Mechanisms of Cl^- Transport

Because Cl^- permeability of the ATL is extremely high, it has been postulated that there are some special mechanisms which accelerate Cl^- transport across this segment.

Evidence for Facilitated Cl^- Transport

Imai and Kokko [35] proposed that Cl^- transport across the rabbit ATL was mediated by facilitated diffusion. This proposition was based on the following three major observations. First, ^{36}Cl flux from the lumen-to-bath exhibited a tendency for saturation as Cl^- concentration was increased. On the other hand, the ^{22}Na flux increased as a linear function of Na^+ concentration. Second, the Cl^- flux was inhibited by Br^-. The inhibitory effect of Br^- was greater when Cl^- concentration was low, suggesting that the inhibition of Cl^- flux by Br^- was roughly competitive in nature. Third, when Ussing's flux ratio analysis was performed, by measuring bidirectional ^{36}Cl fluxes at various diffusion V_T, the flux ratio for Cl^- clearly deviated from the line predicted for simple passive diffusion. These findings suggest that Cl^- transport is mediated by some processes which require interactions of Cl^- with membranes. From these observations, however, we cannot specify the exact mechanism of Cl^- transport.

Effects of Anion Transport Inhibitors

In an attempt to specify the mechanism of Cl^- transport across the ATL, we observed the effects of various anion transport inhibitors on Cl^- transport in the hamster ATL.

Stilbene disulfonate derivatives, such as 4,4'-dithiocyanostilbene-2,2'-disulfonic acid (DIDS) or 4-acetamido-4'-isothiocyanostilbene-2,2'-disulfonic acid (SITS), are known to be highly specific inhibitors for the Cl^-/HCO_3^- antiporter in the red blood cell, the band 3 protein. The apparent high specificity, however, depends on the fact that in red blood cells this is the only protein which is exposed to the cell surface [41]. Therefore, in other biological membranes, their inhibitory effects are not limited to the Cl^-/HCO_3^- antiporter. In the renal tubule they also inhibit $Na^+-3HCO_3^-$ flux. Thus, possible contributions of the K^+-Cl^-, or the $Na^+-K^+-2Cl^-$ cotransporters could be rejected.

Because a transmural NaCl concentration gradient causes diffusion voltage [34–40], the Cl^- transport in the ATL is conductive in nature. Although electrogenic

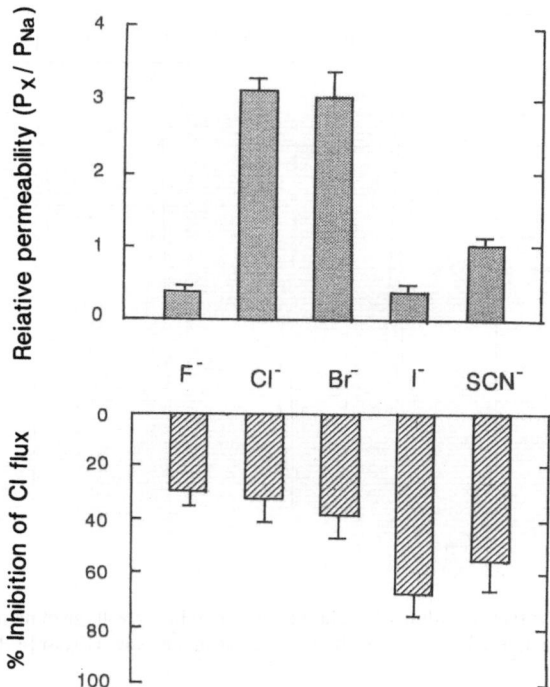

Fig. 7. Halogen permeabilities relative to Cl⁻, measured by simple salt dilution voltage. (*upper panel*), and inhibition of 36Cl flux by halogens (*lower panel*). (Data from Isozaki et al., [62])

antiport or cotransport cannot be ruled out, the mechanisms coupled with major ions, such as HCO_3^-, Na^+, and K^+ are excluded. Thus, by exclusion, we reached the conclusion that a Cl⁻ channel is the most plausible mechanism for Cl⁻ transport across the ATL.

Halogen Selectivity

Recently, Isozaki et al. [62] examined the selectivity of ion permeation across the ATL by measuring the single salt dilution voltage. Figure 7 summarizes halogen permeabilities of this segment, with reference to Na^+. It is clear that this segment is highly permeable to Br⁻, as well as to Cl⁻, but less permeable to I⁻ and to F⁻. By using ³⁶Cl and ¹²⁵I, we measured permeability for Cl⁻ and I⁻ simultaneously, and confirmed that permeability for Cl⁻ was 6 times higher than that for I⁻.

Because Imai and Kokko [35] had previously reported that Br⁻ inhibited Cl⁻ flux, we examined whether other halogens have a similar effect or not. The inhibitory effects of the respective halogens (50 mM) are also shown in Fig. 7. As can be seen in this figure, all halogens and SCN⁻ showed some inhibitory effects. It should be noted that iodine is the most potent inhibitor among these ions, in spite of its low permeability.

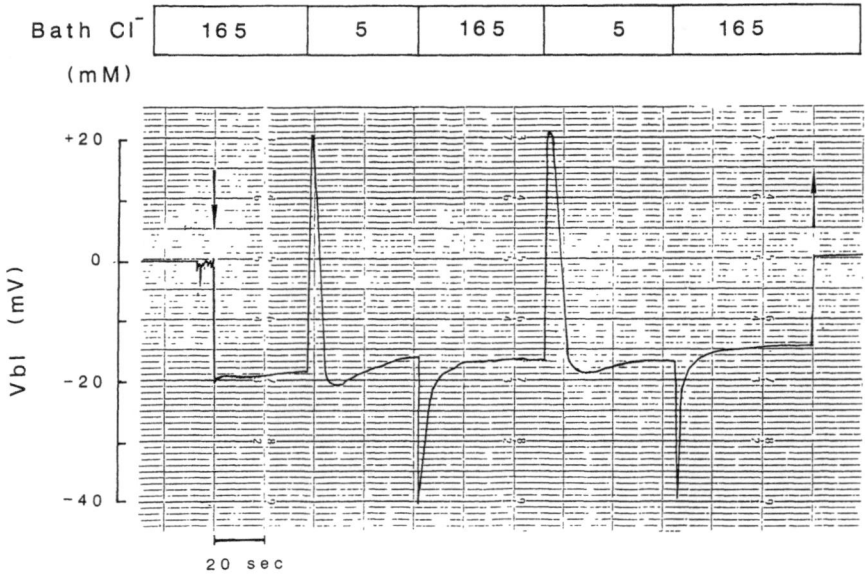

Fig. 8. A representative recording of the basolateral membrane voltage of hamster ATL, showing that Cl⁻ conductance is present in the basolateral membrane. (From [47])

These observations suggest that the putative Cl⁻ channels in the ATL have binding sites which are common to all halogens, but that only Cl⁻ and Br⁻ are permeable.

Route of Cl⁻ Conductance

It is most difficult to answer the question whether Cl⁻ is transported across the transcellular, or the paracellular route, However, success in cell puncture with conventional electrodes by Imai et al. [48] provided a definite answer to this question. In 18 successful impalements V_B was revealed to be -24.5 ± 1.5 mV. As shown in Fig. 8, an abrupt decrease in Cl⁻ concentration in the bath caused transient positive spiky deflection of V_B, indicating that there is a Cl⁻ conductance in the basolateral membrane. The rapid dissipation of the voltage may reflect the fact that Cl⁻ concentration in the cell is rapidly equilibrated with that in ambient solution. When luminal Cl⁻ concentration was decreased, the apical membrane voltage was also deflected. Thus, Cl⁻ conductances exist in series in the apical, as well as in the basolateral, membrane.

Regulation of Cl⁻ Conductance

Because ion channels, in general, are composed of protein, factors which modulate protein conformation may affect the functions of channels. Therefore, we examined the effects of pH, Ca^{2+}, and SH reagents on Cl⁻ conductance in the hamster ATL [38,39,48].

Effects of pH

It is well-known that many ion channels are affected by pH. Usually, acidification of ambient fluid is associated with a decrease in ion transport or conductance. Kondo et al. [38] found that acidification of the bathing fluid sharply decreased relative Cl⁻ conductance, as well as Cl⁻ flux, in the hamster ATL. The P_{Cl}/P_{Na} ratios calculated from salt diffusion voltage were functions of the pH of the bathing or luminal fluid. The affinities for H⁺ binding were pH 5.78 and pH 6.31 at the luminal and the basolateral side, respectively. The slope of Hill's plot was greater than 2, suggesting that there are at least two proton binding sites, or that the proton binding exhibits positive cooperativity.

Effects of Ca²⁺

Ca²⁺ is also known to regulate various channels, including the Cl⁻ channel [49]. The Cl⁻ conductance of the ATL is also regulated by ambient Ca²⁺: a decrease in Ca²⁺ is associated with a decrease in Cl⁻ conductance [39]. Ca²⁺ and proton have mutual interaction in modulating Cl⁻ conductance in the ATL. The mode of the interaction is the uncompetitive type.

Effects of Sulfhydryl Reagents

Kondo and Imai [50] reported that treatment of the ATL with glutaraldehyde selectively inhibited Cl⁻ conductance. Glutaraldehyde is known to cross-link both sulfhydryl and amino groups. Therefore, it is possible that one of these groups of amino acids in the protein moiety of the putative channel may play a critical role in the conductive pathway for Cl⁻. We observed the effects of various SH inhibitors [48], including PCMBS, maleimide, and N-ethyl maleimide (NEM). All these agents showed irreversible inhibitory effects on the Cl⁻ conductance of the ATL.

During the course of this study, we noticed that NEM exhibited a unique dual action on Cl⁻ conductance (Fig. 9). Although an initial application of NEM caused a small suppression of Cl⁻ conductance, elimination of NEM caused further sharp decrease in the conductance, suggesting that NEM caused an irreversible inhibition. However, to our surprise, a second addition of NEM stimulated the conductance. This stimulatory effect of NEM was prevented by dithiothreitol, indicating that the effect is also due to modification of the SH site. The stimulatory effect of NEM was reversible. It was also prevented by NPPB [40], suggesting that the Cl⁻ channel is stimulated by NEM. These observations clearly show that there are at least two distinct regulatory sites, having SH groups, associated with the Cl⁻ channel.

Loci of the Action of Regulating Factors

Because there are two regulatory sites in the channel, as discussed above, we wished to know the modes of action of pH, Ca²⁺, and various transport inhibitors with special reference to these two regulatory sites.

First, we examined whether the stimulatory effect of NEM could be preserved under conditions where the Cl⁻ conductance was inhibited by either low pH or nominally free Ca²⁺ [48]. The experimental protocols were as follows. We observed NaCl

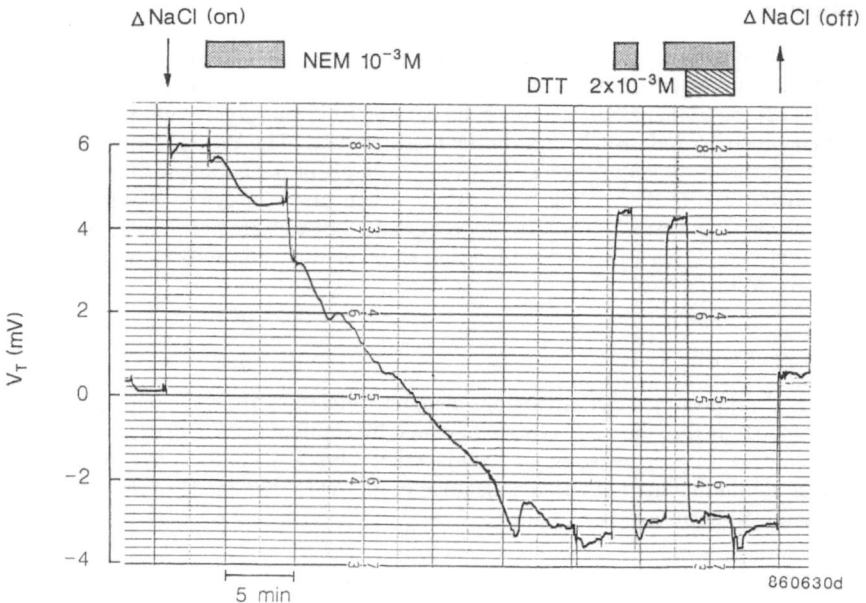

Fig. 9. A representative recording of NaCl diffusion voltage in hamster ATL, showing the dual action of NEM. NEM, N-ethylmaleimide; DTT, dithiothreitol. (From [48])

diffusion voltage as a measure of Cl$^-$ conductance, and the suppressive effects of bath pH 5.8 on the diffusion voltage were observed before and after administration of 1 mM NEM to the bath. After washing NEM from the bath, we observed the stimulatory effect of NEM by applying it again. The stimulatory effect of NEM was also examined when bath pH was 5.8. As for recovery data, the same challenge was repeated, while bath pH was changed to 7.4 again. A similar protocol was conducted, using Ca^{2+}-free bath solution instead of acid pH. The results are summarized in Fig. 10. As clearly shown in this figure, the stimulatory effect of NEM was suppressed markedly when the bath pH was acid, whereas the effect was not prevented by nominally free Ca^{2+}. These observations suggest that the inhibitory site of H$^+$ is located distal to the NEM-stimulating site. On the other hand, the calcium-stimulated site seems to be independent from the NEM-stimulating site.

By using similar protocols, we also examined the sites of action of other inhibitors, such as DIDS and phloretin. The results are summarized in Fig. 11. As shown in the left panel, addition of 1mM DIDS to the bath markedly decreased the diffusion voltage, reflecting the suppression of Cl$^-$ conductance. Under this condition, addition of 1mM NEM caused a stimulatory effect of the same magnitude as that of the second challenge of NEM. On the other hand, in the presence of 1mM phloretin, NEM did not exert any stimulatory effect, as shown in the right panel. These observations support the view that the site of action of DIDS may be the same site at which SH reagents show an irreversible inhibitory effect, whereas the site of action of phloretin is distal to the stimulatory site of NEM.

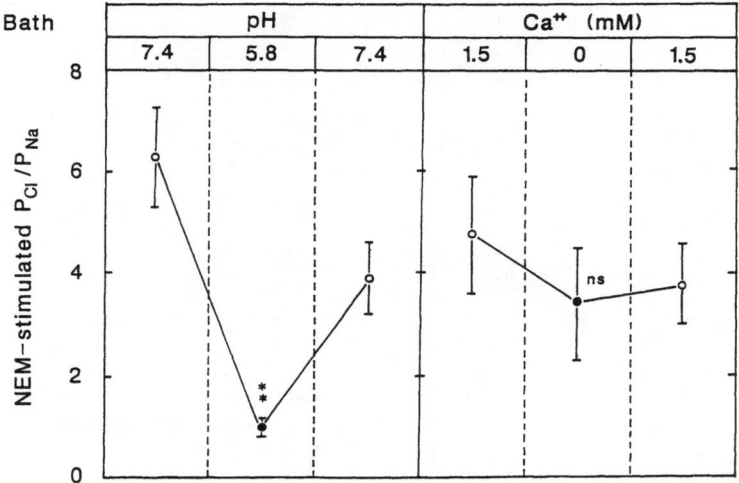

Fig. 10. Effects of pH or Ca^{2+} on N-ethylmaleimide (*NEM*)-stimulated relative Cl^- conductance, as measured by NaCl diffusion voltage. (Data from M. Imai et al. [48])

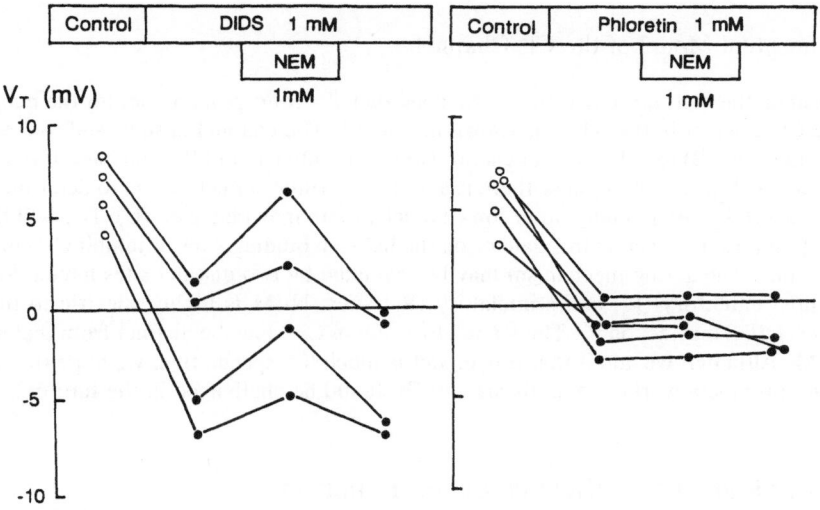

Fig. 11. Effects of DIDD or phloretin on N-ethylmaleimide (*NEM*)-stimualted relative Cl permeability in hamster ATL

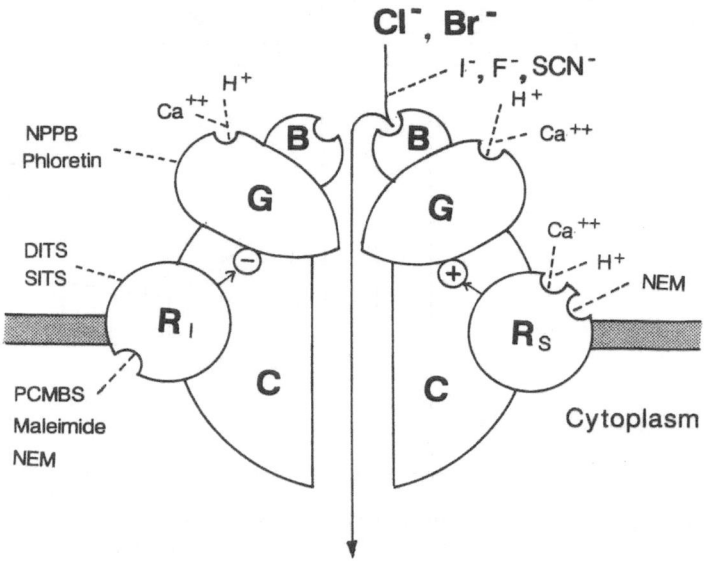

Fig. 12. Conceptual model of the putative Cl⁻ channel in the ATL. B, binding sites; C, channel; G, gates or filters; Ri, inhibitory regulation; Rs, stimulatory regulation

Conceptual Model of the Cl⁻ Channel

Based on the facts discussed above, we constructed a conceptual model for the putative Cl⁻ channel in the ATL, as shown in Fig. 12. The channel is supposed to have binding sites (B) to halogens in general. However, only Cl⁻ and Br⁻ can pass through the channel, probably because there is a barrier or filter in the channel to determine ion selectivity. As in many other ion channels, there may be a gate (G). H⁺, NPPB, and phloretin may act on this gate or on the halogen binding sites to inhibit Cl⁻ conductance. The gating mechanism may be regulated by two distinct sites having SH groups, inhibitory (R_i) and stimulatory (R_S) sites. NEM is highly specific to the latter. DIDS may act on R_i. The stimulatory site of Ca^{2+} may be distinct from that of NEM. Although we admit that this model is much too speculative, we hope that it might provide a working hypothesis, which should be challenged in the future.

Physiological Significance of the Functions of Thin Loop Segments

As a summary of this review, we would like to discuss the physiological significance of thin loop segments very briefly, with reference to three distinct, but somehow interrelated, functions: i.e., 1) the urine concentrating mechanism, 2) K⁺ recycling, and 3) urine acidification.

Urine Concentrating Mechanism

It is needless to say that the thin loop of Henle plays an integral part in the counter-current multiplication system in the renal medulla. Our data clearly show that there is no appreciable active NaCl transport which is sufficient to generate a trans-epithelial NaCl gradient. Rather, we have strong evidence in support of the view that Cl⁻ is transported across the ATL by a special passive mechanism, possibly a Cl⁻ channel. In this regard, the passive diffusion model proposed by Kokko and Rector [51] and by Stephenson [52] may still be relevant. However, computer analysis, based on the transport parameters of the descending limb, showed that, against the hypothesis of the passive model, a significant amount of urea is accumulated in the fluid of the descending limb [53,54]. This would hamper the operation of the pro-posed single effect in the ATL. This situation is unrelated to species difference or to the inter- and intranephron heterogeneity of the descending limb.

Therefore, it is necessary to develop a new version of the passive model, which allows diffusion of both NaCl and urea out of the ATL. We have previously proposed that a single effect could be operating between the compartments of the ATL, the inner medullary collecting duct (IMCD), and capillary networks, if we assume that the low reflection coefficient for urea in the IMCD constitutes an initial driving force which generates a single effect [55]. Although there are considerable disputes about the exact value of the reflection coefficient for urea in the IMCD [56,57], there is no doubt that the osmotic work across the IMCD is operated by the two-solute model [56]. Thus, all passive models should incorporate this single effect. In addition, the special architectural organization of the tubulo-vascular arrangement should also be considered. The internephron heterogeneity in solute permeability properties may be essential for such a three dimensional model. We assume that the SDL may play an important role in the medullary recycling of urea. Furthermore, we should also con-sider the fact that the blood supply of the outer and inner medullar is strictly separate.

K⁺ Recycling

K⁺ reabsorbed in the medullary collecting duct is secreted again into the loop of Henle [33]. It is widely accepted that this K⁺ recycling occurs somewhere in the proximal straight tubule or in the descending limb of Henle's loop [33]. The high K⁺ permeabil-ity in the LDLu may indicate that this segment plays an important role in this phenomenon. In fact, the computer simulation done by Taniguchi et al. [54] sup-ported this hypothesis. Although the high permeability for K⁺ in this segment may be mainly accounted for by the leaky paracellular shunt pathway, the existence of K⁺ conductance in the apical membrane of the LDLu may also be favorable for the secre-tion of K⁺ across this segment.

Urine Acidification

We found that the LDLu has a high capacity for the secretion H⁺ and that it maintains a transmural pH gradient, even though the segment is highly permeable to proton. The physiological significance of the proton secretion is unknown at the present time, because pH in the bend of the loop became less acidic, as compared to the end proximal tubular fluid pH [58]. Therefore, proton secretion in the LDLu may not be directly related to final urine pH. However, it should be noted that Henle's loop may play an important role in the accumulation of ammonia in the renal medulla [59]. Buerkert et al. [60] demonstrated that, in the rat, ammonia secretion occurs somewhere along the proximal straight tubule or descending limb. Good, Knepper, and Burg [61] demonstrated that NH_4^+ is reabsorbed as an ionic form in the thick ascending limb, via Na^+-K^+-$2Cl^-$ cotransport system. These observations are in accordance with the hypothesis that ammonia is accumulated in the renal medulla through the countercurrent multiplication system. Kurtz [31] speculated that acidification of the luminal fluid in the LDLu would shift more of the luminal ammonia to the NH_4^+ form, decrease the luminal NH_3, and would thus favor the non-ionic diffusion of NH_3 into the lumen. Furthermore, it is important to note that the LDLu in hamster is highly permeable to NH_4^+ [28]. Therefore, ionic diffusion, possibly via the paracellular shunt pathway, may also contribute to the medullary recycling of ammonia.

References

1. Kuhn W, Ryffel K (1942) Herstellung konzentrierter Lösungen aus verdünnten durch blosse Membranwirkung. (Ein Modelversuch zur Funktion der Niere). Hoppe Seylers Z Physiol Chem 276:145–178
2. Wirz H, Hargitay B, Kuhn W (1951) Lokalization des Konzentrierungsprozesses in der Niere durch direkte Kryoskopie. Helv Physiol Pharmacol Acta 9:196–207
3. Kuhn W, Ramel L (1959) Aktiver Salztransport als möglicher (und warscheinlicher) Einzeleffekt bei der Harnkonzentrierung in der Niere. Helv Chim Acta 42:628–660
4. Jamison RL, Kritz W (1982) Urinary concentrating mechanism. Structure and function. Oxford, New York
5. Jamison RL, Bennett CM, Berliner RW (1967) Countercurrent multiplication by the thin loops of Henle. Am J Physiol 212:357–366
6. Morgan T, Berliner RW (1968) Permeability of loop of Henle, vasa recta, and collecting duct to water, urea and sodium. Am J Physiol 215:108–115
7. Burg M, Grantham J, Abramow M, Orloff J (1966) Preparation and study of fragments of single rabbit nephrons. Am J Physiol 210:1293–1298
8. Kritz W (1981) Structural organization of the renal medulla: comparative and functional aspects. Am J Physiol 241:R3–R16
9. Bankir L, De Rouffignac C (1985) Urinary concentrating ability: insight from comparative anatomy. Am J Physiol 249:R643–R666
10. Kaissling B, de Rouffignac C, Barrett JM, Kriz W (1975) The structural organization of the kidney of the desert rodent *Psammomys obesus*. Acta Embryol 148:121–143
11. Kriz W, Dietrich J, Hoffman S (1968) Aufbau der Gefassbündel im Nierenmark von Wüstenmäusen (abstract). Naturwissenschaften 50:40
12. Dietrich HJ, Barrett JM, Kriz W, Bulhoff JP (1975) The ultrastructure of thin loop limbs of the mouse kidney. Anat Embryol (Berl) 147:1–13
13. Kriz W, Koepsell H (1974) The structural organization of the mouse kidney. Z Anat Entwicklungsgesch 144:137–163
14. Kritz W, Schnermann J, Koepsell H (1972) The position of short and long loops of Henle in the rat kidney. Z. Anat Entwicklungsgesch 138:301–309
15. Bachman S, Kriz W (1982) Histotopography and ultrastructure of the thin limbs of the loop of Henle in the hamster. Cell Tiss Res 225:111–127
16. Kaissling B, Kritz Z W (1975) Structural organization of the rabbit kidney. Adv Anat Embryol Cell Biol 148:121–143

17. Gottschalk CW, Lassiter WE, Mylle M, Ullrich K, Schmidt-Nielsen B, O'Dell R, Pehling G (1963) Micropuncture study of composition of loop of Henle fluid in desert rodents. Am J Physiol 204:532–535

18. Jamison RL (1968) Micropuncture study of segments of thin loops of Henle in the rat. Am J Physiol 215:236–242

19. Kokko JP (1970) Sodium and water transport in the descending limb of Henle. J Clin Invest 49:1838–1846

20. Miwa T, Imai M (1983) Flow dependent water permeability of the rabbit descending limb of Henle's loop. Am J Physiol 245:F743–F754

21. Abramow M, Orci L (1980) On the "tightness" of the rabbit descending limb of the loop of Henle, physiological and morphological evidence. Int J Biochem 12:23–27

22. Imai M, Hayashi M, Araki M (1984) Functional heterogeneity of the descending limbs of Henle's loop. I. Internephron heterogeneity in the hamster kidney. Pflugers Arch 402:385–392

23. Hebert SC, Andreoli TE (1980) Interactions of temperature and ADH on transport processes in cortical collecting tubules. Am J Physiol 238:F470–F480

24. Berry CA (1985) Characteristics of water diffusion in the rabbit proximal convoluted tubule. Am J Physiol 249:F729–F738

25. Imai M, Yasoshima K, Yoshitomi K (1990) Mechanism of water transport across the upper portion of the descending thin limb of long-looped nephron of hamsters. Pflugers Arch 415:630–637

26. Imai M (1984) Functional heterogeneity of the descending limbs of Henle's loop. II. Interspecies difference among rabbits, rats, and hamsters. Pflugers Arch 402:393–401

27 Imai M, Taniguchi J, Yoshitomi K (1988) Transition of permeability properties along the descending limb of long-loop nephron. Am J Physiol 254:F323–F328

28. Tabei K, Imai M (1986) Permselectivity for cations over anions in the upper portion of the descending limbs of Henle of long loop nephron isolated from hamsters. Pflugers Arch 406:279–384

29. Yoshitomi K, Imai M (1990) Electrophysiological study of the upper part of long descending thin limb (LDLu) (abstract). Kidney Int 37:576A

30. Lopez AG, Amzel LM, Markakis K, Guggino WB (1988) Cell volume regulation by the thin descending limb of Henle's loop. Proc Natl Acad Sci USA 85:2873–2877

31. Kurtz I (1988) Apical and basolateral Na^+/H^+ exchange in the rabbit outer medullary thin descending limb of Henle: Role in intracellular pH regulation. J Membr Biol 106:253–260

32. Koseki C, Matsushima Y, Yoshitomi K, Imai M (1989) Regulation of intracellular pH (pHi) in the upper part of descending limb of long-looped nephron (LDLu): a fluorometric study (abstract). Kidney Int 35:457

33. Jamison RL, Work J, Schafer JA (1982) New pathways for potassium transport in the kidney. Am J Physiol 242:F297–F312

34. Imai M, Kokko JP (1974) Sodium chloride, urea and water transport in the thin ascending limb of Henle. Generation of osmotic gradient by passive diffusion of solutes. J Clin Invest 53:393–402

35. Imai M, Kokko JP (1976) Mechanism of sodium and chloride transport in the thin ascending limb of Henle. J Clin Invest 58:1054–1061

36. Imai M (1977) Function of the thin ascending limb of Henle of rats and hamsters perfused in vitro. Am J Physiol 232:F201–F209

37. Kondo Y, Yoshitomi K, Imai M (1987) Effects of anion transport inhibitors and ion substitution on Cl^- transport in TAL of Henle's loop. Am J Physiol 253:F1206–F1215

38. Kondo Y, Yoshitomi K, Imai M (1987) Effect of pH on Cl^- transport in TAL of Henle's loop. Am J Physiol 253:F1216–F1222

39. Kondo Y, Yoshitomi K, Imai M (1988) Effect of Ca^{2+} on Cl^- transport in thin ascending limb of Henle's loop. Am J Physiol 254:F232–F239

40. Isozaki T, Yoshitomi K, Imai M (1989) Effects of Cl⁻ transport inhibitors on Cl⁻ permeability across hamster ascending thin limb. Am J Physiol 257:F92–F98
41. Wieth JO, Brahm J (1985) Cellular anion transport. In: Seldin DW, Giebisch G (eds) The kidney. Physiology and pathophysiology. Raven, New York, pp 49–89
42. Boron WF, Boulpaep EL (1983) Intracellular pH regulation in the renal proximal tubule of the salamander. Basolateral HCO₃⁻ transport. J Gen Physiol 81:53–94
43. Yoshitomi K, Frömter E (1984) Cell pH of rat proximal tubule in vivo and the conductive nature of peritubular HCO₃⁻ (OH⁻). Pflugers Arch 402:300–305
44. Nelson DJ, Tang JM, Palmer LG (1984) Single-channel recordings of apical membrane chloride conductance in A6 epithelial cells. J Membr Biol 80:81–89
45. Brahm J, Wieth JO (1977) Separate pathways for urea and water and for chloride for chicken erythrocytes. J Physiol (Lond) 266:727–749
46. Wangemann P, Witter M, Di Stefano A, Englert HC, Lang HJ, Schlatter E, Greger R (1986) Cl⁻ channel blockers in the thick ascending limb of the loop of Henle. Structure activity relationship. Pflugers Arch 407:S128–S141
47. Yoshitomi K, Kondo Y, Imai M (1988) Evidence for conductive Cl⁻ pathways across the cell membranes of the thin ascending limb of Henle's loop. J Clin Invest 82:866–871
48. Imai M, Kondo Y, Koseki C, Yoshitomi K (1988) Dual effect of N-ethylmaleimide on Cl⁻ transport across the thin ascending limb of Henle's loop. Pflugers Arch 411:520–528
49. Marty A, Tan VP, Trautmann A (1984) Three types of calcium-dependent channel in rat lacrimal glands. J Physiol (Lond) 357:293–325
50. Kondo Y, Imai M (1987) Effects of glutaraldehyde on renal tubular function. II. Selective inhibition of Cl⁻ transporter in the hamster thin ascending limb of Henle's loop. Pflugers Arch 408:484–490
51. Kokko JP, Rector F Jr (1972) Countercurrent multiplication without active transport in inner medulla. Kidney Int 2:214–223
52. Stephenson JL (1972) Central core model of the renal counterflow system. Kidney Int 2:85–94
53. Pennel JP, Lacy FB, Jamison R (1974) An in vivo study of the concentrating process in descending limb of Henle's loop. Kidney Int 5:337–347
54. Taniguchi J, Tabei K, Imai M (1987) Profiles of water and solute transport along the descending limb: analysis by mathematical model. Am J Physiol 252:F393–F402
55. Imai M, Taniguchi J, Tabei K (1987) Function of thin loops of Henle. Kidney Int 31:565–579
56. Imai M, Taniguchi J, Yoshitomi K (1988) Osmotic work across inner medullary collecting duct accomplished by difference in reflection coefficients for urea and NaCl. Pflugers Arch 412:557–567
57. Chou CL, Sands JM, Nonoguchi H, Knepper MA (1990) Urea gradient-associated fluid absorption with urea = 1 in rat terminal collecting duct. Am J Physiol 258:F1173–F1180
58. DuBose TD Jr, Lucci MS, Hogg RJ, Puccaco LR, Kokko JP, Carter NW (1983) Comparison of acidification parameters in superficial and deep nephron in rats. Am J Physiol 244:F479–F503
59. Good D, Knepper MA (1985) Ammonia transport in the mammalian kidney. Am J Physiol 248:F459–F471
60. Buerkert J, Martin DT (1982) Ammonia handling by superficial and juxtamedullary nephrons in the rat: evidence for an ammonia shunt between the loop of Henle and the collecting duct. J Clin Invest 70:1–12
61. Good DW, Knepper MA, Burg MB (1984) Ammonia and bicarbonate transport by thick ascending limb of rat kidney. Am J Physiol 247:F35–F44
62. Isozaki T, Yoshitomik K, Imai M (in press) Selective ion permeability across thin limb of Henle's loop: interaction of Cl⁻ and other halogens with anion antiport system. Kidney Int

IgA Nephropathy: Recent Views on Pathogenesis and Treatment

HIDETO SAKAI

Chair: J. Stewart Cameron

IgA Nephropathy: Recent Views on Pathogenesis and Treatment

HIDETO SAKAI[1]

SUMMARY. In many parts of the world, IgA nephropathy is one of the most common types of glomerulonephritis. The aim of this lecture is to summarize recent views on the pathogenesis of this disease and to evaluate current treatment in various countries.

The pathogenesis of IgA nephropathy has been investigated primarily in human patients because of the lack of appropriate animal models. It is generally agreed that IgA nephropathy is mediated by circulating IgA-dominant immune complexes which are deposited in the glomeruli. The formation of IgA-dominant immune complexes is likely to be enhanced by genetic factors which promote in vivo production of IgA. The enhancement of IgA production in this disease leads to the formation of various IgA-class autoantibodies. Nonimmunological factors, including various mediators, blood coagulation, and hemodynamic alterations, may cause exacerbation of this disease.

No specific treatment is known to improve the clinical course of IgA nephropathy. Current treatment is aimed at preserving renal functions and stabilizing associated symptoms such as hypertension. The selection of treatment protocols depends on the histopathological findings of renal biopsy specimens, which, so far, provide the most reliable parameters for predicting the prognosis in each patient. The drugs most widely used for treatment of IgA nephropathy are antiplatelet agents. Administration of corticosteroids is more effective for the preservation of renal function in patients with moderate levels of proteinuria than in those with severe proteinuria. Other types of treatment have not been evaluated by multi-center, double-blind studies. Despite relatively high rates of recurrence, transplantation is not contraindicated in the treatment of patients with IgA nephropathy.

[1]Division of Nephrology and Metabolism, Department of Internal Medicine, School of Medicine, Tokai University, Isehara, Kanagawa, 259-11 Japan

Introduction

IgA nephropathy was first reported by Berger and Hinglais [1] in 1968. It is now well known that this disease is one of the most common types of primary glomerulonephritis in many parts of the world. Prognosis of IgA nephropathy is not so benign as initially thought, and approximately 10%–20% of patients with this disease will eventually shift to end-stage renal disease [2]. Specific treatment is currently not available for IgA nephropathy because of lack of knowledge of the precise mechanism of the development and exacerbation of this disease. The aim of this lecture is to summarize recent views on the pathogenesis of this disease and to evaluate current treatment in various countries. The term, "IgA nephropathy," in this lecture is limited to primary IgA nephropathy, because mesangial deposits of IgA are observed in various other diseases [3].

Pathogenesis

Clinical Features

The pathogenesis of IgA nephropathy has been investigated primarily in human patients because of the lack of appropriate animal models. Analysis of clinical features is therefore important in the elucidation of the mechanisms which might be related to the development of this disease.

Age and Sex

It is well known that IgA nephropathy is common in young males, although the age distribution, as well as the ratio of male to female patients with this disease, differs in different countries around the world [2]. The reason for the dominance of IgA nephropathy is unknown. The hyperfunction of IgA-producing B lymphocytes, to be discussed later, might be related to age and to some sex hormones, but there is no direct evidence to support this hypothesis.

Proteinuria and Hematuria

Persistent proteinuria and microscopic hematuria, associated with sporadic macroscopic hematuria, are the main clinical symptoms of IgA nephropathy. It is generally accepted that massive proteinuria is a sign of poor prognosis, although the clinical significance of macroscopic hematuria is yet to be clarified. The precise mechanism which induces occasional macroscopic hematuria is presently unknown.

Persistent Deposition of IgA1 in the Glomeruli

Preponderant deposition of IgA in the mesangial areas, as well as in other parts of the glomeruli, is the major immunohistopathological finding of IgA nephropathy. Intraglomerular deposition of IgA persists for several years or more in the majority of adult patients and in many pediatric patients. An increasing body of evidence suggests that the source of the intra-glomerular IgA is circulating IgA-dominant immune complexes. The reasons for this assumption are as follows: (a) IgA and C3 coexist in the glomerular mesangial areas, as shown by immuno-fluorescence [4], (b) electron-dense deposits are observed in the same area [4], (c) IgA and/or C3 are also observed in the vascular walls of subcutaneous or intramuscular vessels [5], (d) IgA-dominant immune complexes in the circulation are detected by several different techniques [6], (e) IgA nephropathy recurs frequently in allografted kidneys [7], and (f) glomerular IgA disappears rapidly from kidneys with IgA nephropathy when kidneys are transplanted in patients without IgA nephropathy [8].

In most countries, the subclass of IgA deposited in the glomeruli is now regarded as IgA1. The dominance of IgA2 was initially reported by a French group [9], but a subsequent study using monoclonal antibodies indicated that IgA1 is the dominant subclass of intraglomerular IgA [10]. The origin of these IgA1 antibodies is presently unknown. The monoclonarity of intraglomerular IgA was suggested by the dominance of the lambda light chain [11], but deviation in the kappa/lambda ratio has not been confirmed in most countries. It is generally agreed that IgA deposited in the glomeruli does not possess a secretory component. As far as the size and charge of intraglomerular IgA are concerned, anionic polymeric IgA is the dominant molecule, at least in IgA which is deposited in the mesangial areas. In mesangial IgA eluted by acid buffer, the presence of the J chain [12] and molecules of dimeric or even larger size [13], together with relatively negative charge [14], supported the above-mentioned physicochemical characteristics of mesangial IgA. Recently, it was suggested that subepithelial accumulation of proteinaceous materials from the mesangium might result in the degeneration and exfoliation of podocytes, followed by formation of segmental extracapillary lesions or adhesion to Bowman's capsule [15]. In order to elucidate the physicochemical characteristics and clinicopathological significance of IgA in various parts of the glomeruli in this disease, further studies are warranted. The origin of intraglomerular IgA is not fully clarified, but circulating IgA-dominant immune complexes are highly likely to be the source of such IgA, as indicated by the high rate of recurrence of this disease in cadaveric allografted kidneys [7], and the rapid disappearance of IgA from kidneys with IgA nephropathy in recipients with other renal diseases [8]. That these IgA antibodies are not anti mesangial cells and/or their matrix is indicated by the lack of binding of acid-eluted IgA, from renal biopsy specimens of patients with IgA nephropathy, with normal human renal tissues. In situ deposition of some antigen in the glomeruli prior to recurrence of IgA deposition is unlikely, since IgA deposition recurs as early as within one hour.

Geographical Heterogeneity

Immediately after the first report of IgA nephropathy [1], a marked geographical heterogeneity was observed in the prevalence of this disease. IgA nephropathy is frequent in southern European countries such as France, Italy, and Spain, as well as in the Asian-Pacific region, including China, Korea, Singapore, Australia, and Japan [2]. In contrast, this disease is relatively rare in the countries of northern Europe, and in North America and Africa [2]. The differences in the incidence of this disease might be due to racial, rather than environmental, factors, indicated by its heterogenous prevalence in multi-ethnic countries. For example, in the United States, IgA nephropathy is frequent in at least some tribes of American Indians [16], but shows a low incidence in Blacks [17]. There is no clear relationship between IgA nephropathy and HLA antigens [18]. The significance of the alteration in phenotypes of C3 [19] and C4 [20] in the pathogenesis of this disease is presently unknown.

Familial Increase in IgA Production

There has been an increasing number of reports showing the presence of familial increase of both in vivo and in vitro IgA production in this disease. Such familial increase in IgA production suggests the presence of an IgA-specific high responder which might be influenced by some genetic aberrations.

Familial Increase of In Vivo IgA Production

It is well known that more than half of the patients with IgA nephropathy show increased levels of serum IgA. The increased levels of serum IgA were shown to contain a large amount of polymeric IgA1 [21], and isoelectric analysis showed that these larger IgA molecules were negatively charged [22]. It was therefore suggested that the IgA whose levels are increased in the circulation has some common denominators with the IgA in the glomeruli of patients with IgA nephropathy. Increased levels of serum IgA were also observed in some relatives of patients with IgA nephropathy, with or without association of increased levels of IgA-bearing B cells in peripheral blood [23]. Increased levels of peripheral blood IgA-bearing B cells were also confirmed in Spain [24]. The origin of these IgA-bearing B cells in the circulation is presently obscure. However, distribution of isotypes in immunoglobulin-bearing cells in the tonsils from patients with IgA nephropathy [25] was very similar to that observed in peripheral blood, suggesting that some antigenic stimulation in the upper respiratory tract might induce the increased levels of IgA-bearing B cells, which subsequently migrate into the circulation. The increased infiltration of IgA-bearing B cells into tissues was also observed in biopsied specimens of episcleritis in some patients [26], suggesting the presence of systemic vasculitis in this disease.

Familial Increase of In Vitro IgA Production

Familial increase of IgA production has been observed not only in vivo, but also in vitro [27]. It is a matter of controversy, however, whether such an increase is observed in cultures with or without addition of pokeweed mitogens. Details of the references on this aspect have been reviewed elsewhere [28], but it is difficult to compare the results of studies on cell cultures in various laboratories, because of heterogeneity, not only in culture systems, but also in populations of patients examined. The size and subclass of IgA produced in cultured lymphocytes were, at least in patients if not in their relatives, similar to those of IgA deposited in the glomeruli, i.e., polymeric [29] IgA1 [30]. Therefore, it is postulated that IgA-bearing B cells in the circulation might be related to intraglomerular IgA.

Polyclonal Activation of IgA-Producing B Cells

The increased levels of serum IgA observed in patients with IgA nephropathy and in their relatives are probably due to polyclonal IgA, since monoclonal IgA is not found in these subjects. To further confirm this possibility, the kappa/lambda ratio of serum IgA, IgA-bearing B cells, and IgA produced by cultured B cells was examined in patients and their relatives [31]. The results obtained clearly showed that there was no deviation in the kappa/lambda ratio for any of these IgA antibodies. Furthermore, immunization, both of patients with IgA nephropathy [32] and of some of their relatives [31], induced not only an increase in IgA class anti influenza virus antibody, but also an increase in IgA class rheumatoid factor. These results suggested that antigenic stimulation of patients and their families induced not only increases in antigen-specific IgA antibodies, but also simultaneous increases in nonspecific IgA antibodies. These increases in nonspecific IgA antibodies might be responsible for the increase of serum levels of IgA in some patients and their relatives.

Emergence of Various Autoantibodies

Recently, the emergence of various kinds of autoantibodies has been noted in patients with IgA nephropathy, and also, sometimes, in their relatives. These autoantibodies include structural proteins of the glomeruli, such as nuclear protein [33] and collagen [34], and rheumatoid factors [35,36], as well as anti idiotype antibodies [37] and anti F(ab')$_2$ antibodies [38]. The polyclonal expansion of IgA-producing B cells might be responsible for the emergence of these autoantibodies. It is interesting to note that the majority of these antibodies was not restricted to the IgA class but included IgG and IgM to some extent. The polyclonal expansion of B cells in patients with IgA nephropathy might involve various isotypes, although the dominant class was IgA. Furthermore, serum titers of anti nuclear protein in relatives correlated significantly with the severity of tissue damage in renal biopsy specimens from patients [39]. The mechanism of this correlation is presently unknown, but familial increase in auto-antibodies might be related to heterogeneous deposition of IgA in the glomeruli, followed by tissue damage caused by complement activation. As of the time of this writing, however, there is no direct evidence showing the deposition of autoantibodies in the glomeruli of patients with IgA nephropathy. In addition, the emergence of autoantibodies in relatives produces the new question of why these relatives do not seem to have renal diseases, at least as judged by urinalysis without renal biopsy.

Mechanism of Polyclonal Activation of IgA-Producing B Cells

Because IgA is a highly T cell-dependent antibody, altered T cell function has been suspected as a mechanism inducing polyclonal activation of IgA-producing B cells [40]. Decrease in IgA-specific suppressor T cell activity has been observed in patients [41] and in some of their relatives [42]. The decrease in such suppressor T cells was, however, a secondary phenomenon due to activation of IgA-producing B cells, since there was no abnormality in IgA-specific suppressor T cell activity in an identical twin sister of a patient with IgA nephropathy [41]. As far as helper T cells are concerned, there was an elevation in the $CD_4^+/CD8^+$ ratio [43], as well as an increase in IgA-specific helper T cells which have receptors for the Fc portion of IgA (FcαR) (i.e., Tα cells) [44]. The effect of Tα cells on IgA-producing B cells is a matter of controversy. There have been a series of reports showing that both T α cells and FcαR have an inhibitory action in cultures of IgA-producing B cells [45]. The reason for this dichotomy is presently unknown, but addition of IgA to culture systems might induce such inhibitory effects, since all studies showing the inhibitory effects of Tα cells used in vitro addition of IgA, while the studies of helper effects used IgA-free culture media. At least one of the T cell subsets which induce polyclonal activation of IgA-producing B cells is that of IgA-specific switch T cells which specifically convert IgM-producing B cells to IgA-producing B cells. Such IgA-specific switch T cells were first reported by Kawanishi and his associates [46], using a T cell clone from murine Peyer's patches. Subsequently, peripheral blood T cells with FcαR and CD4 antigen (i.e., Tα4 cells) were demonstrated to have IgA-specific switch activity, and these Tα4 cells were significantly increased in patients with IgA nephropathy [47]. Peripheral blood Tα4 cells were also increased in relatives of patients with IgA nephropathy [48], suggesting that these T cells might be responsible for polyclonal activation of IgA-producing B cells in families of patients with this disease.

Isotype switching of immunoglobulins is mediated by the switch region of genes located immediately before heavy chain regions. In the case of IgA, two switch regions (i.e., Sα1 and Sα2) have been recognized to correspond with two subclasses of IgA (i.e., IgA1 and IgA2). The relationship between Tα4 cells and these switch regions is presently unknown, but presumably some cytokines influence these switch regions. Polymorphism of the Sα1 region was reported in European patients with IgA nephropathy [49], while polymorphism of the Sα2 region was observed in Japanese patients [50]. It is presently unknown how these polymorphisms in the switch region induce dominant production of IgA1.

Cytokines responsible for IgA-specific switch activity have not been identified in humans. Interleukin 2 (IL-2), IL-4, IL-5, and IL-6 were proved to induce the expansion of precommitted IgA-producing B cells, but do not induce de novo switch activity. Transforming growth factor β (TGFβ) was demonstrated to be a prospective IgA-specific switch factor in mice [51], but preliminary studies failed to confirm activity in humans (unpublished data).

Impaired Catabolism of IgA

Intraglomerular deposition of IgA in patients with IgA nephropathy might be associated with impaired catabolism of IgA. Decreased function of the reticuloendothelial system [52], as well as the macrophage-monocyte system [53], has been reported. Emergence of blocking factors against Fc receptors has also been reported [54]. It is, however, premature to conclude that impaired clearance is the primary cause of intraglomerular deposition of IgA in this disease, since evidence is lacking for a relationship between the degree of clinical activity of IgA nephropathy, and the degree of impairment in the clearance system.

Search for Antigens

Antigens responsible for the development of IgA nephropathy have been investigated, because this disease is presumed to be mediated by IgA-dominant immune complexes. Numerous candidates for such antigens have been reported, but, in the author's opinion, these candidates should satisfy the following two requirements: (a) the antigen should be observed at the same location as the majority of IgA deposited in the glomeruli, and (b) the antigen should be specifically bound with IgA eluted from the glomeruli of many patients with IgA nephropathy. Elevation of serum antibody titers is not sufficient to prove the pathogenic role of that antigen, because non-specific elevation of various IgA antibodies is likely to be due to polyclonal expansion of IgA-producing B cells in this disease. Presently, there is no antigen which completely satisfies the two requirements listed above. However, a few candidates for such antigens meet these requirements at least partially.

Virus-Like Antigens in the Upper Respiratory Tract

This candidate can satisfy the above requirement (b), but it is not yet proven whether it can meet requirement (a). Many patients with IgA nephropathy show exacerbation of proteinuria and/or hematuria after episodes of upper respiratory infection. It was demonstrated that epithelial cells obtained from the upper respiratory tract showed specific binding with 125-I labelled IgA eluted from the same or allogenic patients with IgA nephropathy [55]. Subsequently, an antigenic substance from the upper respiratory tract was cultured successively in human fibroblasts, suggesting that these antigens were virus-like materials [55]. Recently, polyclonal rabbit antisera against these antigens were produced, and these antisera showed specific binding with the mesangial areas of many patients with IgA nephropathy, without cross reactions with any serum proteins [56]. Further studies, using specific antisera, are warranted in order to identify these virus-like antigens.

Soybean Protein

This candidate satisfies the above requirement (a) but so far it is not known whether soybean protein binds specifically with IgA eluted from the glomeruli of many patients with IgA nephropathy. Various environmental antigens have been observed in some patients with IgA nephropathy, and soybean protein was one of these antigens [57]. The specificity of antisera against soybean has been evaluated, and this antigen was observed in as many as 75% of patients with IgA nephropathy [58]. A combination of several different monoclonal antibodies is required to identify these food antigens in the glomeruli of patients with this disease.

Exacerbating Factors in IgA Nephropathy

Various factors not specific to IgA nephropathy, but more ubiquitous in many renal diseases, have been found to exacerbate this disease. From the clinical standpoint, these factors are important in the management of patients with IgA nephropathy.

Activation of Complement

It has long been a matter of controversy whether IgA-dominant immune complexes in the glomeruli of patients with IgA nephropathy activate the complement component. Recently, however, there is an increasing body of evidence showing the activation of complement, including alternate pathways [59], and evidence showing that the membrane attack complex (MAC) [60] occurs in the glomeruli of patients with IgA nephropathy.

Infiltration of Phagocytic Cells

It is well known that intraglomerular infiltration of phagocytic cells induces progression of tissue damage in many renal diseases. Until recently, however, there has been no evidence showing whether such a phenomenon occurs in IgA nephropathy. Kincaid-Smith et al. [61] reported that polymorphonuclear cells and monocytes infiltrated into the glomeruli of many patients with IgA nephropathy; they thus showed that this phenomenon actually occurred in this disease.

Role of Cytokines

Various cytokines have been demonstrated to induce proliferation of mesangial cells in vitro. Recently, Horii et al. [62], using transgenic mice, demonstrated that interleukin 6 (IL-6) has a potent capacity to proliferate mesangial cells not only in vitro, but also in vivo. They also showed a significant increase in the urinary levels of IL-6 in patients with IgA nephropathy, further suggesting the exacerbating role of IL-6 in this disease.

Blood Coagulation in the Glomeruli

It is well known that intraglomerular coagulation impairs local blood flow and thus causes deterioration of renal functions. The clinical effects of antiplatelet agents such as dipyridamole have been established since the early 1970s [63], and these drugs are now most commonly used for the treatment of IgA nephropathy in many countries.

Hypertension and Microvascular Lesions

Systemic hypertension, with and without associated intraglomerular hypertension, is known as the major factor in the progression of renal dysfunction. The exacerbating roles of hypertension and microvascular lesions have been shown to be related to the progression of IgA nephropathy [64].

Summary of Proposed Pathogenesis

Figure 1 summarizes a proposed model of the pathogenesis of IgA nephropathy. The initial events leading to the development of IgA nephropathy seem to be mediated by various kinds of IgA-dominant immune complexes, which might be induced by some antigenic stimulation in genetic high responders of IgA production. The later events are common in various renal diseases and presumably contribute to the progression of renal damage in this disease.

Treatment

Selection of Therapy

There is no specific treatment for IgA nephropathy. The aim of current treatment is to preserve renal functions and to stabilize associated symptoms such as hypertension. The selection of therapy depends on the prediction of prognosis of individual

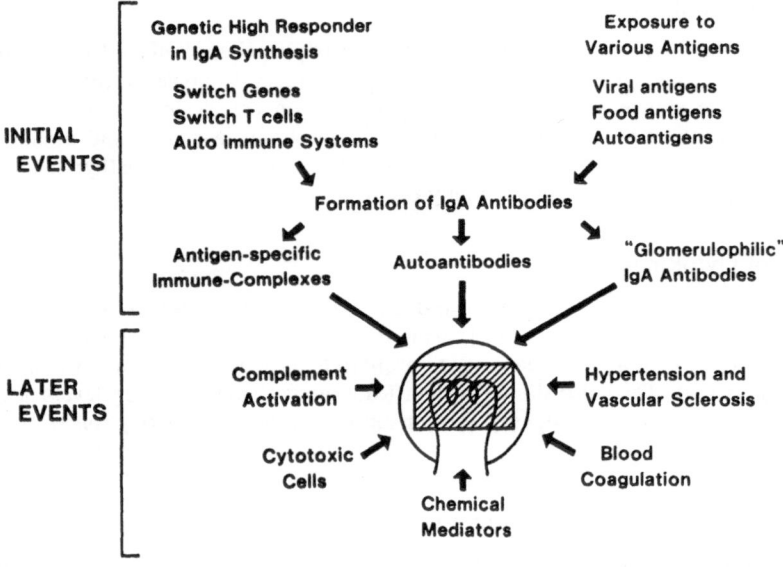

Fig. 1. Pathogenesis of IgA nephropathy (model proposed in 1990). (From [80] with permission)

patients. With respect to parameters for the prediction of prognosis, there are two major streams: (a) one which evaluates multiple factors, including severity of glomerular lesions, proteinuria of more than 2g/day, hypertension, age of more than 35 at onset, and male sex [65], and (b) one which evaluates the single most reliable parameter, which is the severity of glomerular lesions [66]. The common denominator between these two streams is the histopathological findings in renal biopsy specimens. The prognosis of almost all adult patients and the majority of pediatric patients can be predicted by histological findings at the time of the first biopsy, because there will not be much deviation in the degree of tissue damage after the diagnosis. Most institutions around the world classify the histological lesions into several categories, e.g., minimal, slight, moderate, and advanced. No drug therapy is required for the treatment of patients with minimal to slight degree of damage because, with a few exceptions in pediatric patients, most of them remain unchanged during periodic checks. In patients with advanced IgA nephropathy, there is no effective method of preventing renal failure. Therefore, these patients should avoid vigorous immuno-suppressive treatment in order to preserve their general condition in preparation for hemodialysis or allotransplantation. However, all these minimal, slight, and advanced patients need to be treated by appropriate diet, adequate degree of restriction of physical activity, and maintenance of general condition, such as control of hypertension. In addition to this general therapy, administration of drugs will be required in patients with a moderate degree of IgA nephropathy. The prognosis of patients in this category is heterogeneous, but drug therapy is required in all of them because of the lack of a reliable method of predicting their individual prognoses.

Drugs Evaluated by Double Blind Studies

As of the time of this writing, only two drugs have been evaluated by multi-center double-blind studies. These studies, however, were performed in Japan and there are no reports in English. Sixty mg/day of trimetazidine hydrochloride (t.i.d., p.o.) [67] and 300 mg/day of dilazep hydrochloride (t.i.d., p.o.) [68] were found to be effective in the improvement and reduction of proteinuria. One of these drugs, dilazep hydrochloride, has been approved by the Ministry of Health and Welfare of Japan as a drug for treatment of IgA nephropathy. However, double-blind administration of these drugs was performed for only six months, followed by two year follow-ups. Longer periods of double-blind studies were not feasible, for ethical reasons.

Drugs Evaluated by Multi-Center Studies

In many countries, dipyridamole has a relatively long history of use for treatment of IgA nephropathy, but so far no double-blind study has been performed; only multi-center open studies have been performed since 1970 [63]. The clinical effects of these anti platelet agents, i.e., trimetazidine dihydrochloride, dilazep hydrochloride, and dipyridamole, are regarded as similar, although precise scientific comparisons have never been made.

Previously, corticosteroids were used in patients with IgA nephropathy associated with severe proteinuria. Recent studies have shown, however, that steroids are effective in maintaining renal functions in patients with moderate degrees of glomerular lesions associated with a moderate degree of proteinuria, i.e., less than 2 g/day [69]. Similar results have been obtained in an on-going research project of the Ministry of Health and Welfare of Japan (Professor M. Narita, personal communication). In order to establish guidelines for the selection of patients for steroid therapy, further evaluation is warranted.

Drugs and Other Treatment Still in the Experimental Stage

In many countries, nonsteroidal anti inflammatory drugs have been used in patients with various types of chronic glomerulonephritis, but there have been no large-scale studies of this type of drug [70]. Drug-induced gastric irritation and possible increase in serum creatinine levels are still being debated.

The effects of other drugs which interfere with the blood coagulation system have been reported. Defibrination of intraglomerular fibrin deposits by urokinase effected significantly better preservation of renal function for three years, when compared with antiplatelet agents [71]. Use of antiallergic drugs is potentially interesting because of the possible role of allergic reactions in the pathogenesis of IgA nephropathy [72]. Other drugs, such as low dose dopamine [73], danazol [74], and eicosapentaenoic acid [75], showed some limited effects, and further confirmation is warranted.

Coppo et al. [76] have advocated plasmapheresis in the treatment of progressive IgA nephropathy. The experience of Australian groups suggested, however, that this treatment may alter the course of the disease only while treatment continues [77].

Allotransplantation in patients with IgA nephropathy is known to show recurrence rates of more than 50%, but the prognosis of recurrent IgA nephropathy has been regarded as relatively benign [78]. Recently, there have been a few reports showing

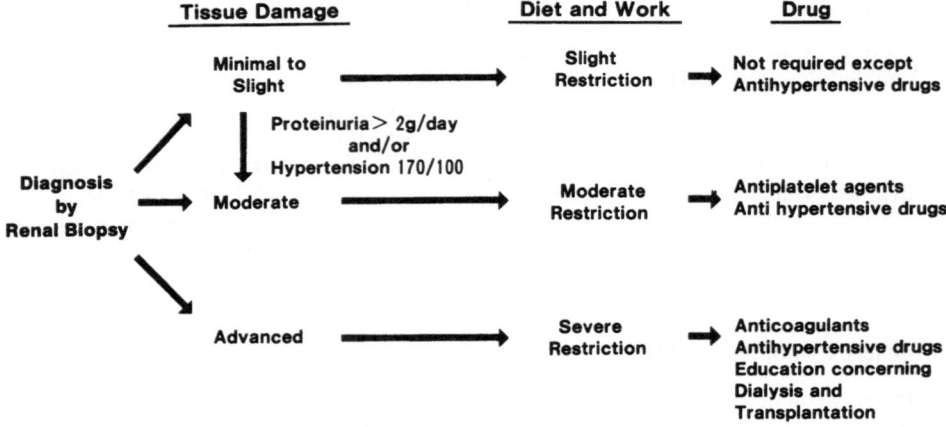

Fig. 2. Treatment of IgA nephropathy (model proposed in 1990)

the progression of recurrent IgA nephropathy to end stage renal disease [79]. However, the rates of progression in transplant patients are relatively low and thus transplantation is not prohibited in the treatment of patients with IgA nephropathy.

Summary of Proposed Treatment

Figure 2 summarizes treatment protocols from recent reports. Selection of treatment should be based on the degree of tissue damage in renal biopsy specimens, although the presence of massive proteinuria and/or hypertension influences the evaluation. Restriction of diet and daily activities will be routine procedure. No drugs are required for patients with a minimal to slight degree of tissue damage. Antiplatelet agents are the drugs of choice in moderate IgA nephropathy. Preservation of general condition and appropriate education are required in patients with severe IgA nephropathy, together with treatment by anticoagulants such as warfarin. Administration of antihypertensive drugs is mandatory if persistent high blood pressure is observed in patients at any stage of IgA nephropathy.

References

1. Berger J, Hingalis N (1968) Les dépôts intercapillaires d'IgA-IgG. J Urol (Paris) 74:694–695
2. D'Amico G (1985) Idiopathic IgA mesangial nephropathy. Nephron 41:1–13
3. Clarkson AR (1987) IgA nephropathy: history, classification, and geographic distribution. In: Clarkson AR (ed) IgA Nephropathy. Martinus Nijhoff, Boston, pp 1–8
4. Berger J (1969) IgA glomerular deposits in renal disease. Transplant Proc 1:939–944
5. Lamperi S, Carozzi S (1979) Skin-muscle biopsy in patients with various nephropathies. Nephron 24:46–50
6. Hall RP, Stachura I, Cason J, Whiteside TL, Lawley TJ (1983) IgA-containing circulating immune complexes in patients with IgA nephropathy. Am J Med 74:56–63

7. Berger J, Yaneva H, Nabarra B, Barbanel C (1975) Recurrence of mesangial deposition after renal transplantation. Kidney Int 7:232–241
8. Sanfilippo F, Croker BP, Bollinger RB (1982) Fate of four cadaveric donor renal allografts with mesangial IgA nephropathy. Transplantation 33:370–376
9. André C, Berthoux FC, André F, Gillon J, Genin C, Sabatier J-C (1980) Prevalence of IgA2 deposits in IgA nephropathies. N Engl J Med 303:1343–1346
10. Conley ME, Cooper MD, Michael AF (1980) Selective deposition of IgA1 in IgA nephropathy, anaphylactoid purpura nephritis, and systemic lupus erythematosus. J Clin Invest 66:1432–1436
11. Lai K-N, Chan KW, Lai FM-C, Ho CP, Yan KW, Lam CWK, Vallnce-Owen J (1986) The immunochemical characterization of the light chains in the mesangial IgA deposits in IgA nephropathy. Am J Clin Pathol 85:548–551
12. Komatsu N, Nagura H, Watanabe K, Nomoto Y, Kobayashi K (1983) Mesangial deposits of J-chain linked polymeric IgA nephropathy. Nephron 33:61–64
13. Tomino Y, Sakai H, Miura M, Endoh M, Nomoto Y (1982) Detection of polymeric IgA in glomeruli from patients with IgA nephropathy. Clin Exp Immunol 49:419–425
14. Monteiro RC, Halbwachs-Mecarelli L, Roque-Barreira MC, Noel L-H, Berger J, Lesavre P (1985) Charge and size of mesangial IgA in IgA nephropathy. Kidney Int 28:666–671
15. Shigematsu H, Kobayashi Y, Hiki Y (1990) Paramesangial destructive lesions in immunoglobulin A nephritis. Ultrastruct Pathol 14:129–139
16. Smith SM, Tung KS (1985) Incidence of IgA-related nephritis in American Indians in New Mexico. Hum Pathol 16:181–184
17. Jennette JC, Wall SD, Wilkman AS (1985) Low incidence of IgA nephropathy in blacks. Kidney Int 28:944–950
18. Egido J, Julian BA, Wyatt RJ (1987) Genetic factors in primary IgA nephropathy. Nephrol Dial Transpl 2:134–142
19. Wyatt RJ, Julian BA, Galla JH, McLean R (1984) Increased frequency of C3 fast alleles in IgA nephropathy. Disease Markers 2:419–428
20. McLean RH, Wyatt RJ, Julian BA (1984) Complement phenotypes in glomerulonephritis: increased frequency of homozygous null C4 phenotypes in IgA nephropathy and Henoch-Schonlein purpura. Kidney Int 26:855–860
21. Valentijn RM, Radl J, Haaijman JJ, Vermeer BJ, Weening JJ, Kaufmann RH, Daha MR, van Es LA (1984) Circulating and mesangial secretory component-binding IgA1 in primary IgA nephropathy. Kidney Int 26:760–766
22. Harada T, Hobby P, Courteau M, Knight JF, Williams DG (1989) Charge distribution of plasma IgA in IgA nephropathy. Clin Exp Immunol 77:211–214
23. Sakai H, Nomoto Y, Arimori S, Komori K, Inouye H, Tsuji, K (1979) Increase of IgA-bearing peripheral blood lymphocytes in families of patients with IgA nephropathy. Am J Clin Pathol 72:452–456
24. Garcia-Hoyo R, Lozano L, Egido J (1987) Immune abnormalities of IgA in six families with IgA nephropathy. In: McGhee JR, Mestecky J, Ogra PL, Beinenstock J (eds) Recent advances in mucosal immunology, Part B. Plenum, New York, pp 1499–1505
25. Béné M-C, Faure G, de Ligney BH, Kessler M, Duheille J (1983) IgA nephropathy: quantitative immunohistomorphometry of the tonsilar plasma cells evidences an inversion of the IgA versus IgG secreting cell membrane. J Clin Invest 71:1342–1347
26. Béné M-C, de Ligney BH, Sirbat D, Faure G, Kessler M, Duheille J (1984) IgA nephropathy: dimeric IgA-secreting cells are present in episcleral infiltrate. Am J Clin Pathol 82:608–611
27. Waldo FB, Beischel L, West CD (1986) IgA synthesis by lymphocytes from patients with IgA nephropathy and their relatives. Kidney Int 29:1229–1233
28. Sakai H (1987) Lymphocyte function in IgA nephropathy. In: Clarkson AR (ed) IgA nephropathy. Martinus Nijhoff, Boston, pp 176–187

29. Egido J, Blasco R, Sancho J, Lozano L, Anchez-Crespo M, Hernando L (1982) Increased rates of polymeric IgA synthesis by circulating lymphoid cells in IgA mesangial glomerulonephritis. Clin Exp Immunol 47:309–316

30. van den Wall Bake AWL, Daha MR, van der Ark A, Hiemstra PS, Radl J, van Es LA (1988) Serum levels and in vitro production of IgA subclasses in patients with primary IgA nephropathy. Clin Exp Immunol 74:115–120

31. Sakai H, Nomoto Y, Tomino Y, Endoh M, Miura M, Suga T (1987) Increases of in vitro and in vivo production of polyclonal IgA in patients and their family members with IgA nephropathy. In: McGhee JR, Mestecky J, Ogra PL, Beinenstock J (eds) Recent advances in mucosal immunology, Part B. Plenum, New York, pp 1507–1514

32. Endoh M, Suga T, Miura M, Tomino Y, Nomoto Y, Sakai H (1984) In vivo alteration of antibody production in patients with IgA nephropathy. Clin Exp Immunol 57:564–570

33. Nomoto Y, Suga T, Miura M, Nomoto H, Tomino Y, Sakai H (1986) Characterization of an acidic nuclear protein recognized by autoantibodies in sera from patients with IgA nephropathy. Clin Exp Immunol 65:513–519

34. Cederholm B, Wieslander J, Bygren P, Heinegard D (1986) Patients with IgA nephropathy have circulating anti-basement membrane antibodies reacting with structures common to collagen I, II, and IV. Proc Natl Acad Sci USA 83:6151–6155

35. Endoh M, Suga T, Sakai H (1985) IgG, IgA, and IgM rheumatoid factors in patients with glomerulonephritis. Nephron 39:330–335

36. Sinico RA, Fornasieri A, Oreni N, Benuzzi S, D'Amico G (1986) Polymeric IgA rheumatoid factor in idiopathic IgA mesangial nephropathy (Berger's disease). J Immunol 137:536–541

37. Gonzalez-Cabrero J, Egido J, Mampaso F, Rivas MC, Hernando L (1989) Characterization of circulating idiotypes containing immune complexes and their presence in the glomerular mesangium in patients with IgA nephropathy. Clin Exp Immunol 76:204–209

38. Schena FP, Pastore A, Ludovico N, Sinico RA, Benuzzi S, Montinaro V (1989) Increased serum levels of IgA1-IgG immune complexes and anti-F(ab')$_2$ antibodies in patients with primary IgA nephropathy. Clin Exp Immunol 77:15–20

39. Nomoto Y, Miura M, Suga T, Endoh M, Tomino Y, Sakai H (1984) Cold reacting anti-nuclear factor (ANF) in families of patients with IgA nephropathy. Clin Exp Immunol 58:63–67

40. Elson CO (1983) T cell specific for IgA switching and for IgA B-cell differentiation. Immunol Today 4:189–190

41. Sakai H, Nomoto Y, Arimori S (1979) Decrease of IgA-specific suppressor T cell activity in patients with IgA nephropathy. Clin Exp Immunol 38:243–248

42. Egido J, Blasco RA, Sancho J, Hernando L (1985) Immunological abnormalities in healthy relatives of patients with IgA nephropathy. Am J Nephrol 5:14–20

43. Chatenoud L, Bach M-A (1981) Abnormalities of T-cell subsets in glomerulonephritis and systemic lupus erythematosus. Kidney Int 20:267–274

44. Sakai H, Endoh M, Tomino Y, Nomoto Y (1982) Increase of IgA specific helper Tα cells in patients with IgA nephropathy. Clin Exp Immunol 50:77–82

45. Yodoi J, Adachi M, Noro N (1987) IgA-binding factors and Fc receptors for IgA: comparative studies between IgA and IgE Fc receptor systems. Int Rev Immunol 2:117–141

46. Kawanishi H, Saltzman LE, Strober W (1983) Mechanism regulating IgA class-specific immunoglobulin production in murine gut-associated lymphoid tissue. 1. T cells derived from Peyer's patches that switch sIgM cells to sIgA B cells in vitro. J Exp Med 157:433–450

47. Sakai H, Miyazaki M, Endoh M, Nomoto Y (1989) Increase of IgA-specific switch T cells in patients with IgA nephropathy. Clin Exp Immunol 78:378–382

48. Miyazaki M (to be published) Abnormalities of cellular immunity in patients with IgA nephropathy and their relatives. Jpn J Med

49. Demaine AG, Rambausek M, Knight JF, Williams DG, Welsh KI, Ritz E (1988) Relation of mesangial IgA glomerulonephritis to polymorphism of immunoglobulin heavy chain switch region. J Clin Invest 81:611–614
50. Miyazaki M (1990) Heterogeneity of the Sα2 region—increased frequency of the heterozygous switch region of IgA2 in patients with IgA nephropathy. In: Sakai H, Sakai O, Nomoto Y (eds) Pathogenesis of IgG nephropathy. HBJ Japan, Tokyo, pp 65–80
51. Coffman RL, Lebman DA, Shrader B (1989) Transforming growth factor β specifically enhances IgA production by lipopolysaccharide-stimulated murine B lymphocytes. J Exp Med 170:1039–1044
52. Bannister KM, Hay J, Clarkson AR, Woodroffe AJ (1984) Fc specific reticulo-endothelial clearance in SLE and glomerulonephritis. Am J Kidney Dis 3:287–292
53. Roccatello D, Coppo R, Piccoli G (1984) Monocyte macrophage system function in primary IgA nephropathy. Contrib Nephrol 40:130–136
54. Roccatello D, Coppo R, Piccoli G, Cordonnier D, Martina G, Rollino C, Picciotto G, Sena LM, Amoroso A (1985) Fc receptors blocking factors in IgA nephropathies. Clin Nephrol 23:159–168
55. Tomino Y, Sakai H, Miura M, Suga T, Endoh M, Nomoto Y, Umehara K, Hashimoto K (1985) Specific binding of circulating IgA antibodies in patients with IgA nephropathy. Am J Kidney Dis 3:149–153
56. Eguchi K, Sakai H, Endoh M, Nomoto Y (1990) Specific antisera against pharyngeal antigens in patients with IgA nephropathy. In: Sakai H, Sakai O, Nomoto Y (eds) Pathogenesis of IgA nephropathy. HBJ Japan, Tokyo, pp 231–246
57. Russell MW, Mestecky J, Julian BA, Galla JH (1986) IgA-associated renal disease: antibodies to environmental antigens in sera and deposition of immunoglobulins and antigens in glomeruli. J Clin Immunol 6:74–78
58. Sato M, Kojima H, Takayama K, Koshikawa S (1988) Glomerular deposition of food antigens in IgA nephropathy. Clin Exp Immunol 73:295–299
59. Wyatt RJ, Kanayama Y, Julian BA, Negoro M, Sugimoto S, Hudson EC, Curd JG (1987) Complement activation in IgA nephropathy. Kidney Int 31:1019–1023
60. Rauterberg EW, Lieberknecht H-M, Wingen A-M, Ritz E (1987) Complement membrane attack (MAC) in idiopathic IgA-glomerulonephritis. Kidney Int 31:820–829
61. Kincaid-Smith P, Nicholls K, Birchall I (1989) Polymorphs infiltrate glomeruli in mesangial IgA glomerulonephritis. Kidney Int 36:1108–1111
62. Horii Y, Iwano M, Suematshu S, Matsusaka T, Matsuda T, Muraguchi A, Yamamoto T, Miyazaki J, Yamamura K, Ishikawa H, Hirano T, Kishimoto T (1990) Interleukin-6 is a growth factor for mouse mesangial cells. In: Sakai H, Sakai O, Nomoto Y (eds) Pathogenesis of IgA nephropathy. HBJ Japan, Tokyo, pp 127–143
63. Kincaid-Smith P, Laver MC, Fairley KF (1970) Dipyridamole and anticoagulants in renal disease due to glomerular and vascular lesions. A new approach to therapy. Med J Aust 1:145–151
64. Katafuchi R, Vamvakas E, Neelakantappa K, Baldwin DS, Gallo GR (1990) Microvascular disease and the progression of IgA nephropathy. Am J Kidney Dis 15:72–79
65. Droz D (1987) IgA nephropathy: clinicopathological correlations. In: Clarkson AR (ed) IgA nephropathy. Martinus Nijhoff, Boston, pp 97–107
66. D'Amico G, Minetti L, Ponticelli C, Fellin G, Ferrario F, Barbiano di Belgioioso G, Duca G (1986) Prognostic indicators in idiopathic IgA mesangial nephropathy. Q J Med New Series 59:363–378
67. Tojo S, Narita M, Miyahara T, Sakai O, Ohono J, Soeda N, Honda N, Nagase M, Sibata M, Orita Y, Ishikawa H, Hara K, Sakuma A (1985) Manseishikyuutaijinen ni taisuru trimetazidine dihydrochloride no rinshokoka. Jin to Toseki 19:1367–1380
68. Tojo S, Honda N, Sibata M, Narita M, Miyahara T, Sakai O, Katoh E, Kida H, Orita Y, Ishikawa H, Hara K, Tanaka T, Takasaki H (1986) Manseishikyuutaijinen ni taisuru AS-05 (Dilazep) no rinshoukouka. Jin to Toseki 20:289–313

69. Kobayashi Y, Hiki Y, Tateno S, Fujii K, Kurokawa A (1990) Indication of steroid therapy in IgA nephropathy (abstract). Proceedings of the XIth international congress of nephrology, July 15-20 1990. Springer, Tokyo Berlin Heidelberg

70. Laurent J, Belghiti D, Bruneau C, Lagrue G (1987) Diclofenac, a nonsteroidal anti-inflammatory drug, decreases proteinuria in some glomerular diseases: A controlled study. Am J Nephrol 7:198-202

71. Miura M, Endoh M, Nomoto Y, Sakai H (1989) Long-term effect of urokinase therapy in IgA nephropathy. Clin Nephrol 32:209-216

72. Sato M, Takayama K, Kojima H, Koshikawa S (1990) Sodium cromoglycate therapy in IgA nephropathy: a preliminary short-term trial. Am J Kidney Dis 15:141-146

73. Beukhof HR, ter Wee PM, Sluiter WJ, Donker AJM (1985) Effect of low-dose dopamine on effective renal plasma flow and glomerular filtration rate in 32 patients with IgA nephropathy. Am J Nephrol 5:267-270

74. Tomino Y, Sakai H, Miura M, Suga T, Endoh M, Nomoto Y (1984) Effect of danazol on solubilization of immune deposits in patients with IgA nephropathy. Am J Kidney Dis 4:135-140

75. Hamazaki T, Tateno S, Shishido H (1984) Eicosapentaenoic acid and IgA nephropathy. Lancet I:1017-1018

76. Coppo R, Basolo B, Giachino O, Rocatelli D, Lajola D, Mazzucco G, Amore A, Piccoli G (1985) Plasmapheresis in a patient with rapidly progressive idiopathic IgA nephropathy: removal of IgA-containing immune complexes and clinical recovery. Nephron 40:488-490

77. Clarkson AR (1987) The treatment of IgA nephropathy. In: Clarkson AR (ed) IgA nephropathy. Martinus Nijhoff, Boston, pp 214-224

78. Berger J, Noel L, Nabarra B (1984) Recurrence of mesangial IgA nephropathy after renal transplantation. Contrib Nephrol 40:195-197

79. Brensilver JM, Mallat S, Scholes J, McCabe R (1988) Recurrent IgA nephropathy in living-related donor transplantation: recurrence or transmission of familial disease? Am J Kidney Dis 12:147-151

80. Sakai H (1990) Pathogenesis of IgA nephropathy. Japn J Clin Immunol 13:307-319

Pathophysiology of Obstructive Nephropathy

SAULO KLAHR

Chair: Shaul G. Massry

Pathophysiology of Obstructive Nephropathy

SAULO KLAHR[1]

SUMMARY. The effects of obstructive uropathy on renal function are the consequence of a variety of factors with complex interactions. Obstruction of the urinary tract decreases glomerular filtration rate (GFR) and renal plasma flow, and modifies tubular function. The decrease in GFR and plasma flow is mediated, in part, by the vasoconstrictors angiotensin II and thromboxane A_2.

A significant infiltration of leukocytes occurs in the kidney following obstruction; furthermore, by abolishing this infiltrate the renal function of the post-obstructed kidney is significantly improved. This indicates that leukocytes have an important role in modulating renal hemodynamics after release of obstruction, whose pathophysiology must now be considered to include an immunological component. Further work is required to define the mechanisms whereby macrophages can influence renal function and to define how the kidney can recruit these cells in such large numbers following obstruction.

Abnormalities in renal tubule function are common in urinary tract obstruction. The major alterations appear to be located in distal segments of the nephron. There is decreased ability to concentrate the urine, the reabsorption of sodium and water is altered, and the secretion of hydrogen and potassium is impaired.

Effects of Obstruction on the Kidney

Urinary tract obstruction has diverse effects on renal function in humans. There is a marked reduction in renal blood flow and glomerular filtration rate, and there are significant changes in renal tubular function [1]. Partial chronic obstruction of the urinary tract can cause progressive atrophy and destruction of nephrons, which may lead to chronic renal insufficiency. Unilateral complete obstruction of urine flow

---

[1]Renal Division, Department of Medicine, Washington University School of Medicine, St. Louis, MO 63110, USA

may be well tolerated for several days; however, if the obstruction persists for more than a week, permanent damage ensues. By the end of three weeks of complete obstruction, recovery of function is usually nil. On the other hand, acute complete bilateral obstruction results in renal failure. Because obstruction is generally a reversible cause of kidney failure, early and accurate diagnosis and prompt treatment are vital to the preservation and restoration of renal function [1].

The clinical manifestations of urinary tract obstructions vary [1]. Complete bilateral obstruction of urine flow is manifested as anuria. Partial obstruction can cause: 1) fluctuating urine output, alternating from oliguria to polyuria; 2) urinary tract infection, usually refractory to treatment; 3) abdominal or flank pain; or 4) unexplained acute or chronic renal failure. Obstruction always must be included in the differential diagnosis of acute renal failure, especially when urine output fluctuates or anuria occurs suddenly.

Pathophysiology of Obstructive Nephropathy

The effects of obstructive uropathy on renal function are the consequence of a variety of factors with complex interactions [2]. Obstruction of the urinary tract has marked effects on glomerular filtration, renal blood flow, and tubular function (see Fig. 1). Studies in experimental animals, using clearance and micropuncture techniques, have examined mainly the effect of acute short-term obstruction of the urinary tract on renal function. The effects of prolonged partial obstruction on renal function are less well characterized.

The Effects of Obstruction on Glomerular Filtration Rate

Glomerular filtration rate decreases progressively after the onset of complete ureteral obstruction [3]. The maintenance of some glomerular filtration following ureteral obstruction is presumably due to: a) the reabsorption of solutes and water along the nephron; b) the ability of the renal tract to dilate; and c) an alteration in renal hemodynamics.

Ureteral obstruction decreases glomerular filtration rate in rats, rabbits, and dogs [2]. After the onset of obstruction, the increased intraureteral pressure is transmitted upward, leading to increased intratubular pressure without a comparable quantitative increase in intraglomerular capillary hydrostatic pressure, resulting in a lower net filtration pressure across the glomerular capillary wall [3]. This appears to be the major factor responsible for the decrease in GFR after the onset of obstruction [3]. However, after 24 hours of obstruction, proximal intratubular pressure returns to normal, or below normal, values in animals with unilateral ureteral obstruction. In animals with bilateral ureteral obstruction, intratubular pressure also decreases, but remains above normal after 24 hours of obstruction [4]. At this time interval both renal plasma flow and intraglomerular capillary pressure are decreased. The decrease in intraglomerular capillary pressure after 24 hours of obstruction accounts for most of the fall in net filtration pressure and diminished single nephron GFR seen in animals with unilateral ureteral obstruction.

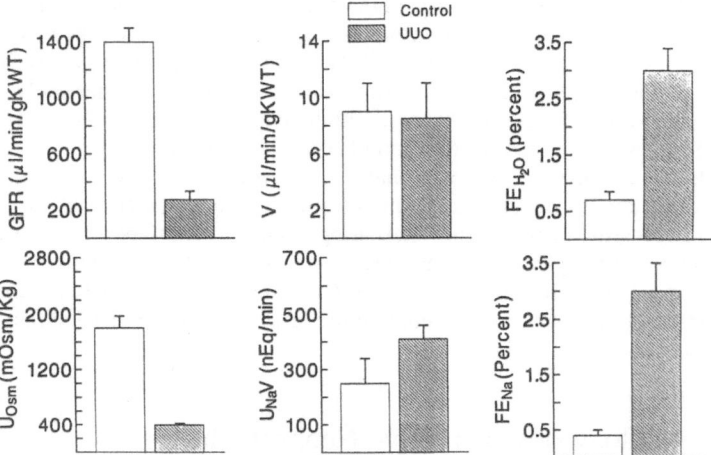

Fig. 1. Renal function after relief of unilateral ureteral obstruction (*UUO*) of 18 hours duration in 6 rats. Values are the mean ± SE for the control untouched kidney (□ and the post-obstructed kidney (■). Both inulin clearance (*GFR*) and urine osmolality (U_{osm}) were significantly lower in the post-obstructed kidney than in the control kidney. There were no significant differences in urine flow (*V*) or absolute sodium excretion ($U_{Na}V$) between the two kidneys. Fractional sodium and water excretion were significantly greater in the post-obstructed kidney than in the control

The decrease in total renal blood flow, due to both afferent and efferent arteriolar vasoconstriction, is accompanied by a fall in plasma flow per nephron, which contributes to the decrease in GFR [2,3]. With acute ureteral obstruction, the decrement in GFR exceeds the fall in renal plasma flow, resulting in a decrease in filtration fraction. This suggests that renal vasoconstriction alone does not account completely for the fall in GFR. Indeed, after relief of obstruction, the ultrafiltration coefficient (K_f) is decreased. This decrement in K_f may be due to a decrease in the total glomerular surface area available for filtration or to a change in the intrinsic permeability characteristics of the glomerular capillary wall. With short-term obstruction (24 hours) total kidney GFR decreases more than single nephron GFR, due to a decrease in the total number of filtering nephrons. Hence, the fall in GFR in acute obstruction is due to a decrement in single nephron GFR and a decrease in the total number of filtering nephrons [2].

Renal Hemodynamics in Animals with Unilateral or Bilateral Ureteral Obstruction

The renal hemodynamics of animals with unilateral or bilateral ureteral obstruction differ [2,3]. Whereas, at 24 hours after unilateral ureteral ligation in rats, the decrease in single nephron GFR is due almost exclusively to a fall in intraglomerular capillary pressure, in rats with bilateral ureteral obstruction both a decrease in intraglomerular capillary pressure and a persistent elevation of intratubular pressure account for the decrease in net filtration pressure. Furthermore, the number of filtering nephrons is greater in animals with bilateral obstruction than in those with unilateral obstruction after 24 hours of ureteral ligation [5]. The mechanisms responsible for these hemodynamic differences between unilateral and bilateral ureteral obstruction have not been elucidated. It has been reported that the levels of circulating atrial peptide, a potent vasodilator, are higher in rats with bilateral ureteral obstruction than in rats with unilateral ureteral obstruction [6]. Atrial peptide causes pre-glomerular vasodilatation and post-glomerular vasoconstriction and has been demonstrated to increase K_f in the isolated perfused glomerular preparation. In addition, the administration of exogenous atrial peptide increases GFR following release of unilateral or bilateral ureteral obstruction [6,7]. Since atrial peptide antagonizes the vasoconstrictive effects of angiotensin II, it is probable that, in vivo, the elevated levels of endogenous atrial peptide in animals with bilateral ureteral obstruction minimize the vasoconstriction that occurs, as compared to animals with unilateral ureteral obstruction.

Role of Vasoactive Compounds

Two major vasoconstrictors, angiotensin II and thromboxane A_2, have a role in the decrease in plasma flow per nephron and in single nephron GFR seen in obstruction [8]. Inhibition of thromboxane A_2 synthesis in rats with ureteral obstruction increases plasma flow per nephron, through decreased vasoconstriction of both afferent and efferent arterioles [8]. Thromboxane may also decrease K_f through mesangial cell contraction [9] and a decrease in the glomerular surface area available for filtration. Although infusion of angiotensin II into normal animals increases net filtration pressure, presumably due to greater vasoconstriction of the efferent than the afferent arteriole, blockade of angiotensin II formation after relief of obstruction increases GFR [8]. This increase in GFR may be due to a greater filtering surface area, since angiotensin II causes mesangial cell contraction [2] and therefore can reduce the total glomerular capillary area available for filtration. In addition, angiotensin II decreases plasma flow per nephron, which also contributes to the fall in single nephron GFR. The central and critical role of these two vasoconstrictors in modulating post-obstructive renal hemodynamics is illustrated (see Fig. 2) by the fact that rats pretreated with both an angiotensin converting enzyme inhibitor and a thromboxane synthase inhibitor prior to obstruction, demonstrate almost normal renal function after release of the obstruction [7].

Vasodilatory prostaglandins such as PGE_2 and prostacyclin, which are produced in increased amounts by the obstructed kidney, may prevent further decrements in GFR by antagonizing the vasoconstrictive effects of thromboxane A_2 and/or angiotensin. Indeed, it has been demonstrated that after release of obstruction in rats, administration of inhibitors of the cyclooxygenase, in the setting of prior inhibition of the thromboxane synthase, leads to a marked decrease in whole kidney GFR and in renal plasma flow [8].

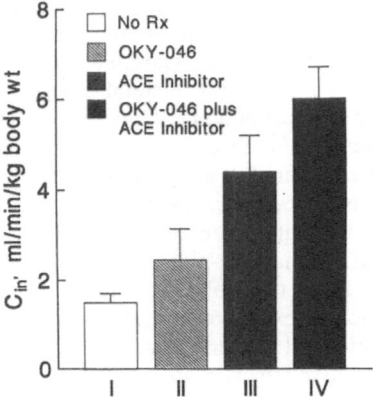

Fig. 2. Inulin clearance values measured 3–4 hours after unilateral release of bilateral ureteral obstruction of 24 h duration in four groups of rats. Values for inulin clearance were significantly greater in rats of group II (pretreated with an inhibitor of thromboxane synthesis), in rats of group III (pretreated with an inhibitor of the angiotensin converting enzyme), and in rats of group IV (treated with both a thromboxane synthase inhibitor and an inhibitor of the angiotensin converting enzyme (ACE), as compared to rats of group I, which were untreated. Notice that the values for inulin clearance in rats of group III are significantly higher than those in group II (P < 0.01), and that the combination of the ACE inhibitor and OKY-046 resulted in the highest values of GFR observed after release of obstruction (group IV). (From [7])

Effects of Obstruction on Renal Plasma Flow

After ureteral ligation, there is an initial increase in renal blood flow, which peaks at 2–3 hours after the onset of obstruction. Subsequently, renal blood flow decreases so that by 5 hours after the onset of obstruction the values are comparable to those seen prior to obstruction [1,2]. Intrinsic myogenic changes in the afferent arteriole, occurring as a consequence of ureteral obstruction, may account for the decrease seen in blood flow. It has been suggested also that the initial increase in renal blood flow to the obstructed kidney is mediated by prostaglandins, presumably prostacyclin [1,2]. Indeed, blockade of prostaglandin synthesis with cyclooxygenase inhibitors completely prevents the increase in ipsilateral blood flow that occurs with obstruction. Also, the exogenous infusion of PGI_2 (prostacyclin) increases blood flow in the obstructed kidney of animals pretreated with cyclooxygenase inhibitors. The increased release of prostaglandins during the initial period of obstruction depends on the de novo synthesis of key enzymes involved in the synthesis of eicosanoids. The activities of both cyclooxygenase and phospholipase A_2 are increased in the obstructed kidney. We have found increased activity of a phosphoethenolamine-specific phospholipase A_2 in isolated glomeruli of rats with ureteral obstruction. This enzyme may be responsible for the release of arachidonic acid from the phospholipid pool. Arachidonic acid in turn serves as the substrate for the synthesis of prostaglandins. The mechanism by which obstruction increases the synthesis and activity of the cyclooxygenase and phospholipase A_2 enzymes is unknown.

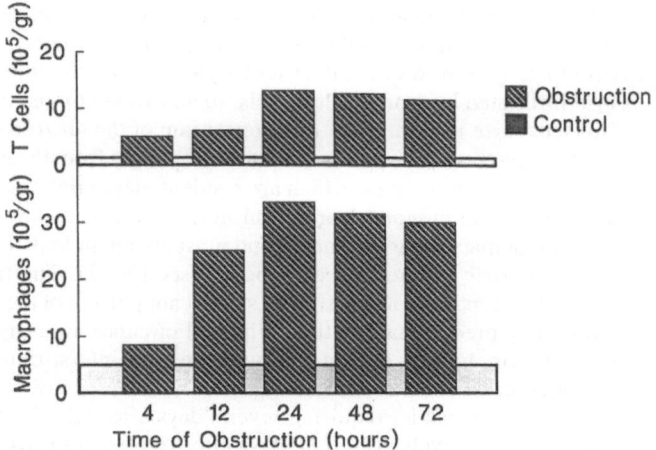

Fig. 3. The T lymphocyte (*upper panel*) and macrophage (*lower panel*) content, expressed as 10^5 cells per gram tissue, of the obstructed kidneys (▨) of rats at different time intervals after the initiation of unilateral obstruction. Control (■) values represent normal kidneys from non-obstructed littermates. Results are expressed as mean ± SE. (From [12])

With more prolonged obstruction, a progressive decrease in renal blood flow occurs, such that by 24–48 hours after the onset of obstruction, renal plasma flow is only 30%–40% of the values obtained prior to ureteral ligation [1,2]. In addition, 12–24 hours after the onset of obstruction there is a marked increase in the synthesis of thromboxane A_2 by the kidney. Thromboxane A_2 is a powerful vasoconstrictor, which may be responsible, in part, for the increased renal vascular resistance and decreased renal blood flow observed at later stages of obstruction [1,2].

Role of Infiltrating White Blood Cells in the Decrement in GFR and Renal Plasma Flow

In the 1970s it was found that a proliferation of interstitial fibroblasts and an infiltration of mononuclear cells occurred in the renal parenchyma of rabbits with chronic ureteral obstruction [10]. Subsequently, this leukocyte infiltrate was linked to the increase in prostaglandin E_2 production by the chronically hydronephrotic rabbit kidney [11]. It was also postulated, but not proven, that the infiltration of the renal parenchyma by mononuclear cells may underlie the augmented release of thromboxane A_2 and prostaglandin E_2 in response to bradykinin or endotoxin [11].

We have examined the initial phases of cell infiltration in a model of acute ureteral obstruction [12]. We found that a leukocyte influx is one of the earliest responses of the kidney to ureteral obstruction. The infiltrate was observed within 4 hours of obstruction, but its peak response occurred at 24 hours, after which a plateau was observed (Fig. 3). The leukocytes did not appear to represent a destructive infiltrate. They formed distinctive rings around tubular cells, particularly in distal tubules [12].

It is known that normal kidneys have small numbers of resident leukocytes, predominantly macrophages, in the renal cortex, mainly in the glomeruli. The normal medulla is completely devoid of resident leukocytes. In obstruction, however, the medulla is also infiltrated by mononuclear cells, to an extent comparable to that of the cortex. This leukocyte infiltration of the interstitium of the obstructed kidney was associated with a relative depletion of resident macrophages from the glomeruli. The fate of these glomerular leukocytes, which are resident mesangial macrophages, has not been elucidated. The mononuclear cell infiltrate present in the obstructed kidney consists mainly of macrophages. The second most abundant leukocytes are T lymphocytes of the cytotoxic suppressor cell subclass (see Fig. 3). The fact that T lymphocytes of the helper type do not constitute a significant portion of the infiltrate, despite the fact that they predominate in the peripheral circulation, suggests some degree of selectivity. B-lymphocytes are not present in the renal interstitium. Neutrophils are also absent from this infiltrate.

The infiltrate is slowly reversible, requiring several days after release of obstruction to revert to near normal levels [12]. Two days after release of obstruction, the macrophage content of the cortical interstitium appeared to increase modestly and then to fall to near normal levels by six days after release of the obstruction. In contrast, the T lymphocytes in the cortex diminish rapidly, to less than 20% of their values, during obstruction and two days after release of the ureteral ligation, with a further decrement noted four days later. However, a small increase in both cell populations, as compared to normal kidneys, was noted as long as a week after release of obstruction.

We also examined the functional significance of this leukocyte infiltration. The kinetics of arrival of the macrophages and leukocytes correlates temporally with the decline in glomerular filtration rate. As mentioned above, following the onset of obstruction there is an initial increase in renal blood flow, mediated by prostaglandins, which declines after 4 hours. At 24 hours, values for renal plasma flow are between 40%–70% of those observed prior to obstruction. The mechanism underlying this progressive vasoconstriction appears to be augmented production of thromboxane A_2. The chronically obstructed kidney displays an enhanced ability to metabolize arachidonic acid [1,2,11], and thromboxane synthase activity is increased. Inhibition of thromboxane synthase dramatically improves postobstructive renal hemodynamics and partially reverses the renal vasoconstriction that occurs with acute ureteral obstruction [7,8].

To examine the potential role of the infiltrating cells in the decrease in GFR and renal plasma flow seen with ureteral obstruction, we studied rats that underwent total body radiation prior to ureteral obstruction [13]. Irradiation abolished the leukocyte infiltration observed in the kidney after 24 hours of obstruction. Irradiation had no effect on renal morphology or function in normal rats. In contrast, elimination of the infiltrate by prior irradiation of the rats with bilateral ureteral obstruction decreased thromboxane B_2 excretion in the urine and significantly improved renal hemodynamics in the post-obstructed kidney [13]. This implies that the infiltrating leukocytes contribute to the hemodynamic changes observed in the post-obstructed kidney. We propose that the leukocytic infiltrate is, in part, responsible for the decline in GFR and renal plasma flow seen after obstruction, possibly via the production of vasoactive prostanoids such as thromboxane A_2. Indeed, it is of note that renal plasma flow, which increases for the first few hours after obstruction, only begins to decline at about 4 hours after obstruction, at a time when the leukocyte infiltrate is becoming evident.

Eliminating the leukocyte infiltrate from the renal parenchyma does not, however, return the function of the post-obstructed kidney to normal. This suggests that leukocyte-independent mechanisms are also present. It is also clear that the elimination of the infiltrating macrophages by prior irradiation does not reduce the excretion of thromboxane B_2 in the urine to baseline levels. This is consistent with obstruction causing enhanced production of this vasoactive prostanoid by structures intrinsic to the kidney, such as glomerular epithelial or mesangial cells [14]. Such leukocyte independent sources of thromboxane A_2 may also be capable of modulating renal hemodynamics [1,2].

We have found recently that glomeruli isolated from animals with bilateral ureteral obstruction produce greater quantities of prostaglandin E_2 (PGE$_2$), 6-keto PGF$_{1\alpha}$, the stable metabolite of prostacyclin, and thromboxane B_2, the stable metabolite of thromboxane A_2, than glomeruli isolated from kidneys of normal animals [14]. Since there is a depletion of endogenous macrophages from the glomeruli of the obstructed kidney, it is clear that the increased synthesis of thromboxane B_2 by isolated glomeruli is related to its production by an intrinsic glomerular cell. Most likely this reflects increased production of thromboxane A_2 by mesangial cells, although this has not been established in the obstructed model. In addition, we found that this increased synthesis of prostanoids by isolated glomeruli was restored to levels comparable to those seen in normal kidneys when the animals were pretreated with an ACE inhibitor prior to the onset of ureteral obstruction [14]. This suggests that endogenous angiotensin II has an important role in the increased synthesis of prostanoids found in isolated glomeruli from rats with bilateral ureteral obstruction. The most likely explanation for these results may be a marked stimulation of phospholipase A_2 and/or cyclooxygenase by angiotensin II in glomeruli from rats with bilateral ureteral obstruction. Therefore, the increased thromboxane excretion in the urine of animals with bilateral ureteral obstruction may have two origins: increased production by intrinsic glomerular cells, as well as production by macrophages that invade the renal parenchyma during obstruction.

Although the available data indicate that leukocytes may promote, or directly contribute to, a locally enhanced production of thromboxane A_2, it has not been established whether or not other substances or factors released by infiltrating macrophages modulate epithelial cell function. What contribution, if any, the accompanying suppressor T lymphocytes present in the infiltrate make to the renal response to obstruction requires further characterization. Finally, the nature of the stimulus coupling urinary tract obstruction to the appearance of a leukocyte infiltrate in the renal parenchyma has not been completely defined. Initial experiments indicate the release of a chemoattractant substance by the obstructed kidney. The nature of this chemoattractant agent has not been completely elucidated, although preliminary observations suggest that it is a lipid substance [15].

Polymorphonuclear leukocytes and monocytes are present in the renal interstitium of rabbits subjected to three days of ureteral obstruction. The obstructed kidney, when perfused ex vivo, exhibits an exaggerated increase in the elaboration of eicosanoids in response to bradykinin and the chemotactic peptide, N-formilmethionil-leucil-phenylalanine. Essential fatty acid deficiency (i.e., deprivation of ω-6-fatty acids) attenuated the elaboration of eicosanoids by the obstructed kidney perfused ex vivo. It also prevented the increase in the activities of microsomal cyclooxygenase and thromboxane synthase seen after three days of ureteral occlusion. Fatty acid deficiency also attenuated the influx of macrophages into the kidney, an effect that was attributed to inhibition of the synthesis of leukotriene B_4, which is a known chemoattractant for monocytes [16].

The long-term effects of this immunological infiltrate on renal function and structure remain to be defined. However, focal segmental glomerulosclerosis is a common histological finding in patients with ureteropelvic obstruction [17]. This focal segmental glomerulosclerosis was present in areas closely associated with intense interstitial and periglomerular inflammation. It could be envisioned that growth factors released by invading leukocytes have a role in the development and progression of fibrotic and sclerotic changes that occur in the chronically obstructed kidney [18]. It is, therefore, likely that the cellular infiltrate may contribute to the renal damage and to the progressive decrease in renal function observed with chronic urinary tract obstruction.

Recovery of Renal Function after Release of Ureteral Obstruction

The extent to which GFR recovers after release of ureteral obstruction depends on the duration of the obstruction. This has been studied in both the dog and the rat. In the dog, serial measurements of GFR have been made after one week of complete ureteral obstruction [1,2]. Assuming the glomerular filtration rate for each kidney was half that of the whole animal prior to ureteric ligation, immediately after release of the obstruction GFR averaged 25% of ipsilateral control values and 16% of the concurrent values for the contralateral kidney, the latter having undergone a compensatory increase in function. Follow-up studies revealed an increase in the GFR of the obstructed kidney and a decline in the GFR of the normal kidney, with values stabilizing at 2 months. In no case was there complete functional recovery of the obstructed kidney, and at 2 years the GFR of the experimental kidney remained 50% below the simultaneous value obtained for the contralateral kidney. These changes in glomerular filtration rate were paralleled by decrements in effective renal plasma flow, as assessed by the clearance of paraaminohippurate, consequently filtration fraction did not change.

In the rat, a permanent decrease in GFR occurs if ureteral obstruction is present for more than 72 hours [9]. Complete recovery of glomerular filtration rate is seen 7–9 days after release of shorter periods (less than 30 hours) of obstruction [2,3]. Although this would suggest that short-term obstruction is completely reversible and that most of the decrease in GFR is functional, there is evidence to suggest that the "normalization" in filtration rate may not be a consequence of a homogenous recovery in the single nephron GFR (SNGFR) of all nephrons. In post-obstructed kidneys calculations of total glomerular filtration rate, based on determinations of surface nephron SNGFR, yielded values that were greater than those obtained from clearance measurements [1,2]. This may be explained by the fact that, using Hansen's technique, 40% of superficial nephrons (those accessible to micropuncture) were found to be filtering immediately following release of the obstruction, whereas only 12% of juxtamedullary nephrons were filtering, suggesting a selective loss of juxtamedullary nephrons [1,2]. Subsequent studies indicated that 3–6 hours after release of unilateral ureteral obstruction of 24 hours duration, GFR values are one-sixth of those observed prior to ligation of the ureter. With time there is an increase in the GFR, such that by days 14 and 60 after the release of obstruction, values for GFR in the post-obstructed kidney are comparable to those in the contralateral untouched kidney [19]. However, when SNGFR and the number of filtering nephrons were determined, using a modification of Hansen's technique, a decrease in the total number of filtering nephrons was found in the post-obstructed kidney, such that only 85% of the nephrons in this kidney were filtering, compared to 100% in the contralateral kidney. The normalization of whole kidney GFR was therefore at the expense of hyperfiltration (increase in SNGFR) in the remaining functional nephrons, and there was a permanent decrement in the total number of functional nephrons. The mechanism responsible for this permanent loss of nephrons following ureteral obstruction remains to be defined, as does its long-term significance in terms of the development of chronic renal failure in patients with obstructive uropathy.

Alterations in Tubular Function

Abnormalities in renal tubule function are common in urinary tract obstruction [1,2]. The major alterations appear to be located in distal segments of the nephron. There is a concentrating defect, the reabsorption of sodium and other solutes such as phosphorus, magnesium and calcium is altered, and the secretion of hydrogen and potassium is impaired.

Sodium and Water Reabsorption

The absolute amount of sodium excreted by the post-obstructed kidney after release of unilateral ureteral obstruction differs little from that excreted by the contralateral untouched kidney [1,2]. However, fractional sodium excretion is greater in the post-obstructed kidney, due to the marked fall in GFR. In addition, fractional water excretion is increased and the ability to concentrate the urine is markedly impaired, with a maximal osmolality of 300–400 mOsm reported in the rat [1,2,20]. Micropuncture experiments after release of unilateral ureteral obstruction in rats have shown that fractional reabsorption of salt and water is increased in proximal segments of surface nephrons of the post-obstructed kidney [20]. This contrasts with the marked decrease in salt and water reabsorption in juxtamedullary nephrons [20]. Calculations, based on analysis of fluid collected from the bend of the loop of Henle in the post-obstructed kidney, suggest a marked decrease in salt and water reabsorption in proximal segments of juxtamedullary nephrons. In addition, due to a decrease in medullary tonicity, related at least in part to decreased reabsorption of sodium chloride in the thick ascending limb during obstruction, there is a marked fall in the abstraction of water from the descending limb which traverses the medulla [20]. As a consequence, water delivery to the bend of the loop of Henle of juxtamedullary nephrons is significantly increased in the post-obstructed kidney, when compared with the contralateral kidney of the same animals. Despite a decrease in the filtered load of sodium in the post-obstructed kidney, the absolute excretion of this cation is comparable to that in the contralateral control kidney. This is, presumably, due to decreased sodium reabsorption in the proximal tubule and thick ascending limb of juxtamedullary nephrons [21]. The increased excretion of water may be related not only to decreased reabsorption in juxtamedullary nephrons, but also to a marked decrease in the response to antidiuretic hormone at the level of the cortical collecting duct. Indeed, it has been demonstrated that water permeability, in response to an osmotic gradient and antidiuretic hormone, is markedly decreased in in vitro perfused cortical collecting tubules isolated from kidneys of rabbits obstructed for 4 or 24 hours [21,22].

Following relief of obstruction, the ability to concentrate the urine is impaired to a greater extent than the ability to dilute the urine. Dilution of the urine occurs mainly in the thick ascending limb of Henle's loop, due to greater reabsorption of solute than water in this nephron segment. The differential impairment of concentration and dilution suggests that factors other than decreased reabsorption of solute by the thick ascending limb of Henle have a role in the concentrating defect. One such factor may be the relative increase in papillary blood flow in obstruction, which, combined with an overall decrease in glomerular filtration rate in deep nephrons, would lead to solute depletion in the medullary interstitium.

In summary, decreases in medullary tonicity are, presumably, due to: 1) decreased removal of solute from the thick ascending limb of Henle's loop; 2) decrease in the total number of juxtamedullary nephrons; 3) washout of solutes from the medulla, due to increased medullary blood flow; and 4) decreased hydrosmotic response of the cortical collecting duct to antidiuretic hormone. All these factors contribute to the concentrating defect seen after release of obstruction.

The quantitative excretion of sodium and water is somewhat different after unilateral release of bilateral ureteral obstruction. In this setting, sodium and water reabsorption in proximal segments of surface nephrons is decreased, in contrast with the increased reabsorption observed after release of unilateral ureteral obstruction. Consequently, after unilateral release of bilateral ureteral obstruction, proximal delivery of salt and water to more distal segments is augmented. Part of this increased natriuresis and diuresis could be attributed to urea excretion [23]. Urea retained during the period of bilateral obstruction is excreted in the urine after release of obstruction and acts as an osmotic agent, promoting salt and water excretion. However, the osmotic diuresis due to urea does not account quantitatively for all the natriuresis and diuresis seen after relief of bilateral obstruction [23]. Therefore, other factors may be important. Recent observations indicate that the plasma levels of atrial peptide are elevated in animals with bilateral ureteral obstruction, but not in those with unilateral ureteral obstruction. Indirect evidence, using heparin, which has been shown to antagonize some of the biological effects of atrial peptide, indicates that atrial peptide may play a role in the increased natriuresis and diuresis observed after relief of bilateral ureteral obstruction [6]. Data in patients also indicate that the levels of atrial peptide are increased in obstruction and that these plasma levels decrease after relief of obstruction.

Defective Urinary Acidification

Acid excretion is impaired after release of bilateral or unilateral ureteral obstruction in both humans and experimental animals [1,2]. Falls and Stacy noted a urine pH of 7.2 and bicarbonate wasting in a patient with post-obstructive diuresis in a solitary kidney. This patient also did not acidify his urine adequately after ammonium chloride loading. Following recovery of renal function the acidification defect disappeared. This patient had decreased proximal reabsorption of bicarbonate during the post-obstructive diuresis. However, most studies suggest that a distal renal tubular acidosis with inability to lower the urine pH to normal minimum values in response to acidemia is much more common in patients with urinary tract obstruction [1,2]. This acidifying defect seems to be reversible in the majority of patients. However, in certain patients the acidifying defect may persist. Berlyne found that after a brief ammonium chloride load 6 of 7 patients with chronic hydronephrosis could not acidify their urine to pH values below 5.3. However, in two patients the acidification defect was corrected several weeks following relief of obstruction. Better et al. described urine pHs of 6.5–7.5 in the post-obstructed kidney of a patient with complete unilateral ureteral obstruction of three months' duration. After ammonium chloride loading, the urine pH from the post-obstructed kidney fell from 6.7 to 5.7, while the contralateral kidney had a normal response.

An acidifying defect similar to that seen in humans can be elicited after ureteral obstruction in both the rat and the dog [1,2]. In this setting, urine pH from the post-obstructed kidney of rats was greater than 7 and was not influenced by an acid load. Bicarbonate titration studies and micropuncture studies revealed no decrease in proximal reabsorption of bicarbonate after release of unilateral ureteral obstruction, when compared to sham-operated animals. In the post-obstructed kidney, urine pCO_2 values remained low after bicarbonate loading. These data suggest that the acidifying defect observed after release of unilateral ureteral obstruction is due either to decreased hydrogen secretion in the distal tubule of surface nephrons and the collecting duct, or to marked alterations in the reabsorption of bicarbonate in juxtamedullary nephrons. Laski and Kurtzman [24], using perfused nephron segments from rabbits with ureteral obstruction, found a decrease in JT_{CO_2} that was detected earlier in perfused medullary collecting duct segments. Only later was there a slight fall in JT_{CO_2} in cortical segments. These data suggest that the initial defect in acidification occurs in medullary segments. Sabbatini and Kurtzman [25], using an indirect method, have evaluated the activity of H-ATPase in microdissected segments of rat nephrons obtained 24 hours after the onset of urinary tract obstruction. In animals with acute ureteral obstruction, NEM-sensitive ATPase activity was markedly reduced. In the cortical collecting duct, NEM-sensitive ATPase activity fell significantly, but to a lesser degree than was observed in the medullary collecting duct. If, indeed, NEM-sensitive ATPase is an adequate measure of hydrogen ATPase, this finding suggests that in obstruction there is an abnormality in acidification in the cortical collecting duct, but that the major defect in acidification is located at the level of the medullary collecting duct.

Using monoclonal antibodies to the 31 kilodalton subunit of the hydrogen ATPase, Purcell and associates [26] have demonstrated a decrease in the apical staining for hydrogen ATPase in intercalated cells of rats with ureteral obstruction. This decrease in staining suggests a loss, or removal, of hydrogen ATPase from the apical border of intercalated cells during the period of obstruction. Three–five days after release of obstruction of 24 h duration, the staining for hydrogen ATPase in the apical border was normal; this was accompanied by values of urine pH in the post-obstructed kidney similar to those observed in the contralateral untouched kidney. These data, then, would suggest that a decreased number of hydrogen ATPase pumps in the apical surface of intercalated cells are responsible for the acidifying defect that occurs with ureteral obstruction. The mechanism underlying the removal of H^+ pumps from the apical membrane of acid-secreting cells remains to be determined.

Abnormal Potassium Excretion

Hyperkalemic distal renal tubular acidosis has also been found in patients with chronic obstructive uropathy [27]. At all levels of glomerular filtration rate, the fractional excretion of potassium was less in patients with obstructive uropathy than in patients with comparable degrees of renal insufficiency due to a garden variety of renal diseases. Hyperkalemic-hyperchloremic acidosis has been described in a series of patients with urinary tract obstruction [27]. Three major mechanisms were uncovered that may explain the development of hyperkalemic-hyperchloremic acidosis in individuals with obstructive uropathy: 1) a selective deficiency of aldosterone secretion, probably secondary to diminished production of renin by the kidney, hyporeninemic hypoaldosteronism; 2) a defect in renal hydrogen secretion, with inability to lower urine pH maximally in the presence of systemic acidosis and decreased urinary excretion of both ammonium and titratable acid (type IV distal renal tubular acidosis); and 3) a combination of these two defects. It is possible that part of the defect may relate to a decreased sensitivity of the distal tubule to the kaliuretic effect of aldosterone. Batlle and coworkers [27] have suggested that a defect in sodium reabsorption in the distal nephron results in a decrease in the intraluminal negative potential difference. This voltage-dependent defect could contribute to the diminished secretion of both hydrogen ion and potassium. This defect, of course, may be due, in part, to an altered response to the action of aldosterone of this nephron segment during obstruction.

Pathological Changes in the Obstructed Kidney and Mechanisms of Nephron Destruction

Complete ureteral occlusion produces progressive dilatation of the renal pelvis during the first few weeks. There is perirenal and periureteral edema. The kidney weight increases due to edema, although the renal tissue, per se, atrophies. After 4–8 weeks, parenchymal weight decreases, due to atrophy which is greater than the intrarenal edema. The obstructed kidney appears dark blue with scattered areas of ischemia, wedges of congestion, necrosis, and some frank infarcts [1].

The microscopic changes of hydronephrosis have been studied in experimental animals. During the first few days after the onset of obstruction, there is flattening of the papilla with pronounced dilatation of the distal nephron [1,28]. The proximal tubules initially undergo dilatation and then slowly atrophy [1,28]. After the first week of obstruction, the dilated collecting tubules also show atrophy and necrosis. By two weeks, there is progressive dilatation of the collecting and distal tubules and atrophy of the proximal tubule epithelial cells. After 4 weeks of obstruction, there is a 50% decrease in the medullary thickness, with continued atrophy and dilatation of distal and collecting tubules. The cortex is thinner with marked atrophy of the proximal tubules. After 8 weeks of obstruction, only a thin parenchymal strip remains, consisting primarily of connective tissue and small sclerotic glomeruli.

Proliferation of medullary interstitial cells has been noted by the fifth day of obstruction [10]. There are also chronic interstitial inflammatory changes, which are more severe than glomerular changes. Ultimately, however, glomeruli become hyalinized in a pattern not dissimilar from that seen in nephrosclerosis. It should be emphasized, however, that chronic obstruction results predominantly in an interstitial disease, with relative preservation of glomerular structures.

Recently, Tanner and Evan [29] have examined glomerular and proximal tubular morphology after single nephron obstruction, utilizing a wax block. The anatomical changes found after obstruction of single nephrons resembled those seen after ureteral obstruction. There was nephron atrophy and there were glomerular changes. The latter developed at a later time than the tubular changes. The major glomerular abnormalities, after one month of obstruction, were reduced diameter, decreased number and size of capillaries, fusion of epithelial cell foot processes, thickened basement membrane of Bowman's capsule, and periglomerular fibrosis. The changes seen in the proximal tubule with prolonged single nephron blockade or urinary tract obstruction include a loss of apical microvilli, decreased cell height, simplification of basolateral membranes, and a reduction in the number of mitochondria. There is widening of the interstitial space and thickening of the tubular basement membrane. When single nephrons were obstructed, the morphological changes were circumscribed to that nephron and no ultrastructural abnormalities were seen in adjacent nephrons. After one day of obstruction, the morphological changes seen in the tubule upstream or downstream to the block were quite different. Severe injury occurred in downstream segments, whereas changes in upstream segments were modest. These differences in morphology may be due to the interruption of tubule fluid flow to the downstream segments.

The mechanisms underlying the development of nephron atrophy and nephron destruction following urinary tract obstruction have not been established, but three interrelated changes may have a role: 1) decreased blood flow; 2) disuse atrophy; and 3) infiltration of the renal parenchyma by leukocytes.

When single nephrons are obstructed, glomerular blood flow to such nephrons decreases. Glomerular blood flow decreases by 35% after 24 h of obstruction and by 70% after one week of obstruction [29]. Similar changes in blood flow are observed in animals with ureteral obstruction. Blood flow to the kidney is markedly decreased after one month of obstruction. The markedly decreased size of the glomerulus at this time is consistent with a pronounced decrease in perfusion. Increased local production of angiotensin II and thromboxane A_2 may play a role in the decreased blood flow to the glomerulus [1,2,14]. Peritubular capillary flow may be reduced with prolonged tubule obstruction and may contribute to the morphological changes. However, Tanner and Evan [29] did not observe cell necrosis, which is commonly seen with severe ischemia. On the other hand, the metabolic demands of the obstructed tubule may be less, due to a decrease in the filtered load of sodium as GFR declines. Therefore, the oxygen supply to a blocked nephron might be adequate for its metabolic needs. A reduction in blood flow alone may not be sufficient to account for the development of nephron atrophy.

Disuse atrophy [28] may account, at least in part, for the involution of the glomerular and tubular units. If the filtered load decreases, the tubular transport of solutes and water falls. The decreases in cell size and number of mitochondria are consistent with a decrease in tubular transport of solutes. The potential mechanisms linking changes in renal tubular transport to changes in cell structure are unknown.

Invading leukocytes may also play a role in the morphological changes observed. As early as a few hours after obstruction, T lymphocytes and macrophages are present in the kidney [12]. Tanner and Evan [29] also observed neutrophils and lymphocytes in the glomerulus and near the tubules during single nephron obstruction. Cells were associated only with blocked nephrons. The stimulus causing accumulation of inflammatory cells is not known. It may be related to the release of a chemoattractant by the kidney. The presence of inflammatory cells with urinary tract obstruction is characteristic of this disorder. Such cells, particularly macrophages, are known to release proteases, other enzymes, and cytokines, and to produce oxygen derived free radicals [30]. These and other chemical agents may damage the nephron. Stimulated macrophages produce increased amounts of thromboxane A_2 and other prostanoids, which can also affect blood flow [30]. Infiltrating leukocytes may stimulate the proliferation of fibroblasts and cause increased deposition of collagen and mucopolysaccharides in the interstitium. This may increase the diffusion distances between tubular cells and capillaries, causing impaired oxygen delivery to the tubular cells and subsequent tubule atrophy [28]. Therefore, infiltrating leukocytes may have an important role in the nephron atrophy that occurs with prolonged urinary tract obstruction.

Acknowledgments. The original work cited in this manuscript was supported by U.S.P.H.S. NIDDK Grants DK-09976, DK-07126, and DK-40321.

The author thanks Ms. Pat Verplancke for her assistance in the preparation of this manuscript.

References

1. Klahr S, Harris KPG (to be published) Obstructive nephropathy. In: Seldin DW, Giebisch G (eds) The kidney, 2nd Edn. Raven, New York
2. Klahr S, Harris KPG, Purkerson ML (1988) Effects of obstruction on renal function. Pediatr Nephrol 2:34–42
3. Wright FS (1982) Effects of urinary tract obstruction on glomerular filtration rate and renal blood flow. Semin Nephrol 2:5–16
4. Dal Canton A, Corradi A, Stanziale R, Maruccio G, Migone L (1979) Effects of 24-hour ureteral obstruction on glomerular hemodynamics in rat kidney. Kidney Int 15:457–462
5. Buerkert J, Martin D (1983) Relation of nephron recruitment to detectable filtration and recovery of function after release of ureteral obstruction. Proc Soc Exp Biol Med 173: 533–540
6. Purkerson ML, Blaine EH, Stokes TJ, Klahr S (1989) Role of atrial peptide in the natriuresis and diuresis that follows relief of obstruction in the rat. Am J Physiol 256:F583–F589
7. Purkerson ML, Klahr S (1989) Prior inhibition of vasoconstrictors normalizes GFR in postobstructed kidneys. Kidney Int 35:1305–1314
8. Yarger WE, Shocken DD, Harris RH (1980) Obstructive nephropathy in the rat: possible roles for the renin-angiotensin system, prostaglandins, and thromboxanes in postobstructive renal function. J Clin Invest 65:400–412
9. Mene P, Dunn MJ (1986) Contractile effects of TxA_2 and endoperoxide analogues on cultured rat glomerular mesangial cells. Am J Physiol 251:F1029–F1035

10. Nagle RB, Johnson ME, Jervis HR (1976) Proliferation of renal interstitial cells following injury induced by ureteral obstruction. Lab Invest 35:18–22
11. Okegawa T, Jonas PE, DeSchryver K, Kawasaki A, Needleman P (1983) Metabolic and cellular alterations underlying the exaggerated renal prostaglandin and thromboxane synthesis in ureter obstruction in rabbits. Inflammatory response involving fibroblasts and mononuclear cells. J Clin Invest 71:81–90
12. Schreiner G, Harris KPG, Purkerson ML, Klahr S (1988) The immunological aspects of acute ureteral obstruction: Immune cell infiltrate in the kidney. Kidney Int 34:487–493
13. Harris KPG, Schreiner GF, Klahr S (1989) Effect of leukocyte depletion on the function of the postobstructed kidney in the rat. Kidney Int 36:210–215
14. Yanagisawa H, Morrissey J, Morrison AR, Klahr S (1990) Role of angiotensin II in eicosanoid production by isolated glomeruli from rats with bilateral ureteral obstruction. Am J Physiol 258:F85–F93
15. Rovin BH, Harris KPG, Morrison A, Klahr S, Schreiner GF (1990) Renal cortical release of a specific macrophage chemoattractant in response to ureteral obstruction. Lab Invest 63:213–220
16. Spaethe SM, Freed MS, De Schryver-Kecskemeti K, Lefkowith JB, Needleman P (1988) Essential fatty acid deficiency reduces the inflammatory cell invasion in rabbit hydronephrosis resulting in suppression of the exaggerated eicosanoid production. J Pharmacol Exp Ther 245:1088–1094
17. Steinhardt GF, Ramon G, Salinas-Madrigal L (1988) Glomerulosclerosis in obstructive uropathy. J Urol 140:1316–1318
18. Davis BB, Thomason D, Zenser TV (1983) Renal disease profoundly alters cortical interstitial cell function. Kidney Int 23:458–464
19. Bander SJ, Buerkert JE, Martin D, Klahr S (1985) Long-term effects of 24-hour unilateral ureteral obstruction on renal function in the rat. Kidney Int 28:614–620
20. Yarger WE, Buerkert J (1982) Effect of urinary tract obstruction on renal tubular function. Semin Nephrol 2:17–30
21. Hanley MJ, Davidson K (1982) Isolated nephron segments from rabbit models of obstructive nephropathy. J Clin Invest 69:165–174
22. Campbell HT, Bello-Reuss E, Klahr S (1985) Hydraulic water permeability and transepithelial voltage in the isolated perfused rabbit cortical collecting tubule following acute unilateral ureteral obstruction. J Clin Invest 75:219–225
23. Purkerson ML, Klahr S (1984) Protein intake conditions the diuresis seen after relief of bilateral ureteral obstruction in the rat. Proc Soc Exp Biol Med 177:62–68
24. Laski ME, Kurtzman NA (1989) Site of the acidification defect in the post-obstructed collecting tubule. Miner Electrolyte Metab 15:195–200
25. Sabatini S, Kurtzman NA (1990) Enzyme activity in obstructive uropathy: basis for salt wastage and the acidification defect. Kidney Int 37:79–84
26. Purcell H, Harris KPG, Lim I, Klahr S, Gluck S (1989) Mechanisms of the acidifying defect after release of unilateral ureteral obstruction (abstract) Kidney Int 35:461
27. Batlle DC, Arruda JAL, Kurtzman NA (1981) Hyperkalemic distal tubular renal acidosis associated with obstructive uropathy. N Engl J Med 304:373–380
28. Møller JC, Jorgensen TM, Mortensen J (1986) Proximal tubular atrophy: qualitative and quantitative structural changes in chronic obstructive nephropathy in the pig. Cell Tiss Res 244:479–491
29. Tanner GA, Evan AP (1989) Glomerular and proximal tubular morphology after single nephron obstruction. Kidney Int 36:1050–1060
30. Nathan CR (1987) Secretory products of macrophages. J Clin Invest 79:319–326

Very Long-Term Dialysis

YOSHIHEI HIRASAWA

Chair: Belding H. Scribner

Very Long-Term Dialysis

YOSHIHEI HIRASAWA[1]

In this presentation, I would like to report our clinical results of long-term dialysis and discuss present problems. In the past 24 years, 1650 patients have been treated chronically by dialysis in our hospitals and satellite hospitals; 480 patients have died. The cumulative survival rate was 62% in the 10th year after starting dialysis therapy and 50% in the 20th year after starting dialysis therapy.

The main causes of death were cardiac (33%), infectious (21%), cerebro-vascular (18%), gastrointestinal (8%), and malignant (7%) diseases. The death rate due to cerebro-vascular disease and cancer increased in patients who had been on dialysis for longer than 10 years. Reflecting the progress of therapy, the survival rate in young patients has risen remarkably in the past 10 years.

Therapeutic progress has overcome many complications that occur frequently in patients receiving long-term dialysis treatment. These complications are hepatitis, pericarditis, peripheral neuropathy, dialysis hypersensitivity (ethylene oxide allergy), aluminum intoxication, and others. Recently, rHuEOP treatment of anemia has also been achieved.

However, it became clear that dialysis amyloidosis, a new complication, was occurring frequently in long-term dialysis patients. Among our patients, carpal tunnel syndrome and arthropathy, deriving from dialysis amyloidosis, began to appear from about the 8th year of dialysis therapy, and the complication rate rose with prolongation of dialysis, reaching about 50% in the 20th year of therapy.

In order to prevent dialysis amyloidosis, in the past 5 years we have performed hemodialysis with endotoxin-free bicarbonate-dialysate and with dialyzers which we have found to be extremely effective in the elimination of B_2 microglobulin (B_2M). Endotoxin concentration in dialysate was always below 20pg/ml, and the highest levels of serum β_2M of the patients were maintained within 20–40mg/l. It is interesting to note that in the last two years a decrease has been observed in the incidence of carpal tunnel syndrome, bone cyst formation, and arthropathy.

[1]Shinrakuen Hospital, 1-27 Nishi Ariake-machi, Niigata, 950-21 Japan

The pathogenesis of dialysis amyloidosis is unknown, therefore long-term observation is necessary to judge whether or not these measures are useful. If the correction of hyper β_2 microglobulinemia is effective in the prevention of dialysis amyloidosis, the administration of hemofiltration (HF) or hemodiafiltration (HDF) would be significant, and the development of on line HF or HDF would be an important factor.

In spite of the administration of active vitamin D, an increase in the incidence rate of secondary hyperparathyroidism has been observed in long-term dialysis patients. About 60% of our patients who had been on dialysis treatment for over 10 years had an abnormal rise of serum parathyroid hormone, and about 10% of those patients underwent parathyroidectomy. Pulse therapy with $1,25(OH)_2D_3$ was effective against hyperparathyroidism in many patients. However, it was often difficult to proceed with this therapy because of the development of hypercalcemia.

A better method for prevention of hyperparathyroidism would be the clinical administration of a drug that has a suppressive action on the parathyroid without enhancing hypercalcemia. Further, the development of a phosphate-binder that does not cause hypercalcemia is important.

Acceleration of vascular caldification is a conspicuous phenomenon in long-term dialysis patients. Since the cause of vascular calcification is assumed to be partly related to a disorder of Ca and P metabolism, the progress of therapy against secondary hyperparathyroidism may decrease the incidence of vascular calcification.

At present, 328 patients (127 in our hospital and 201 in our satellite hospitals) are being treated by dialysis which has lasted over 10 years. Twenty-six of them have a dialysis history of over 20 years, and 138 of them have been on dialysis for 15–20 years. Of these 328 patients, 40.5% are receiving night-time dialysis, 50.5% are on day-time dialysis, and 9.0% are on dialysis during hospitalization, due to complications. Almost all patients on night-time dialysis are engaged in full-time occupations. About half of the patients on day-time dialysis work as housewives or have part-time jobs.

Although some problems remain to be solved, I believe that we have been able to achieve excellent results through dialysis treatment, in terms both of prolongation of life and of rehabilitation.

Mechanisms of Na⁺, Cl⁻, and HCO₃⁻ Transport in the Proximal Tubule

Mechanisms of Na^+, Cl^-, and HCO_3^- Transport in the Proximal Tubule

PETER S. ARONSON

Chair: Gerhard Giebisch

Mechanisms of Na+, Cl-, and HCO3- Transport in the Proximal Tubule

PETER S. ARONSON[1]

Introduction

The general purpose of this lecture/chapter is to provide an overview of the mechanisms mediating Na+, Cl-, and HCO3- transport in the proximal tubule of the mammalian kidney. Because this topic is so broad, attention will be focussed on four main issues concerning transport across the membranes of the proximal tubule cell: 1) mechanisms of acid secretion across the luminal membrane; 2) mechanisms of base exit across the basolateral membrane; 3) mechanisms of Cl- entry across the luminal membrane; and 4) mechanisms for Cl- exit across the basolateral membrane. For each of these topics, the properties of the major transport pathways determined largely (but not exclusively) on the basis of studies on isolated membrane vesicles will be correlated with the physiological roles of these same pathways as determined on the basis of studies on the intact tubule. Finally, a summary attempting to integrate these subcellular mechanisms into the overall functioning of the intact proximal tubule will be presented. Literature citations will be representative, rather than comprehensive, due to the time/space limitations imposed on this lecture/chapter.

Mechanisms of Acid Secretion Across the Luminal Membrane

The first mechanism to be described that was capable of mediating the uphill secretion of H+ across the luminal membrane of the proximal tubule cell was Na+-H+ exchange, which was demonstrated by Murer et al. in brush border membrane vesicles isolated from rat renal cortex [1]. We confirmed the presence of a Na+-H+ exchanger in rabbit renal brush border membrane vesicles [2], and then used this experimental preparation to define several properties of this transport system [2-8].

[1]Section of Nephrology, Department of Medicine, Yale School of Medicine, New Haven, CT 06510, USA

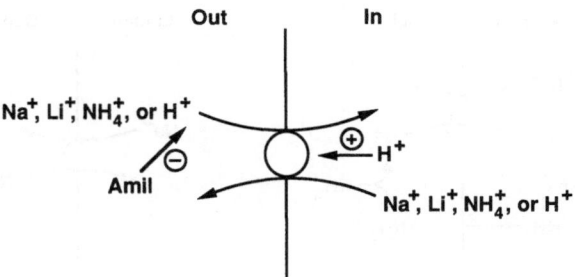

Fig. 1. Schematic model of the Na⁺-H⁺ exchanger. Amil, amiloride

We found that Li^+ and NH_4^+ competitively inhibited Na^+ uptake, suggesting that these cations might also be substrates for transport by this pathway [3,8]. Indeed, we demonstrated that in addition to Na^+-H^+ exchange, the system could also mediate Li^+-H^+ exchange, Na^+-Na^+ exchange and Na^+-NH_4^+ exchange [2,3,7]. External H^+ could compete for binding with external Na^+, Li^+, and NH_4^+ [7]. Amiloride was identified as an inhibitor of this pathway [2,4,8] that competed at the external site shared by Na^+, Li^+, and H^+ [4,7,8]. Internal H^+, in addition to serving as a substrate for transport, was found to be a potent allosteric activator of the Na^+-H^+ exchanger [6].

Taken together, our studies supported the model illustrated in Fig. 1, indicating that the Na^+-H^+ exchanger behaves as if it could bind any one of four cations – Na^+, H^+, Li^+, or NH_4^+ – on one side of the membrane and exchange the cation for any one of the same four cations on the opposite side of the membrane. The model also indicates that external amiloride acts as a competitive inhibitor and that internal H^+ acts as an allosteric activator. This model predicts at least two transport modes – namely, external Na^+ for internal H^+ exchange, and external Na^+ for internal NH_4^+ exchange – whereby the Na^+-H^+ exchanger could mediate secondary active acid secretion across the luminal membrane driven by the inward Na^+ gradient that is normally present due to the active extrusion of Na^+ across the basolateral membrane via the Na^+, K^+-ATPase.

Since the initial description of the Na^+-H^+ exchanger, additional mechanisms for acid secretion across the luminal membrane of the proximal tubule cell have been

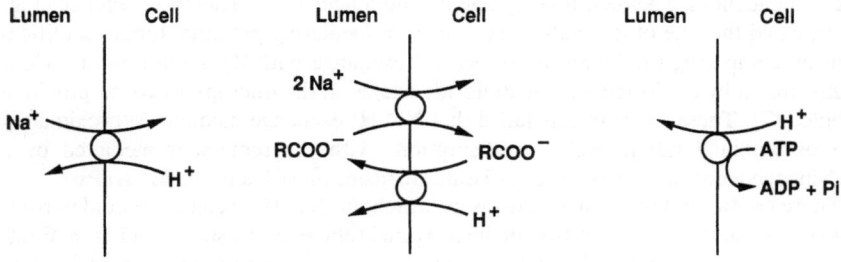

Fig. 2. Mechanisms of acid secretion across the luminal membrane of the proximal tubule cell

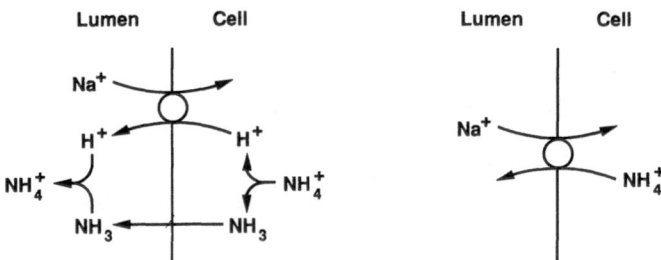

Fig. 3. Possible mechanisms of NH_4^+ secretion across the luminal membrane of the proximal tubule cell

described, as illustrated in Fig. 2. A Na^+-cotransport system for the secondary active reabsorption of monocarboxylates like lactate was first described by Barac-Nieto and Kinne in renal brush border membrane vesicles [9]. When we found that the brush border membrane also contained a separate pathway mediating H^+-organic anion cotransport (indistinguishable from organic anion-OH^- exchange) [10,11], we postulated that Na^+-coupled monocarboxylate uptake followed by H^+-coupled monocarboxylate backflux might be a mechanism for uphill H^+ secretion [12]. That such a mechanism could actually mediate acid extrusion from the proximal tubule cell was demonstrated by Nakhoul and Boron [13]. However, the contribution of this mechanism to transtubular acid secretion under physiologic conditions could not be detected by Geibel and coworkers [14].

The existence in brush border membrane vesicles of an ATPase activity that might be involved in acid-base transport was first reported by Kinne-Saffran and Kinne [15]. Controversy persisted as to whether this activity was mitochondrial or endosomal, rather than brush border, in origin. However, Burkhardt and colleagues have recently provided strong evidence that a H^+-ATPase coexists on the brush border membrane with the Na^+-H^+ exchanger [16].

What is the relative proportion of acid secretion that is mediated by Na^+-H^+ exchange versus the H^+-ATPase in the intact proximal tubule under physiologic conditions? Multiple studies have shown that $\geq 80\%$ of acid secretion in the proximal tubule is Na^+-dependent and/or dependent on operation of the Na^+, K^+-ATPase [12], seeming to argue that the Na^+-H^+ exchanger mediates almost all of proximal tubule acid secretion. But, given the recent evidence that base exit from the proximal tubule cell is Na^+-dependent (see below), this argument is no longer valid. Therefore, Preisig et al. reevaluated the role of the Na^+-H^+ exchanger in mediating proximal tubule acidification by comparing the inhibition of Na^+-H^+ exchange with the inhibition of HCO_3^- reabsorption by amiloride and an amiloride analog in the microperfused rat proximal tubule [17]. These workers concluded that Na^+-H^+ exchange mediates approximately 2/3 of proximal tubule HCO_3^- reabsorption, with the remainder mediated by a Na^+-independent, amiloride-insensitive mechanism, most likely the H^+-ATPase.

There are two potential mechanisms by which the Na^+-H^+ exchanger could participate in mediating NH_4^+ secretion in the proximal tubule, as illustrated in Fig. 3. First, by virtue of its being the principal pathway for active H^+ secretion across the luminal membrane, the Na^+-H^+ exchanger would acidify the lumen, thereby providing a favorable gradient for secretion of NH$_4^+$ by nonionic diffusion of NH$_3$. Second, as predicted by the membrane vesicle studies described above [3], the Na$^+$-H$^+$ exchanger might be capable of mediating direct Na$^+$-NH$_4^+$ exchange. Nagami has recently provided important evidence supporting the concept that direct Na$^+$-NH$_4^+$ exchange via the Na$^+$-H$^+$ exchanger contributes importantly to net secretion of NH$_4^+$ produced in proximal tubule cells [18]. He measured total NH$_4^+$ production and the portion of the produced NH$_4^+$ that was actually secreted into the lumen of isolated and perfused proximal tubules of the mouse. When operation of the Na$^+$-H$^+$ exchanger was inhibited by changing the luminal perfusate to one containing a reduced Na$^+$ concentration and amiloride, total NH$_4^+$ production was unchanged, but luminal NH$_4^+$ secretion was virtually abolished. Additional experiments demonstrated that this inhibition of luminal NH$_4^+$ secretion by inhibiting the function of the Na$^+$-H$^+$ exchanger could not be attributed to a change in luminal pH secondarily affecting nonionic diffusion of NH$_3$. Thus, these data strongly supported the notion that direct Na$^+$-NH$_4^+$ exchange can occur on the Na$^+$-H$^+$ exchanger, as predicted by the vesicle studies.

Mechanisms of Base Exit Across the Basolateral Membrane

Boron and Boulpaep identified a stilbene-sensitive, electrogenic Na$^+$-HCO$_3^-$ cotransport system that mediates the coupled transfer of Na$^+$, HCO$_3^-$ and net negative charge across the basolateral membrane of the isolated, perfused proximal tubule of the salamander [19]. We confirmed the presence of this transporter in basolateral membrane vesicles isolated from the rabbit renal cortex [20], and then used this experimental preparation to define several properties of this transport system [20–23].

One issue we examined was the stoichiometry of the Na$^+$-HCO$_3^-$ cotransporter [21]. When the membrane potential is approximated by the Nernst potential for K$^+$, as in the presence of the K$^+$ ionophore valinomycin, equilibrium thermodynamics predicts that the Na$^+$-HCO$_3^-$ cotransport system should come to equilibrium and mediate no net flux when:

$$\frac{[Na^+]_i}{[Na^+]_o} = \left(\frac{[HCO_3^-]_o}{[HCO_3^-]_i}\right)^n \left(\frac{[K^+]_o}{[K^+]_i}\right)^{n-1}$$

where n is the HCO$_3^-$:Na$^+$ stoichiometry [21]. Our experimental approach was to impose transmembrane Na$^+$, HCO$_3^-$, and K$^+$ gradients of varying magnitude and direction, and then to measure the net flux of Na$^+$ over the subsequent short interval. In this way, we could determine the conditions for equilibrium of the transport system and thereby calculate n. The data indicated that the stoichiometry of the Na$^+$-HCO$_3^-$ cotransporter is 3 HCO$_3^-$:Na$^+$, or a thermodynamically equivalent process. Studying rat proximal tubules by in situ microperfusion, Yoshitomi et al. also estimated that the HCO$_3^-$:Na$^+$ stoichiometery is 3:1, based on comparison of the fall in both intracellular Na$^+$ activity and intracellular pH that occurred in response to a sudden reduction of peritubular HCO$_3^-$ concentration [24].

It should be emphasized that although the preceding results were consistent with a cotransport stoichiometry of 3 HCO$_3^-$ per Na$^+$, they were equally consistent with

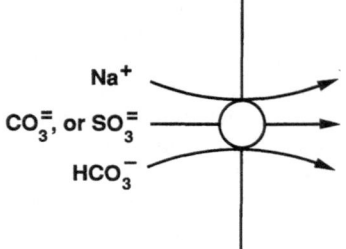

Fig. 4. Schematic model of the Na^+-HCO_3^- cotransporter

any transport process in which there is the net transfer of 3 equivalents of base, 1 Na^+, and 2 negative charges per transport event. Therefore, the purpose of the next series of experiments was to define the actual ionic mechanism of the Na^+-HCO_3^- cotransport system [22]. We found that the rate of Na^+ influx into basolateral membrane vesicles was stimulated as a function of $[CO_3^{2-}]$ at constant $[HCO_3^-]$, suggesting that CO_3^{2-} is a substrate for the Na^+-HCO_3^- cotransporter. The presence of a divalent anion site was confirmed by the finding that SO_3^{2-} but not SO_4^{2-} could compete with CO_3^{2-} and could itself be cotransported with Na^+. Importantly, Na^+-SO_3^{2-} cotransport was demonstrable only in the presence of HCO_3^-, indicating that in addition to the divalent anion site there must be a HCO_3^- site whose occupancy is mandatory for operation of the transport system. As illustrated in Fig. 4, the results of these experiments suggested that CO_3^{2-} can interact with the Na^+-HCO_3^- cotransporter at a site shared by SO_3^{2-}, and that HCO_3^- interacts at a separate site. Electrogenic cotransport of 3 equivalents of base per Na^+ would then occur by 1:1:1 coupled fluxes of Na^+, CO_3^{2-}, and HCO_3^-.

The exquisite HCO_3^- dependence of this transporter suggested to us that there might be an important interaction between carbonic anhydrase and the Na^+-HCO_3^- cotransporter. We therefore examined whether inhibition of carbonic anhydrase with acetazolamide would affect operation of the Na^+-HCO_3^- cotransporter in basolateral membrane vesicles [23]. We found that concentrations of acetazolamide up to 0.6 mM added to the external solution and preloaded into the vesicles had virtually no effect when Na^+ influx was measured in the presence of a directly imposed inward HCO_3^- gradient. This result indicated that carbonic anhydrase is not directly involved in mediating transport through the Na^+-HCO_3^- cotransporter. We then tested whether carbonic anhydrase in the basolateral membrane vesicles could be rate limiting for Na^+-HCO_3^- cotransport under conditions where HCO_3^- was being generated or consumed.

In the presence of a CO_2/HCO_3^- buffer system, but in the absence of an initial HCO_3^- gradient, Na^+ influx was stimulated by an outward NH_4^+ gradient. This stimulation of Na^+ influx by an outward NH_4^+ gradient was significantly inhibited by 0.6 mM acetazolamide, suggesting that acetazolamide blocked the ability of the NH_4^+ gradient to generate an inward HCO_3^- gradient. In the presence of an inward HCO_3^- gradient, Na^+ influx was inhibited by an inward NH_4^+ gradient. The magnitude of this inhibition of Na^+ influx was reduced by 0.6 mM acetazolamide, suggesting that acetazolamide blocked the ability of NH_4^+ to collapse the inward HCO_3^- gradient. Similarly, Na^+ influx in the presence of an inward HCO_3^- gradient was

Lumen   **Cell**   **Interstitium**

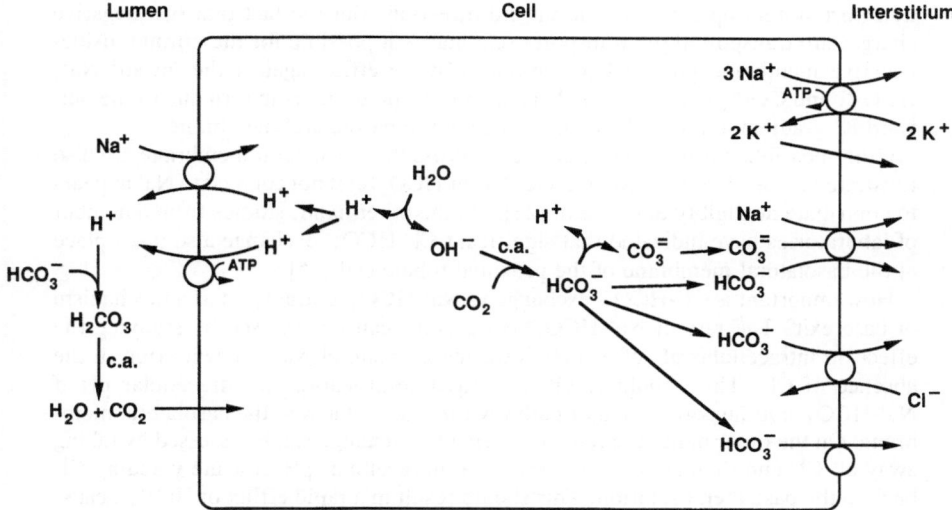

Fig. 5. Model of the proximal tubule cell emphasizing possible mechanisms of base exit across the basolateral membrane. c.a., carbonic anhydrase

inhibited by an outward acetate gradient, and this inhibition was reduced by acetazolamide. Thus, acetazolamide caused either inhibition or stimulation of Na⁺ uptake depending on the conditions with respect to pH and HCO₃⁻ gradients. These results indicated that the operation of the Na⁺-HCO₃⁻ cotransporter is markedly, although indirectly, dependent on the activity of carbonic anhydrase.

The physiological role of the Na⁺-HCO₃⁻ cotransporter in the process of proximal tubule acidification is illustrated in Fig. 5. Secretion of H⁺ across the luminal membrane occurs principally by Na⁺-H⁺ exchange with an additional contribution from a H⁺-ATPase. Secretion of H⁺ via recycling of monocarboxylates is not shown. It should be emphasized that membrane vesicle studies have clearly shown that both the Na⁺-H⁺ exchanger and the H⁺-ATPase can operate in the absence of CO₂/HCO₃⁻. Thus, the effect of luminal membrane H⁺ secretion is to split water and liberate OH⁻ in the cell. As just discussed, the Na⁺-HCO₃⁻ cotransporter can transport base only in the form of HCO₃⁻ and CO₃²⁻, which are generated within the cell or at the basolateral membrane by the action of carbonic anhydrase. Thus, the essential role of intracellular and/or basolateral membrane carbonic anhydrase is to convert OH⁻ to the forms of base that can exit the cell via the Na⁺-HCO₃⁻ cotransporter. This leads to the prediction that inhibition of carbonic anhydrase should prevent base exit.

The stoichiometry of the Na⁺-HCO₃⁻ cotransporter is important for understanding why this system normally functions in the direction of mediating base exit from the cell. Under physiologic conditions, a large Na⁺ gradient is directed inward across the basolateral membrane; the pH and HCO₃⁻ concentration in the cell are slightly lower than in the interstitial fluid. Thus, inward Na⁺, HCO₃⁻, and CO₃²⁻ gradients favor this transport system operating in the inward direction. But the fact that two negative charges are transported per transport cycle makes it possible for the normal inside-negative membrane potential membrane to drive efflux against the inward Na^+, HCO_3^-, and CO_3^{2-} gradients [24]. This membrane potential is in turn due to the outward K^+ gradient and high K^+ conductance of the basolateral membrane.

Other possible mechanisms of base exit across the basolateral membrane are also illustrated in Fig. 5. Simple conductive OH^- or HCO_3^- exit not coupled to Na^+ appears to contribute negligibly to base exit [25]. On the other hand, studies from a number of laboratories have indicated that significant Cl^--HCO_3^- exchange also takes place at the basolateral membrane of the proximal tubule cell [25].

How important is Cl^--HCO_3^- exchange vs Na^+-HCO_3^- cotransport as a mechanism of base exit? The rate of Na^+-HCO_3^- cotransport can be assessed by studying the effect on intracellular pH of acutely lowering basolateral Na^+ concentration in the absence of Cl^-. This should result in a rapid acidification of intracellular pH if Na^+-HCO_3^- cotransport is a major pathway for base exit across the basolateral membrane. On the other hand, the rate of Cl^--HCO_3^- exchange can be assessed by taking away all Cl^- and then studying the effect on intracellular pH of acutely adding Cl^- back to the basolateral solution. This should result in a rapid efflux of HCO_3^-, causing acidification of intracellular pH if Cl^--HCO_3^- exchange is a major pathway for base efflux across the basolateral membrane. Experiments of this type were carried out by Alpern and Chambers in the rat proximal tubule [26]. Lowering basolateral Na^+ caused a much greater drop in intracellular pH by operation of the Na^+-HCO_3^- cotransporter, compared to the very small effect of peritubular Cl^- in causing intracellular acidification by operation of the Cl^--HCO_3^- exchanger. Thus, these studies indicated that Na^+-HCO_3^- cotransport is far and away the predominant mechanism for base exit across the basolateral membrane of the proximal tubule cell. Recent evidence suggests that Cl^--HCO_3^- exchange may play a more important role in mediating base exit across the basolateral membrane in the S_3 segment of the proximal tubule [27].

Given that Na^+-HCO_3^- cotransport is the predominant mechanism of base exit through most of the proximal tubule, is its operation dependent on a functional interaction with carbonic anhydrase as predicted by the membrane vesicle studies? This issue was studied by Sasaki and Marumo [28]. These workers measured intracellular pH and stimulated efflux of HCO_3^- through the Na^+-HCO_3^- cotransporter by either lowering peritubular HCO_3^- or by lowering peritubular Na^+. In both cases, the operation of the Na^+-HCO_3^- cotransporter, as reflected by its causing intracellular acidification, was markedly inhibited by acetazolamide. These findings confirm the vesicle studies, indicating an important role for cytoplasmic and/or basolateral membrane carbonic anhydrase in providing transportable substrate, namely HCO_3^- and CO_3^{2-}, for the Na^+-HCO_3^- cotransport system.

Mechanisms of Cl^- Entry Across the Luminal Membrane

As will be discussed in more detail later, there is a passive driving force for Cl^- reabsorption via the paracellular pathway all along the proximal tubule. However, studies from a number of laboratories have indicated that there must also be a component of

Fig. 6. Model of NaCl entry across the luminal membrane by Cl$^-$-formate exchange in parallel with Na$^+$-H$^+$ exchange and nonionic diffusion of formic acid

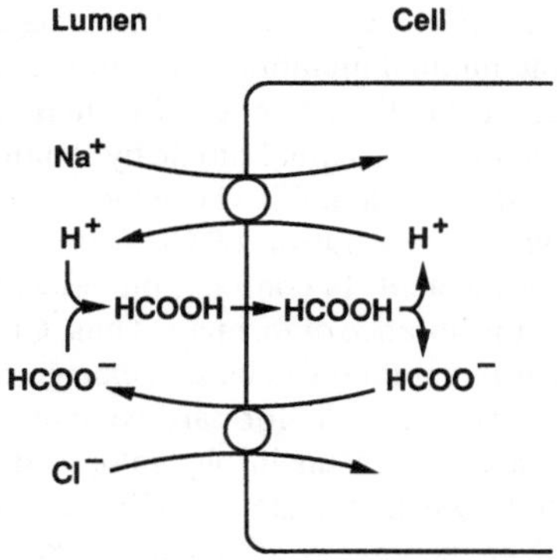

transcellular Cl$^-$ reabsorption as well [29]. Because intracellular Cl$^-$ in the proximal tubule cell is above electrochemical equilibrium, Cl$^-$ entry must occur by an uphill mechanism.

Using rabbit brush border membrane vesicles we could find no evidence for Na$^+$-Cl$^-$ or Na$^+$-K$^+$-2Cl$^-$ cotransport [30] as found in other nephron segments. We therefore tested for the presence of anion exchange processes that might account for uphill Cl$^-$ transport across the luminal membrane [31]. We initially tested whether outward gradients of HCO$_3^-$, or well-known organic anions like acetate, would stimulate Cl$^-$ uptake, compared to the inert anion gluconate. Disappointingly, we found that outward gradients of neither HCO$_3^-$ nor acetate were particularly effective in stimulating Cl$^-$ uptake. Surprisingly, an outward gradient of formate caused a much more appreciable stimulation of Cl$^-$ uptake, suggesting the presence of a Cl$^-$-formate exchange process. Confirming the presence of a Cl$^-$-formate anion exchanger, we found that imposing an outward Cl$^-$ gradient stimulated the uphill transport of formate. An outward Cl$^-$ gradient did not stimulate the uptake of acetate, confirming the selectivity of this transport process for formate.

Clearly, given the low concentrations (0.2–0.5 mM) of formate found in biological fluids, not much Cl$^-$ could be reabsorbed in exchange for formate unless there was a mechanism to recycle formate across the luminal membrane. Since formate was known to cross lipid bilayers fairly well by nonionic diffusion, we proposed the model illustrated in Fig. 6 for the role of Cl$^-$-formate exchange in mediating Cl$^-$ entry across the luminal membrane. According to this model, H$^+$ secretion, which largely occurs by Na$^+$-H$^+$ exchange, would generate an inward H$^+$ gradient across the luminal membrane. This would then drive filtered formate into the cell by nonionic diffusion of formic acid. In the more alkaline environment of the cell, the formic acid would dissociate to form H$^+$ and formate. The resulting outward formate gradient could then drive uphill Cl$^-$ uptake by Cl$^-$-formate exchange. Formate would continually recycle by nonionic diffusion; the net process is formate-catalyzed NaCl entry.

This model makes several testable predictions. First, if the Na$^+$-H$^+$ exchanger is blocked with amiloride, adding back luminal Cl$^-$ to a Cl$^-$-free luminal solution should cause cell acidification by the parallel operation of Cl$^-$-formate exchange and nonionic diffusion of formic acid. Indeed, if Cl$^-$-formate exchange, rather than

$Cl^--HCO_3^-$ exchange, is the predominant mechanism for Cl^--base exchange across the luminal membrane, the effect of luminal Cl^- on intracellular pH should be much greater in the presence of formate than in its absence. This prediction was tested in the rabbit proximal tubule by Baum [32]. He found that intracellular pH significantly acidified when Cl^- was added to the lumen in the presence of formate, consistent with the operation of Cl^--formate exchange in parallel with nonionic diffusion of formic acid. In contrast, the effect of Cl^- on intracellular pH was very much smaller in the absence of formate. Thus, Cl^--formate exchange is the major pathway for luminal membrane Cl^--base exchange, as predicted by the vesicle studies.

Given that Cl^--formate exchange is the major pathway for Cl^--base exchange, does it actually result in physiologically significant NaCl transport into and across the cell? One manifestation of increased NaCl entry across the luminal membrane would be an increase in cell volume. We tested this prediction in isolated and perfused proximal tubules of the rabbit [33]. In the absence of Cl^-, adding a phyisological concentration of formate to the luminal perfusate (0.5 mM) induced a small increase in cell volume, presumably due to uptake of Na^+-formate by nonionic diffusion of formic acid in parallel with Na^+-H^+ exchange. In the presence of Cl^-, formate induced a much larger increase in cell volume, as predicted if formate catalyzes NaCl entry across the brush border membrane. Accordingly, this experiment suggested that a physiological formate concentration actually can induce significant net NaCl entry across the luminal membrane of the proximal tubule cell.

But does this NaCl entry across the luminal membrane, induced by formate, actually stimulate transtubular NaCl transport? To answer this question, we measured Jv, the rate of volume reabsorption, under conditions of low HCO_3^-, where Jv would reflect the rate of isotonic NaCl reabsorption in isolated perfused proximal tubules of rabbit [34]. We found that adding physiological formate concentrations to the lumen and bath caused a significant and reversible stimulation of Jv, indicating that Cl^--formate exchange actually does contribute importantly to transtubular Cl^- reabsorption. Acetate could not mimic the effect of formate, confirming the selectivity for formate determined in the vesicle studies. However, a significant Jv was observed even in the absence of added formate, despite the symmetrical conditions with no measurable transtubular potential difference, and thus no passive driving force for Cl^- reabsorption. This suggested either that the tubule may produce formate endogenously, or that additional pathways for Cl^- entry across the luminal membrane must exist.

We therefore screened for additional anion exchange modes of Cl^- transport [35]. When outward gradients of various organic anions were tested for their ability to stimulate ^{36}Cl uptake, we found that only oxalate significantly stimulated Cl^- uptake. Imposing a large outward Cl^- gradient stimulated the uphill accumulation of oxalate, confirming the presence of a Cl^--oxalate exchange process. In contrast, an outward Cl^- gradient had virtually no effect on SO_4^{2-} uptake, and an outward SO_4^{2-} gradient had minimal effect on Cl^- uptake, confirming that SO_4^{2-} does not share this pathway.

However, an outward SO_4^{2-} gradient stimulated uphill oxalate uptake, and an outward oxalate gradient stimulated uphill SO_4^{2-} uptake, indicating the presence of another anion exchange pathway, shared by oxalate and SO_4^{2-}, that was similar to, if not identical with, that present in basolaeral membrane vesicles [36]. These and additional studies led us to conclude that at least three distinct anion exchangers were present on the brush border membrane of the proximal tubule, as illustrated in Fig. 7.

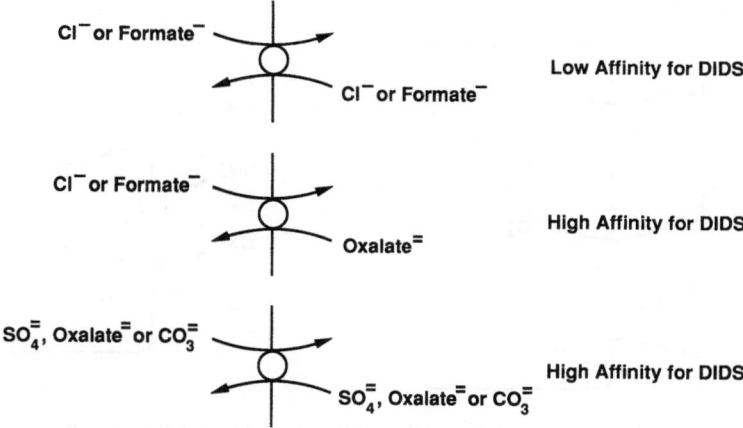

Fig. 7. Summary of properties of three luminal membrane anion exchangers

One exchanger, the Cl$^-$-formate exchanger, can perform electroneutral monovalent anion exchange using formate or Cl$^-$ as substrates, but has little or no affinity for divalent anions such as oxalate or SO$_4^{2-}$. This system is sensitive to inhibition only by relatively high, near mM, concentrations of disulfonic stilbenes like DIDS. A separate transporter, the Cl$^-$-oxalate exchanger, can exchange the monovalent anion Cl$^-$ or formate for oxalate but cannot exchange monovalent anions for each other or for SO$_4^{2-}$. By virtue of exchanging a monovalent for a divalent anion, this system is electrogenic. The Cl$^-$-oxalate exchanger is sensitive to relatively low micromolar concentrations of DIDS. Finally, a third anion exchanger was present that could exchange any pair of divalent anions among SO$_4^{2-}$, oxalate, and CO$_3^{2-}$. This system was electroneutral, had no affinity for Cl$^-$, and was highly sensitive to inhibition by DIDS.

The possible role of the Cl$^-$-formate exchanger in mediating Cl$^-$ entry across the brush border membrane has already been discussed. For Cl$^-$-oxalate exchange to likewise contribute importantly to luminal Cl$^-$ entry, there would need to be a mechanism present to recycle oxalate from lumen to cell. There are at least two possible mechanisms by which this third exchanger, the SO$_4^{2-}$-oxalate-CO$_3^{2-}$ exchanger, could serve that function, as shown in Fig. 8. First, consider that every two cycles of the Na$^+$-H$^+$ exchanger would generate an intracellular CO$_3^{2-}$. The resulting outward gradient of CO$_3^{2-}$ could drive uphill oxalate uptake via CO$_3^{2-}$-oxalate exchange. The resulting outward oxalate gradient could then drive Cl$^-$ entry via Cl$^-$-oxalate exchange. In this scheme, oxalate would recycle, and the net effect would be Na$^+$-coupled Cl$^-$ entry with a 2 Na$^+$:Cl$^-$ stoichiometry.

Alternatively, the process of Na$^+$-SO$_4^{2-}$ cotransport known to be present in the brush border membrane [37] leads to the cell uptake of SO$_4^{2-}$ and the generation of an outward SO$_4^{2-}$ gradient. This outward SO$_4^{2-}$ gradient could then drive oxalate uptake via SO$_4^{2-}$-oxalate exchange. The resulting outward oxalate gradient could then drive Cl$^-$ entry via Cl$^-$-oxalate exchange. Again, oxalate would recycle, and the net effect

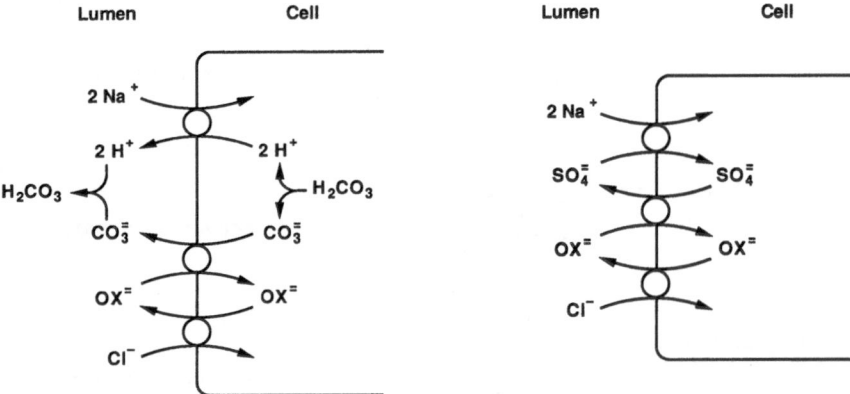

Fig. 8. Possible mechanisms for Cl⁻ entry across the luminal membrane by Cl⁻-oxalate exchange

would be Na⁺-coupled Cl⁻ entry with a 2 Na⁺:Cl⁻ stoichiometry. These potential mechanisms have not yet been tested in the intact tubule.

Mechanisms of Cl⁻ Exit Across the Basolateral Membrane

At least three different mechanisms for Cl⁻ exit across the basolateral membrane have been proposed, as illustrated in Fig. 9. One possibility is Cl⁻ exit through a Cl⁻ conductive pathway not coupled to the movement of any other ions. Since Cl⁻ is above electrochemical equilibrium in the proximal tubule cell, there is a passive driving force favoring Cl⁻ exit through any such Cl⁻ conductance present in the basolateral membrane. Studies from several groups have suggested that the Cl⁻ conductance of the basolateral membrane of the proximal tubule cell is negligibly small and cannot contribute significantly to Cl⁻ exit [38–40]. However, recent electrophysiologic studies by Welling and O'Neill [41], and our measurements of KCl movement across the basolateral membrane as manifested by cell volume changes [42], have suggested that the basolateral membrane Cl⁻ conductance is volume-activated. The increased cell volume induced by formate, as discussed above,

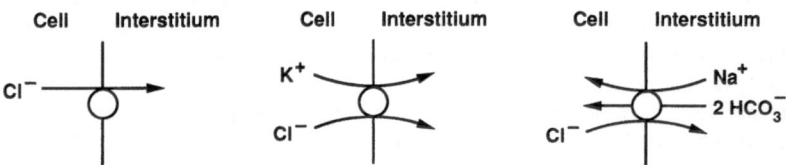

Fig. 9. Possible mechanisms of Cl⁻ exit across the basolateral membrane of the proximal tubule cell

might then activate the Cl⁻ conductance so that it becomes a major mechanism for Cl⁻ exit under physiologic conditions.

Alternatively, studies by Sasaki and co-workers have indicated that two electroneutral mechanisms, namely K^+-Cl^- cotransport and Na^+-dependent Cl^--HCO_3^- exchange, are present at the basolateral membrane of the rabbit proximal straight tubule [40,43]. Similar evidence has been presented by Ishibashi, Rector, and Berry for the rabbit proximal convoluted tubule [44]. These workers found that changes in peritubular K^+ caused changes in intracellular Cl^- activity as predicted for a K^+-Cl^- cotransport process. Membrane vesicle studies have conflicted concerning the presence of K^+-Cl^- cotransport [45,46]. Under physiologic conditions, the electrochemical gradients for both K^+ and Cl^- are directed outward across the basolateral membrane so that this pathway will mediate Cl^- efflux.

Intracellular Cl^- was also found to respond to changes in peritubular Na^+ and HCO_3^- consistent with the presence of a Na^+-dependent Cl^--HCO_3^- exchanger [43,44]. Membrane vesicle studies have conflicted concerning the presence of Na^+-dependent Cl^--HCO_3^- exchange [20,46,47]. This is a transport process that moves Na^+ and two equivalents of base in one direction, in exchange for Cl^- in the opposite direction. Under physiologic conditions, the inward Na^+ gradient would provide the driving force for this system to operate in the direction shown. How much of Cl^- exit occurs by this or any other pathway is at present not clear and is a topic of active investigation in several laboratories.

Summary of Proximal Tubule Transport Processes

The principal mechanisms for transcellular Na^+, Cl^-, and HCO_3^- transport in the mammalian proximal tubule are illustrated in Fig. 10. The most important primary active transport process is, of course, the Na^+ pump, which uses the free energy of ATP hydrolysis to extrude Na^+ and take up K^+ across the basolateral membrane. Most of the K^+ taken up by the pump recycles out across the basolateral membrane. The resulting inward Na^+ gradient is then used to drive the cotransport systems for organic solutes such as glucose and amino acids. There are really multiple distinct cotransport systems that are lumped together in Fig. 10 only for simplicity. Sugars and amino acids driven into the cell by Na^+ cotransport exit passively across the basolateral membrane. The current of Na^+ across the cell associated with Na^+ cotransport of organic solutes generates a lumen-negative transtubular potential difference in the early proximal tubule that drives a small amount of passive Cl^- reabsorption through the paracellular pathway [48].

H^+ is secreted largely by Na^+-H^+ exchange, with some additional contribution from the H^+-ATPase and possibly from recycling of monocarboxylates, a mechanism that is not illustrated. The HCO_3^- formed in the cell exits largely via Na-HCO_3^- cotransport, with perhaps a small contribution from Cl^--HCO_3^- exchange, that becomes more appreciable relative to Na^+-HCO_3^- cotransport in S_3. The overall process of acidification results in HCO_3^- reabsorption. In addition to the well-known role of luminal membrane carbonic anhydrase, intracellular and/or basolateral carbonic anhydrase is critically important for presenting base in a transportable form to the base exit mechanisms, particularly the Na^+-HCO_3^- cotransporter.

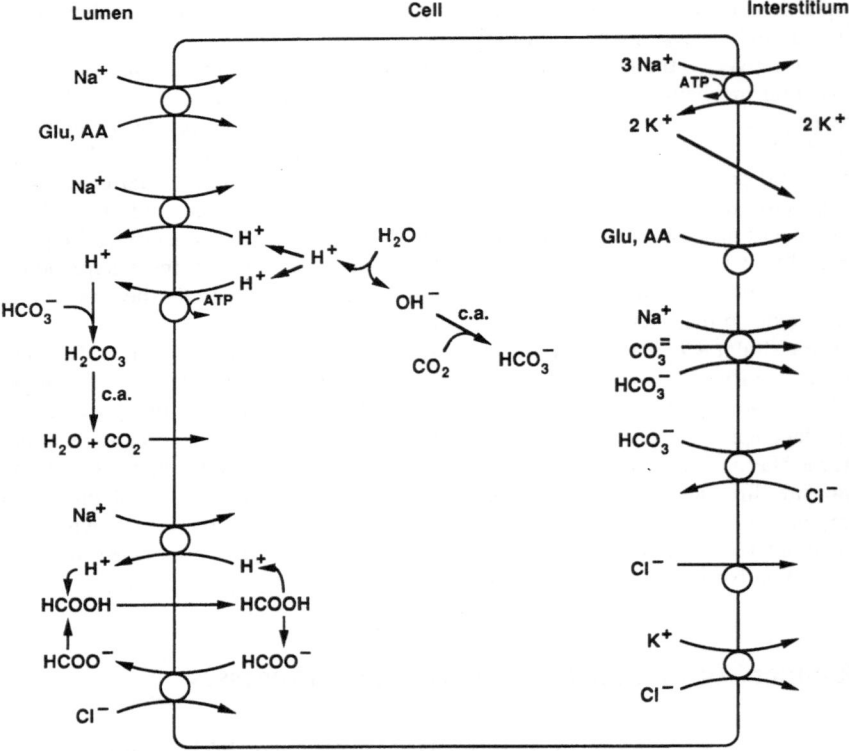

Fig. 10. Summary of the principal mechanisms for transcellular Na^+, Cl^- and HCO_3^- transport in the proximal tubule. c.a., carbonic anhydrase; AA, amino acid; Glu, glucose

In the early proximal tubule there is probably very little Cl^- transport via the Cl^--formate exchanger, because the luminal pH is not yet acid enough to permit efficient recycling of formic acid. In studies not discussed above, we found that NaCl transport catalyzed by formic acid recycling can occur in S_1, but depends critically on an acid luminal pH [34]. However, as acidification and HCO_3^- reabsorption proceed along the course of the proximal tubule, the lumen pH does become more acid, formic acid recycling would be facilitated, and Na^+-Cl^- entry via the Cl^--formate exchanger would then occur in parallel with the Na^+-H^+ exchanger. Whether other luminal membrane pathways, such as Cl^--oxalate exchange, which is not illustrated here, contribute to Cl^- entry is not known. The relative contributions of various Cl^- exit mechanisms are also unclear. It is possible that due to the increased cell volume resulting from Na^+-coupled organic solute entry and from formate-induced NaCl entry, the basolateral Cl^- conductance becomes sufficiently activated to mediate an important fraction of Cl^- exit. Alternatively, Cl^- exit may be largely by K^+-Cl^- cotransport, or by the Na^+-dependent Cl^--HCO_3^- exchanger that is not illustrated.

In any event, one consequence of the luminal pH dependence of Na$^+$-Cl$^-$ transport via the formate-dependent mechanism may be the preferential HCO$_3^-$ reabsorption that occurs in the early proximal tubule. The resulting isotonic water reabsorption causes luminal Cl$^-$ concentration to rise. An outward Cl$^-$ concentration gradient then develops across the proximal tubule. Passive resorption of Cl$^-$ can then occur through the paracellular pathway, generating a lumen-positive transtubular potential difference that can drive a component of passive Na$^+$ reabsorption as well [48]. The net effect of this additional passive NaCl reabsorption is to increase the amount of total Na$^+$ and Cl$^-$ that can be reabsorbed per ATP hydrolyzed by the Na$^+$, K$^+$-ATPase.

It should be clear that the Na$^+$-H$^+$ exchanger plays a critical role in mediating both HCO$_3^-$ and Cl$^-$ reabsorption in the proximal tubule. For this reason, considerable recent attention has focussed on the regulation of Na$^+$-H$^+$ exchange activity in the proximal tubule by hormones and neurotransmitters involved in Na$^+$ and volume homeostasis, such as angiotensin II, alpha adrenergic agonists, and dopamine.

Acknowledgment. Work in the author's laboratory has been supported by NIH Grants DK-33793 and DK-17433.

References

1. Murer H, Hopfer U, Kinne R (1976) Sodium/proton antiport in brush-border-membrane vesicles isolated from rat small intestine and kidney. Biochem J 154:597–604
2. Kinsella JL, Aronson PS (1980) Properties of the Na$^+$-H$^+$ exchanger in renal microvillus membrane vesicles. Am J Physiol 238:F461–F469
3. Kinsella JL, Aronson PS (1981) Interaction of NH$_4^+$ and Li$^+$ with the renal microvillus membrane Na$^+$-H$^+$ exchanger. Am J Physiol 241:C220–C226
4. Kinsella JL, Aronson PS (1981) Amiloride inhibition of the Na$^+$-H$^+$ exchanger in renal microvillus membrane vesicles. Am J Physiol 241:F374–F379
5. Kinsella JL, Aronson PS (1982) Determination of the coupling ratio for Na$^+$-H$^+$ exchange in renal microvillus membrane vesicles. Biochim Biophys Acta 689:161–164
6. Aronson PS, Nee J, Suhm MA (1982) Modifier role of internal H$^+$ in activating the Na$^+$-H$^+$ exchanger in renal microvillus membrane vesicles. Nature 299:161–163
7. Aronson PS, Suhm MA, Nee J (1983) Interaction of external H$^+$ with the Na$^+$-H$^+$ exchanger in renal microvillus membrane vesicles. J Biol Chem 258:6767–6771
8. Mahnensmith RL, Aronson PS (1985) Interrelationships among quinidine, amiloride and lithium as inhibitors of the renal Na$^+$-H$^+$ exchanger. J Biol Chem 260:12586–12592
9. Barac-Nieto M, Murer H, Kinne R (1980) Lactate-sodium cotransport in rat renal brush border membranes. Am J Physiol 239:F496–F506
10. Blomstedt JW, Aronson PS (1980) pH gradient-stimulated transport of urate and para-aminohippurate in dog renal microvillus membrane vesicles. J Clin Invest 65:931–934
11. Guggino SE, Martin GJ, Aronson PS (1983) Specificity and modes of the anion exchanger in dog renal microvillus membrane vesicles. Am J Physiol 244:F612–F621
12. Aronson PS (1983) Mechanisms of active H$^+$ secretion in the proximal tubule. Am J Physiol 245:F647–F659
13. Nakhoul NL, Boron WF (1988) Acetate transport in the S3 segment of the proximal tubule and its effect on intracellular pH. J Gen Physiol 92:395–412
14. Geibel J, Giebisch G, Boron WF (1989) Effects of acetate on luminal acidification processes in the S3 segment of the rabbit proximal tubule. Am J Physiol 257:F586–F594

15. Kinne-Saffran E, Kinne R (1974) Presence of bicarbonate-stimulated ATPase in the brush border microvillus membrane of the proximal tubule. Proc Soc Exp Biol Med 146:751–753

16. Turrini F, Sabolic I, Zimolo Z, Moewes B, Burckhardt G (1989) Relation of ATPases in rat renal brush-border membranes to ATP-driven H^+ secretion. J Membr Biol 107:1–12

17. Preisig PA, Ives HE, Cragoe EJ Jr, Alpern RJ, Rector FC Jr (1987) Role of the Na^+/H^+ antiporter in rat proximal tubule bicarbonate absorption. J Clin Invest 80:970–978

18. Nagami GT (1988) Luminal secretion of ammonia in the mouse proximal tubule perfused in vitro. J Clin Invest 81:159–164

19. Boron WF, Boulpaep EL (1983) Intracellular pH regulation in the renal proximal tubule of the salamander. Basolateral HCO_3^- transport. J Gen Physiol 81:53–94

20. Grassl SM, Aronson PS (1986) Na^+/HCO_3^- cotransport in basolateral membrane vesicles isolated from rabbit renal cortex. J Biol Chem 261:8778–8783

21. Soleimani M, Grassl SM, Aronson PS (1987) Stoichiometry of Na^+-HCO_3^- cotransport in basolateral membrane vesicles isolated from rabbit renal cortex. J Clin Invest 79:1276–1280

22. Soleimani M, Aronson PS (1989) Ionic mechanism of Na^+-HCO_3^- cotransport in rabbit renal basolateral membrane vesicles. J Biol Chem 264:18302–18308

23. Soleimani M, Aronson PS (1989) Effects of acetazolamide on Na^+-HCO_3^- cotransport in basolateral membrane vesicles isolated from rabbit renal cortex. J Clin Invest 83:945–951

24. Yoshitomi K, Burckhardt B-Ch, Frömter E (1985) Rheogenic sodium-bicarbonate cotransport in the peritubular cell membrane of rat renal proximal tubule. Pflugers Arch 405:360–366

25. Preisig PA, Alpern RJ (1989) Basolateral membrane H-OH-HCO_3 transport in the proximal tubule. Am J Physiol 256:F751–F765

26. Alpern RJ, Chambers M (1987) Basolateral membrane Cl/HCO_3 exchange in the rat proximal convoluted tubule. J Gen Physiol 89:581–598

27. Kurtz I (1989) Basolateral membrane Na^+/H^+ antiport, Na^+/base cotransport, and Na^+-independent Cl^-/base exchange in the rabbit S_3 proximal tubule. J Clin Invest 83:616–622

28. Sasaki S, Marumo F (1989) Effects of carbonic anhydrase inhibitors on basolateral base transport of rabbit proximal straight tubule. Am J Physiol 257:F947–F952

29. Schild L, Giebisch G, Karniski L, Aronson PS (1986) Chloride transport in the mammalian proximal tubule. Pflugers Arch 407(Suppl 2):S156–S159

30. Seifter JL, Knickelbein R, Aronson PS (1984) Absence of Cl-OH exchange and Na-Cl cotransport in rabbit renal microvillus membrane vesicles. Am J Physiol 247:F753–F759

31. Karniski LP, Aronson PS (1985) Chloride/formate exchange with formic acid recycling: a mechanism of active chloride transport across epithelial membranes. Proc Natl Acad Sci USA 82:6362–6365

32. Baum M (1988) Effect of luminal chloride on cell pH in rabbit proximal tubule. Am J Physiol 254:F677–F683

33. Schild L, Aronson PS, Giebisch G (1990) Effects of apical membrane Cl^--formate exchange on cell volume in rabbit proximal tubule. Am J Physiol 258:F530–F536

34. Schild L, Giebisch G, Karniski LP, Aronson PS (1987) Effect of formate on volume reabsorption in the rabbit proximal tubule. J Clin Invest 79:32–38

35. Karniski LP, Aronson PS (1987) Anion exchange pathways for Cl^- transport in rabbit renal microvillus membranes. Am J Physiol 253:F513–F521

36. Kuo S-M, Aronson PS (1988) Oxalate transport via the sulfate-HCO_3 exchanger in rabbit renal basolateral membrane vesicles. J Biol Chem 263:9710–9717

37. Lücke H, Stange G, Murer H (1979) Sulfate-ion/sodium-ion cotransport by brush-border membrane vesicles from rat kidney cortex. Biochem J 182:223–229

38. Bello-Reuss E (1982) Electrical properties of the basolateral membrane of the straight portion of the rabbit proximal renal tubule. Am J Physiol 326:49–63

39. Cardinal J, Lapointe J-Y, Laprade R (1984) Luminal and peritubular ionic substitutions

and intracellular potential of the rabbit proximal convoluted tubule. Am J Physiol 247:F352–F364

40. Sasaki S, Ishibashi K, Yoshiyama N, Shiigai T (1988) KCl cotransport across the basolateral membrane of rabbit renal proximal straight tubule. J Clin Invest 81:194–199

41. Welling PA, O'Neill RG (1990) Cell swelling activates basolateral Cl and K conductances in rabbit proximal tubule. Am J Physiol 258:F951–F962

42. Schild L, Aronson PS, Giebisch G (to be published) Basolateral transport pathways for K$^+$ and Cl$^-$ in the rabbit proximal tubule: effects on cell volume. Am J Physiol

43. Sasaki S, Yoshiyama N (1988) Interaction of chloride and bicarbonate transport across the basolateral membrane of rabbit proximal straight tubule. Evidence for sodium coupled chloride/bicarbonate exchange. J Clin Invest 81:1004–1011

44. Ishibashi Y, Rector FC Jr, Berry CA (1990) Chloride transport across the basolateral membrane of rabbit proximal convoluted tubules. Am J Physiol 258:F1569–F1578

45. Eveloff J, Warnock DG (1987) K-Cl transport systems in rabbit renal basolateral membrane vesicles. Am J Physiol 252:F883–F889

46. Grassl SM, Holohan PD, Ross CR (1987) Cl$^-$-HCO$_3^-$ exchange in rat renal basolateral membrane vesicles. Biochim Biophys Acta 905:475–484

47. Chen P-Y, Verkman AS (1988) Sodium-dependent chloride transport in basolateral membrane vesicles isolated from rabbit proximal tubule. Biochemistry 27:655–660

48. Rector FC Jr (1983) Sodium, bicarbonate, and chloride absorption by the proximal tubule. Am J Physiol 244:F461–F471

Biology of Acid-Base Transport in Distal Urinary Epithelia

PHILIP R. STEINMETZ

Chair: Claude Amiel

Biology of Acid-Base Transport in Distal Urinary Epithelia

Philip R. Steinmetz[1]

SUMMARY. The biology of acid-base transport in distal urinary epithelia is reviewed under four headings: 1) The major function of urinary acidification is based in α intercalated cells or carbonic anhydrase cells. The α cells secrete H⁺ into the urinary compartment by means of a vacuolar H^+-ATPase located at the apical cell membrane. Structure-function studies reveal that the number of pumps in an apical membrane position varies with acid-base conditions via a mechanism of exocytosis and endocytosis. The basolateral membrane of the α cell contains $Cl-HCO_3$ exchangers, which closely resemble the red cell band 3 protein, and parallel conductive Cl channels. The high transport rates achieved by α cells appear to be a function of the efficient packing of H^+-ATPase molecules in the apical membrane. 2) The function of bicarbonate secretion is confined to a small population of β intercalated cells and is less well understood. β cell function is observed in turtle urinary bladder and in the cortical segments of the mammalian collecting duct. The apical membrane of the β cell contains a $Cl-HCO_3$ exchanger that differs from the basolateral one of the α cell. Transport is driven by a basolateral H^+-ATPase. 3) The sodium transporting cells of the distal nephron usually contain basolateral Na/H antiporters involved in the regulation of intracellular pH. In some segments an apical Na/H antiporter may contribute to vectorial H⁺ secretion. 4) Overall acid-base transport in the distal nephron is a complex function of the geometry of the transporting systems and the availability of proton acceptors.

Introduction

The last decade has seen rapid expansion of our understanding of acid-base transport in the kidney: perfusion studies of tubule segments, studies of individual cell types by electrophysiologic and fluorescence techniques, structure-function studies of

---

[1]Division of Nephrology, University of Connecticut School of Medicine, Farmington, CT 06032, USA

model epithelia of turtle and toad bladder and of mammalian collecting duct (CD), and, most recently, immunocytochemical studies of transport proteins and purification and cDNA cloning of several major transporters. We have characterized many new acid-base transporters and we have learned about the remarkable diversity of structure and function along the nephron.

For this lecture I focus on urinary acidification by the tight urinary epithelia of the distal nephron and of the turtle and toad bladder, which are responsible for the final regulation of H^+ excretion and which are equipped to maintain steep pH gradients and to respond to acid-base changes and to hormonal control. At one time during the early years of nephrology, the great "black box" period of kidney physiology, it was thought that there was *one* major mechanism for proximal HCO_3 reabsorption and *one* for distal acidification.

Now we know all too well how several hundred million years of evolution have left us with great complexity, reflecting a long history of adaptations to new demands. On the *one hand* we have learned to accept this complexity, on the other we keep encountering some remarkably similar arrangements in the cellular organization of acid-base transporter, and we find that the transport proteins being used have barely changed over more than a hundred million years and that the same transporters are used in different cells, tissues, and species. A good transporter will be used over and over again. Therefore we can still come up with general models for the major transport functions. For example, the major system for distal urinary acidification is contained in the α type intercalated or carbonic anhydrase-rich cells of turtle bladder and of collecting duct. In some segments these α cells function as pure H^+ secretors. Much has been learned about the acid-base transporters at their apical and basolateral cell membranes and about the organization and regulation of H^+ secretion. The first part of this review will be devoted to this system. The next part will deal with the so-called β cell system, which is less well understood and is confined to only a small population of cells in turtle bladder and to only one segment, the cortical segment, in the rabbit CD. This HCO_3-secreting cell population is quite interesting, even if it is not always operative. The third topic deals with the acid-base function of the Na-transporting cells, such as the principal cells (PC) and inner medullary collecting duct (IMCD) cells. Here, we have to distinguish between "housekeeping" functions and net transepithelial transport of acid or base. By looking at the prototypes of these functions I hope to avoid generating a long catalogue of different transport systems in different places of the nephron. At the end, I shall present a brief survey of the regulation of the major acid-base transporters and the importance of proton acceptors in net acid excretion.

α Cell Function of H^+ Secretion

Physiologic Studies in Turtle Bladder

The initial studies of the flat sheet preparation of turtle urinary bladder reflected, primarily, the function of H^+ secretion in the α type carbonic anhydrase cells. The epithelium was treated as a black box. Physiologic studies revealed that H^+ secretion is *not directly* dependent on Na transport. There is only indirect electrical coupling, so that H^+ secretion is accelerated by lumen-negative PD. Serosal addition of HCO_3

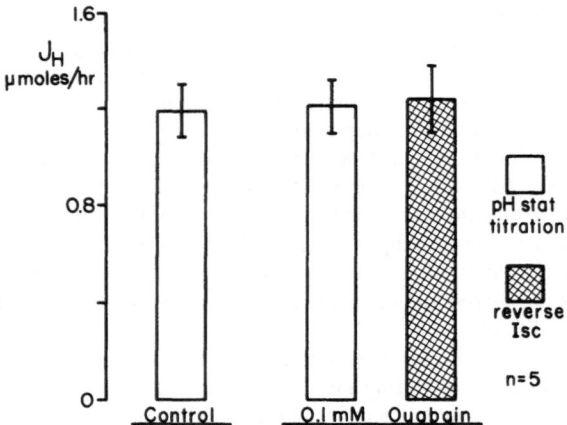

Fig. 1. Failure of ouabain to inhibit H⁺ secretion (J_H) at constant p CO_2. The reverse short-circuit current (*Isc*) is approximately equal to the pH state rate. (From [8] with permission)

caused a marked reduction in net acid secretion if Cl⁻ was present in luminal solution. The discovery of an electroneutral Cl-HCO_3 exchange transport system complicated the model system for some time until this complication itself became the subject of study, i.e., the existence of two polarities of acid-base transport in the same epithelium.

Figure 1 shows that H⁺ secretion in the short-circuited state is unaffected by inhibition of Na⁺ transport. In fact, the Isc in presence of ouabain is equivalent to the pH stat rate, indicating that all of the H⁺ secretion occurs with transfer of charge. In support for the electrogenicity of H⁺ secretion is, also, the fact that H⁺ secretion is not dependent on the presence of other electrolytes: Na⁺ and K⁺ are not required. Cl⁻ is required in trace amounts only on the serosal side, presumably for the exit step of HCO_3^-.

H⁺ secretion continues under anaerobic conditions. In the absence of O_2 the transport of H⁺ becomes critically dependent on glucose as a substrate. It turns out that H⁺ transport is tightly coupled to metabolism. In this example, two H⁺ are transported for each lactate produced anaerobically and this stoichiometry is preserved when the transport rate is manipulated by inhibitors or an opposing electrochemical potential gradient for protons. These studies [1], and others by Beauwens and Al Awqati [2], indicate that the apical cell membrane is very tight to H⁺ ions. In contrast, the basolateral cell membrane has a very high HCO_3^- permeability.

Structure-Function Studies Reveal Different Cell Types

The studies by Rosen [3], Husted et al. [4], and Stetson and Steinmetz [5,6] led first to the distinction between granular and carbonic anhydrase-rich (CA) cells and, later, to the distinction of α and β type CA cells in turtle bladder. Gluck et al. [7] described the stimulation of exocytosis by CO_2, which could account for the remarkable apical area changes of the CA cells reported by Husted et al. [4]. The reader is referred

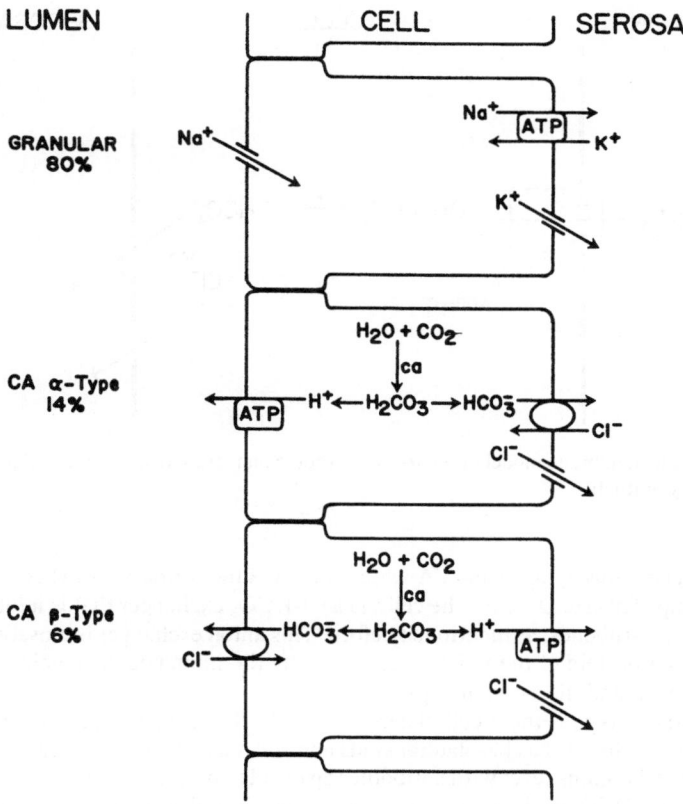

Fig. 2. The major cell types correspond to major transport functions in turtle urinary bladder and, probably, in certain other tight urinary epithelia, such as the cortical segment of the collecting duct (CD). CA, carbonic anhydrase. (From [8] with permission)

to references [5,6,8] for a more detailed description of the structure-function studies that form the basis for the three cell types shown in Fig. 2. These cell types are comparable to those of the cortical collecting duct (CCD).

The cell type constituting the majority is the granular or principal cell, which absorbs Na and is capable of secreting K in the cortical segment. The acid-base functions of this cell appear to be confined to intracellular pH regulatioin. It has a Na/H antiporter in the basolateral membrane (not shown), which probably does not participate in vectorial transport. The next cell type is the α CA cell which, in turtle bladder, makes up about 14% of total cell number. It is common in the outer medullary collecting duct (OMCD), where it is the only type of acid-base transporting cell. In the absence of Na^+ transport this cell dominates the transport functions of turtle bladder and OMCD. It produces a lumen positive PD, is inhibited by acetazolamide, and has a remarkable apical membrane that can be expanded by fusion of subapical membrane vesicles or shrunk by retrieval of apical membrane and formation of reserve

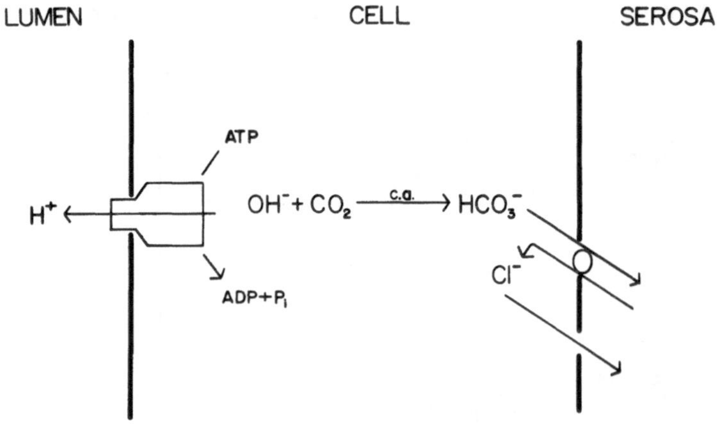

LUMEN   CELL   SEROSA

Fig. 3. Double membrane model of the α-type carbonic anhydrase (*c.a.*) or intercalated cell of tight urinary epithelia

vesicles. It contains cytoplasmic CA which catalyzes the formation of HCO_3^- behind the H^+ pump. This HCO_3^- exits the cell via a $Cl-HCO_3$ exchanger that is inhibited by the disulfonic stilbenes, as mentioned before. This anion exchanger is closely related to the band 3 protein of the red cell, as shown by the immunocytochemical studies of Drenckhahn and his associates [9].

The third cell type is the β cell. There is considerable evidence that it is involved in HCO_3^- secretion. It has basolateral studs and rod-shaped particles and, in the rat, the basolateral regions react with antibodies against H^+-ATPase. Under ordinary conditions, the $Cl-HCO_3$ exchange transport by the β cells is electroneutral, a one for one exchange. The basolateral H^+-ATPase is thought to be the primary active transport process. A parallel Cl^- conductance permits the overall exchange to operate electroneutrally. The apical $Cl-HCO_3$ exchanger, however, fails to react with red cell band 3 antibodies and is not easily inhibited by disulfonic stilbenes. Hence, it differs substantially from the basolateral exchanger of the cells. I shall come back to the β cell later. For now, we may conclude that the functions of Na^+ absorption, H^+ secretion and HCO_3^- secretion are based in different cell types in turtle bladder and in certain segments of CD.

Organization of α Cell: Apical Membrane

Figure 3 is focussed on the α cell: this is the double membrane model. H^+ transport by the apical pump is tightly coupled to ATP hydrolysis. The work of Dixon and Al Awqati [10] in turtle bladder was based on this coupling and first suggested that the pump of urinary acidification was a reversible H^+-translocating ATPase. Subsequent studies, by Gluck and his associates, in turtle bladder and bovine medulla have led to characterization of the ATPase as an electrogenic H^+-ATPase that is inhibited by NEM and DCCD and that differs from the mitochondrial ATPase. Immunoaffinity purification of the bovine ATPase by Gluck and Caldwell [11] has defined the

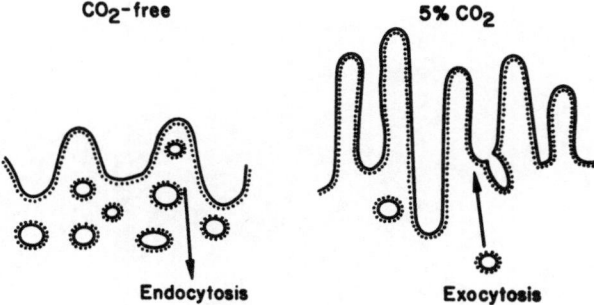

Fig. 4. Schematic representation of apical membrane coated with studs. CO_2 stimulation of H^+ secretion is associated with expansion of the apical area of α cells, by a mechanism of exocytosis

ATPase as a vacuolar H^+-ATPase with a molecular weight of about 580000 dalton and about 10 different subunits. Immunocytochemical studies with antibodies against the 70 and 56 kD subunits of the H^+-ATPase demonstrate that the ATPase is localized at the cytoplasmic regions below the apical microplicae, where high magnification electron microscopy reveals a stud-like coating of the cytoplasmic leaflet of the apical membrane [12,13]. The studs are stalked spheres about 10 nM long and about 9 nM in their widest diameter. The new lines of evidence now available strongly suggest that the studs correspond to the catalytic units of the H^+-ATPase molecules.

In Fig. 4 the response of the "studded" apical membrane to CO_2 is shown. In turtle bladder, the apical membrane of the microplicae and the membrane vesicles have roughly the same density of studs. In the absence of CO_2 (left), the apical membrane is shrunk and there are many membrane vesicles coated with studs in the cytoplasm. The pumps are in a reserve position and don't contribute to transepithelial transport. If CO_2 is added, these vesicles fuse with the apical membrane in a matter of minutes, expand the apical surface, and increase the number of pumps in position. This expansion was quantitated by morphometric measurements by Stetson and Steinmetz [6].

The planar surface area of individual α cells increased from 28 ± 2 to 65 ± 4 μm^2 after CO_2 addition. The degree of folding also increased, so that the total folded area increased more than fourfold. These comparisons were made in paired bladder halves fixed in Ussing chambers after H^+ secretion rates had been measured. The density of rod-shaped particles (RSP) on freeze fracture replicas of the apical membrane was also determined. In turtle and toadbladder, as well as in the CD, RSPs are seen in the same cell membranes and membrane vesicles as the studs. The two, however, are observed with different techniques and represent different structures. The studs appear to represent catalytic units of the H^+ ATPase within the cytoplasm and the RSP are a linear array of 2 or 3 spherical units representing intramembrane components, possibly transmembrane components of the ATPase. Hence, a RSP may represent 2 or 3 pumps or a multiple thereof. Since we had estimated the total area of apical membrane and had freeze fracture studies of several α cell apical membranes at low and high CO_2, we estimated the total number of RSP and compared it with the total H^+ transport rates for the same tissues. Because of the small sample of α cell

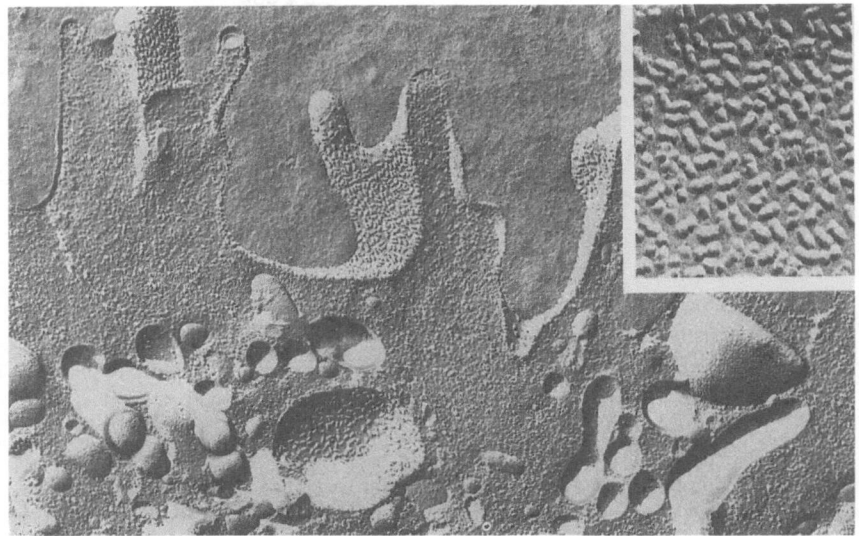

Fig. 5. Freeze-fracture electron micrograph of the apical membrane of an α-type carbonic anhydrase cell. Numerous *rod-shaped particles* are shown on the protoplasmic phase of apical microplicae and certain cytoplasmic vesicles. *Inset* reveals higher magnification of rod-shaped particles. (From [5] with permission)

fractures we couldn't be sure that CO_2 increased the density of RSP, but it was clear that the total area and the total number of RSP in an apical position was increased about five-fold, while the transport rate increased nine-fold. Taken together, these studies suggest that a large part, about 60%, of the CO_2 induced increase in H^+ secretion is accounted for by an increased number of pumps at the apical membrane of the α cells.

Figure 5 shows a freeze fracture surface of the apical cell membrane of an α cell. Note numerous RSP on the protoplasmic face. Each RSP consists of 2 or 3 spherical subunits of 12 nM diameter (Inset). A major question is how RSPs on freeze fracture relate to studs on transmission electron microscopy (TEM). The simplest arrangement would be that in which each spherical subunit in a RSP was linked to a cytoplasmic stud. On the average, there were about 3000 RSP/μm^2 or 7500 spherical subunit/μm^2. This estimate is not very different from that made by Brown, Hartwig, and Gluck [12] in α cells of toadbladder, for studs. These authors used a rapid freezing method, in which they sheared away the apical membrane of the cytoplasm and obtained a beautiful view of the studs on the cytoplasmic side of the membrane. They found a density of studs in toadbladder of about 16000/μm^2, which is about twice the density of the spherical subunits in RSP. Whether the spherical subunits are linked to one or two studs, and whether they actually represent transmembrane channels or some other structural characteristic of the way pumps are packed in the membrane, is not known.

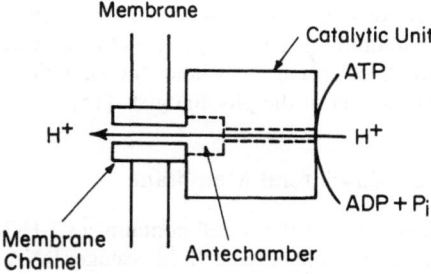

Fig. 6. A physiologist's working model for an ATP-driven proton pump. The pump complex consists of a membrane channel and a catalytic unit, linked via an antechamber that serves as a buffer compartment. (From [15] with permission)

In the near future these questions may be resolved by means of high resolution electron microscopy. According to our estimates, the average transport rate per RSP in turtle bladder at room temperature was 200 protons per s, or 80 per spherical subunit. That would be 80 or 40 per s per pump, depending on the number of pumps associated.

To return to the double membrane model of the αcell. The primary active transport step at the apical membrane is a H^+-ATPase. Based on the monomer assumption of 2 1/2 studs per RSP, the pump number at the apex of an αcell varies between 1 1/2 million and 6 million, as a function of CO_2 tension. Changes in pump number constitute a major way of regulating the transport rate. Aside from the H^+ pumps, there are few transporters or channels detectable in the apical cell membrane under ordinary conditions. Old studies on the coupling between transport and metabolism in bladder and more recent electrophysiologic studies, carried out in the outer medullary collecting duct by Koeppen [14], indicate that the apical membrane is very tight to ions, including protons.

As a result of this tightness, the rate of H^+ secretion (J_H) during secretion against pH gradients is a function of the active component of H^+ transport. Since apical areas do not change during acute luminal pH changes, the J_H vs Δ pH relation reflects the intrinsic properties of the H^+ pump (or of a given population of H^+ pumps). Transport stops at an opposing Δ pH of 3 U or a PD of 180 mV. At favorable gradients the transport rate reaches a maximal value. Andersen et al. [15] were able to simulate the observed J_H vs Δ pH relation by means of a set of assumptions about kinetic factors and a two component model of the H^+ pump complex. As shown in Fig. 6, their working model consisted of a catalytic unit where translocation of H^+ was coupled to ATP hydrolysis and a passive transmembrane channel linked to the catalytic unit through a buffer compartment (antechamber). Over the last few years, the biochemical studies of Gluck and Caldwell [11] and Stone and coworkers [16] have provided important new information about the subunit structure of vacuolar H^+-ATPase. The immunopurification studies of Gluck and coworkers have characterized the vacuolar ATPase of kidney medulla as a large protein of about 580 kD. There appear to be 3 subunits of 70 kD where ATP is bound during its hydrolysis and where NEM may inhibit. A smaller subunit of 56 kD is part of the catalytic unit and the structure of this unit has been highly conserved all the way from the archaebacteria to the mammalian kidney. The transmembrane channel appears to be formed by 6 copies of a 15 kD subunit which binds DCCD. On the whole, the subunit structure is consistent with the two component model of the physiologists [15].

Organization of α Cell:Basolateral Membrane

The basolateral cell membrane of the α cell contains a Cl-HCO_3 exchanger that is closely related to the band 3 protein of red cell. Messenger RNA studies of the kidney anion exchanger indicate that this exchanger is close to the red cell exchanger, except for a series of amino acids at the aminoterminal end. In any event, the α cells of turtle bladder, OMCD, and CCD contain a band 3-like exchanger in their basolateral membrane, as judged from immunocytochemical studies by Drenckhahn et al. [9], Schuster [17], and Verlander et al. [18], and as judged from the traditional response to stilbenes and Cl-removal. It is of interest that the turnover rate of the anion exchanger is much higher than that of the H^+ pump, so that a cell with 5 million H^+ pumps may only require some 50000 exchangers. Recent studies of cell attached patches have revealed the existence of high conductance Cl^- channels with possible transport rates well over a million/s. For the sake of comparison, that α cell would require only a small number, less than 50, of Cl channels in its basolateral membrane to accommodate the recycling of Cl^-. I have mentioned the intrinsic regulation of the H^+ pump rate by $\Delta \tilde{\mu}H$ and the regulation of the pump number by CO_2. At the basolateral membrane, the activity of Cl channels would directly affect the transfer of negative charge and, thereby, $\Delta \tilde{\mu}H$ across the apical membrane. In some α cells, the basolateral membrane may also contain Na/H antiporters. These antiporters are in the wrong position for vectorial H^+ secretion, but may play a role when the cell is acid loaded.

β Cell Function of HCO_3 Secretion

The next major transport function is HCO_3^- secretion by β cells. Renal tubular secretion of HCO_3 was first described in the 1950s, in the alligator. In the early 1970s, when Leslie, Schwartz, and I [19] found an electroneutral transport system for HCO_3^- secretion in turtle bladder, we were afraid that the system might be a reptilian peculiarity that would complicate the model. Subsequently, McKinney and Burg [20] and others showed a similar transport system in rabbit CCD. Following the discovery of two subtypes of carbonic anhydrase cells [5,21] with opposite functional polarities, this system has received considerable attention. Figure 7 shows a double membrane model for the β cell of turtle bladder operating under ordinary conditions, that is, without stimulation by cAMP. The net rate of HCO_3^- secretion equals the net rate of Cl-absorption and both rates are independent of sodium transport. H^+ pumps are located at the basolateral cell membrane, along with parallel Cl^- channels. For each H^+ ion extruded, a HCO_3^- ion is generated and subsequently secreted into the urine via a neutral Cl-HCO_3 exchanger. The Cl entering across the apical membrane exits through conductive basolateral channels, so that the overall exchange operation remains neutral. The ultrastructural and immunocytochemical evidence for baso-

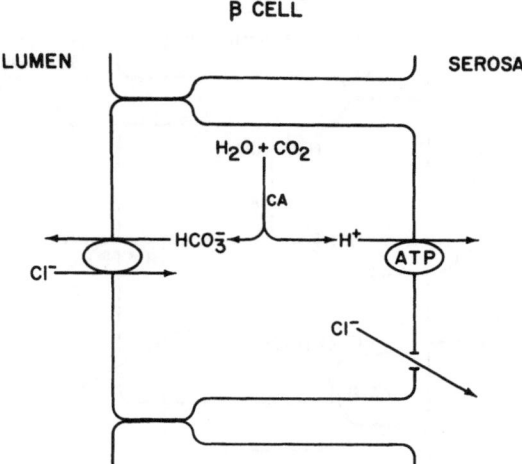

Fig. 7. Cellular organization of electroneutral HCO$_3$ secretion in β carbonic anhydrase (*CA*) cell

lateral H$^+$ pumps is compelling, but the nature of the apical Cl-HCO$_3$ exchanger remains to be clarified. The apical exchanger differs from the basolateral one in that antibodies to various parts of the band 3 protein have failed to react with it [9,17] and in that it is relatively resistant to inhibitors, as shown by Kohn et al. [22]. As you can see, the β cell is not a simple mirror reversal of the α cell. In turtle bladder, the electroneutral model for HCO$_3^-$ secretion is modified and HCO$_3^-$ secretion is stimulated by maneuvers that increase cAMP, such as phosphodiesterase inhibitors and certain peptides.

Cyclic AMP introduces an apical anion conductance for Cl$^-$ and, to some extent, for HCO$_3^-$ (Fig. 8). Total HCO$_3^-$ secretion is increased as an electrogenic component of HCO$_3^-$ secretion is added. A Cl ion entering the cell on the exchanger has two options. It can recycle across the apical membrane or it can exit across the basolateral membrane. In turtle bladder, the basolateral exit rate and therefore the neutral component, is decreased. Studies by Stetson [23] suggest that cAMP may cause selective addition of Cl$^-$ channels to the apical membrane. Activation or insertion of Cl channels by cAMP is also a mechanism for anion secretion in other epithelia, such as tracheal and intestinal epithelia. In turtle bladder, cAMP increases HCO$_3$ secretion and has little effect on H$^+$ secretion, so that the combined effect is usually one of reducing net acid secretion. In the rabbit CCD, it appears that electroneutral rather than the electrogenic HCO$_3$ secretion is increased [17], an effect somewhat different from that in turtle bladder. Furthermore, there appear to be species differences among the mammalian CCDs studied. It should not be surprising that the overall effects of cAMP vary among tissues. Not only are there different cell types and different prevalences of α or β cells, but also, within a single cell type, cAMP may cause activation of Cl channels in different cell membranes. In this example, apical activation decreases transcellular Cl absorption, whereas

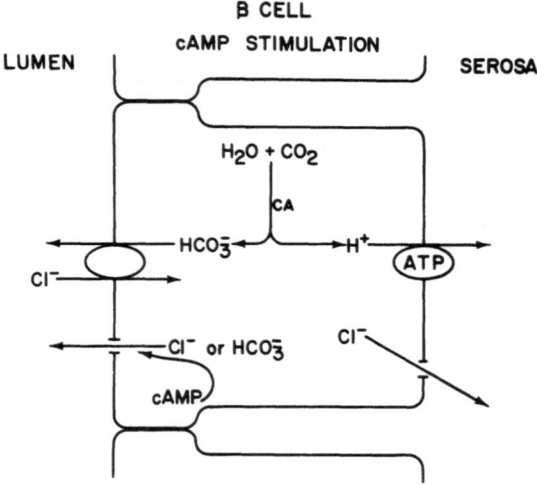

Fig. 8. Stimulation of electrogenic HCO_3^- secretion by cAMP in β carbonic anhydrase (*CA*) cell

basolateral activation might increase Cl absorption, depending on the initial conditions. It is clear that activation (used as an operational term) of Cl channels may have potent effects on the transport rate and on the electrogenicity of acid-base transport, but it is also clear that such effects depend very much on the precise membrane sites being activated.

In terms of β cell function, it is well to remember that this cell is found in very limited regions of the collecting duct system. β cells are confined to the cortical segments of the collecting duct. Their numbers, furthermore, depend on the acid-base condition of the animal. In rabbits on an alkaline ash diet, the majority of intercalated cells (IC) have a functional polarity of β cells. Schwartz, Barasch, and Al-Awqati [24] showed that acid loading would reverse the functional polarity of these intercalated cells to the H^+ secreting α form, as judged from their pH response to basolateral Cl removal. In turtle bladder, β cells make up about a third of the intercalated cells and the α and β forms appear to maintain a relatively stable polarity. For example, turtle α or β cells are clearly unipolar, as judged from their ultrastructure, i.e., cytoplasmic studs and rod-shaped intramembrane particles are either on one or the other pole, i.e., more than 95% are on the apical side in α cells and more than 95% are on the basolateral side in β cells. However, in rabbit CCD, one finds these elements on both poles, with one pole having a greater abundance than the other. The rabbit IC may be described as bipolar. It is likely that the adoptive response of the IC of rabbit CCD does not involve a complete reversal of all transporters between the two poles, but rather some remodelling that shifts the bulk of the H^+-ATPase molecules to the other cell membrane by some means of vesicular traffic. According to current models, the basolateral Cl^- conductance stays in place; the fate of the Cl-HCO_3 exchanger in this reversal remains poorly understood.

Acid-Base Function of Sodium-Transporting Cells

The third topic deals with acid-base transport in Na transporting cells. The granular cells transport Na and their O_2 consumption is not affected by carbonic anhydrase inhibition, as shown by Schwartz and coworkers in turtle bladder [25]. Conversely, the carbonic anhydrase rich cells are not affected by ouabain, in terms of either O_2 consumption or transport. Hence, vectorial acid-base transport and sodium transport appear to be separated into different cells in turtle bladder. In the CD the separation of function is less clear and varies with the segments.

In general, the intercalated cells of the CD contain both carbonic anhydrase and Na, K-ATPase, as shown by Ridderstrale et al. [26] in the rabbit. Electrophysiologic studies, however, by Koeppen [14] have shown that the OMCD intercalated and inner stripe cells behave like H^+ secreting cells. They have extremely high apical membrane resistances without detectable Na conductances and their basolateral membranes have Cl conductances, instead of the usual K conductances of principal cells. The separations between H^+ transport and Na transport become unclear in other segments of the CD. For example, in the initial segment of the IMCD, α cell function and Na reabsorption may well coexist in the same cells. Brown et al. [13] demonstrated H^+-ATPase in the apical regions of the cells of this segment. Since the vacuolar H^+-ATPase dates back to the primitive archaebacteria, it appears that H^+ pumps preceded the development of Na^+ pumps by a long period. In some instances, the H^+-ATPases continued to serve as the primary plasma membrane pumps, in other instances they became incorporated in Na^+ transporting cells.

Aside from incorporating H^+ pumps for vectorial transport, Na^+ transporting cells have acid-base transporters for housekeeping functions. These transporters have been defined, to an important extent, by means of fluorescence techniques for intracellular pH. For example, all Na-transporting cells that have been studied in the collecting duct appear to contain basolateral Na/H antiporters which play a role in the recovery from an acid load, but are in the wrong position to contribute to H^+ secretion into the urine. In some more proximal segments, like the thick ascending limb of Henle's loop and the distal convoluted tubule, there appear to be apical Na/H antiporters which resemble the antiporters of the proximal tubule and do contribute to H^+ secretion. The principal cells of the CCD may also contain a basolateral Cl/HCO_3 exchanger, as described by Weiner and Hamm [27]. The basolateral Cl/HCO_3 exchanger and Na/H antiporter are involved primarily in intracellular pH regulation.

Overall Function of Distal Urinary Acidification

How is distal urinary acidification integrated? Asking the question, we tend to assume that the processes are part of a system that is completely determined. This assumption goes back to Laplace, who believed in a universe that operates like clockwork. If you know all components and their initial conditions and all laws, you can predict all events. The problem for urinary acidification is that the components interact with each other and rarely can be measured simultaneously under identical conditions. Also, the rules underlying these interactions are not precisely known. Hence, we end up with a lot of isolated systems that can't be simply added up to get the whole

State-of-the-Art Lectures

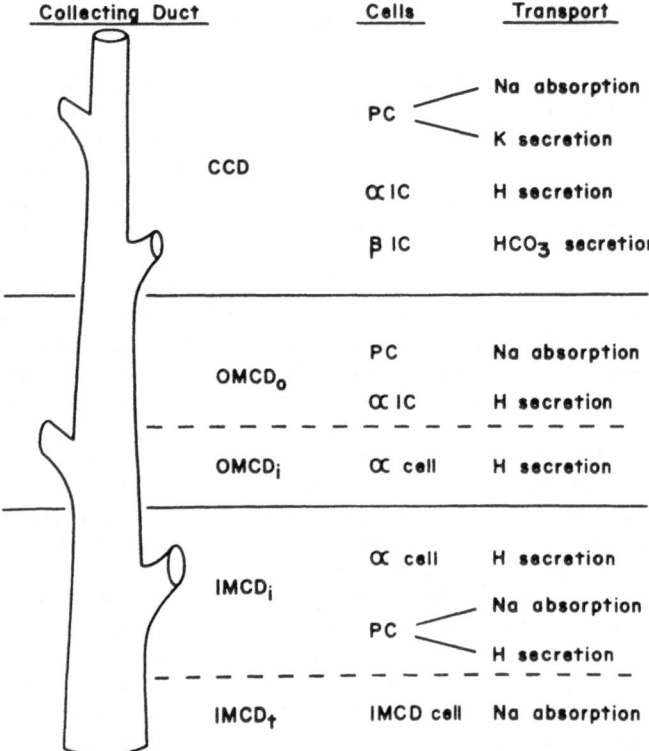

Fig. 9. Major transepithelial transport processes in collecting duct (*CD*). CCD, cortical CD; OMCD$_o$, outer stripe of outer medullary CD; OMCD$_i$, inner stripe of OMCD; IMCD$_i$ and IMCD$_t$, initial and terminal segments of inner medullary CD; PC, principal cell; IC, intercalated cell

system in vivo. Often, subsystems have their own evolutionary history, which bears little relation to acid-base transport. The best thing to do is to characterize each system (as we have always done) and to recognize the common, as well as the local, features, and to determine the context in which they should be taken within the overall system. Now that we work at the cellular and molecular level we need fewer black boxes, but we need more storage boxes to place the numerous local data and bits of incomplete knowledge into. Each student of urinary acidification must find the best simplification for his or her vantage point.

Figure 9 provides such a simplification of the collecting duct system. The fluid enters the cortical collecting duct (CCD) through connecting tubules, which are similar to the CCD. Much of the filtered HCO$_3$ has been reabsorbed in the proximal tubule (PT). In the thick ascending limb of Henle's loop and in the distal convoluted tubule this reabsorption is continued by transporters similar to those of the PT, namely an apical Na/H antiporter and, probably, a basolateral Na3(HCO$_3$) cotransporter. The filtered HCO_3 is nearly reabsorbed by the time the CD begins contributing to net acid excretion.

The CCD is extremely versatile. The principal cells reabsorb Na and secrete K, at rates regulated by aldosterone. The intercalated cells secrete H^+ in cells with predominant α polarity and HCO_3^- in cells with predominant β polarity. This is the only segment where HCO_3^- secretion has been observed. None has been found beyond the cortical segment. The cortical segments also respond to K^+ depletion with increased K-ATPase activity of an ouabain resistant variety. Whether this ATPase is a H^+/K^+ ATPase or a Na^+/K^+ ATPase in a storage or ouabain resistant form, remains to be further explored. The regulation of acid-base transport is also versatile. Acute increases in peritubular HCO_3^- increase HCO_3^- secretion. Slower HCO_3^- loading increases the β polarity of IC cells and, thereby, the IC capacity to secrete HCO_3^-. Increases in CO_2 tension stimulate H^+ secretion under some, but not all, conditions. Aldosterone increases H^+ secretion via the voltage effect of stimulated Na^+ transport, as well as directly by some unspecified increase in H^+ pumps. Maneuvers increasing cellular cAMP tend to increase HCO_3^- secretion and, thereby, reduce any net H^+ secretion. Several peptide hormones such as VIP, glucagon, and, in some species, isoproterenol, stimulate HCO_3^- secretion. The catecholamines may stimulate both α and β cells, with the net outcome depending on the initial conditions. Paillard and Bishara [28] and Schuster and [17] have recently reviewed this field.

The OMCD is less versatile, but may serve as a better prototype for the study of H^+ secretion and α cell function. All intercalated cells of this segment are cells with a clearly unipolar organization. It has not been possible to bring about a polarity reversal by alkali loading. Na^+-transporting cells dominate in the outer stripe. In the less aerobic inner stripe, most cells behave as α cells secreting H^+. Their electrophysiology is one of H^+ secretion, with the typical basolateral Cl conductance and almost no apical ion conductance. H^+ secretion in this segment is stimulated directly by aldosterone. It is also regulated by CO_2 and HCO_3 in the expected directions.

The IMCD has been studied in vivo by microcatherization and perfusion, as well as in vitro, in culture preparations. The initial IMCD contains an apical membrane H^+-ATPase, as shown by Brown et al. [13]. Carbonic anhydrase is also present in the initial, but *not* in the terminal segments. The initial segment contributes to urinary acidification through H^+ secretion by apical H^+ pumps, a function comparable to α cell function. This segment, as well as the terminal segment, also contains Na/H antiporters. Their cellular distribution is not well characterized. In principle, an apical antiporter might contribute to urine acidification when concentration gradients are favorable, i.e., when the urine concentration of Na^+ is high and that of H^+ is low.

These are the main segments and functions along the CD system. In the overall system, the bulk of distal H^+ secretion is performed by α cells or α-like cells. As we have discussed, the regulation of H^+ secretion is a function, first, of the size of the H^+ pump population facing the lumen, and second, of the electrochemical potential difference for protons, $\Delta \tilde{\mu}H$, across the apical membrane. The intrinsic properties of the H^+ pumps are such that the pumps stop pumping as the pH gradient or the $\Delta \tilde{\mu}H$ approaches 3 pH units. The importance of the negative feedback inhibition of H^+ secretion cannot be overestimated. Significant net acid excretion can be achieved only if H^+ acceptors are available in the lumen. In the CD, ammonia and ammonium are the major buffer pair. Recent studies by Good and Knepper [29] have clarified the ways by which NH_3 and NH_4 ion accumulate within the medullary interstitium. They have shown how the transport of NH_4 ion is an important component of total ammonium transport in the proximal tubule and the thick ascending limb of Henle's loop. Once the NH_4^+ and NH_3 have accumulated within the interstitium, however, the diffusible NH_3 continues to play an old-fashioned role as a major proton acceptor within the lumen. This H^+ acceptor allows the H^+ pumps to secrete H^+ ions without self inhibition. Impaired H^+ secretion or impaired availability of ammonia can lead to a renal tubular acidosis.

Much less is known about the pathophysiology of HCO_3^- secretion. In principle, the β cells could play a role in preventing a dietary alkalosis. Since the apical exchanger is regulated by the luminal Cl^- concentration, reduced HCO_3^- secretion could contribute to Cl depletion alkalosis.

To conclude, despite the remarkable heterogeneity observed within distal urinary epithelia, we can recognize distinct cellular and molecular mechanisms that are central to acid-base transport and we can understand many of the principles by which they are regulated. Over the next few years, our knowledge of the major transport proteins—the H^+-ATPase, the kidney-related anion exchangers, and the Cl channels—is likely to expand. We shall learn more about the way these proteins are targeted to their membrane sites and the way they are expressed and regulated.

Acknowledgment. This work was supported by NIH research grant DK-30693.

References

1. Steinmetz PR, Husted A, Mueller A, Beauwens R (1981) Coupling between H^+ transport and anaerobic glycolysis in turtle urinary bladder: effects of inhibitors of H^+ ATPase. J Membr Biol 59:27–34
2. Beauwens R, Al-Awqati Q (1976) Active H^+ transport in the turtle urinary bladder: coupling of transport to glucose oxidation. J Gen Physiol 68:421–439
3. Rosen S (1972) Localization of carbonic anhydrase activity in turtle and toad urinary bladder mucosa. J Histochem Cytochem 20:696–702
4. Husted RF, Mueller AL, Kessel RG, Steinmetz PR (1981) Surface characteristics of carbonic-anhydrase rich cells in turtle urinary bladder. Kidney Int 19:491–502
5. Stetson DL, Steinmetz PR (1985) α- and β-types of carbonic anhydrase-rich cells in turtle bladder. Am J Physiol 249 (Renal Fluid Electrolyte Physiol 18):F553–F565
6. Stetson DL, Steinmetz PR (1986) Correlation between apical intramembrane particles and H^+ secretion rates during CO_2 stimulation in turtle bladder. Pflugers Arch 407(Suppl 2):S80–S84
7. Gluck S, Cannon C, Al Awqati Q (1982) Exocytosis regulates urinary acidification in turtle bladder by rapid insertion of H^+ pumps into the luminal membrane. Proc Natl Acad Sci USA 79:4327–4331
8. Steinmetz PR (1986) Cellular organization of urinary acidification. Am J Physiol 251 (Renal Fluid Electrolyte Physiol 20):F173–F187
9. Drenckhahn D, Oelmann M, Schaaf P, Wagner M, Wagner S (1987) Band 3 is the basolateral anion exchanger of dark epithelial cells of turtle urinary bladder. Am J Physiol 252 (Cell Physiol 21):C570–C574
10. Dixon TE, Al-Awqati A (1979) Urinary acidification in turtle bladder is due to a reversible proton-translocating ATPase. Proc Natl Acad Sci USA 76:3135–3138

11. Gluck S, Caldwell J (1988) Proton-translocating ATPase from bovine kidney medulla:partial purification and reconstitution. Am J Physiol 254:F71–F79
12. Brown D, Gluck S, Hartwig J (1987) Structure of the novel membrane-coating material in proton-secreting epithelial cells and identification as an H$^+$-ATPase. J Cell Biol 105:1637–1648
13. Brown D, Hirsch S, Gluck S (1988) Localization of a proton pumping ATPase in rat kidney. J Clin Invest 82:2114–2126
14. Koeppen BM (1985) Conductive properties of the rabbit outer medullary collecting duct:inner stripe. Am J Physiol 248 (Renal Fluid Electrolyte Physiol 17):F500–F506
15. Andersen OS, Silveira JEN, Steinmetz PR (1985) Intrinsic characteristics of the proton pump in the luminal membrane of a tight urinary epithelium. The relation between transport rate and Δ $\bar{\mu}$H. J Gen Physiol 86:215–234
16. Stone DK, Crider BP, Xie XS (1990) Structure of vacuolar proton pumps. Semin Nephrol 10:159–165
17. Schuster VL (1990) Bicarbonate reabsorption and secretion in the cortical and outer medullary collecting tubule. Semin Nephrol 10:139–147
18. Verlander JW, Madsen KM, Low PS, Allen DP, Tisher CC (1988) Immunocytochemical localization of band 3 protein in the rat collecting duct. Am J Physiol 255 (Renal Fluid Electrolyte Physiol 24):F115–F125
19. Leslie BR, Schwartz JH, Steinmetz PR (1973) Coupling between Cl$^-$ absorption and HCO$_3$ secretion in turtle urinary bladder. Am J Physiol 255:610–617
20. McKinney TD, Burg MB (1978) Bicarbonate secretion by rabbit cortical collecting tubules in vitro. J Clin Invest 61:1421–1427
21. Stetson DL, Beauwens R, Palmisano J, Mitchell PP, Steinmetz PR (1985) A double-membrane model for urinary bicarbonate secretion. Am J Physiol 249 (Renal Fluid Electrolyte Physiol 18):F546–F552
22. Kohn OF, Mitchell PP, Steinmetz PR (1990) Characteristics of apical Cl-HCO$_3$ exchanger of bicarbonate-secreting cells in turtle bladder. Am J Physiol 258:F9–F14
23. Stetson DL (1989) Turtle urinary bladder:regulation of ion transport by dynamic changes in plasma membrane area. Am J Physiol 257:R973–R981
24. Schwartz GJ, Barasch J, Al-Awqati Q (1985) Plasticity of functional epithelial polarity. Nature 318:368–371
25. Schwartz JH, Bethencourt D, Rosen S (1982) Specialized function of carbonic anhydrase-rich and granular cells of turtle bladder. Am J Physiol 242 (Renal Fluid Electrolyte Physiol 11):F627–F633
26. Ridderstrale Y, Kashgarian M, Koeppen B, Giebisch G, Stetson D, Ardito T, Stanton B (1988) Morphological heterogeneity of the rabbit collecting duct. Kidney Int 34:655–670
27. Weiner ID, Hamm LL (1990) Regulation of intracellular pH in the rabbit cortical collecting tubule. J Clin Invest 85:274–281
28. Paillard M, Bichara M (1989) Peptide hormone effects on urinary acidification and acid-base balance: PTH, ADH, and glucagon. Am J Physiol 256:F973–F985
29. Good DW, Knepper MA (1990) Mechanisms of ammonium excretion:role of the renal medulla. Semin Nephrol 10:166–173

Osmolytes and Cell Osmoregulation in the Kidney

F.X. BECK, K. THURAU, M. SCHMOLKE,
and W.G. GUDER

Chair: Tadao Niijima

Osmolytes and Cell Osmoregulation in the Kidney

F.X. Beck, K. Thurau[1], M. Schmolke, and W.G. Guder[2]

Summary. The cells of the renal papilla are subject to widely varying extracellular osmolalities. In antidiuresis these cells are surrounded by hypertonic fluids, while in diuresis interstitial solute concentrations decline to levels comparable to those of the renal cortex. Papillary cells adapt to these extreme variations in extracellular tonicity by modulating the intracellular concentrations of small organic osmoeffectors (osmolytes), such as trimethylamines (glycerophosphorylcholine, betaine) and polyols (sorbitol, inositol). Variations in the intracellular concentrations of these osmolytes are accomplished by transmembrane net movement of water (cell swelling or shrinkage), by regulation of release and/or uptake of osmoeffectors via specific transmembrane transport pathways, and by changes in the intracellular synthesis of these organic compounds. These adaptive mechanisms allow intracellular electrolyte concentrations to remain relatively constant, despite extreme fluctuations in extracellular salinities. Accumulation of nonperturbing, organic osmolytes rather than inorganic electrolytes at high extracellular tonicities avoids the deleterious effects of elevated electrolyte concentrations on intracellular macromolecules. In addition, some of these osmolytes (trimethylamines) are assumed to counteract the adverse effects of high urea concentrations on the structure and function of cell proteins.

Introduction

The osmolality of the body fluids is maintained within narrow limits by the adequate response of the kidney to alterations in the organism's water balance. When water intake exceeds non-renal water loss and dilution of the body fluids develops, the kidney excretes the excess water, without major changes in solute excretion, by forming a hypoosmotic urine. On the other hand, during water shortage, the solutes to be

[1]Physiologisches Institut der Universität und [2]Institut für Klinische Chemie, Städtisches Krankenhaus München-Bogenhausen, 8000 Munich, Federal Republic of Germany

eliminated by the kidney are excreted in as small a volume of water as possible—hyperosmotic urine is produced.

The stability of the body fluids' osmolality contrasts sharply with the extreme variability of the renal medulla's solute concentrations. In antidiuresis, osmolalities many times higher than plasma osmolality prevail in the papilla, while in a state of diuresis papillary solute concentrations are decreased almost to isotonicity [1]. The cells of the renal medulla are thus subject to extreme changes in extracellular osmolality. In addition to this osmotic challenge, these cells are endangered by high urea concentrations in antidiuresis. This solute, which in the presence of antidiuretic hormone readily equilibrates across inner medullary cell membranes, may adversely affect the structure and function of cell proteins at these very high concentrations [2]. During the past few years concepts have emerged which allow us to explain how medullary cells are able not only to cope with extreme water stress, but also how they may escape the deleterious effects of high intracellular urea concentrations.

The study of intracellular electrolyte concentrations, in the rat renal papilla in antidiuresis, provided one of the first clues for the dominant role that organic osmolytes play in medullary cell osmoadaptation [3,4]. Using electron microprobe analysis on freeze-dried cryosections of the papillary tip, intracellular electrolyte concentrations were obtained which did not differ fundamentally from those of cells surrounded by isotonic fluids, such as proximal tubule cells [3,4]. These observations contrasted with earlier studies in which high sodium chloride concentrations, measured in medullary cells in antidiuresis, were assumed to balance the high extracellular salt concentrations (for review see [1]). Since, in antidiuresis, urea can be assumed to distribute freely across cell membranes, it is virtually certain that this substance does not impose any major osmotic stress on medullary cells. The finding of low cell sodium and chloride concentrations [3,4] implied that the high interstitial salt concentrations had to be balanced osmotically by equivalent concentrations of osmotically active substances, not directly detectable by electron microprobe analysis. For this phenomenon the term "osmotic gap" was coined (Fig. 1) [4]. Already at that time, it was clear that at least part of this gap could be filled by some organic osmoeffector, the so-called organic osmolytes.

Three classes of organic compounds must be considered as potential intracellular osmolytes: amino acids and their derivatives, methylamines, such as glycerophosphorylcholine and betaine, and polyols, such as sorbitol and inositol.

Although substantial amounts of amino acids and their derivatives (often assessed as ninhydrin-positive substances) have been demonstrated in the renal papilla, it is uncertain whether this group of osmolytes contributes significantly to cellular osmoadaptation, because high concentrations of amino acids have also been measured in extracellular compartments of the papilla [5]. In addition, information on the effect of alterations in the diuretic state on papillary amino acid contents is conflicting. While Law and Turner observed the concentrations of ninhydrin-positive substances to increase in papillary cells on exposure to hypertonic bathing solutions [6], Gullans and coworkers were unable to demonstrate any effect of water deprivation on papillary levels of ninhydrin-positive substances in vivo [7].

Analyses of the intrarenal distribution of glycerophosphorylcholine, betaine, sorbitol, and inositol have shown that substantial amounts of these osmolytes are present in the papillary tip in antidiuresis [8–12]. Since it is reasonable to assume that these compounds are located mainly in the intracellular compartment (see

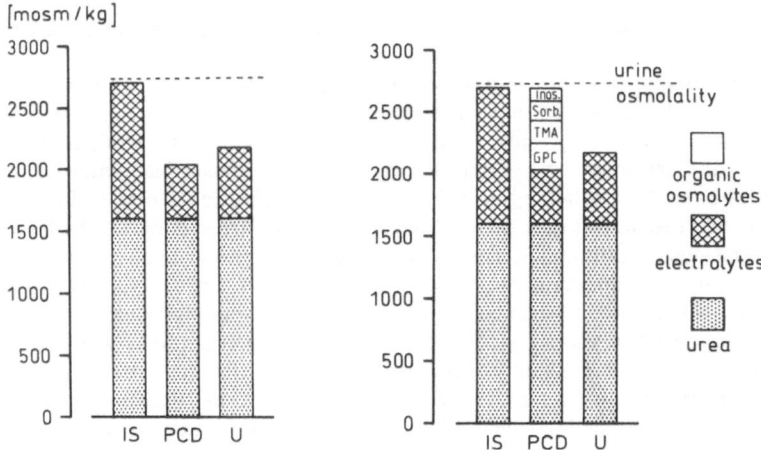

Fig. 1. Contribution of different osmoeffectors to total solute concentrations in the interstitium (*IS*), papillary collecting duct cells (*PCD*) and urine (*U*) in antidiuresis. The urea concentration and osmolality measured in the urine are assumed to exist in all tissue compartments. The contribution of inorganic electrolytes to total osmolality is assumed to be twice the sum of the sodium and potassium concentrations in a given compartment. The intracellular concentrations of glycerophosphorylcholine (*GPC*), other trimethylamines (*TMA*, mainly betaine), sorbitol (*sorb.*), and inositol (*inos.*) were calculated from total tissue contents of organic osmolytes, assuming the intracellular compartment to comprise 40% of papillary volume. (Adapted from [13])

below), and since the intracellular compartment comprises about 40% of total papillary tissue volume, estimates of intracellular concentrations of these organic osmolytes can be obtained [1,13]. These calculations suggest that most of the intracellular osmotic gap can be accounted for by trimethylamines and polyols (Fig. 1) [1,13].

Electron microprobe studies have also shown that the electrolyte concentrations of tubule cells in the inner stripe of the outer medulla are very similar to those of cortical tubule cells [14]. These results were taken to indicate that these cells achieve osmotic equilibrium with their hypertonic environment by accumulating organic osmolytes [1,14], as do inner papillary cells. Since the predominant osmolytes in the outer medulla are inositol and betaine (see below), it seems reasonable to assume that these osmoeffectors play a dominant role in the osmoadaptation of renal tubule cells located in the outer medulla.

Intrarenal Distribution of Organic Osmolytes During Different States of Diuresis

Methylamines

Glycerophosphoryl Choline (Fig. 2)

An analysis, by Ullrich and Pehling in the mid-fifties, of the spatial distribution of phosphorus-containing substances in the kidney showed the tissue content of an acid

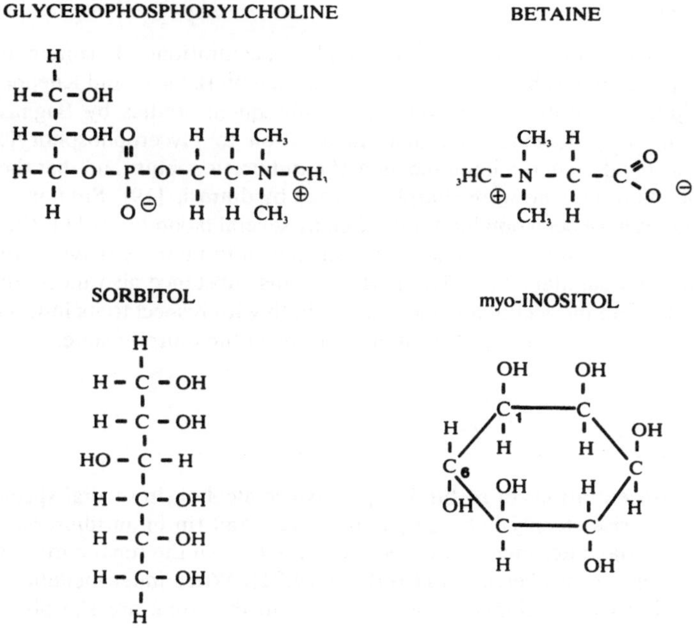

GLYCEROPHOSPHORYLCHOLINE   BETAINE

```
    H
    |
  H-C-OH
    |
  H-C-OH O      H  H  CH₃                 CH₃ H
    |    ||      |  |  |                    |   |      O
  H-C-O - P-O -C-C-N-CH₃             ₃HC - N - C - C⁄
    |    |      |  |  |  ⊕                ⊕ |   |     ⊙O
    H    O⊖     H  H  CH₃                 CH₃ H
```

SORBITOL   myo-INOSITOL

```
      H
      |
  H - C - OH                         OH    OH
      |                               |     |
  H - C - OH                   H      C₁----C      OH
      |                        |  ⁄   |     |   \  |
  HO - C - H                   C₆     H     H     C
      |                        |  \   OH    H  ⁄  |
  H - C - OH                   OH     C-----C     H
      |                               |     |
  H - C - OH                          H    OH
      |
  H - C - OH
      |
      H
```

Fig. 2. Structural formulae of four types of organic osmolytes

soluble phosphorus compound to increase steeply between the outer medulla and the papillary tip in antidiuresis [15]. The remarkable concentration gradient of this substance was greatly attenuated during water diuresis [15]. Three years later this substance was identified by Schimassek, Kohl, and Bücher as glycerophosphorylcholine [8]. An important role in the osmotic adaptation of papillary cells was ascribed to glycerophosphorylcholine by these authors [8]. Several studies conducted on different species have, since then, confirmed these early observations of steeply increasing concentrations of glycerophosphorylcholine along the cortico-papillary axis in antidiuresis [8–12,16–17]. This gradient is markedly attenuated during states associated with low urine osmolalities [9,11,15–17]. Hence, glycerophosphorylcholine meets two requirements of an intracellular osmolyte, namely, that tissue glycerophosphorylcholine contents rise in parallel with tissue osmolality between cortex and papillary tip and that they are changed appropriately by the diuretic state.

Several lines of evidence suggest that glycerophosphorylcholine is restricted to the intracellular compartment. Urine concentrations of glycerophosphorylcholine are very low, as are the phosphorus concentrations of both the interstitial and intravascular compartments of the papilla [3,4,9]. These extracellular spaces are thus excluded from containing substantial amounts of glycerophosphorylcholine. In addition, intracellular phosphorus concentrations are high and are closely related to interstitial sodium concentration [3]. Finally, in isolated papillary collecting ducts, glycerophosphorylcholine has been found in concentrations similar to those of tissue homogenates of total papillae [9,10,12].

Betaine (Fig. 2)

Using ^{14}N nuclear magnetic resonance, high concentrations of trimethylamines, other than glycerophosphorylcholine, were detected by Balaban and Knepper in the inner medulla of antidiuretic rabbits [18]. Subsequent studies by Bagnasco and coworkers directly demonstrated that, in addition to glycerophosphorylcholine, betaine was abundant in the inner medulla of antidiuretic rabbits and that these high tissue contents of betaine were sharply reduced by diuresis [19]. Similar results in various species have been obtained since then by several laboratories [11,17,20–22]. In addition, tissue levels of betaine have been shown to increase between the outer medulla and the papillary tip [11,23]. Hence, this substance also meets the basic requirements of an intracellular osmoeffector, both with respect to its intrarenal distribution pattern and in its response to alterations in the diuretic state.

Polyols

Sorbitol (Fig. 2)

The tissue concentrations of sorbitol, a polyhydric alcohol, in several species have been shown to rise steeply between papillary base and tip in antidiuresis (Fig. 3) [10–12,21]. In the outer medulla, tissue levels are low; in the renal cortex, sorbitol frequently even escapes detection [10–12,17,19,21]. When inner medullary osmolality is diminished by diuresis, sorbitol levels in this zone are sharply reduced [10–12,19–22]. A preferential intracellular localization of sorbitol can be inferred from the observation that papillary collecting ducts isolated from hydropenic rats contain high concentrations of sorbitol [10,12,24].

Inositol (Fig. 2)

The intrarenal distribution of inositol, a cyclic polyol, contrasts markedly to that of the trimethylamines and sorbitol, since the highest tissue contents of inositol are found in the outer, rather than in the inner medulla [11,12,17,25]. In fact, inositol levels tend to decrease between papillary base and tip. In most species investigated, though not in all [17], inositol levels in the papilla are significantly reduced by diuresis [11,12,20,22,25].

Metabolism and Transmembrane Transport of Organic Osmolytes

Trimethylamines

Glycerophosphorylcholine

Glycerophosphorylcholine is thought to be liberated from phosphatidylcholine (lecithin) via the sequential action of phospholipase(s) A [13,26]. A second, direct metabolic pathway, in which choline is transferred from cytidinediphosphocholine to glycerophosphate [13] is less likely, since isolated rat papillary collecting duct cells incorporate inorganic phosphate into phosphatidylcholine before the label appears in the glycerophosphorylcholine pool [27]. In addition, while biosynthesis of glycerophosphorylcholine is slow and exhibits a considerable time lag after addition of its

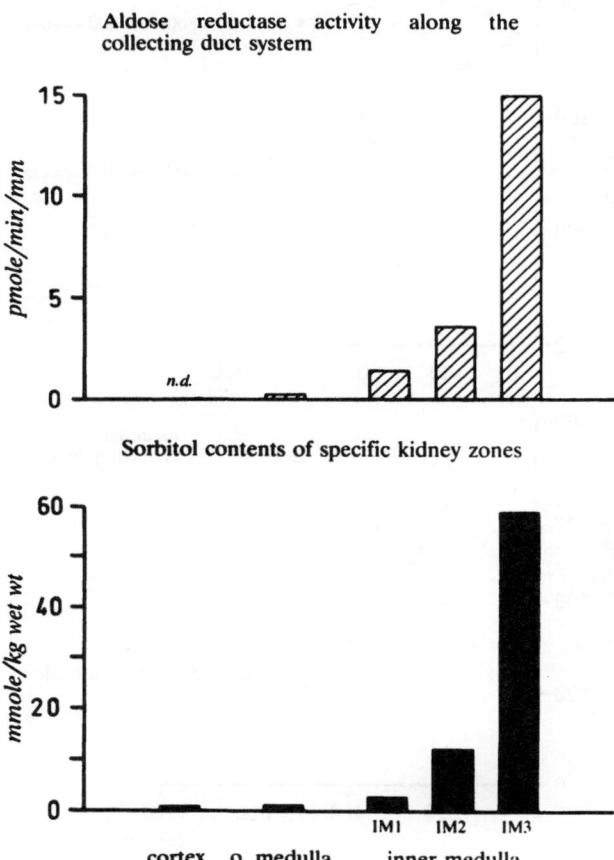

Fig. 3. Distribution of aldose reductase activity along the rat collecting duct system (*upper panel*). Sorbitol contents of different kidney zones (rat, antidiuresis) are shown *below*. (Adapted from [10,35])

precursors, the precursor choline is rapidly incorporated into tubular phospholipids [27]. The glycerophosphorylcholine degrading activity of papillary tissue has been shown to be low and not to be activated by diuresis [9]. On the other hand, isolated papillary collecting duct cells rapidly release glycerophosphorylcholine, without signs of osmotic cell rupture, when extracellular tonicity is reduced (Fig. 4) [12]. Available evidence thus suggests that the fall of the intracellular contents of glycerophosphorylcholine induced by diuresis is not due to enhanced intracellular degradation, but rather to activation of efflux into the extracellular compartment. At present, it is unclear whether uptake of glycerophosphorylcholine from the extracellular compartment into papillary cells contributes to the intracellular glycerophosphorylcholine pool. Likewise, information on the mechanisms mediating

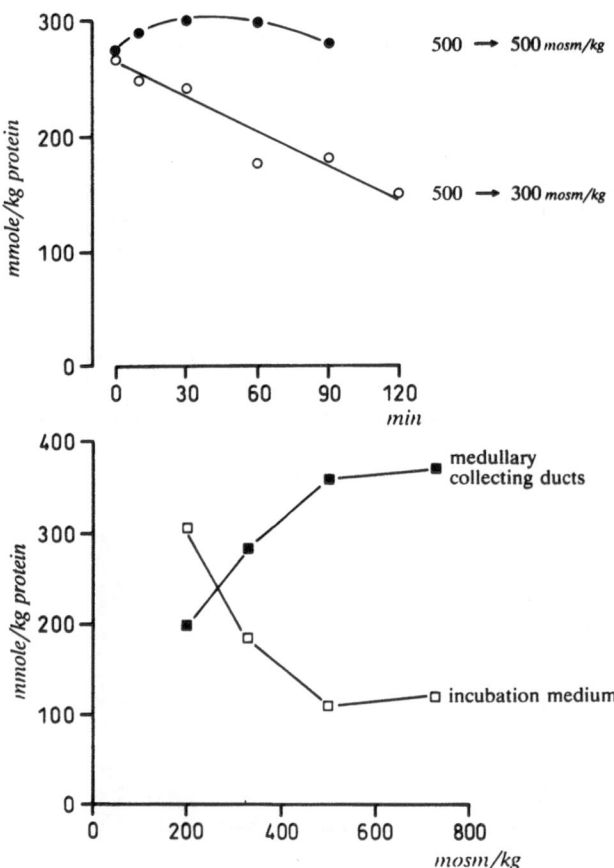

Fig. 4. Glycerophosphorylcholine contents of isolated papillary collecting ducts after transfer from hypertonic (500 mosm/kg) to isotonic (300 mosm/kg) incubation media (*upper panel*). Glycerophosphorylcholine contents of isolated collecting ducts and of the incubation media, measured after incubation (90 minutes) at different osmolalities, are shown in the *lower panel*. (Adapted from [12])

intracellular accumulation of glycerophosphorylcholine during the transition from diuresis to antidiuresis (reduced efflux enhanced uptake, enhanced liberation from phosphatidylcholine) is also scarce.

Betaine

Betaine is synthesized from choline via betaine aldehyde, a reaction which proceeds in mitochondria and is catalyzed by choline dehydrogenase and by betaine aldehyde dehydrogenase [26,28]. In the rabbit nephron, betaine synthesis has been found in proximal (S_3) and inner medullary tubules, but not in the thick ascending limb or in cortical and outer medullary collecting tubules. In accordance with these observations, betaine formed in vivo from labeled choline is rapidly accumulated in inner medulla and cortex in antidiuresis [29]. Grossmann and Hebert have shown choline dehydrogenase to be present in the inner medulla [28]. During chronic hypernatremia this enzyme was moderately stimulated in the medulla, but much more so in the cortex [28]. The uptake of the precursor choline into isolated papillary collecting ducts proceeds via a specific, sodium-independent transmembrane transport pathway [30]. This entry step is not stimulated by incubation in hypertonic bathing media [30], suggesting that modulation of choline uptake does not play a major role in regulating intracellular betaine levels, at least during acute changes of papillary osmolality. On the other hand, transport systems have been described which mediate uptake of betaine into renal tubule cells against steep transmembrane concentration gradients. This specific betaine transport has been shown in cortical tubule cells and in Madin-Darby canine kidney (MDCK) cells, a permanent line of renal tubule cells. Nakanishi and coworkers were able to demonstrate that a major portion of betaine uptake in MDCK cells is sodium-dependent and activated by chronic incubation in hypertonic media [31]. This raises the possibility that betaine synthesized in cortical tubules is taken up into medullary cells during hypertonic stress.

The response of intracellular betaine to decreasing extracellular concentrations of poorly permeable solutes has, as yet, not been studied directly in cells of the renal papilla. Investigations addressing this problem have, however, been performed on MDCK cells kept chronically in media of high tonicity. After switching the incubation medium from hypertonic to isotonic, betaine efflux from these cells rose significantly, while betaine uptake into the cells gradually declined [32].

Polyols

Sorbitol

Sorbitol is synthesized from glucose by the action of aldose reductase, and further metabolized to fructose by sorbitol dehydrogenase [13,26,33]. Glucose is taken up by papillary collecting duct cells via a sodium-independent mechanism, similar to that found in the basolateral membranes of proximal tubule cells [34]. Both enzymes of the sorbitol pathway, aldose reductase and sorbitol dehydrogenase, have been found in the renal inner medulla. Aldose reductase is present in all nephron segments of the renal medulla, as well as in the epithelium lining the papilla [33,35]. Studies on single nephron segments by Sands and coworkers have shown the activity of aldose reductase to increase steeply toward the tip of the papilla along both the collecting duct system (Fig. 3) and the thin descending and ascending limbs [35]. On the other hand, sorbitol dehydrogenase activity is much lower in the terminal papillary collecting duct than in proximal tubules [35]. These observations suggest that cell sorbitol contents may be regulated by changing aldose reductase, rather than sorbitol dehydrogenase, activity.

The sharp fall of tissue sorbitol contents in the inner medulla, seen after the transition from an antidiuretic to a diuretic state, is most likely due to rapid efflux of sorbitol out of medullary cells. Evidence for this has been obtained from in vitro experiments on isolated papillary collecting ducts, which demonstrate that sorbitol is rapidly released from the collecting duct cells when transferred from hypertonic to isotonic media [12,24]. Since the release of intracellular marker molecules, such as lactate dehydrogenase or ATP, was not increased by this experimental maneuver [12,24], this enhanced exit of sorbitol is not due to osmotic rupture of the cell membrane. The adaptation of intracellular sorbitol levels to acute alterations in extracellular tonicity is thus mainly achieved by alteration in sorbitol permeability of these cells. Changes in sorbitol efflux were not seen when urea was used to vary the osmolality of the incubation media [12].

The production of sorbitol, however, was not affected by acute reduction of extracellular solute concentration. Similarly, furosemide diuresis for 2 hours also failed to change aldose reductase activity [22]. The amount of aldose reductase mRNA in the papilla of the diuretic rats in this study, was, however, significantly reduced [22]. In agreement with these results, aldose reductase activities are diminished in the papilla of diabetes insipidus rats, in which interstitial tonicities are chronically low compared with normal rats [22]. The concept that cells in the renal medulla adjust their intracellular sorbitol levels to altered extracellular solute concentrations by rapid changes in cell sorbitol permeability and slow modulation of sorbitol synthesis is supported by observations on papillary cells in culture. In these cells, reduction of extracellular tonicity from 500 to 300 mosm/kg leads to rapid sorbitol efflux within a few minutes and to a slow fall of aldose reductase activity during the next few days [36].

One of the variables determining the production of sorbitol by inner medullary collecting duct cells is the glucose concentration of the incubation fluid [10,12]. It is, thus, not surprising that very high sorbitol levels are observed in the inner medulla of diabetic rats [23,37]. Grunewald and Kinne have shown that these high sorbitol contents are not due only to increased glucose availability, but are due also to enhanced aldose reductase activity in the inner medulla of diabetic rats [37]. Despite augmented capacity for sorbitol production, sorbitol permeability is not increased in these cells. This imbalance of sorbitol production and sorbitol release may contribute to necrosis of the inner medulla, which is a late complication in diabetes.

Inositol

The cyclic polyol, inositol, is an essential precursor of inositol-containing phospholipids and of inositolpolyphosphates which act as second messengers in a variety of cells. Inositol derives from D-glucose via three consecutive enzymatic steps: Myoinositol 1-phosphate synthase acts on glucose-6-phosphate to form L-myo-inositol 1-phosphate. This is utilized subsequently by myo-inositol 1-phosphate phosphatase to produce myo-inositol [13,26]. Inositol can also be liberated from phosphatidylinositol via D-inositol 1-phosphate [26]. Up to now, it is, however, not completely clear whether intracellular accumulation of inositol in the outer and inner medulla occurs via these pathways. There is evidence that inositol can be catabolized to CO_2 via the glucuronate-xylulose pathway in the cortex and medulla, but not in the papilla [13].

On the other hand, specific uptake mechanisms for inositol have been demonstrated in MDCK cells. These transport pathways are activated by chronic incubation in hypertonic or inositol-free media, and they accomplish sodium-dependent inositol uptake against steep transmembrane inositol gradients [38]. If a similar transport system is also responsible for inositol uptake in renal medullary cells in vivo, the increase in extracellular sodium concentration during the transition from a diuretic to an antidiuretic state may help to achieve steep transmembrane inositol gradients.

Inositol is rapidly released from isolated papillary collecting duct cells on transfer from hypertonic incubation medium to a medium of lower tonicity [12]. Inositol efflux appears to proceed via specific pathways and appears not to be caused by osmotic rupture of cell membranes, since the release of marker molecules for cellular integrity, such as ATP or lactate dehydrogenase, was not increased by reducing extracellular tonicity [12]. Similar observations have been made in MDCK cells [32].

The major regulatory mechanisms responsible for the adjustment of intracellular inositol levels appear to be the appropriate modulation of inositol efflux and uptake. While changes in inositol permeability appear to constitute the short-term response to altered extracellular tonicity, alterations in inositol uptake become effective only after long-term perturbation of extracellular tonicity.

Information on the signals which trigger the increase or decrease of intracellular levels of organic osmolytes is scanty. Antidiuretic hormone, an obvious candidate, is probably not involved directly in the regulation of intracellular osmolytes, since studies on Brattleboro rats have shown that there is a considerable delay between the rise in urine osmolality and the increase of osmolytes in the papillary tissue [39]. In addition, accumulation of osmolytes in MDCK cells, in response to elevated extracellular tonicity, is partially inhibited by antidiuretic hormone [40]. The induction of aldose reductase has been studied in greater detail in a line of renal cells derived from the papillary surface epithelium. In these cells, expression of aldose reductase correlated with an increase in cell potassium concentration, but even better with an increase in the sum of intracellular sodium plus potassium concentrations [41]. This observation suggests that a rise in intracellular ionic strength may play an important role in the regulation of sorbitol production. Another variable influencing intracellular accumulation of sorbitol is the concentration of glucose in the extracellular compartment. In several studies, a clear correlation between extracellular glucose concentration and cell sorbitol levels was demonstrated [12,37]. Recent evidence suggests that increased intracellular calcium activities may contribute to the release of sorbitol from papillary collecting duct cells after hypotonic stress [42].

Even less is known about the factor which regulate intracellular levels of inositol and methylamines. Uptake of sorbitol, betaine, and inositol is modulated by the intracellular concentration of the respective osmolyte. When high intracellular concentrations of these osmolytes are reached, the uptake (inositol, betaine) or the production (sorbitol) slows [23,31,38,43]. It is conceivable, that, as for aldose reductase, the uptake of osmolytes or their precursors depends in some way on intracellular ionic strength. Such a betaine uptake system is well characterized in bacteria. This transporter contributes significantly to the osmotic adaptation of these cells to hypertonicity. The expression of a gene (proU) which codes for this betaine transporter is greatly stimulated by increased cell potassium concentrations [44].

Response of Inner Medullary Cells to Hyper- and Hypotonic Stress

Changes in intracellular concentrations of organic osmolytes may, however, be caused not only by changing the amount of intracellular organic osmoeffectors, but also by changing the amount of cell water. Electron microprobe studies on freeze-dried cryosections show the volume of papillary cells to increase when interstitial tonicity decreases [4]. Water shifts across the cell membranes, which are associated with dilution or passive concentration of intracellular osmoeffectors, may thus contribute to the osmotic adaptation of medullary cells. Moreover, these cell volume changes seem to persist in vivo for prolonged periods, because they could still be observed several hours after the onset of diuresis [4]. Complete volume regulation was, however, seen in isolated perfused papillary collecting ducts [45]. In these studies, elevation of extracellular tonicity induced cell shrinkage and subsequent restoration of cell volume by uptake of sodium and chloride via parallel Na-H-and Cl-HCO$_3$-exchangers [45]. The volume regulatory decrease was dependent on the presence of ADH in the peritubular bathing solution. On the other hand, complete volume regulation after hyperosmotic stress was not observed in a cell line derived from the papillary surface epithelium [41] and in the renal papillary surface epithelium in vitro [46].

The response of medullary cells to environmental hypertonic stress may thus comprise three phases. First, osmometric water efflux into the extracellular compartment produces cell shrinkage, with passive concentration of intracellular inorganic and organic osmoeffectors. Second, the subsequent activation of sodium and chloride uptake mechanisms favors restoration of cell volume. Enhanced entry of sodium can be assumed to stimulate active pump-mediated Na-K-exchange, so that in this phase increased amounts of intracellular potassium chloride primarily mediate cell osmoadaptation. Cell volume recovery in vivo is probably incomplete, so that cell concentrations of organic osmolytes may already be elevated at this stage, due to persistent moderate cell shrinkage. In the third phase, transport or/and metabolic pathways of organic osmolytes are modulated so as to attain increased cell levels of these osmoeffectors. This allows reduction of monovalent electrolyte concentrations to steady state values — thereby achieving full osmotic adaptation.

Lowering extracellular tonicity is associated with cell swelling and concomitant dilution of intracellular osmoeffectors. Subsequent stimulation of potassium chloride efflux may accomplish partial volume recovery. Even at this stage, exit of organic osmolytes may participate in the adaptive response. The final osmotic adjustments are achieved by appropriate modulation of those transport and metabolic pathways responsible for setting the intracellular levels of organic osmolytes.

Functional Advantages of Organic Osmolytes

For the cells of the renal medulla, the strategy of accumulating organic osmolytes, rather than inorganic electrolytes, in antidiuresis is advantageous in several respects [1,2].

First, high concentrations of inorganic electrolytes are known to perturb the structure and function of proteins [2]. This is well known from in vitro experiments, in which specific functional properties of enzymes, such as affinities and maximal turnover rates, are greatly diminished by increasing salt concentrations in the incubation medium. These adverse effects on enzyme function can be avoided if the solute concentration is increased by the addition of organic osmolytes, such as betaine, glycine, or trimethylamine oxide, rather than inorganic electrolytes.

Due to these non-perturbing properties, these osmoeffectors have been termed "compatible" osmolytes.

The second advantage concerns the role of urea. In antidiuresis, a major portion of total intracellular osmolality in the papilla is made up by urea. In the rat, for instance, urea concentrations of 1500 mmole/l or more are observed at the tip of the papilla [1]. These urea concentrations are high enough to destabilize protein structure and severely impair protein function. Trimethylamines have been shown to counteract this destabilizing effect of urea [2]. Trimethylamines, thus, may serve not only as *compatible* osmoeffectors, but also as *counteracting* osmoeffectors. Although the underlying mechanism is not completely understood, the most popular view is that these trimethylamines stabilize hydrogen bonds and are thus able to impair the weakening of these intramolecular bonds by urea. The native state of proteins is thus conserved and the unfolding of proteins is impeded.

Finally, the ability of renal papillary cells to respond to increased extracellular salt concentrations, with accumulation of organic osmolytes, allows the retention of low cell sodium concentrations. This is important because many transmembrane transport pathways, such as Na-H- and Na-Ca-exchange, rely on steep transmembrane sodium gradients. It is thus likely that high intracellular sodium concentrations would compromise cell proton and cell calcium homeostasis. In addition, intracellular accumulation of certain organic osmolytes themselves, such as betaine and inositol, is sodium-dependent and thus relies on steep transmembrane sodium gradients (see above).

Finally, it should be remembered that, in vivo, the alterations of extracellular tonicity during the transition from diuresis to antidiuresis, and vice versa, are gradual, rather than abrupt. This implies that the different phases of cell osmoadaptation in the papilla, enumerated above, are most likely not strictly separated, but may represent a continuum of states, in which activation and/or suppression of transport pathways for inorganic electrolytes and organic osmolytes, as well as metabolism of organic osmolytes, occurs in a coordinate and well balanced manner.

Acknowledgments. Studies carried out in the authors' laboratories were supported by grants from the Deutsche Forschungsgemeinschaft (Be 963/2-2, 2-3; Gu 82/3-2, 3-3).

References

1. Beck FX, Dörge A, Thurau K (1988) Cellular osmoregulation in renal medulla. Renal Physiol Biochem 11:174–186
2. Yancey PH, Clark ME, Hand SC, Bowlus RD, Somero GN (1982) Living with water stress: evolution of osmolyte systems. Science 217:1214–1222
3. Beck F, Dörge A, Rick R, Thurau K (1984) Intra- and extracellular element concentrations of rat renal papilla in antidiuresis. Kidney Int 25:397–403
4. Beck F, Dörge A, Rick R, Thurau K (1985) Osmoregulation of renal papillary cells. Pflügers Arch 405:S28–S32
5. Dantzler WH, Silbernagl S (1988) Amino acid transport by juxtamedullary nephrons: distal reabsorption and recycling. Am J Physiol 255:F397–F407
6. Law RO, Turner DPJ (1987) Are ninhydrin-positive substances volume-regulatory osmolytes in rat renal papillary cells? J Physiol 386:45–61

7. Gullans SR, Blumenfeld JD, Balschi JA, Kaleta M, Brenner RM, Heilig CW, Hebert SC (1988) Accumulation of major organic osmolytes in rat renal inner medulla in dehydration. Am J Physiol 255:F626–F634

8. Schimassek H, Kohl D, Bücher T (1959) Glycerylphosphorylcholine, die Nierensubstanz "Ma-Mark" von Ullrich. Biochem Z 331:87–97

9. Wirthensohn G, Beck FX, Guder WG (1987) Role and regulation of glycerophosphoryl-choline in rat renal papilla. Pflügers Arch 409:411–415

10. Wirthensohn G, Lefrank S, Guder WG, Beck FX (1987) Studies on the role of glycerophosphorylcholine and sorbitol in renal osmoregulation. In: Kovacevic Z, Guder WG (eds) Molecular nephrology: biochemical aspects of kidney function. Walter de Gruyter, Berlin, pp 321–327

11. Yancey PH, Burg MB (1989) Distribution of major organic osmolytes in rabbit kidneys in diuresis and antidiuresis. Am J Physiol 257:F602–F607

12. Wirthensohn G, Lefrank S, Schmolke M, Guder WG (1989) Regulation of organic osmolyte concentrations in tubules from rat renal inner medulla. Am J Physiol 256: F128–F135

13. Beck FX, Dörge A, Thurau K, Guder WG (1990) Cell osmoregulation in the countercur-rent system of the renal medulla: The role of organic osmolytes. In: Beyenbach KW (ed) Cell volume regulation, comp physiol. Karger, Basel, pp 132–158

14. Beck FX, Dörge A, Ring T, Sauer M (1989) Element composition of tubule cells in the inner stripe of the renal outer medulla. Miner Electrolyte Metab 15:144–149

15. Ullrich KJ, Pehling G (1956) Über das Vorkommen von Phosphorverbindungen in ver-schiedenen Nierenabschnitten und Änderungen ihrer Konzentration in Abhängigkeit vom Diuresezustand. Pflügers Arch 262:551–561

16. Philippson C (1964) Der Gehalt an Glycerylphosphorylcholin und Glycerylphosphoryl-äthanolamin von Nierenmark und Nierenrinde hochreiner Wistarratten während forcierter Wasserdiurese und extrem langer Durst-Antidiurese. Pflügers Arch 280:30–37

17. Yancey PH (1988) Osmotic effectors in kidneys of xeric and mesic rodents: corticomedul-lary distributions and changes with water availability. J Comp Physiol 158:369–380

18. Balaban RS, Knepper MA (1983) Nitrogen-14 nuclear magnetic resonance spectroscopy of mammalian tissues. Am J Physiol 245:C439–C444

19. Bagnasco S, Balaban R, Fales HM, Yang YM, Burg M (1986) Predominant osmotically active organic solutes in rat and rabbit renal medullas. J Biol Chem 261:5872–5877

20. Wolff SD, Stanton TS, James SL, Balaban RS (1989) Acute regulation of the predominant organic solutes of the rabbit renal inner medulla. Am J Physiol 257:F676–F681

21. Chambers ST, Kunin CM (1987) Osmoprotective activity for Escherichia coli in mam-malian renal inner medulla and urine. Correlation of glycine and proline betaines and sor-bitol with response to osmotic loads. J Clin Invest 80:1255–1260

22. Cowley BD, Ferraris JD, Carper D, Burg M (1990) In vivo osmoregulation of aldose reduc-tase mRNA, protein, and sorbitol in renal medulla. Am J Physiol 258:F154–F161

23. Guder WG, Beck FX, Schmolke M (1991) Organic compounds in renal volume regulation. Proceedings of the XIth Congress of nephrology, July 15–20 1990. Springer, Tokyo Berlin Heidelberg.

24. Grunewald RW, Kinne RKH (1989) Intracellular sorbitol content in isolated rat inner medullary collecting duct. Pflügers Arch 414:178–184

25. Cohen MA, Hruska KA, Daughaday WH (1982) Free myo-inositol in canine kidneys: selective concentration in the renal medulla. Proc Soc Exp Biol Med 169:380–385

26. Wolff SD, Balaban RS (1990) Regulation of the predominant renal medullary organic solutes in vivo. Annu Rev Physiol 52:727–746

27. Schmolke M, Bornemann A, Guder WG (to be published) Distribution and regulation of organic osmolytes along the nephron. In: Koide H, Endou H, Kurokawa K (eds) Cell biol-ogy of nephron heterogeneity: fine structure and functions. Karger, Basel

28. Grossman EB, Hebert SC (1989) Renal inner medullary choline dehydrogenase activity: characterization and modulation. Am J Physiol 256:F107-F112
29. Eng J, Berkowitz BA, Balaban RS (to be published) Renal distribution and metabolism of [^{2}H$_9$]choline. A^{2}H NMR and MRI study. NMR Biomed
30. Bevan C, Kinne RKH (1990) Choline transport in collecting duct cells isolated from the rat renal inner medulla. Pflügers Arch 417:324-328
31. Nakanishi T, Turner RJ, Burg MB (1990) Osmoregulation of betaine transport in mammalian renal medullary cells. Am J Physiol 258:F1061-F1067
32. Nakanishi T, Burg MB (1989) Osmoregulatory fluxes of myo-inositol and betaine in renal cells. Am J Physiol 257:C964-C970
33. Terubayashi H, Sato S, Nishimura C, Kador PF, Kinoshita JH (1989) Localization of aldose and aldehyde reductase in the kidney. Kidney Int 36:843-851
34. Grunewald RW, Kinne RKH (1988) Sugar transport in isolated rat kidney papillary collecting duct cells. Pflügers Arch 413:32-37
35. Sands JM, Terada Y, Bernard LM, Knepper MA (1989) Aldose reductase activities in microdissected rat renal tubule segments. Am J Physiol 256:F563-F569
36. Bagnasco S, Murphy HR, Bedford JJ, Burg MB (1988) Osmoregulation by slow changes in aldose reductase and rapid changes in sorbitol flux. Am J Physiol 254:C788-C792
37. Grunewald RW, Kinne RKH (1989) Sorbitol metabolism in inner medullary collecting duct cells of diabetic rats. Pflugers Arch 414:346-350
38. Nakanishi T, Turner RJ, Burg MB (1989) Osmoregulatory changes in myoinositol transport by renal cells. Proc Natl Acad Sci USA 86:6002-6006
39. Schmolke M, Beck FX, Guder WG (1989) Effect of antidiuretic hormone on renal organic osmolytes in Brattleboro rats. Am J Physiol 257:F732-F737
40. Heilig CW, Brenner BM, Yu ASL, Kone BC, Gullans SR (1990) Modulation of osmolytes in MDCK cells by solutes, inhibitors, and vasopressin. Am J Physiol 259:F653-F659
41. Uchida S, Garcia-Perez A, Murphy HR, Burg M (1989) Signal for induction of aldose reductase in renal medullary cells by high external NaCl. Am J Physiol 256:C614-C620
42. Bevan C, Theiss C, Kinne RKH (1990) Role of Ca^{2+} in sorbitol release from rat inner medullary collecting duct (IMCD) cells under hypoosmotic stress. Biochem Biophys Res Comm 170:563-568
43. Moriyama T, Garcia-Perez A, Burg MB (1989) Osmotic regulation of aldose reductase protein synthesis in renal medullary cells. J Biol Chem 264:16810-16814
44. Epstein W (1986) Osmoregulation by potassium transport in Escherichia coli. FEMS Microbiol Rev 39:73-78
45. Sun A, Hebert SC (1989) Rapid hypertonic cell volume regulation in perfused inner medullary collecting duct. Kidney Int 36:831-842
46. Sands JM, Knepper MA, Spring KR (1986) Na-K-Cl cotransport in apical membrane of rabbit renal papillary surface epithelium. Am J Physiol 251:F475-F484

The Pathogenesis of Tubulointerstitial Nephritis

PETER S. HEEGER, GUNTER WOLF
and ERIC G. NEILSON

Chair: Priscilla Kincaid-Smith

The Pathogenesis of Tubulointerstitial Nephritis

PETER S. HEEGER, GUNTER WOLF, and ERIC G. NEILSON[1]

SUMMARY. Tubulointerstitial nephritis is a common form of both acute and chronic renal disease in humans. Over the last 12 years we have been studying the pathogenic mechanisms involved in tubulointerstitial nephritis, using several animal models which are similar to distinct forms of human interstitial injury. The immunopathogenesis of tubulointerstitial nephritis can be arbitrarily divided into three phases. The afferent, or antigen recognition phase, involves expression of the nephritogenic antigen, recognition and presentation of the nephritogenic antigen in the context of appropriate MHC determinants, and circumvention of the usual mechanisms of tolerance. The immunoregulatory phase consists of multiple counter-regulatory events, both humoral and cell-mediated, that influence the amplitude and qualitative nature of the immune response. The final, effector, phase includes the various mechanisms directly responsible for tubulointerstitial injury and subsequent fibrosis. Additionally, once the immune response has been initiated, a number of factors can influence the progression of tubulointerstitial injury toward end stage renal disease.

Introduction

Tubulointerstitial nephritis accounts for up to 15% of cases of acute renal failure, and as many as 25% of cases of chronic renal failure have been ascribed to the long term sequelae of this disease [1,2]. Additionally, interstitial inflammation and subsequent fibrosis occur in most forms of renal failure resulting in end stage renal disease, regardless of the primary etiology. The significance of this form of renal disease is underscored by morphometric correlations suggesting that changes in tubular function and glomerular filtration rate correlate more strongly with histologic deteriora-

[1] Renal-Electrolyte Section of the Department of Medicine, and the Cell Biology and Immunology Graduate Groups, University of Pennsylvania, Philadelphia, PA 19104–6144, USA

Table 1. Immune mechanisms of tubulointerstitial nephritis

Immune mechanism	Animal model	Human disease
Immune deposit disease	NZB/W mouse or immunization with Tamm-Horsefall protein	Systemic lupus erythematosis Sjögren's syndrome Planted antigens Drugs Infections
Anti-TBM disease	Anti-TBM models in rats, mice, and guinea pigs	Drugs Idiopathic Renal transplantation Anti-GBM disease
Primarily cell-mediated disease	Spontaneous TIN in kdkd mice	Infections Drugs Pyelonephritis Medullary cystic disease Idiopathic

tion of interstitial architecture than with changes in glomerular structure. Our laboratory has long been interested in elucidating the pathogenic mechanisms involved in the initiation, regulation, expression, and progression of tubulointerstitial nephritis, and it is the purpose of this report to summarize some of our views. Due to space limitations, many of the references cited herein are recent, fully referenced review articles.

Although virtually all forms of human tubulointerstitial nephritis probably have an immune basis regardless of etiology, most of the information on pathogenesis of this disease comes from animal models [1–3]. There are three distinct immunohistological forms that can be recognized (Table 1). First, immune deposits, usually formed in situ through the reaction of antibodies with planted antigen, can mediate the inflammatory response. Preformed circulating immune complexes preferentially deposit in the glomerulus, and are not commonly implicated as causative in tubulointerstitial nephritis. Subsequent to immune complex deposition, activation of complement, and infiltration by polymorphonuclear leukocytes and lymphocytes eventually result in interstitial fibrosis. Animal models providing insight into this form of tubulointerstitial nephritis include the NZB/W mouse, as well as mice immunized with Tamm-Horsfall protein [3]. In humans, tubulointerstitial nephritis associated with immune deposits has been observed with lupus erythematosus and Sjögren's syndrome, and accompanies various forms of glomerulonephritis [2,3].

Secondly, anti-tubular basement membrane (anti-TBM) antibodies can promote tubulointerstitial nephritis. Anti-TBM disease can be induced in mice, rats, and guinea pigs following immunization with heterologous renal tubular antigens [3,4]. After 2 weeks, circulating antibodies and a linear deposition of IgG along the TBM can be observed by immunofluorescence. Later, mononuclear cells infiltrate the tubulointerstitium and progressive interstitial fibrosis ensues. Although both the humoral and cell-mediated arms of the immune system are activated in all forms of anti-TBM disease, the relative contribution of these arms toward disease expression varies between the different models studied [1–3]. Anti-TBM disease may occur in humans as a complication of drug therapy, infection, after renal transplantation, following Goodpasture's syndrome, or in an idiopathic form [2].

Finally, polymorphonuclear and mononuclear cell infiltration can occur in the absence of antibody deposition. Spontaneous tubulointerstitial nephritis in the kdkd mouse is an experimental model of this cell-mediated injury [5]. Similar lesions are found in human tubulointerstitial disease after chronic obstructive pyelonephritis and hydronephrosis, and in medullary cystic disease [2].

The pathogenesis of tubulointerstitial nephritis can be arbitrarily divided into three general phases [1,6]. Antigen recognition, the afferent phase, begins with the loss of tolerance to self-antigens, and loss of the genetically determined ability to respond to foreign antigens. The second immunoregulatory phase comprises protective processes that influence the amplitude and qualitative nature of the immune response. The final efferent, or effector, phase includes the mechanisms directly responsible for producing interstitial damage. These processes, as well as factors influencing disease progression once established, will be discussed in the ensuing sections.

Antigen Recognition Phase

Initiation of an autoimmune response requires the overcoming of protective mechanisms that result in tolerance to self-antigens. Tolerance to one's own parenchymal tissues can occur through failure of antigen to properly associate with MHC molecules on the surface of antigen presenting cells, through clonal deletion in the thymus or peripheral clonal anergy of self-reactive T cells, or through the action of specific suppressor cells [1].

Target antigen

The first and foremost factor in overcoming tolerance is that the inciting antigen must be present, and must be accessible to the immune system. The antigen may be endogenous, or may result from exposure to exogenous agents. Infectious agents (particularly viruses), can provide appropriate target antigens through molecular mimicry, or may damage interstitial tissues through toxic mechanisms and thereby expose novel immunogenic antigens [7]. Drugs can also act as hapten bridges to the tubulointerstitium, and can target the immune response towards previously unrecognized self-antigens [1].

The target antigen of murine anti-TBM disease is called 3M-1 [8]. It was recently identified as a glycoprotein with a molecular weight of 30–48 Kd, and can be localized to the lateral site of proximal tubular basement membrane. This nephritogenic antigen is expressed in an autosomal dominant pattern and is controlled by a single group of genes which are independent of the MHC, but closely linked to the gene for albinism on the first linkage group [9]. Using a monoclonal anti-3M-1 antibody, a closely related antigen with a similar molecular weight was isolated from the kidney of a human patient, suggesting significant evolutionary conservation [10]. Not all mammals tested have an accessible form of this antigen, however. Lewis rats, a strain not susceptible to anti-TBM disease following immunization with heterologous renal tubular antigen, do not bind anti-TBM antibodies in a linear pattern [3]. These animals develop circulating serum anti-TBM antibodies, however, and in vitro collagenase solubilization of the TBM preparations uncovers anti-TBM binding, implying that the reactive epitopes are normally sequestered from the immune system.

Additionally, 3M-1 may be absent in certain humans, explaining the development of anti-TBM disease after kidney transplantation (the recipient does not express the antigen but is given a graft that does, resulting in an immune response) [2]. Recently, screening of a cDNA expression library from murine proximal tubule cells has resulted in the isolation of a unique family of isoforms with transcripts of 1.7–1.9 kb, encoding the 3M-1 antigen [11]. These genes, and their transcripts, can be localized to tubular epithelium by in situ hybridization (E.G. Neilson unpublished observations). A synthetic peptide deduced from the cDNA framework region binds anti-3M-1 monoclonal antibodies and can function as specific antigen for a 3M-1 reactive helper T cell line (E.G. Neilson unpublished observations).

MHC Determinants

Effector T-cells recognize their target antigen in the context of specific MHC-determinants, thus defining genetic restriction. Murine anti-TBM disease, for example, is genetically restricted, and maps, in an autosomal dominant fashion, to H-2K^{s} [12]. The induction of anti-TBM disease, or its aberrant expression in normally non-susceptible animals, also depends on the visibility of MHC class II determinants. These have traditionally been localized to the surface of macrophages, dendritic cells, or B lymphocytes. More recently, however, it has been appreciated that epithelial cells (including renal tubular cells) can act as antigen-secreting, as well as antigen-presenting, cells, and may express class II MHC molecules under certain conditions. We have shown in an in vitro system that a proximal tubular cell line secreting the 3M-1 target antigen (MCT cells) can present this self-antigen to syngeneic T helper cells in the context of class II MHC determinants [13,14]. Furthermore, treatment of MCT cells with γ-interferon increases the expression of class II molecules on the cell surface [14]. Interestingly, exogenous interferon treatment of a mouse strain that is normally not susceptible to anti-TBM disease converts this mouse to a susceptible strain. On the other hand, anti-tubular basement membrane antibodies, which bind to tubular epithelium, protectively down regulate the transcription and subsequent surface expression of class II MHC determinants on tubular cells [14]. The regulation of MHC class II determinants in the kidney is closely modulated by the immune repertoires expressing interstitial disease.

Other Factors

Despite the presence and accessibility of a target antigen and its association with the appropriate MHC molecule, other factors may lead to tolerance, and inhibit the expression of disease. Clonal deletion of specific reactive T cells during ontogeny could theoretically prevent the autoimmune response. There are, however, no major detectable differences yet, other than genetic restriction and selected cell phenotype, in the recognition properties of the T cell repertoires in mice that are susceptible or nonsusceptible to anti-TBM disease [1]. In addition, there is no evidence that clonal anergy, the inability of a T cell clone to react to an appropriately recognized antigen-MHC complex, plays a role in the susceptibility to anti-TBM disease.

Tolerance, of course, can also be overcome through the effects of regulatory T lymphocytes. Suppressor T cells can actively inhibit the activation of specific helper or effector T cells, despite their appropriate recognition of the antigen-MHC complex.

Since suppression is also an important immunoregulatory mediator, relevant examples will be discussed in the next section.

Immune Regulatory Phase

Activation of the nephritogenic T and B cell repertoires is normally self-limited by specific down regulatory events. These regulatory events are controlled either by complementary interactions in the immune repertoire, or by the immunologic visibility of the target antigen. In anti-TBM disease, helper T cells responding to tubulointerstitial antigens (after circumventing the above mentioned mechanisms of tolerance) induce the differentiation of nephritogenic effector T cells and anti-TBM antibody secreting B cells, and are thus central participants in these immunoregulatory events [1].

In Brown Norway rats, anti-TBM antibody production and cell-mediated events are quantitatively and temporally related to the expression of disease [1,3]. It has been demonstrated in our laboratory that an anti-idiotypic humoral immune response can modulate the idiotypic humoral and cell-mediated responses in this model [3,15]. Exogenous anti-idiotypic antibodies decrease the delayed-type hypersensitivity (DTH) response to renal tubular antigen, as well as limit disease progression, even if administered two weeks after initial immunization. Rats that are not susceptible to anti-TBM disease develop their own anti-idiotypic network upon immunization, which prevents disease [3]. The Brown Norway rat, however, does not normally develop an anti-idiotype response. This is due to the emergence of a specific suppressor cell that inhibits clonal expansion of these T and B cells. Idiotypically marked humoral and cell-mediated (anti-renal tubular antigen) responses thus go unchecked, leading to disease expression [1,3,15]. Additionally, a suppressor network can be induced in Brown Norway rats through immunization with renal tubular antigen and incomplete Freund's adjuvant. The induced suppressor cells have a cross-reactive idiotype to anti-TBM antibodies, and are able to specifically decrease production of anti-TBM antibodies, as well as abrogate disease progression [3].

The regulatory events involved in murine anti-TBM disease are somewhat analogous (Fig. 1). Antibody quality and quantity, however, do not differ between susceptible and nonsusceptible strains of mice. As discussed in the previous section, however, anti-TBM antibodies can down regulate the transcription of MHC class II molecules, and therefore decrease the immunologic visibility of available antigen. The important role of cell-mediated immune responses operating in anti-TBM disease was largely worked out in mice [1]. An antigen-specific, I-A restricted, CD4+ helper T cell (Th) emerges first, and is an essential mediator of subsequent events [16]. This helper cell induces both a CD4+ and a CD8+ effector cell (Te) early in the immune response of both susceptible and nonsusceptible mice [1]. The CD4+ effector cells recognize antigen in vitro, are class II restricted, but have difficulty normally recognizing relevant tubular antigen locally within the kidney. These cells preferentially emerge in nonsusceptible mouse strains [1]. The nephritogenic class I restricted CD8+ effector cell emerges in susceptible strains and directly causes disease. Nonsusceptible mice have such CD8+ effector cells, but their clonal expansion is inhibited by other regulatory T cells residing in the immune system [1]. These CD8+, I-J+ suppressor cells (Ts) prevent the emergence of the CD8+ effector cells.

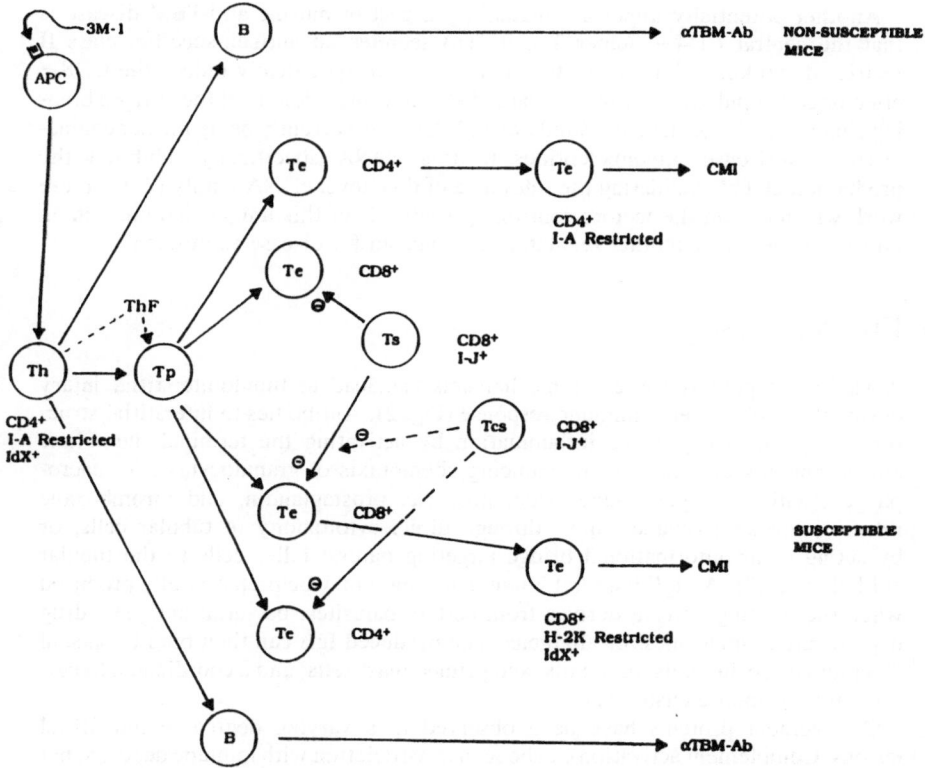

Fig. 1. Development of the immune response in murine anti-TBM disease. See text for explanation. APC, antigen presenting cell; B, B lymphocyte; Th, helper T lymphocyte; ThF, helper
factor; Tp, undifferentiated precursor T lymphocyte; Te, effector T lymphocyte; Ts, suppressor
T lymphocyte; Tcs, contrasuppressor T lymphocyte; CMI, cell mediated immune response;
IdX+, idiotype +

In susceptible mice, the disease-protective suppressor cells are subverted, in turn, by
CD8+, class I restricted contrasuppressor cells (Tcs), allowing immune injury to
occur [17]. Immune regulation of effector T cell preference thus critically determines
susceptibility to the development of anti-TBM disease [1,17].

Suppression is also an important influence on the expression of disease in the kdkd
mouse model of tubulointerstitial nephritis. The kdkd mouse is a congenic subline of
the CBA/Ca mouse, and is uniquely susceptible to a spontaneous, CD8+ T cell-
mediated, autosomally dominant tubulointerstitial nephritis [1]. The nonsusceptible
wild-type CBA/Ca mouse contains, in its immune system, a specific suppressor T cell
that inhibits activation of the CD8+ effector cell, and thus prevents the expression
of disease [1,18]. In the kdkd mouse, this suppressor cell, in turn, is inhibited by a
specific contrasuppressor cell, thus facilitating clonal expansion of the CD8+ effector cell, and allowing expression of disease [17,18].

Another potentially important regulatory aspect of murine anti-TBM disease is that the central CD4+ helper T cell (Th) secretes an antigen-specific, class II restricted cytokine, T helper factor (ThF), that can specifically induce the CD8+ effector cell population to cause disease [19]. Molecular cloning of the antigen binding chain of ThF has yielded a family of cDNA that is currently being further characterized. Antisense oligonucleotides to this cDNA specifically inhibited the production of ThF, validating the relevance of this novel cDNA family [20]. Future work will focus on the factors controlling synthesis of this unique cytokine, in an effort to understand another regulatory mechanism for disease expression.

Effector Phase

A variety of potential effector mechanisms can lead to tubulointerstitial injury during the nephritogenic immune response (Fig. 2). Antibodies to interstitial structures may directly produce inflammation by activating the terminal membrane attack complex of complement, inducing chemotaxis of granulocytes and macrophages (with subsequent superoxide, protease, prostaglandin, and thromboxane release), invoking tubular injury through direct cytotoxicity of tubular cells, or by acting as an informational bridge targeting natural killer cells to the tubular epithelium [1,2]. An IgE humoral immune response may be preferentially produced when the inciting antigen derives from certain parasites, bacterial antigens, drug hapten-carrier molecules, or allergens. The produced IgE can then bind to special receptors on eosinophils, basophils, and primed mast cells, and a coordinated hypersensitivity response ensues [1].

Complement proteins have been observed to a varying degree in interstitial lesions. Complement activation can be seen in association with immune deposits, but it has also been occasionally observed when the nephritogenic process does not involve a humoral response. Exact mechanisms of activation under these circumstances are not fully worked out, but there is evidence that increased renal ammoniagenesis can activate complement [21]. Interstitial injury is not dependent on complement activation, however, in that C4 and C5 deficient animals can develop interstitial nephritis [1].

The hallmark of interstitial nephritis is the presence of mononuclear cells, mostly T cells, macrophages, and occasionally, eosinophils [1]. Effector T cells can induce delayed-type hypersensitivity responses with the release of inflammatory lymphokines, or they can directly produce cell-mediated cytotoxicity. Recently, a class I restricted CD8+ effector T cell line has been established in culture, and future work will further elucidate this cell's mechanism of cytotoxicity [22]. Additionally, T cells release a variety of lymphokines (including epidermal growth factor, transforming growth factor β, platelet derived growth factor, interleukins 1-6 (IL1-6), tumor necrosis factor, and others), that modulate the growth and biosynthesis of extracellular matrix in tubular epithelium and fibroblasts, as well as mediate the regenerative and hypertrophic responses of remnant epithelial tissue [23]. All of these factors can modulate procollagen deposition in the tubulointerstitial microenvironment, either through an increase in de novo procollagen biosynthesis, or through a decrease in proteolytic degradation. In addition, supernatants derived from cultured class II restricted T helper cells can influence the secretion of various

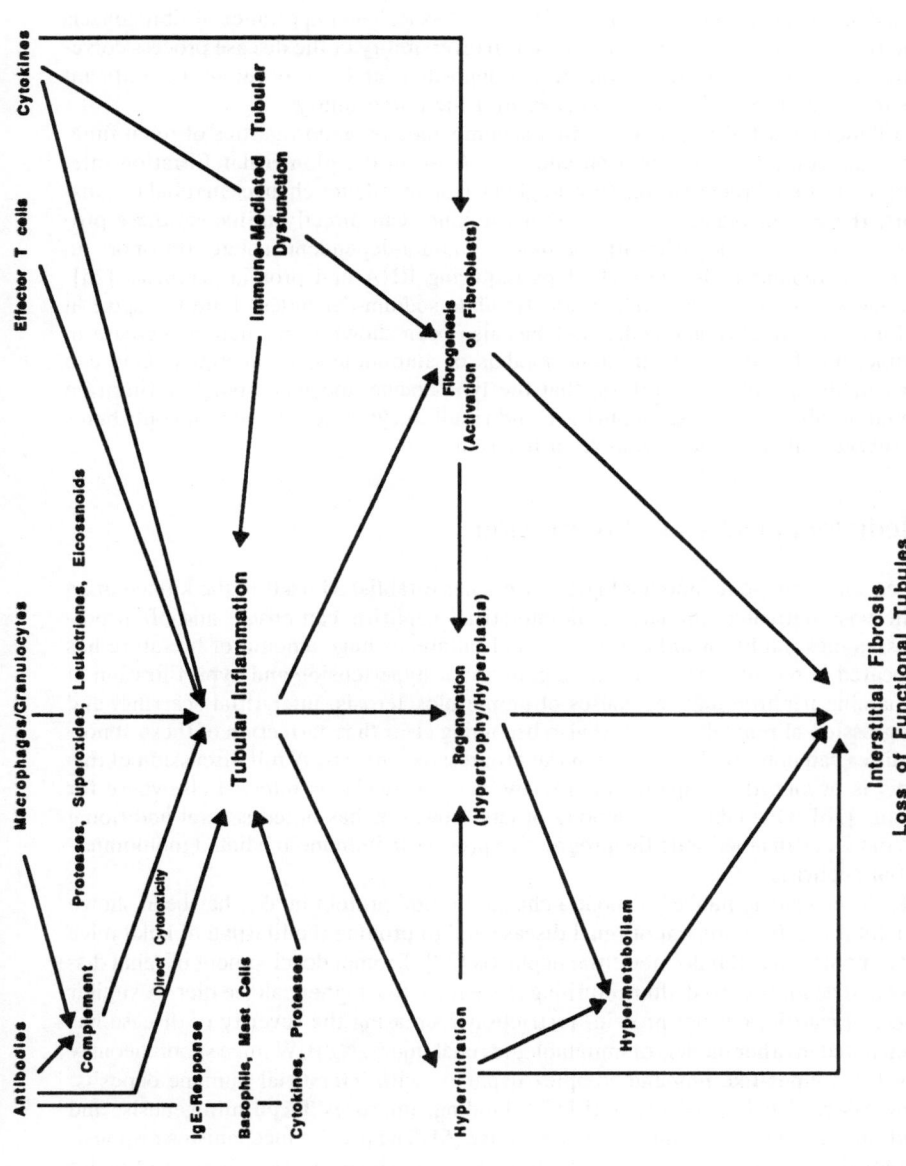

Fig. 2. Overview of the different effector mechanisms causing tubular injury, with interstitial fibrosis culminating in permanent loss of functional tubules

procollagens from tubular cells and interstitial fibroblasts [24]. More recent studies suggest that this effect is mediated through the aforementioned T helper factor (E.G. Neilson unpublished observations). The growth response itself may also lead to hypermetabolism of tubular cells, ultimately resulting in oxygen deprivation and the transformation of functional tubules into scar tissue. The importance of fibrogenesis and scar formation cannot be overstated. Irreversibility of the disease process correlates with the amount of fibrous tissue deposited, and can occur to a significant degree in as short a time as 7–10 days after the initial injury.

Tubulointerstitial nephritis is often accompanied by abnormalities of renal function, including sodium retention and a decrease in the glomerular filtration rate. Although altered renal plasma flow might be responsible for changes in tubular transport, there is increasing evidence that cytokines can directly influence these processes. IL-1 can significantly enhance sodium-dependent solute transport in proximal tubular cells, through steps requiring RNA and protein synthesis [25]. Similarly, tumor necrosis factor can stimulate sodium-dependent fluid transport in cultured proximal tubule cells. IL-1 has also been shown to mediate a decrease in glomerular filtration rate in some models of autoimmune renal injury. One can reasonably speculate, therefore, that the lymphocyte and macrophage infiltration found in tubulointerstitial nephritis could result in cytokine release that contributes to subsequent abnormalities in renal function.

Mediators of Disease Progression

Once a nephritogenic immunologic process has established itself in the kidney of an otherwise untreated animal, tubulointerstitial nephritis can ensue, and often progresses inexorably toward end-stage renal failure. A huge amount of literature has appeared in recent years concerning glomerular hypertension and hyperfiltration of remaining nephron units as causes of glomerulosclerosis, interstitial scarring, and progression of renal disease. It is also becoming clear that correction of these abnormalities can potentially slow down the progressive process. A full discussion of this topic is beyond the scope of this review, and the reader is referred elsewhere for details [26]. Our laboratory, among others, however, has noted several additional factors that can ameliorate the progressive process in immune-mediated tubulointerstitial nephritis.

Reduced caloric intake, without a change in total protein intake, has been shown to inhibit the development of renal disease and to prolong the lifespan of kdkd mice with spontaneous tubulointerstitial nephritis [27]. Prompt development of renal disease and death occurred after returning these mice to a higher calorie diet. A similar effect of calorie, but not protein, restriction decreasing the severity of disease has been noted in other models of immunologic renal injury. NZB/W mice spontaneously develop a lupus-like immune complex nephritis with interstitial immune deposits. Low calorie feeding reduces anti-DNA binding, improves T cell mitogenesis, and leads to less severe renal disease in these mice [6]. The precise mechanisms responsible for the preservation of renal function through calorie restriction are still under investigation.

A low protein diet, independent of caloric intake, can also favorably influence the outcome of immune-mediated renal disease. A low protein diet (3% versus 27%) at the time of immunization prevented the development of anti-TBM disease in rats, and stabilized histology and renal function in animals with already established disease [28]. This effect was most likely caused by nonspecific inhibition of T cell function, because DTH reactions to antigen were blunted in the 3% group. Other potential mechanisms for the protective effect of low protein diet include a decrease in glomerular hypertension, an alteration of mitochondrial oxygen consumption, and a modulation of tubular cell metabolism, all resulting in preservation of injured tubuloepithelial cells.

Furthermore, it has been shown that primary nonimmunological lesions, such as an acute reduction in renal mass, can lead to the stimulation of tubular ammoniagenesis by remnant nephrons, subsequent complement activation, and the production of chronic tubulointerstitial nephritis [21]. A protein restricted diet would, therefore, reduce the dietary acid load, decrease ammoniagenesis, and inhibit the nonspecific activation and deposition of complement in the renal tubulointerstitium.

Hyperlipidemia and hypercholesterolemia have been shown to contribute to the progression of glomerular renal disease in several animal models, but such a role in immune-mediated tubulointerstitial nephritis has yet to be proven [29]. Animals fed a high-cholesterol diet frequently do develop foam cells in the tubulointerstitium. Although the origin of foam cells is unknown, they appear to have characteristics of monocytes and macrophages, and can produce reactive oxygen intermediates which may be directly toxic to the tubular epithelium. The occurrence of foam cells has also been described in human tubulointerstitial nephritis, but the relevance of these cells in the pathogenesis of disease is presently unknown [2].

Our laboratory has also been interested in the disease abrogating effect of prostaglandin E_1 (PGE_1) treatment on tubulointerstitial nephritis. Administration of PGE_1 at the time of immunization delayed development of murine anti-TBM disease and diminished the DTH response in SJL mice. When begun on day 7 after immunization, however, this effect was not seen, suggesting that the immunosuppressive effect of PGE_1 occurs during the period of CD8 + nephritogenic effector T cell induction [30]. Further in vitro analysis revealed that PGE_1 led to the release of a nonspecific suppressor factor from T cells. Murine IL-1 was then shown to inhibit this PGE_1 suppressive effect [30]. When started during the first week after immunization, PGE_1 treatment also inhibited the development of acute and chronic inflammation in Brown Norway anti-TBM disease [3].

Conclusions and Future Directions

The immunopathogenesis of tubulointerstitial nephritis involves a complex interaction of genetic, immunologic, and environmental factors that determine initiation, development, and progression of disease in a given individual. The disease process proceeds through the expression and recognition of the nephritogenic antigen, the selection of an appropriate helper, effector, and regulatory T cell repertoire, the production of anti-TBM antibody, and finally, the various effector mechanisms responsible for tubular injury, fibrosis, and scarring. The next step in furthering our understanding of the pathogenesis of tubulointerstitial nephritis will be the molecular characterization of the various events in the disease process, with the ultimate goal of modifying these molecular interactions so as to prevent or attenuate the disease.

Acknowledgments. Original work in the authors' laboratory was supported by grants from the National Institute of Health (AR-20553, DK-30280, and DK-41110). Dr. Heeger is a recipient of a National Research Service Award (DK-08446) from the National Institutes of Health. Dr. Wolf is a recipient of a fellowship from the Boehringer Ingelheim Funds, Stuttgart, Federal Republic of Germany. Dr. Neilson is the recipient of an Established Investigator Award (85-108) from the American Heart Association and its Pennsylvania affiliates.

References

1. Neilson EG (1989) Pathogenesis and therapy of interstitial nephritis. Kidney Int 35:1257–1270
2. Neilson EG, Clayman MD, Kelly CJ (1989) The immunopathogenesis of interstitial nephritis. In: Massry S, Glassock R (eds) Textbook of nephrology, 2nd edn. Williams and Wilkins, Baltimore, pp 578–584
3. Wilson CB (1989) Study of the immunopathogenesis of tubulointerstitial nephritis using model systems. Kidney Int 35:938–953
4. Neilson EG, Phillips SM (1979) Cell-mediated immunity in interstitial nephritis. I. T lymphocyte systems in nephritic guinea pigs: the natural history and diversity of the immune response. J Immunol 123:2373–2380
5. Neilson EG, McCafferty E, Feldman A, Clayman MD, Zakheim B, Korngold R (1984) Spontaneous interstitial nephritis in kdkd mice. I. An experimental model of autoimmune renal disease. J Immunol 133:2560–2565
6. Kelly CJ, Haverty T, Neilson EG (1989) Control of the nephritogenic immune response. In: Wilson CB, Brenner BM, Stein JH (eds) Contemporary issues in nephrology. Churchill Livingstone, New York, pp 35–57 (Immunopathology of renal disease, vol 18)
7. Cameron JS (1989) Immunologically mediated interstitial nephritis: primary and secondary. Adv Nephrol 18:207–248
8. Clayman MD, Martinez-Hernandez A, Michaud L, Alper R, Mann R, Kefalides NA, Neilson EG (1985) Isolation and characterization of the nephritogenic antigen of anti-tubular basement membrane disease. J Exp Med 161:290–305
9. Neilson EG, Gasser DL, McCafferty E, Zakheim B, Phillips SM (1983) Polymorphism of genes involved in anti-tubular basement membrane disease in rats. Immunogenetics 17:55–65
10. Claymann MD, Michaud L, Brentjens J, Andres GA, Kefalides NA, Neilson EG (1986) Isolation of the target antigen of human anti-tubular basement membrane antibody-associated interstitial nephritis. J Clin Invest 77:1143–1147
11. Neilson EG, Sun MJ, Emergy J, Kelly C, Haverty T, Clayman M, Cooke NE (1989) Molecular cloning of the 3M-1 nephritogenic antigen. Kidney Int 35:358
12. Neilson EG, Phillips SM (1982) Murine interstitial nephritis. I. Analysis of disease susceptibility and its relationship to pleiomorphic gene products defining both immune response genes and a restrictive requirement for cytotoxic T cells at H-2^K. J Exp Med 155:1075–1085
13. Haverty TP, Kelly CJ, Hines WH, Amenta PS, Watanabe M, Harper RA, Kefalides NA, Neilson EG (1988) Characterization of a renal tubular epithelial cell line which secretes the autologous target antigen of autoimmune experimental interstitial nephritis. J Cell Biol 107:1359–1368
14. Haverty TP, Watanabe M, Neilson EG, Kelly CJ (1989) Protective modulation of class II MHC gene expression in tubular epithelium by target antigen-specific antibodies. Cell-surface directed down-regulation of transcription can influence susceptibility to murine tubulointerstitial nephritis. J Immunol 143:1133–1141

15. Neilson EG, Zakheim B (1983) T cell regulation, anti-idiotypic immunity, and the nephritogenic immune response. Kidney Int 24:289–302
16. Neilson EG, McCafferty E, Mann R, Michaud L, Clayman M (1985) Murine interstitial nephritis. III. The selection of phenotypic (Lyt and L3T4) and idiotypic T cell preferences by genes in Igh-1 and H-2^k characterizes the cell-mediated potential for disease expression: susceptible mice provide a unique T cell repertoire in response to tubular antigen. J Immunol 134:2375–2382
17. Kelly CJ, Neilson EG (1988) Contrasuppression in autoimmunity. Immunol Res 7:56–66
18. Kelly CJ, Neilson EG (1987) Contrasuppression in autoimmunity. Abnormal contrasuppression facilitates expression of nephritogenic effector T cells and interstitial nephritis in kdkd mice. J Exp Med 165:107–123
19. Hines WH, Mann RA, Kelly CJ, Neilson EG (1990) Murine interstitial nephritis IX. Induction of the nephritogenic effector T cell repertoire with an antigen-specific T cell cytokine. J Immunol 144:75–83
20. Saad T, Mandelbrot D, Sun MJ, Kelly CJ, Hines WH, Neilson EG (1990) Isolation of the cDNA for the antigen binding chain of a helper T cell factor in murine interstitial nephritis. Kidney Int 37:430
21. Nath KA, Hostetter MK, Hostetter TH (1985) Pathophysiology of chronic tubulointerstitial disease in rats. Interactions of dietary acid load, ammonia, and complement component C3. J Clin Invest 76:667–675
22. Meyers CM, Kelly CJ (1990) An antigen specific CTL line transfers interstitial nephritis and is cytotoxic to antigen expressing tubular epithelial cells. Kidney Int 37:423
23. Wolf G, Neilson EG (to be published) Molecular mechanisms of tubulointerstitial hypertrophy and hyperplasia. Kidney Int
24. Neilson EG, Jimenez SA, Phillips SM (1980) Cell-mediated immunity in interstitial nephritis. II: T lymphocytes-mediated fibroblast proliferation and collagen synthesis: An immune mechanism for renal fibrogenesis. J Immunol 125:1708–1714
25. Schreiner GF, Kohan DE (1990) Regulation of renal transport processes and hemodynamics by macrophages and lymphocytes. Am J Physiol 258:F761–F767
26. Klahr S, Schreiner G, Ichikawa I (1988) The progression of renal disease. N Engl J Med 318:1657–1666
27. Fernandes G, Yunis EJ, Miranda M, Smith J, Good RA (1978) Nutritional inhibition of genetically determined renal disease and autoimmunity with prolongation of life in kdkd mice. Proc Natl Acad Sci USA 75:2888–2892
28. Agus D, Mann R, Cohn D, Michaud L, Kelly C, Clayman M, Neilson EG (1985) Inhibitory role of dietary protein restriction on the development and expression of immune-mediated antitubular basement membrane-induced tubulointerstitial nephritis in rats. J Clin Invest 76:930–936
29. Keane WF, Kasiske BL, O'Donnell MP (1988) Hyperlipidemia and the progression of renal disease. Am J Clin Nutr 47:157–160
30. Kelly CJ, Zurier RB, Krakauer KA, Blanchard N, Neilson EG (1987) Prostaglandin E$_1$ inhibits effector T cell induction and tissue damage in experimental murine interstitial nephritis. J Clin Invest 79:782–789

Lipids and the Pathogenesis of Kidney Disease

JOHN F. MOORHEAD

Chair: Roscoe R. Robinson

Lipids and the Pathogenesis of Kidney Disease

JOHN F. MOORHEAD[1]

SUMMARY. The nephrotic syndrome presents clinically with a pattern of proteinuria, edema, albuminuria, hypoalbuminemia, and hyperlipidemia. Despite, or perhaps because of, familiarity with the syndrome, its possible implications for the progression of renal disease have been neglected. However, a large amount of information has been accumulated from animal models in the last decade, which, in aggregate, strongly suggests an important role for abnormalities of lipid metabolism in progressive renal disease. This review considers the metabolic background against which some of the pathological changes in animal models of nephrotic syndrome take place. Analogies between glomerular disease and atherosclerosis are discussed in the context of cellular pathology, the cardiovascular complications of nephrosis, and the relative protection of females from atherosclerosis. The role of lipid lowering drugs is discussed in relation to disease prevention in animal models. Reference is made to the role of excess eicosanoid synthesis in glomerular disease. Lack of information on the value or otherwise of long term lipid lowering therapy in patients with proteinuria, hyperlipidemia, and progressive renal disease emphasizes the need for long term studies of lipid lowering therapy in these patients.

Introduction

The clinicopathological components of the nephrotic syndrome are very familiar. An initial glomerular injury, usually unrecognized, leads to proteinuria, edema, hypoproteinemia, hyperlipidemia, and lipoproteinuria. These are the cardinal clinicopathological features of the nephrotic syndrome, however initiated. This review will explore the mechanisms by which hyperlipidemic glomerular injury may take place, and will examine some of the difficulties which are likely to occur in the interpretation and prevention of lipoprotein induced disease in man.

---

[1]Department of Nephrology, The Royal Free Hospital, Hampstead, London, NW3 2QG, UK

In 1982 we proposed that lipoproteins could be a cause of progressive kidney disease [1]. This hypothesis suggested that any (possibly self-limiting) condition which resulted in albuminuria and hyperlipidemia could establish secondary self perpetuating renal damage, with further loss of protein in the urine and continued inappropriate liver synthesis of lipoprotein. The excess circulating lipoprotein would then both cause and maintain further glomerular injury, so perpetuating the cycle. Other risk factors, such as continued activity of immune processes, increased glomerular pressure, and dietary factors, would continue to contribute to glomerular disease unless independently controlled. It is not yet certain how all these factors combine to produce irreversible glomerular damage. However, much experimental evidence has accumulated since 1982 which implicates lipids in the pathogenesis of progressive renal disease, and a review of this complex process is therefore timely.

Historical Evidence

Nephrotic hyperlipidemia has, until recently, been regarded as an epiphenomenon having little relevance to the pathogenesis of the underlying kidney disease. There has, however, been considerable interest in hyperlipidemia, both as a secondary metabolic phenomenon and for the abundant deposits of lipid in renal tissue in patients with nephrotic syndrome. Virchow [2] characterized lipid deposition in the kidney as "fatty metamorphosis" and Munk first described the plasma lipid abnormalities of the nephrotic syndrome in 1913 [3]. In their study of diabetic kidneys, Kimmelstiel and Wilson noted the presence of fat in some glomeruli [4], and subsequently Wilens et al. [5] reported that in diabetics glomerular lipidosis occurred only with glomerular sclerosis. The presence of glomerular lipid in 75% of sclerotic diabetic kidneys was reported by Hartroft [6] who, interestingly, also suggested for the first time that elevated intraglomerular pressure might contribute to glomerular lesions. French et al. [7] showed that feeding a 1% cholesterol diet to guinea pigs caused severe glomerular disease with cholesterol crystals in glomerular capillaries and intraglomerular proliferation of monocytes, a finding confirmed by Al-Shebeb in guinea pigs and New Zealand rabbits [8]. The first observation that abnormalities of lipid metabolism might be linked to glomerular disease in man was made by Gjone [9] in a report of the rare familial condition of lecithin:cholesterol acyl transferase (L:CAT) deficiency. Charlesworth and Edwards [10] suggested that hypertriglyceridemia was a risk factor in the outcome of renal transplantation in man. This concept was later supported in animal work by Edwards [11], who showed that pre-existing hyperlipidemia inhibited normal healing in female Sprague-Dawley rats with aminonucleoside nephrotic syndrome. In this study, high fat diets accelerated glomerular disease and lipid lowering drugs reduced proteinuria and glomerulosclerosis. Pavlovic et al. [12] observed that increased dietary fat prolonged proteinuria in the acute phase of puromycin aminonucleoside (PAN) nephrosis. An interesting animal model of hyperlipidemic renal disease is the obese Zucker rat, which is insulin resistant, hyperphagic, and hyperlipidemic, and develops heavy proteinuria and glomerular sclerosis [13]. Its lean litter mates do not develop hyperlipidemia and renal disease. Kasiske et al. [14], using clofibrate in these animals, confirmed Edwards' observation that lipid lowering effectively reduced proteinuria [15].

Pathological and Metabolic Background

The nephrotic syndrome is characterized by a striking increase in plasma lipoproteins. The liver cell secretes excess very low density lipoprotein (VLDL) which is carried in the circulation by apo-B100. Removal of fatty acids and trial-glycerol from this particle gives rise to low density lipoprotein (LDL), which carries apo-B100 throughout its normal 36-hour life cycle. In the nephrotic syndrome, increased concentrations of apo-B are partly due to increased secretion of VLDL, the stimulus for which is low plasma albumin concentration. Despite this clear clinical correlation, the precise signal at a cellular level which causes lipoprotein secretion, rather than albumin synthesis alone, has not been elucidated. In vitro, relative increases in the viscosity of the culture medium, obtained by the addition of compounds of widely differing mass concentration and osmolarity, have been shown to inhibit VLDL secretion from rat hepatocytes [16]. It has also been shown that apo-B secretion by HepG2 cells is influenced in a dose-dependent manner by albumin in the culture medium, although no change in the level of apo-B mRNA occurred when apo-B output was modulated [17]. In man, plasma oncotic pressure, but not plasma viscosity, has been shown to influence total plasma cholesterol concentration.

The excess synthesis of lipoprotein is accompanied by slower than normal metabolism in the peripheral circulation [18]. The turnover rate of VLDL and LDL is prolonged for several reasons, which include decreased activity of two enzymes, lipoprotein lipase (LPL) and lecithin: cholesterol acyl transferase (L:CAT). Reduction in LPL activity may be due to a combination of inhibition and urinary loss of cofactors. L:CAT activity is reduced both as a result of urinary losses of co-factors associated with high density lipoprotein (HDL), and as a result of product inhibition caused by reduction in plasma albumin concentration, since albumin is responsible for removing the reaction product, lysolecithin, thus allowing the reaction to continue.

Since the glomerulus may be damaged by immunological, toxic, hemodynamic, and other insults, it seems, a priori, unlikely that it should be always protected from high concentrations of lipoproteins. However, glomerular disease does not occur (as far as is known) in primary hyperlipidemia. This may reflect a need for a combination of two predisposing conditions, prior glomerular vascular injury and a hyperlipidemic response to proteinuria. However, the absence of data on renal function in primary hyperlipidemias could also reflect failure to investigate. It is not known, for example, whether microproteinuria exists in hyperlipidemias, or whether such patients have an increased risk of developing renal diseases. The characteristics of the glomerular microcirculation may also have a role. For example, the mesangium is focused at the glomerular stalk and the small area it presents to the circulating plasma may reduce its susceptibility to circulating lipoproteins.

Comparisons with atheromatous disease in other parts of the vascular system have given rise to useful speculation that some glomerular diseases have much in common with atherosclerosis.

Analogies with Atherosclerosis

The fact that glomerulosclerosis and atherosclerosis occur in widely different anatomical sites need not preclude or deter interpretation along similar lines. Many of the requirements for atherosclerosis are satisfied by the cellular and metabolic conditions found in hyperlipidemic renal disease. Although elevated LDL is not regularly accompanied by renal disease, it is not known whether the normal glomerulus is ever susceptible to LDL damage. It is more likely that damage is initiated by some other agent, commonly immunological, and then sustained by the resulting hyperlipidemia. In fact, the details of the pathogenesis of progressive disease, as proposed [1], coincided to some extent with those proposed at that time for atherosclerosis [19]. The proposed pathogenesis of atherosclerosis in blood vessels bears similarities to that suggested for glomerulosclerosis. Thus endothelial injury, and lipid infiltration, are basic requirements. LDL is proposed as the endothelial damaging agent, with monocytes being attached to endothelium and infiltrating the subendothelial tissue. Leary [20] was the first to suggest that monocytes were implicated in the pathogenesis of the atherosclerotic lesion, and Ross [19], more recently, observed that monocytes interact with altered endothelium, penetrating subendothelial areas and accumulating lipid to form the foam cells which constitute part of the atherosclerotic plaque. Smooth muscle cells may also cause free radical damage to LDL and then internalize the altered lipoprotein, becoming foam cells.

The Role of the Macrophage

The macrophage is important in the pathogenesis of atherosclerosis, and may have a similar role in glomerular disease. The combination of endothelial injury by glomerular inflammatory processes, followed by neutrophil and macrophage influx, is probably a common event in certain forms of glomerulonephritis. The transformation of bone marrow derived monocytes into lipid laden macrophages (foam cells) takes place in vivo by the internalization of cholesterol ester from plasma lipoproteins. This occurs via the scavenger receptors, of which there are three, one of which prefers acetyl LDL, one oxidized LDL, the third binding both. As in atheromatous plaques, there are probably several glomerular mechanisms for the modification of LDL which allow its uptake by the macrophage. Acetylation, which increases the net negative charge of the lipoprotein, is mimicked by oxidation of unsaturated fatty acids into oxides and aldehydes which then attach to lysines of apoB-100, increasing its negative charge. A second method, oxidation of LDL by macrophages, occurs in response to several stimuli, including IgG and IgA immunoglobulins, and can be prevented by the antioxidant probucol. Finally, oxidized LDL can combine in vitro with proteoglycan [21] and collagen, forming a complex which may independently promote foam cell formation. The charge and conformational changes in LDL induced by these reactions preclude normal LDL receptor-mediated clearance. Since the macrophage is unable to clear cholesterol, it accumulates as droplets in the cytoplasm, forming the foam cell. The uptake of oxidized LDL by the macrophage may stimulate it to produce growth factors, cytokines, and other mediators capable of stimulating collagen synthesis and proliferation of mesangial cells. The combined effect of these changes would eventually produce irreversible scarring in the glomerular tuft.

Does evidence exist that these processes might take part in progressive glomerular disease? Monocytes are involved in the pathogenesis of several renal diseases in man, including focal glomerulosclerosis. Cotran [22] drew attention to the presence of monocytes in glomerular proliferative lesions. In studies of rabbit nephrotoxic serum nephritis, Thomson et al. [23] reported that macrophages accumulated in damaged glomeruli and infiltrated Bowman's space.

It would be surprising if the activity of infiltrating glomerular monocytes exposed to trapped LDL differed substantially from their behavior in the more familiar atherosclerotic plaque. In fact, experimental evidence now supports a link between the presence of glomerular monocytes, hyperlipidemia and glomerulosclerosis. Early experiments in guinea pigs fed a 1% cholesterol diet showed striking glomerular monocyte infiltration, associated with glomerular sclerosis, glomerular fat droplets, an increase in mesangial cells and fiber, and macrophage-like cells [7]. On the other hand, Grond et al. [24] found no excess of monocytes in male Wistar rats with chronic puromycin aminonucleoside (PAN) nephrosis after 20 weeks of weekly injections of PAN. This negative result may have been due to the late stage of the examination, since others have reported that, in rabbit nephrotoxic serum nephritis, macrophages have disappeared by 40 days [23]. The removal of macrophages from the glomeruli of rabbits with acute serum sickness by anti macrophage serum resulted in both a profound reduction in proteinuria and only mild histological lesions. It has recently been shown that essential fatty acid deficiency (EFAD) depletes Sprague-Dawley rat glomeruli of resident macrophages [25]. Using this information in hyperlipidemic PAN nephrosis, Diamond [26] showed that glomerular macrophages, glomerular sclerosis, and proteinuria are all reduced, and that the late chronic phase of PAN is ameliorated. In experiments in which 17β-ethinyl-estradiol was given to uninephrectomized obese Zucker rats, it was observed that improvement in glomerular disease was accompanied by significant reductions in plasma cholesterol, glomerular macrophages, and in vitro glomerular eicosanoid synthesis (J.F. Moorhead, submitted for publication).

The Role of the Mesangial Cell

The principal sites in which lipoprotein trapping may occur in injured glomeruli are the mesangium and the basement membrane. In physiological conditions in vitro, apo-B basic residues enable receptor binding to mesangial cells in culture, so promoting internalization. But the mesangial cell is also susceptible to lipoprotein damage. Thus, it was found that rat mesangial cells were killed in vitro by LDL in a concentration-dependent fashion [27]. Others have shown that this toxicity is mediated more efficiently by oxidized LDL, which may be present under conditions of local inflammation and monocyte ingress. In addition, mesangial cells, like the smooth muscle cells with which they share some characteristics, proliferate in vitro when stimulated appropriately by LDL [27]. Furthermore, infiltrating macrophages produce mediators which stimulate mesangial cell proliferation. Together, these observations may explain why mesangial hypercellularity and scarring is found in several models of nephritis. Lipoproteins may be captured by charge affinity in basement membrane glycosaminoglycans. ApoB binds, in vivo and in vitro, to collagen, and in vitro to heparan sulfate glycosaminoglycans (HSGAG) [21], a major constituent of the glomerular basement membrane (GBM). This binding may be enhanced by the reported presence in the GBM of a 130Kd residue with sequence homology to the LDL receptor [28]. Thus, apo-B alone may exert its pathological effects by neutralizing glomerular charge, added to which the combination of LDL-GAG, referred to previously, may permit internalization by macrophages.

Cardiovascular Complications

Since the postulated lesions of lipoprotein-mediated glomerular disease and athero-sclerosis have a similar pathological basis it would be expected that extrarenal atherosclerosis would be recognized frequently in persistent proteinuria. The few studies which have examined ischemic heart disease and nephrotic syndrome have, in general, supported an association. Elevation of plasma lipids has been claimed as a risk factor in nephrotics [29], and has been reported to have caused premature atherosclerosis in a five-year-old child [30]. Mallick and Short [31] concluded that patients with persisting heavy proteinuria appear to be at substantial risk of developing ischemic heart disease. Wass et al. [32], in a study of 159 patients of whom more than 25% had minimal change disease, were less confident of a connection, but their paper was difficult to interpret. The report of the European Dialysis and Transplant Association (EDTA) for 1978 revealed a dramatically higher death rate from cerebrovascular accident (CVA) for patients on regular dialysis programs, suggesting, perhaps, that a substantial number of dialysis patients acquire their vascular disease while their renal function is declining and before dialysis starts.

Gender

Females are relatively protected from atherosclerosis, and it follows that any consideration of hyperlipidemia and progression of renal disease should include the contribution of gender. It is noteworthy that animal models of glomerular disease often make the distinction clear. For example, male Munich-Wistar rats develop heavy proteinuria and nephrotic syndrome while females do not [33], and in an immune complex model of nephritis, proteinuria is more severe in males [34]. Further, glomerulosclerosis after subtotal nephrectomy is less severe in female rats [35]. One possible non-hormonal, cholesterol related, explanation for these sex differences may be the operation of the mevalonate 'shunt.' Mevalonate, a precursor of cholesterol, is metabolized by normal rat kidney, but to a lesser extent in females than in males. More mevalonate is therefore available for cholesterol metabolism in males than in females with significant renal disease. This may result in more lipoprotein being available to damage the glomeruli of male rats.

In man, two studies of patients with renal impairment, one of mixed pathogenesis [36] and the other in membranous nephropathy [37], reported a male-female ratio of 2:1. In a follow-up study of 139 patients with idiopathic membranous glomerulonephritis, Murphy et al. [38] reported that the patients whose renal function deteriorated were mainly nephrotic males. Hopper et al. [37], in a study of 100 patients with membranous nephropathy, found that this form of nephropathy was less frequent and more benign in women. On the other hand, immune reactivity is greater in females than in males, possibly due to down regulation of T-cell function and stimulation of B-cell function by estrogens [39].

This decreased susceptibility may account for the fact that renal failure programs care for fewer females than males. Carlsten and coworkers' study [39] cited polycystic kidney disease, but similar observations have been made in IgA nephropathy [40], although sex distribution in this group of conditions is not uniform worldwide [41]. Also, there are gender-dependent differences in age-specific changes of renal function, so that while renal function declines in males continuously [42], in the female it begins to decline gradually after the menopause. There is some evidence that renal disease in general is more common in men than in premenopausal women, and that this difference is not present before the menarche.

Could some of this difference be accounted for by protection from abnormalities of lipid metabolism in females with proteinuria and hyperlipidemia? Perhaps the protection of normal premenopausal women from atherosclerosis extends to lipid abnormalities in women with the nephrotic syndrome. Females with renal failure seem to be relatively immune from the cardiovascular complications of renal failure. For example, The 1987 European Dialysis and Transplant Association study of cardiovascular complications of renal failure found that the myocardial death rate was twice as high in males than in females. Whether this effect could have been influenced by estrogens in women or by androgens in men is unknown: we are ignorant of the effects of physiological concentrations of estrogens in human renal diseases. In comparing male and female disease, it should be remembered that the combination of relatively small effects in amelioration of disease in females and aggravation in males would combine to accentuate differences, necessitating caution in the interpretation of results.

Proteinuria and Hyperlipidemia: a Neglected Association

Proteinuria is recognized as an important feature of progressive disease, often being used as a direct measure of the effect of treatment or experiment. There are strong relationships between proteinuria and serum albumin, and between serum albumin and plasma cholesterol concentrations (Figs. 1,2). Warwick et al. [43] confirmed an association between proteinuria, LDL cholesterol, and plasma triglyceride, and in their study the absolute synthetic rate of LDL was also strongly correlated with proteinuria. Proteinuria correlates closely with deterioration of renal function, and reduction of proteinuria by administration of low protein diets may be associated with slowing of the rate of progression [44]. In IgA nephropathy, reputedly the most common worldwide form of glomerular disease, four independent indicators of poor outcome include proteinuria and glomerulosclerosis [41]. By inference, deterioration or improvement in renal function could have been caused by changes in plasma lipoproteins. Unfortunately, no large studies of proteinuria have related glomerular disease to changes in plasma lipids. Gross obesity has been reported to cause the nephrotic syndrome [45] and has been associated with focal segmental glomerular sclerosis. Recently, a number of cases of apo-E associated proteinuric lipoprotein glomerulopathy have been reported from Japan, and further developments of this work are awaited with great interest. Aside from these special cases, there is a consensus that most glomerular diseases which are accompanied by proteinuria have a worse prognosis than non-proteinuric renal

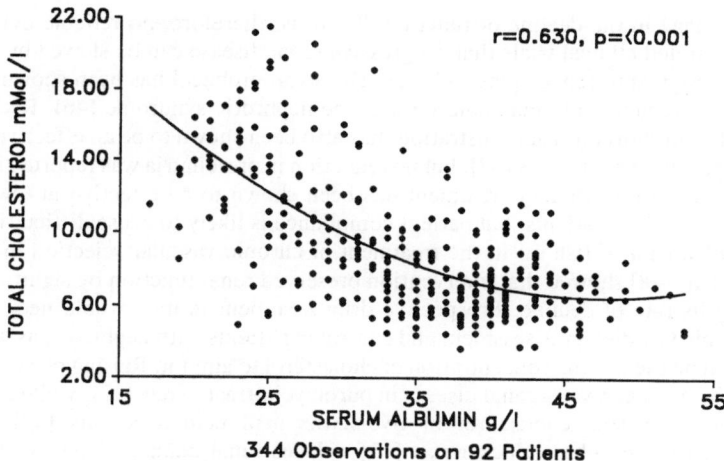

Fig. 1. The relationship between plasma cholesterol and serum albumin in nephrotic patients

diseases; it is likely that lipoprotein-mediated damage contributes to progression in some or all of these conditions.

Lipid Lowering

The few clinical studies of lipid lowering in the progression of renal disease have been short term and uncontrolled. Existing long term studies have concentrated on factors such as hypertension and the role of dietary protein, and have usually begun

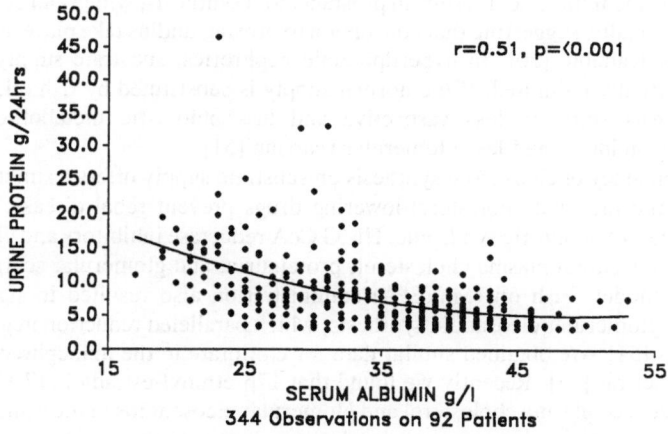

Fig. 2. The relationship between proteinuria and serum albumin in nephrotic patients

at a late stage in the decline of function. There is, therefore, no reliable evidence from controlled clinical trials that progressive renal disease can be slowed by drugs or diets designed to reduce plasma lipids. However, probucol has been shown to be effective in reducing plasma cholesterol in the nephrotic syndrome [46]. Recently, synvinolin, in short term administration, has also been shown to be an effective lipid lowering agent in nephrotics [47], but no reduction in proteinuria was reported in this uncontrolled study. Dietary treatment has been shown to be effective in lowering lipids in transplant patients, but patient compliance is likely to cause difficulties. In a controlled trial of fish oil in the treatment of chronic vascular rejection in man, Sweny et al. [48] showed that intervention preserved renal function by significantly reducing its rate of decline. Prospective drug treatment in man would need to be accompanied by dietary assessment and control in patients with nephrosis, as well as a decision on the plasma concentration of cholesterol to aim for. Raising plasma cholesterol by diet aggravates renal disease in puromycin-treated rats [12], while dietary reduction of plasma cholesterol in five-sixths nephrectomized rats [49] or in uninephrectomized obese Zucker rats [13] reduces renal damage. Dietary enrichment with eicosapentaenoic acid reduces renal disease, proteinuria, and mortality in murine lupus nephritis.

An important question relates to the timing of intervention. At present, there is little evidence favoring any particular time for diet or drug intervention and such questions will be resolved only by well designed clinical trials. In animals, evidence from many studies suggests that prevention or very early intervention is effective.

Renal Eicosanoids

Renal eicosanoid synthesis may have an important role in the mediation of some of the phenomena discussed here. Eicosanoid synthesis requires the presence of C_{20} unsaturated fatty acids in unesterified form before prostaglandin synthesis can take place. The source of free acids may be cholesterol esters, triglycerides, or phospholipids, from which they are freed by the actions of phospholipases. Perfusion of organs with arachidonic acid results in prostaglandin synthesis, which can be blocked pharmacologically, suggesting that conversion to prostaglandins take place as soon as substrate is available [50]. In hyperlipidemic nephrotics, substrate supply is presumably virtually unlimited. If the normal supply is substituted by fish oil, eicosanoid synthesis shifts to less vasoactive and less phlogistic metabolites, with decreased proteinuria and less glomerular scarring [51].

The dependency of eicosanoid synthesis on substrate supply offers a simple explanation for the fact that cholesterol-lowering drugs prevent renal disease in some animal models of nephrotic syndrome. HMG CoA reductase inhibitors and clofibrate [52] both reduce total plasma cholesterol, proteinuria, and glomerular scarring in a Zucker rat model. Fish oil (MaxEPA) administration also resulted in significant lowering of glomerular eicosanoid synthesis, which paralleled reduction in glomerular sclerosis [51]. We obtained similar data for clofibrate in the uninephrectomized (UNx) Zucker rat [13]. Recently we found that 17β-ethinyl-estradiol (17-EE), dramatically reduced plasma cholesterol and glomerular eicosanoids in the same model. These findings offer encouragement for the argument that therapeutic lowering of plasma cholesterol in man may also be beneficial to the kidney.

Conclusions

Clinical and experimental evidence available to date permits the following broad conclusions. In experimental animal models of non immune mediated nephrotic syndrome, treatment which lowers plasma lipoprotein cholesterol, diverts eicosanoid synthesis to less active metabolites, or deprives the animal of essential fatty acids, ameliorates renal disease. On the other hand, feeding saturated fat either delays recovery, in the case of PAN nephrosis, aggravates disease. In immune mediated systems, e.g., murine systemic lupus erythematosus (SLE), the renal disease is largely prevented by unsaturated fatty acid feeding.

To summarize the evidence to date, the glomerular structures susceptible to lipoprotein mediated injury are the mesangium, the basement membrane, and the resident and infiltrating glomerular monocytes. Lipoprotein (apoB-100) may damage the glomerular basement membrane directly or may damage it after peroxidation by activated macrophages. Lipid peroxidation results in foam cell formation via the macrophage scavenger receptors, with further glomerular and interstitial damage resulting from activated macrophages. The glomerular injury is perpetuated by continued exposure to lipoproteins. Comparisons with systemic atherosclerosis have helped to explain many of the glomerular abnormalities found in glomerulosclerosis.

References

1. Moorhead JF, Chan MK, El-Nahas M, Varghese Z (1982) Lipid nephrotoxicity in chronic progressive glomerular and tubulo-interstitial disease. Lancet II:1309–1312
2. Virchow R (1860) A more precise account of fatty metamorphosis. London, Churchill, pp 342–366
3. Munk F (1913) Klinische diagnostik der degenerativen nierenerkrankungen. Z Clin Med 78:1–52
4. Kimmelstiel P, Wilson C (1936) Intercapillary lesions in the glomeruli of the kidney. Am J Pathol 12:83–98
5. Wilens SL, Elster SK, Baker JP (1951) Glomerular lipidosis in intercapillary glomerulosclerosis. Ann Intern Med 24:592–607
6. Hartroft WS (1955) Fat emboli in glomerular capillaries of choline deficient rats and of patients with diabetic glomerulosclerosis. Am J Pathol 31:381–391
7. French SW, Yamanaka W, Ostwald R (1967) Dietary induced glomerulosclerosis in the guinea pig. Arch Pathol Lab Med 83:204–210
8. Al-Shebeb T, Frohlich J, Magil AB (1988) Glomerular disease in hypercholesterolemic guinea pigs: A pathogenetic study. Kidney Int 33:498–507
9. Gjone E, Blomhoff JP, Skarbovik AJ (1974) Possible association between an abnormal low density lipoprotein and nephropathy in lecithin cholesterol acyltransferase deficiency. Clin Chim Acta 54:11–18
10. Charlesworth JA, Edwards KDG (1974) Relation of hypertriglyceridemia to kidney transplant dysfunction and rejection, and response to antilymphocyte globulin therapy. Prog Biochem Pharmacol 9:107–120
11. Edwards KDG (1981) Controversies in nephrology. New York, Masson, pp 3–15
12. Pavlovic NM, Malik S, Chan MK, Z Varghese, Persaud JW, Moorhead JF (1984) The influence of high fat diet on the proteinuria in puromycin induced nephrotic syndrome in rats. Clin Sci 66:26P

13. Wheeler DC, Nair DR, Singh GS, Persaud J, Sweny P, Varghese Z, Moorhead JF (1988) Lipid-lowering therapy reduces proteinuria in the uninephrectomised obese Zucker rat. Nephrol Dial Transplant 3:533
14. Kasiske BL, O'Donnell, Keane WF (1986) The lipid lowering agent clofibric acid reduces glomerular injury in obese Zucker rats. Clin Res 34:600A
15. Zucker LM (1965) Hereditary obesity in the rat associated with hyperlipemia. Ann NY Acad Sci 131:447–458
16. Yedgar S, Weinstein DB, Patsch W, Schonfeld G, Casanada FE, Steinberg D (1982) Viscosity of culture medium as a regulator of synthesis and secretion of very low density lipoproteins by cultured hepatocytes. J Biol Chem 257(5):2188–2192
17. Pullinger CR, North JD, Teng BB, Rifici VA, De Brito AER, Scott J (1989) The apolipoprotein B gene is constitutively expressed in HepG2 cells: regulation of secretion by oleic acid, albumin, and insulin, and measurement of the mRNA half-life. J Lipid Res 30:1065–1077
18. Moorhead JF, Wheeler DC, Varghese Z (1989) Glomerular structures and lipids in progressive renal disease. Am J Med 87:12N–20N
19. Ross R (1986) The pathogenesis of atherosclerosis – an update. N Engl J Med 314:488–500
20. Leary T (1941) The genesis of atherosclerosis. Arch Pathol Lab Med 32(4):507–555
21. Iverius PH (1972) The interaction between human plasma lipoproteins and connective tissue glycosaminoglycans. J Biol Chem 247(8):2607–2613
22. Cotran RS (1978) Monocytes, proliferation, and glomerulonephritis. J Lab Clin Med 92:837–840
23. Thomson NM, Holdsworth SR, Glasgow EF, Atkins RC (1979) The macrophage in the development of experimental crescentic glomerulonephritis. Am J Pathol 94:223–240
24. Grond J, Van Goor H, Erkelens DW, Elema JD (1986) Glomerular sclerotic lesions in the rat. Virchows Arch [Cell Pathol] 51:521–534
25. Lefkowith JB, Schreiner G (1987) Essential fatty acid deficiency depletes rat glomeruli of resident macrophages and inhibits angiotensin II - induced eicosanoid synthesis. J Clin Invest 30:947–956
26. Diamond JR (1990) Effects of dietary interventions on glomerular pathophysiology. Am J Physiol 27:F1–F8
27. Wheeler DC, Persaud J, Kingstone D, Sweny P, Varghese Z, Moorhead JF (1989) Receptor mediated binding of human low density lipoprotein (LDL) to rat mesangial cells in vitro (abstract) Kidney Int 35:439
28. Pietromonaco SF, Farquhar MG (1989) Identification and characterization of a cDNA encoding the core protein of heparin sulfate proteoglycans from the rat glomerular basement membrane (abstract). Kidney Int 35:163
29. Alexander JH, Schapel GJ, Edwards KDG (1974) Increased incidence of coronary heart disease associated with combined elevation of serum triglyceride and cholesterol concentrations in the nephrotic syndrome in man. Med J Aust 2:119–122
30. Kallen RJ, Brynes, Aronson AJ, Lichtig C, Spargo BH (1977) Premature coronary atherosclerosis in a 5-year-old with corticosteroid-refractory nephrotic syndrome. Am J Dis Child 131:976–980
31. Mallick NP, Short CD (1981) The nephrotic syndrome and ischemic heart disease. Nephron 27:54–57
32. Wass VJ, Chilvers C, Jarrett RJ, Cameron JS (1979) Does the nephrotic syndrome increase the risk of cardiovascular disease? Lancet II:664–667
33. Remuzzi A, Puntorieri S, Mazzoleni A, Remuzzi G (1988) Sex related differences in glomerular ultrafiltration and proteinuria in Munich-Wistar rats. Kidney Int 34:481–486
34. Gretz N, Zeier M, Geberth S, Strauch M, Ritz E (1989) Is gender a determinant for evolution of renal failure? A study in autosomal dominant polycystic kidney disease. Am J Kidney Dis 14:178–183

35. Lombet JR, Adler SJ, Anderson PS, Nast CC, Olsen D, Glassock RJ (1988) Sex vulnerability in the subtotal nephrectomy (Nx) model of glomerulosclerosis (abstract). Kidney Int 33:378
36. Hunt LP, Short D, Mallick NP (1988) Prognostic indicators in patients presenting with the nephrotic syndrome. Kidney Int 34:382–388
37. Hopper JJR, Trew PA, Biava CG (1981) Membranous nephropathy:its relative benignity in women. Nephron 29:18–24
38. Murphy BF, Fairley KF, Kincaid-Smith PS (1988) Idiopathic membranous glomerulonephritis:long term follow up in 139 cases. Clin Nephrol 30:175–181
39. Carlsten H, Holmdahl R, Tarkowski A, Nilsson LA (1989) Oestradiol- and testosterone-mediated effects on the immune system in normal and autoimmune mice are genetically linked and inherited as dominant traits. Immunology 68:209–214
40. D'Amico G, Imbasciati E, Belgioioso GB, Bertoli S, Fogazzi G, Ferrario F, Fellini G, Ragni A, Colasanti G, Minetti L, Ponticell C (1985) Idiopathic IgA mesangial nephropathy. Medicine 64(1):49–60
41. D'Amico G (1987) The commonest glomerulonephritis in the world. IgA nephropathy. Q J Med 64:709–727
42. Lindeman RD, Tobin J, Shock W (1985) Longitudinal studies on the rate of decline in renal function with age. J Am Geriatr Soc 33:278–285
43. Warwick GL, Caslake MJ, Boulton-Jones JM, Dagen M, Packard CJ, Shepherd J (1990) Low-density lipoprotein metabolism in the nephrotic syndrome. Metabolism 39:187–192
44. El Nahas AM, Masters-Thomas A, Brady SA, Farrington K, Wilkinson V, Hilson AJW, Varghese Z, Moorhead JF (1984) Selective effect of low protein diets in chronic renal diseases. Br Med J [Clin Res] 289:1337–1342
45. Weisinger JR, Kempson RL, Eldridge FL, Swenson RS (1974) The nephrotic syndrome: a complication of massive obesity. Ann Intern Med 81:440–447
46. Appel G, Gelfand J, Kunis C, Blum C (1985) Treatment of hyperlipidemia of the nephrotic syndrome: a controlled trial (abstract). Kidney Int 270:131
47. Rabelink AJ, Erkelens DW, Hene RJ, Joles JA (1988) Effects of simvastatin and cholestyramine on lipoprotein profile in hyperlipidaemia of nephrotic syndrome. Lancet II:1335–1337
48. Sweny P, Wheeler DC, Lui SF, Amin NS, Moorhead JF, Jeremy JY, Mikhailidis DP, Varghese Z, Fernando ON, et al. (1989) Dietary fish oil supplements preserve renal function in renal transplant recipients with chronic vascular rejection. Nephrol Dial Transplant 4:1070–1075
49. Kasiske BL, O'Donnell MP, Daniels F, Keane WF (1985) The lipid lowering agent clofibric acid ameliorates renal injury in the 5/6 nephrectomy model of chronic renal failure. Clin Res 33:488A
50. Walker LA, Frolich JC (1987) Renal prostaglandins and leukotrienes. Rev Physiol Biochem Pharmacol 107:1–72
51. Wheeler DC, Nair DR, Persaud JW, Varghese Z, Moorhead JF (1990) Dietary fatty acid intake influences progression of glomerulosclerosis in the obese Zucker rat (abstract). Kidney Int 37:524
52. Kasiske BL, O'Donnell MP, Cleary MP, Keane WF (1988) Treatment of hyperlipidemia reduces glomerular injury in obese Zucker rats. Kidney Int 33:667–672

Symposia

Immunological and Cellular
Mechanisms of Glomerulonephritis

Chair: William G. Couser (USA)
Leishi Li (China)

Glomerular Injury Induced by the C5b-9 Membrane Attack Complex of Complement

WILLIAM G. COUSER[1]

SUMMARY. Strong evidence implicates the assembly and glomerular epithelial cell membrane insertion of C5b-9 in mediating proteinuria in experimental membranous nephropathy. The cellular basis for this effect may involve cell activation by sublytic concentrations of C5b-9, resulting in release at the epithelial cell interface of inflammatory mediators. Potential mediators released by the epithelial cell may include oxidants, proteases or prostaglandins. Epithelial cell detachment from underlying basement membrane may also be involved. Further studies to define the cellular basis of the C5b-9 effect are required.

The intracellular processing and excretion of C5b-9 into the urinary space by glomerular epithelial cells under antibody and C5b-9 attack has led to studies showing that elevated urinary C5b-9 is a sensitive marker of on-going deposition of antibody to epithelial cell membrane antigens in the rat. The presence of elevated urinary C5b-9 in a subset of human patients with membranous nephropathy suggest that a similar mechanism may be operative in this disease.

Introduction

Considerable progress has been made in recent years in clarifying the mechanisms by which glomerular immune deposits induce tissue injury [1]. This has included recognition that the role of complement in the mediation of glomerular disease, which was clearly established in the 1960s [2], includes not only generation of chemotactic factors such as C5a which lead to neutrophil localization, but also the formation of the C5b-9 membrane attack complex of complement which inserts into the lipid bilayer of glomerular cell membranes and leads to a non-inflammatory type of renal lesion [3]. In this paper, I will present briefly the evidence in support of a role for the C5b-9

[1]Division of Nephrology, University of Washington, Seattle, WA 98195, USA

complex in glomerular disease and review what little is currently known of the cellular mechanism for this effect. This subject has been reviewed in more detail elsewhere [4, 5].

The human glomerular disease in which this mechanism is most likely operative is membranous nephropathy, but a role is probable in other lesions as well, particularly if subepithelial immune deposits are present [5].

Evidence for C5b-9 Mediated Proteinuria in Experimental Membranous Nephropathy

The first evidence for C5b-9 induced glomerular injury derived from studies of the mediation of proteinuria in the passive Heymann nephritis (PHN) model of MN in rats. PHN is induced by injection of a heterologous antibody to a proximal tubular brush border fraction termed FxlA. Studies by several laboratories over the past decade have demonstrated that the subepithelial immune complex deposits which develop in PHN form in situ [6,7] due to IgG antibody reacting with antigens on the membrane of the GEC. The best characterized of these at the present time is GP330 [8]. These antigen-antibody complexes activate complement producing glomerular deposits of the C5b-9 membrane attack complex, but the antigen-antibody complexes themselves are patched, capped, and shed from the cell surface by mechanisms requiring an intact GEC cytoskeleton to form the discontinuous subepithelial immune complex deposits characteristic of MN [9,10]. In PHN, proteinuria develops four to five days after antibody injection, when sufficient IgG has deposited to induce injury; it is morphologically indistinguishable from MN in man, in that no circulating effector cells or other inflammatory changes are present [11,12]. Despite the lack of inflammatory changes, however, studies in which rats were depleted of complement with cobra venom factor during the five days required for proteinuria to develop, demonstrated that complement-depletion totally abolished proteinuria in PHN without altering antibody deposition [12]. We speculated that this lesion involved a glomerular effect of C5b-9 rather than generation of chemotactic or opsonic factors such as C5a, the only complement-mediated mechanism previously implicated in glomerular injury.

A macromolecular complex, C5b-9 results from proteolytic cleavage of C5 to generate C5b, which then combines with C6 and C7 to form the C5b6,7 complex, an amphophilic molecule which has binding sites for the lipid bilayer of cell membranes (reviewed in 13). With binding of C8 and multiple C9 molecules, the C5b-9 complex inserts into the lipid bilayer of cell membranes [13]. A protective mechanism for C5b-9 injury may be afforded by plasma S-protein (vitronectin), which results in formation of SC5b-7 complexes which can bind C8 and C9 but cannot insert into cell membranes and are therefore considered inactive [14]. Membrane insertion of C5b-9 results in rapid lysis of non-nucleated cells such as erythrocytes, but lysis of nucleated cells is much more difficult to achieve.

Confirmation that C5b-9 assembly is critical in the mediation of proteinuria in PHN has been provided now by studies in the intact animal, in the isolated perfused kidney, and in isolated glomeruli. In intact rats, selective depletion of C6 to prevent assembly of C5b-9 can be maintained throughout the four to five day period required for proteinuria to develop following antibody injection [15]. Selective C6 depletion prevents glomerular assembly of C5b-9 complexes, as detected by staining for C5b-9 neoantigens, and abolishes the development of proteinuria without altering glomerular deposition of antibody or C3. In the isolated perfused rat kidney, proteinuria does not develop when antibody deposition occurs in the presence of serum deficient in C6 or C8, but appears immediately following addition of normal serum containing all complement components [16]. In collaboration with Dr. Virginia Savin, we have recently shown, in the isolated rat glomerulus, that glomerular permeability to albumin, reflected by changes in the reflection coefficient for albumin (which is calculated from the volumetric response in isolated glomeruli to changes in oncotic pressure gradient), is increased within 10 minutes in normal glomeruli exposed to anti Fx1A antibody IgG and normal serum as a complement source *in vitro* [17]. No change in permeability is induced by antibody in the presence of C6 or C7 deficient serum [17]. Since the principal biologic function of C6, C7, and C8 is the assembly of the C5b-9 membrane attack complex, these studies provide convincing evidence that proteinuria in experimental MN induced by antibody to GEC antigen is mediated by C5b-9 in the intact animal, the isolated perfused kidney, and the isolated glomerulus.

A role for C5b-9 has also been established in mediating injury in MN induced by other mechanisms. In the autologous phase of PHN where injury results from antibody reacting with previously deposited but sub-nephritogenic quantities of antibody to GEC, injury also appears to be C5b-9 mediated in the intact animal [18,19] and in the isolated perfused kidney [20]. Similar results are obtained when subepithelial deposits form in situ, due to localization of cationic antigens and antibodies to them. Thus the onset of proteinuria is delayed in genetically C6 deficient rabbits with cationic BSA induced serum sickness, compared to normal controls, despite comparable amounts of glomerular immune complex deposits [21]. Rats selectively depleted of C6 develop significantly less proteinuria in response to a nephritogenic quantity of cationic IgG containing immune complexes, compared to controls [22]. Evidence for a nephritogenic role for C5b-9 has also been obtained in models of anti-GBM nephritis in rabbits [23,24].

Cellular Basis for C5b-9 Effect

The cellular basis for the C5b-9 effect has not been defined. To better understand this process we developed a monoclonal antibody directed against a C9 neoantigen present only in the assembled rat C5b-9 complex [25]. This antibody stains PHN glomeruli in a pattern similar to staining for IgG and similar to that reported in human MN and other diseases by Falk and others [26]. Immunoultrastructural studies in PHN, utilizing this reagent, demonstrate early C5b-9 localization in subepithelial deposits and along the surfaces of the GEC membrane, particularly in regions of clathrin coated pits where the putative GP330 antigen is expressed [27]. The cell bound C5b-9 then undergoes endocytosis and is transported through the GEC in large multivesicular bodies before being exocytosed into the urinary space [27]. This is in contrast to the cellular handling of antigen-antibody complexes which are primarily patched and capped and then shed from the cell surface where they form granular deposits that become non-covalently bound to the GBM (Reviewed in

[10]). Several authors have demonstrated S protein in subepithelial immune deposits in MN [28]. This finding has prompted comment that the glomerular C5b-9 deposits are inactivated, cannot insert into cell membranes, and are therefore not likely to be pathogenic. We believe this is probably the case with SC5b-9 deposits, which remain extracellularly with the immune complex and may represent most of the glomerular C5b-9. However, freeze-fracture studies in early PHN reveal clusters of large 200–250 A intramembrane particles, which compare in size and appearance to membrane inserted C5b-9 [27]. Although these active, membrane-inserted complexes may represent a small fraction of the total glomerular C5b-9 deposits, they appear to be sufficient to cause disease.

Despite these advances in understanding the role of C5b-9 in the mediation of MN, the cellular consequences of C5b-9 attack on the GEC remain poorly understood. There appear to be both structural and functional consequences of GEC C5b-9 attack. The structural changes are predominantly an increase in thickness of the GBM, due primarily to an accumulation of laminin along the outer surface and in the characteristic spikes projecting from the subepithelial surface [29,30]. This process progresses to glomerulosclerosis resulting from an accumulation of normal extracellular matrix components, predominantly type IV collagen [31]. Functional changes in the barrier to protein filtration consist of the development of large pore defects [32] which appear to represent areas of GEC detachment from underlying basement membrane [33]. At present it is unclear what the relationship is, if any, between the structural and functional changes in the basement membrane.

One possibility for the C5b-9 effect might be that C5b-9 induces an abnormality in GEC production of laminin or other constituents of the basement membrane, resulting over time in a persistent remodeling of the basement membrane structure, with altered barrier function. Hansch et al. have reported a several-fold increase in production of type IV collagen by rat GEC following C5b-9 attack [34], but no studies of laminin production have appeared. However, the alteration which occurs in glomerular permeability in experimental MN induced by C5b-9 can develop in minutes in the isolated kidney and glomerulus and therefore seems unlikely to result from an alteration in matrix component metabolism.

As in non-inflammatory lesions induced by antibody alone, GEC detachment appears to underlie the permeability defect in MN as well [33]. Thus, a C5b-9 induced alteration in expression or function of integrins, or the matrix components to which they bind, might lead to epithelial cell detachment and proteinuria. One study showed no alteration in expression or distribution of a beta one integrin in human MN [35]. However, other integrins and cell membrane receptors have not been explored.

A third mechanism by which C5b-9 might be pathogenic at the cellular level may involve cell activation, with release of potentially toxic inflammatory mediators by the GEC itself. Although membrane insertion of C5b-9 leads to lysis of non-nucleated cells such as erythrocytes, nucleated cells are relatively resistant to C5b-9 attack and may actually be stimulated by this [14]. With respect to GEC, Quigg et al. have shown that antibody to GEC membrane, in the presence of sublytic concentrations of complement, induces non-cytolytic injury, as evidenced by the release of low molecular weight intracellular markers and formation of membrane vesicles similar to those excreted in the urine in PHN [36]. Sublytic C5b-9 attack also results in increased intracellular calcium, activation of phospholipase C, increased levels of

IP2, IP3, diacyl glycerol, and phosphatidic acid, with release of arachidonic acid, $PGF_2\alpha$, and thromboxane [37,38]. Enhanced prostaglandin production by GEC following sublytic C5b-9 attack has also been reported by Hansch [39]. Similar changes occur in mesangial cells in response to C5b-9 [40]. This phenomenon of C5b-9 induced cell activation could result in release, at the GBM-GEC interface, of several cell-derived substances. Three potential inflammatory mediators warrant consideration: prostaglandins, oxidants, and proteinases.

With respect to prostaglandins, Cybulsky et al. reported a reduction in C5b-9 mediated proteinuria in the isolated perfused kidney when a thromboxane synthesis inhibitor was employed [41]. Two groups have demonstrated a reduction in proteinuria with indomethacin in models of MN [42,43], although these results may in part reflect a reduction in glomerular filtration rate [43]. We have demonstrated, in PHN rats, a marked increase in glomerular PGE_2 and thromboxane production by glomeruli that was complement dependent and may have derived from the GEC [44]. However, administration of a thromboxane synthesis inhibitor, which reduced glomerular thromboxane production by over 80%, had no effect on C5b-9 induced proteinuria in PHN [44] or in another model of MN induced with cationized IgG which is believed to be C5b-9 mediated [22,45]. Thus it seems unlikely that alterations in GEC prostaglandin metabolism account directly for the altered permeability to protein induced by C5b-9.

A second possible GEC-derived mediator would be reactive oxygen species. Oxidants including H_2O_2, superoxide anion, and hydroxyl radical have all been implicated in various forms of inflammatory renal injury [46]. Adler et al. have shown that C5b-9 can directly stimulate cultured mesangial cells to produce H_2O_2 and superoxide anion [14]. Although oxidant production by the GEC is relatively low, three studies have described a beneficial effect of administration of the hydroxyl radical scavengers DMSO and dimethylthiourea (DMTU) on proteinuria in PHN [47–49]. Moreover, a beneficial effect of the iron chelating agent deferoxamine suggests participation of the Haber-Weiss reaction to form hydroxyl radical [49]. However, a direct effect of C5b-9 on GEC oxidant production remains to be documented.

A final potential candidate for a GEC derived mediator would be a GBM-degrading proteinase. From our laboratory, preliminary evidence exists for the production of a proteinase with type IV collagenase activity by GEC. A stimulation of proteinase production by sublytic C5b-9 attack could lead to an immediate and non-inflammatory type of glomerular lesion such as that seen in early MN.

Urinary C5b-9 Excretion as an Index of Disease Activity in Membranous Nephropathy

The observation that membrane inserted C5b-9 is transported intracellularly and exocytosed into the urinary space prompted us to develop a sensitive ELISA assay for both rat and human C5b-9 in urine. In the rat, urinary C5b-9 excretion is elevated only when subepithelial deposits result from antibody to the GEC membrane, and C5b-9 excretion in urine is not seen in a variety of other experimental immune glomerular diseases with comparable glomerular C5b-9 deposits, or in non-immune proteinuric glomerular lesions [3,50]. In the rat, urinary C5b-9 excretion closely parallels disease activity (on-going glomerular immune deposit formation). Within hours of the onset of antibody deposits C5b-9 excretion is increased in both the heterologous and autologous phases of PHN and before proteinuria appears; C5b-9 excretion ceases promptly when antibody deposition is halted by transplanting a nephritic kidney to a normal host [19,50]. Of interest, glomerular C3 deposition follows a very similar course and may also serve as a marker of disease activity [19,51]. Similar results have been obtained in the autologous immune complex nephritis (active Heymann nephritis) model [51].

We have attempted to extend these observations in the experimental animal to study MN in man with some success. In studies of 148 patients with proteinuric glomerular diseases, elevated urinary C5b-9 (analyzed as differences from expected values based on urinary C5 excretion) was found in only nine (of 40) patients with idiopathic MN and in four (of six) patients with lupus MN, and not in a variety of other diseases with comparable levels of proteinuria, or in controls [52]. These findings have now been confirmed by Coupes et al. [53]. Patients with elevated urinary C5b-9 values were generally studied earlier in the course of disease and had higher levels of urine protein excretion than MN patients with normal urinary C5b-9 values, findings consistent with a greater likelihood of disease activity in high C5b-9 excretors [52]. These results imply that, in at least one subset of patients with idiopathic and lupus MN, the disease mechanism is analogous to the autoimmune process involving antibody to the GEC defined in the Heymann models in rats and that GEC membrane insertion of C5b-9 also takes place in man. Urinary C5b-9 excretion may serve as a useful marker of immune disease activity in MN in the absence of an assay for the pathogenic antibody.

References

1. Couser WG (1985) Mechanisms of glomerular injury in immune-complex disease (nephrology forum). Kidney Int 28:569–583
2. Cochrane CG, Unanue E, Dixon FJ (1965) A role of polymorphonuclear leukocytes and complement in nephrotoxic nephritis. J Exp Med 122:99–110
3. Couser WG, Baker PJ, Adler S (1985) Complement and the direct mediation of immune glomerular injury: A new perspective (editorial review). Kidney Int 28:879–890
4. Cybulsky AV, Quigg RJ, Salant DJ (1988) Role of the complement membrane attack complex in glomerular injury. In: Wilson CB, Brenner BM, Stein J (eds) Contemporary issues in nephrol, vol 18. Churchill Livingston, New York, pp 57–86
5. Couser WG, Abrass CK (1988) Pathogenesis of membranous nephropathy. Annu Rev Med 39:517–530
6. Van Damme BJC, Fleuren GJ, Bakker WW, Vernier RL, Hoedemaeker Ph.J (1978) Experimental glomerulonephritis in the rat induced by antibodies directed against tubular antigens. V. Fixed glomerular antigens in the pathogenesis of heterologous immune complex glomerulonephritis. Lab Invest 38:502
7. Couser WG, Steinmuller DR, Stilmant MM, Salant DJ, Lowenstein LM (1978) Experimental glomerulonephritis in the isolated perfused rat kidney. J Clin Invest 62:1275
8. Kerjaschki D, Farquhar MG (1982) The pathogenic antigen of Heymann nephritis is a membrane glycoprotein of the renal proximal tubular brush border. Proc Natl Acad Sci USA 79:5557–5561
9. Camussi G, Brentjens JR, Noble B, Kerjaschki D, Malavasi F, Roholt OA, Farquhar MG, Andres G (1985) Antibody-induced redistribution of Heymann's antigen on the surface of

cultured glomerular visceral epithelial cells: Possible role in the pathogenesis of Heymann glomerulonephritis. J Immunol 135:2409

10. Brentjens JR, Andres GA (1989) Interaction of antibodies with renal cell surface antigens. Kidney Int 35:954–968

11. Salant DJ, Darby C, Couser WG (1980) Experimental membranous glomerulonephritis in rats. Quantitative studies of glomerular immune deposit formation in isolated glomeruli and whole animals. J Clin Invest 66:71–81

12. Salant DJ, Belok S, Madaio MP, Couser WG (1980) A new role for complement in experimental membranous nephropathy in rats. J Clin Invest 66:1339–1350

13. Muller-Eberhard HJ (1988) Molecular organization and function of the complement system. Annu Rev Biochem 57:321–347

14. Adler S, Baker PJ, Johnson RJ, Ochi RF, Pritzl P, Couser WG (1986) Complement membrane attack complex stimulates production of reactive oxygen metabolites by cultured rat mesangial cells. J Clin Invest 77:762–767

15. Baker PJ, Ochi RF, Schulze M, Johnson RJ, Campbell C, Couser WG (1989) Depletion of C6 prevents development of proteinuria in experimental membranous nephropathy in rats. Am J Pathol 135:185–194

16. Cybulsky AV, Quigg RJ, Salant DJ (1986) The membrane attack complex in complement-mediated glomerular epithelial cell injury: Formation and stability of C5b-9 and C5b-7 in rat membranous nephropathy. J Immunol 137:1511–1516

17. Savin VJ, Johnson RJ, Couser WG (1990) Antibody induced complement activation increases albumin permeability of isolated rat glomeruli (abstract). Kidney Int 37: 430

18. Adler S, Salant DJ, Dittmer JE, Rennke HG, Madaio MP, Couser WG (1983) Mediation of proteinuria in membranous nephropathy due to a planted glomerular antigen. Kidney Int 23:807–815

19. Pruchno CJ, Burns MW, Schulze M, Johnson RJ, Baker PJ, Couser WG (1989) Urinary excretion of C5b-9 reflects disease activity in passive Heymann nephritis. Kidney Int 36:65–71

20. Cybulsky AV, Rennke HG, Feintzeig ID, Salant DJ (1986) Complement-induced glomerular epithelial cell injury. Role of the membrane attack complex in rat membranous nephropathy. J Clin Invest 77:1096–1107

21. Groggel GC, Adler S, Rennke HG, Couser WG, Salant DG (1983) Role of the terminal complement pathway in experimental membranous nephropathy in the rabbit. J Clin Invest 72:1948–1957

22. Ochi RF, Johnson RJ, Baker PJ, Adler S, Couser WG (1986) C6 depletion diminishes proteinuria in experimental membranous nephropathy induced by an exogenous antigen (abstract). Kidney Int 29:287

23. Groggel GC, Salant DJ, Darby C, Rennke HG. Couser WG (1985) Role of the terminal complement pathway in the heterologous phase of anti-glomerular basement membrane nephritis in the rabbit. Kidney Int 27:643–651

24. Tipping PG, Boyce NW, Holdsworth SR (1989) Relative contributions of chemo-attractant and terminal components of complement to anti-glomerular basement membrane (GBM) glomerulonephritis. Clin Exp Immunol 78:444–448

25. Perkinson DT, Baker PJ, Couser WG, Johnson RJ, Adler S (1985) Membrane attack complex deposition in experimental glomerular injury. Am J Pathol 120:121–128

26. Falk RJ, Dalmasso AP, Kim Y, Tsai CH, Scheinman JI, Gewurz H, Michael AF (1983) Neoantigen of the polymerized ninth component of complement. Characterization of a monoclonal antibody and immunohistochemical localization in renal disease. J Clin Invest 72:560–573

27. Kerjaschki D, Schulze M, Binder S, Kain R, Ojha PP, Susani M, Horvat R, Baker PJ, Couser WG (1989) Transcellular transport and membrane insertion of the C5b-9 membrane attack complex of complement by glomerular epithelial cells in experimental membranous nephropathy. J Immunol 143:546–552

28. Bariety J, Hinglais N, Bhakdi S, Mandet C, Rouchon M, Kazatchkine MD (1989) Immuno-histochemical study of complement S protein (Vitronectin) in normal and diseased human kidneys: relationship to neoantigens of the C5b-9 terminal complex. Clin Exp Immunol 75:76–81

29. Fukatsu A, Matsuo S, Killen PD, Martin GR, Andres GA, Brentjens JR (1988) The glomerular distribution of type IV collagen and laminin in human membranous glomerulonephritis. Hum Pathol 19:64–68

30. Matsuo S, Brentjens JR, Andres G, Foidart J-M, Martin GR, Martinez-Hernandez A (1986) Distribution of basement membrane antigens in glomeruli of mice with autoim-mune glomerulo-nephritis. Am J Pathol 122:36–49

31. Adler S, Striker LJ, Striker LJ, Striker GE, Perkinson DT, Hibbert J, Couser WG (1986) Studies of progressive glomerular sclerosis in the rat. Am J Pathol 123:553–562

32. Shemesh O, Ross JC, Deen WM, Grant GW, Myers BD (1986) Nature of the glomerular capillary injury in human membranous glomerulopathy. J Clin Invest 77:868–877

33. Schneeberger EE, O'Brien A, Grupe WE (1979) Altered glomerular permeability in Munich-Wistar rats with autologous immune complex nephritis. Lab Invest 40:227–235

34. Torbohm I, Schonermark M, Wingen A-M, Berger B, Rother K, Hansch GM (1990) C5b-8 and C5b-9 modulate the collagen release of human glomerular epithelial cells. Kidney Int 37:1098–1104

35. Kerjaschki D, Ojha PP, Susani M, Horvat R, Binder S, Hovorka A, Hillemanns P, Pytela R (1989) A β_1-integrin receptor for fibronectin in human kidney glomeruli. Am J Pathol 134:481–489

36. Quigg RJ, Cybulsky AV, Jacobs JB, Salant DJ (1988) Anti-Fx1A produces complement-dependent cytotoxicity of glomerular epithelial cells. Kidney Int 34:43–52

37. Cybulsky AV, Salant DJ, Quigg RJ, Badalamenti J, Bonventre JV (1989) Complement C5b-9 complex activates phospholipases in glomerular epithelial cells. Am J Physiol 257:F826–F836

38. Cybulsky AV, Bonventre JV, Quigg RJ, Lieberthal W, Salant DJ (1990) Cytosolic calcium and protein kinase C reduce complement-mediated glomerular epithelial cell injury. Kid-ney Int 38:803–811

39. Hansch GM, Betz M, Gunther J, Rother KO, Sterzel B (1988) The complement membrane attack complex stimulates the prostanoid production of cultured glomerular epithelial cells. Int Arch Allergy Appl Immunol 85:87–93

40. Lovett DH, Hansch G-M, Goppelt M, Resch K, Gemsa D (1987) Activation of glomerular mesangial cells by the terminal membrane attack complex of complement. J Immunol 138:2473–2480

41. Cybulsky AV, Lieberthal W, Quigg RJ, Rennke HG, Salant DJ (1987) A role for thrombox-ane in complement-mediated glomerular injury. Am J Pathol 128:45–51

42. Zoja C, Benigni A, Verroust P, Ronco R, Bertane T, Remuzzi G (1987) Indomethacin reduces proteinuria in passive Heymann nephritis in rats. Kidney Int 31:1335–1343

43. Kirschenbaum MA, Liebross BA, Serros ER (1985) Effect of indomethacin on proteinuria in rats with autologous immune complex nephropathy. Prostaglandins 30:295–303

44. Stahl RAK, Adler S, Baker PJ, Chen Y-P, Pritzl PM, Couser WG (1987) Enhanced glomerular prostaglandin formation in experimental membranous nephropathy. Kidney Int 31:1126–1131

45. Thaiss F, Germann PJ, Kahf S, Schoeppe W, Helmchen U, Stahl RAK (1989) Effect of thromboxane synthesis inhibition in a model of membranous nephropathy. Kidney Int 35:76–83

46. Johnson RJ, Klebanoff SJ, Couser WG (1988) Oxidants in glomerular injury. In: Wilson CB, Brenner BM, Stein J (eds) Contemporary issues in nephrology, vol 18. Churchill Livingston, New York, pp 87–110

47. Lotan D, Kaplan BS, Fong JSC, Goodyer PR, DeChadarevian J-P (1984) Reduction of protein excretion by dimethyl sulfoxide in rats with passive Heymann nephritis. Kidney Int 25:778–788
48. Kaplan BS, Milner LS, Lotan D, Mills M, Goodyer PR, Fong JSC (1986) Interaction of dimethyl sulfoxide and nonsteroidal anti-inflammatory agents in passive Heymann's nephritis. J Lab Clin Med 107:425–430
49. Shah SV (1988) Evidence suggesting a role for hydroxyl radical in passive Heymann nephritis in rats. Am J Physiol 254:F337–F344
50. Schulze M, Baker PJ, Perkinson DT, Johnson RJ, Ochi RF, Stahl RA, Couser WG (1989) Increased urinary excretion of C5b-9 distinguishes passive Heymann nephritis in the rat. Kidney Int 35:60–68
51. Pruchno CJ, Burns MW, Schulze M, et al. (to be published) Urinary excretion of the C5b-9 membrane attack complex of complement is a marker of immune disease activity in autologous immune complex nephritis. Am J Pathol
52. Schulze M, Donadio JV, Pruchno CJ, et al. (to be published) Elevated urinary excretion of the complement C5b-9 complex in a subset of patients with membranous nephropathy. N Engl J Med

Platelets in Immune Mediated Glomerular Disease

RICHARD J. JOHNSON[1]

SUMMARY. Platelets are recognized for their role in hemostasis, but may also act as proinflammatory cells capable of releasing vasoactive, chemotactic, proliferative, and proteolytic factors or enzymes. Platelet activation and localization to glomeruli can be demonstrated in numerous experimental and human glomerular diseases, especially in diseases associated with endothelial cell or mesangial cell injury. Proposed roles for platelets in glomerular injury include initiating glomerular thrombosis, facilitating immune complex deposition, modulating hemodynamic changes and mediating glomerulosclerosis. We have recently demonstrated a critical requirement for platelets in neutrophil-mediated glomerulonephritis. The mechanism may involve an augmentation of neutrophil injury by the platelet or platelet products. Platelets also mediate mesangial cell proliferation in immune complex nephritis. The effect involves a platelet-mediated induction of platelet-derived growth factor (PDGF) and PDGF-receptor synthesis by the mesangial cell, and is also associated with the acquisition by the mesangial cell of a smooth muscle phenotype. Thus, the platelet has important and diverse roles in glomerular inflammation. Platelets can mediate direct effects, such as in the formation of platelet-fibrin thrombi, but may effect glomerular inflammation indirectly via their ability to interact with neutrophils and glomerular mesangial cells.

Platelets as Inflammatory Effector Cells

The blood platelet is well-recognized for having a major role in hemostasis and thrombosis. It is becoming increasingly evident that the platelet, like the neutrophil and monocyte, may also function as an inflammatory effector cell independent of its role in coagulation. Platelets contain numerous inflammatory mediators within their alpha, and dense granules, as well as within lysosomes, and can release their contents

---

[1]Division of Nephrology, Department of Medicine, University of Washington, Seattle, WA 98195, USA

Table 1. Platelet products important in inflammation

Adhesive proteins: Fibrinogen, fibronectin, von-Willebrand factor, thrombospondin, GMP140
Lipid mediators: Thromboxane A_2, lipoxygenase products, platelet activating factor (PAF)
Cationic proteins: β-thromboglobulin, platelet factor 4, platelet basic protein, connective tissue activating peptide III
Degrading enzymes: Heparanase, neutral proteinases, acid hydrolases
Vasoactive amines: Histamine, serotonin
Adenine nucleotides: ADP, ATP
Growth factors: Platelet derived growth factor (PDGF), transforming growth factor-β (TGF-β), epidermal growth factor/TGF-α, hepatocyte growth factor, endothelial cell growth factor, and interleukin I (IL-1)
Oxidants: Superoxide anion (O_2^-), H_2O_2
Anti-inflammatory products: α-1 antiproteinase, α-2 macroglobulin, superoxide dismutase, catalase, glutathione peroxidase, adenosine

following stimulation. Platelet releasates contain vasoactive, thrombogenic, chemotactic, proliferative, and proteolytic factors/enzymes (Table 1) [1]. Platelets, like leukocytes, can undergo chemotaxis, phagocytosis, degranulation, and generate cytotoxicity. Platelets do not contain an NADPH oxidase (which is present in neutrophils), but nevertheless are capable of generating small quantities of oxidants via both the cycloxygenase and lipoxygenase pathways [2]. Platelet generation of oxidants may mediate killing of various parasites as well as cultured endothelial cells [3,4]. Platelets can generate C5a (via platelet chemotactic factor) and can release terminal complement components that participate in additional C5b-9 formation [1,5]. Finally, platelets and megakaryocyte can endocytose plasma components, including IgG, and can subsequently release these components at sites of inflammation [6].

Platelet Participation in Glomerular Diseases

Platelets and platelet antigens have been described in glomeruli in numerous experimental glomerular diseases, particularly diseases associated with endothelial [7,8] or mesangial cell [9,10] injury. Platelets and platelet antigens can also be documented in glomeruli in a wide variety of human glomerular diseases, including IgA nephropathy, diffuse proliferative lupus nephritis, hemolytic uremic syndrome, and membranoproliferative glomerulonephritis (GN) [11]. In many of these diseases evidence for systemic platelet activation is often present, and is manifested by decreased platelet survival, the presence of platelet release products in plasma, and occasionally, thrombocytopenia [12,13].

Mechanisms for Platelet Localization and Activation in GN

The mechanisms responsible for the platelet localization are probably the consequence of the cellular injury and subsequent exposure of the subendothelium and basement membrane. It is known that *collagen fragments* can act as a strong chemotactic stimulus for platelets [14]. Another chemoattractant for platelets may be *platelet activating factor (PAF)*. Ito, Andres, and colleages have reported that the influx of platelets and neutrophils in glomeruli of rabbits with hyperacute transplant rejection may be due to the release by damaged glomerular cells of PAF, which can be detected in high levels in the renal veins of these animals [15]. In addition, activated neutrophils may cause intraglomerular platelet aggregation and activation by releasing oxidants that inactivate local ADPase within the glomerular capillary wall, resulting in increased concentrations of ADP [16]. This is consistent with our observation that glomerular endothelial cell and mesangial cell injury secondary to neutrophil oxidants produced by the myeloperoxidase-hydrogen peroxide reaction results in a marked influx of platelets [7].

Recently we have also reported an important *role for complement* in platelet localization in a model of subendothelial immune complex nephritis (the con A model) [8], and in the model of mesangial proliferative GN induced by anti-Thy 1 antibody [10]. Using ^{111}In-labeled platelets, we were able to demonstrate significant platelet accumulation in glomeruli, which in the con A model peaked with over 5000 platelets per glomerulus 10 minutes after disease induction [8]. Rats with con A GN that were depleted of complement with cobra venom factor had minimal glomerular platelet localization [8]. It is possible that the complement-dependent platelet localization results from tissue injury by the terminal membrane attack complex of complement [17]. It is also possible that the platelets are responding to complement activation products. It is known, for example, that guinea pig platelets can be activated by C3a and C5a [18]. The mechanism does not appear to be due to complement-mediated neutrophil localization. At least for the con A model, the initial platelet influx precedes the neutrophil localization and occurs despite profound leukocyte depletion [8].

Once localized, platelet activation ensues, with a change in shape from discoid to round, the formation of filopodia, and the centralization of granules. Platelet aggregation occurs secondary to a conformational change in the cell surface glycoprotein GPIIb-GPIIIa, allowing the platelet to bind fibrinogen which acts as an interconnecting link between platelets. Platelets also adhere to exposed areas of basement membrane and subendothelium, by utilizing the GPIb receptor to bind to von Willebrand factor. Immune adherence mechanisms may also be operative, resulting in the direct binding of the platelet to immune complexes by the platelet Fc receptor (primarily in primates) or by the CR1 receptor (as in rabbits and rats) [1]. Human platelets also have CR2, CR3, and CR4 receptors, but their functional significance remains to be established. Platelet activation is also associated with a "release" reaction in which the platelets discharge numerous mediators from alpha, dense, and lysosomal granules into the extracellular space.

Roles for the Platelet in Immune Mediated Glomerular Injury

The platelet has been proposed to have several important roles in immune mediated glomerular injury. The first major role ascribed to the platelet was to *facilitate immune complex deposition* in glomeruli in acute serum sickness [19]. The proposed mechanism involves antigen binding to IgE-sensitized basophils, followed by release from the basophil of PAF [20,21]. PAF causes platelet activation with the release of vasoactive amines and cationic proteins that subsequently mediate an increase in glomerular permeability, thus facilitating immune complex deposition [20,21]. Platelets may also mediate *glomerular thrombosis* [22]. Platelets, when activated, expose phospholipids on their cell surfaces which act as a matrix for coagulation reactions, providing binding sites for activated coagulation factors and generating prothrombinase activity that accelerates the formation of thrombin [23]. Platelets can also potentiate tissue factor production by monocytes and endothelial cells [24,25]. This latter observation is important, as recent experimental data strongly suggests that monocyte-macrophage release of tissue factor may be responsible for fibrin deposition in several glomerular diseases [26]. We have also reported that platelet depletion markedly reduces fibrin deposition in the con A model of subendothelial immune complex nephritis [27]. Platelets may also *modulate glomerular hemodynamics*, particularly by the release of vasoactive substances, such as thromboxane, that can mediate a significant reduction in the glomerular filtration rate (GFR). Other platelet products can also mediate mesangial cell contraction, and thus potentially modulate GFR; these include PDGF, PAF, and histamine [28]. Platelets have also been proposed to have a role in *glomerulosclerosis*. Platelet infiltration and thrombosis may precede glomerulosclerosis both in experimentally mediated glomerular injury [29,30] and in lupus nephritis in man [31]. Anti-platelet agents have also been reported to inhibit the glomerulosclerosis that develops following renal ablation [32,33]. A potential mechanism may involve release by the platelet of transforming growth factor (TGF)-β, which can induce mesangial cells to produce collagen, fibronectin, and heparan sulfate proteoglycans [34,35].

Recently we have performed studies on two additional roles for the platelet in glomerular injury; specifically, that of *augmenting neutrophil-mediated injury*, and that of *mediating mesangial cell proliferation and activation*. These studies are summarized below.

Platelets are Required for Neutrophil-Mediated Glomerular Injury

Early in our studies we were impressed by the frequent coexistence of platelets and neutrophils in glomeruli of both human and experimentally-induced glomerular diseases [8]. Platelets and neutrophils have been noted to co-localize in numerous inflammatory conditions, including the Arthus reaction, the Shwartzman reaction, hyperacute transplant rejection, and in various inflammatory skin lesions. Studies by Henson in the late 1960s demonstrated that in passive cutaneous anaphylaxis in rabbits both platelets and neutrophils were required for injury to occur [36]. The importance of platelets in neutrophil-mediated injury was further demonstrated by Ward et al. who reported that platelet depletion could prevent neutrophil-mediated injury in a rat model of the adult respiratory distress syndrome [37].

To investigate a potential interaction of the platelet and neutrophil in immune glomerular injury, we performed platelet depletion studies in the neutrophil and complement-dependent model of immune complex nephritis induced with concanavalin A (con A) and anti-con A antibody [27]. Platelet depletion completely prevented proteinuria in this model. The decrease in albuminuria could not be attributed to differences in blood or glomerular neutrophil counts, complement, or glomerular antibody binding.

It is possible that the mechanism involves an additive effect of platelets and neutrophils in mediating glomerular injury. As shown in Table 1, platelets can release a variety of mediators that could, theoretically, mediate changes in glomerular permeability. For example, the release of platelet cationic proteins, which could bind to anionic sites present in the glomerular basement membrane (GBM) could thus neutralize the charge barrier [20,21]. PAF can also induce direct changes in vascular permeability [20]. Platelets can contain the endoglycosidase, heparanase, which can degrade glycosaminoglycans such as the heparan sulfate component of heparan sulfate proteoglycan [38]. Kanwar and colleagues have reported that intrarenal perfusion of heparanase will lead to increased glomerular permeability to protein [39]. Platelets can also release oxidants and proteases, although the quantities are small relative to the neutrophil or monocyte [1,3,4].

Although it is possible that the platelet and neutrophil mediated effects are additive, we believe that a more likely mechanism involves an interaction of these two cell types within the glomerulus. Platelets and/or platelet products can, under certain conditions, augment neutrophil adherence, aggregation, CR3 expression, phagocytosis, degranulation, oxidant release, and cytotoxicity [1]. Platelets can also interact with neutrophils to potentiate PAF production, augment leukotriene B_4 formation, and generate new eicosanoids [1]. However, platelets or platelet products have also been reported to inhibit certain neutrophil functions, due to the presence within the platelet of anti-proteinases, adenosine, glutathione peroxidase, and other anti-inflammatory substances (Table 1). The complexity of the platelet-neutrophil interaction can be appreciated when one considers the multiple proinflammatory (as well as anti-inflammatory) mediators/substances that both cells can release. Nevertheless, the observation that both platelets and neutrophils are required for proteinuria to develop in the con A model of nephritis suggests an important synergy of these two cells in glomerular inflammation.

Role of Platelets in Glomerular Cell Proliferation

Studies in several experimental models of glomerular disease, including "Arthus"-type nephritis [30,40] and the glomerular injury induced by the myeloperoxidase system [7] have shown that these diseases are characterized by an initial platelet infiltration followed by endothelial cell or mesangial cell proliferation. Whereas these studies suggest an important association of platelets with glomerular cell proliferation, the first demonstration that platelets actually mediated the cell proliferation was reported by Cattell, who noted that platelet-depleted rats with Habu snake venom-induced glomerular injury had significantly less glomerular hypercellularity [9].

We examined the role of platelets in a rat model of GN induced with antibody to the Thy 1 antigen present on the mesangial cell membrane [41]. This model results in acute complement-dependent mesangiolysis (i.e., mesangial cell loss with dissolution of mesangial matrix) followed by marked hypercellularity in mesangial areas [17]. Because the hypercellularity represents both endogenous glomerular cell proliferation and leukocyte infiltration, we identified proliferating cells by immunostaining tissue sections for the proliferating cell nuclear antigen (PCNA) [41]. PCNA is an auxiliary protein to DNA polymerase δ that is expressed during the cell cycle from late G1 until the M phase (peaking during the S phase) [42]. In addition, double immuno-labeling was performed in which tissue sections were stained for both PCNA and the common leukocyte antigen (CD45). This was performed because some leukocytes may have recently proliferated in the marrow prior to localizing in the glomerulus, and also because certain leukocyte populations, such as monocytes and lymphocytes, can proliferate at sites of inflammation. Thus, double immuno-labeling allowed us to distinguish proliferating glomerular cells (i.e., PCNA+, CD45-) from proliferating cells of bone marrow origin (PCNA+, CD45+). Utilizing these special methods, we were able to demonstrate that platelet depletion significantly reduced *glomerular cell proliferation*, independent of effects on glomerular antibody binding or complement levels.

There are several potential mechanisms by which the platelet could mediate glomerular cell proliferation. First, proliferation could be mediated by the direct release of platelet growth factors such as PDGF. Activated platelets have also been reported to express interleukin (IL)-1 on their cell surfaces [43]. It is also possible that the platelet mechanism is indirect, and involves a platelet-mediated induction of monocyte-macrophages or glomerular cells to release their own growth factors. Alternatively, the platelet mechanism could involve induction of the mesangial cell to upregulate growth factor receptors that would increase responsiveness of the mesangial cell to growth factor action.

In this regard an important growth factor is PDGF. Not only is it a major growth factor present in platelets, but it is capable of inducing mesangial cell proliferation [44]. Mesangial cells will also produce their own PDGF when they are exposed to a variety of growth factors (including PDGF), thus providing for a potential autocrine-mediated amplification of the proliferative stimulus [45].

Role of PDGF in Mesangial Proliferative GN

Gesualdo et al. recently reported that PDGF A-chain and B-chain mRNA were markedly elevated in whole kidney RNA from mice with an experimental IgA nephropathy [46]. However, studies using whole kidney RNA do not distinguish between PDGF mRNA of tubular or glomerular origin. Kidney epithelial cells in culture can express PDGF B-chain mRNA [47].

Recent studies by H. Iida and others in our laboratory have provided evidence that mesangial cell proliferation in anti-Thy 1 GN is associated with markedly increased gene expression for PDGF A and B chain in *glomerular RNA* extracts [48]. *In situ* hybridization has allowed us to identify individual cells that are expressing PDGF B chain mRNA in mesangial regions of glomeruli of these diseased rats (unpublished work).

The identification of the cells expressing PDGF B-chain protein in the rat model of anti-Thy 1 GN has been further studied by immunostaining. Double-immunostaining with a monoclonal antibody to the PDGF B-chain and to α-smooth muscle actin suggests that the majority of cells expressing PDGF are also α-smooth muscle actin positive [48]. This suggests that the majority of cells expressing PDGF B-chain are mesangial cells (see below).

An increase in gene and protein expression for PDGF β receptor in glomeruli also occurs in the anti-Thy 1 model of mesangial proliferative GN [48]. Immunostaining with a polyclonal antibody to the PDGF receptor β-subunit strongly suggests that the PDGF-R is expressed by mesangial cells. A similar upregulation of the PDGF-R β protein has also been reported in various types of mesangial proliferative nephritis in man [49].

Rats with anti-Thy 1 GN that were platelet depleted had significantly reduced PDGF and PDGF receptor gene and protein expression [48]. This suggests that one mechanism for platelet-mediated proliferation may be to induce mesangial cells to produce their own PDGF and PDGF receptors. This would allow for an autocrine-mediated amplification of the initial proliferative stimulus.

Platelet-Mediated Mesangial Cell Activation

We also have recent data that the platelet-mediated mesangial cell proliferation in anti-Thy 1 GN is associated with a phenotypic change of the mesangial cell to assume smooth muscle-like features. Specifically, there appears to be de novo expression of α-smooth muscle actin, by proliferating mesangial cells, that is mediated by platelets and complement [50]. Thus, platelets not only mediate mesangial cell proliferation, but they may also modulate changes in mesangial cell phenotype that may be potentially significant in active GN.

Conclusion

The platelet is a diverse cell that may play a major role in many forms of glomerular injury. One of the major roles may be to augment neutrophil-mediated injury of the glomerular capillary wall. Also important is the role of the platelet in inducing mesangial cell proliferation and activation. This mechanism may involve a platelet mediated stimulation of mesangial cells to produce PDGF that can act as an autocrine growth factor. Further studies are needed to determine the potential benefits of therapy designed to inhibit platelet activation in glomerulonephritis.

Acknowledgments. The author would like to acknowledge Dr. H. Iida, Dr. A. Yoshimura, and Dr. D.F. Bowen-Pope for their important contributions on the PDGF studies, and also Dr. W.G. Couser and Dr. C.E. Alpers for their valuable advice and suggestions.

Support for these studies was provided by U.S. Public Health Service grants DK-39068, DK-40802, and by research grants from the Northwest Kidney Foundation and the Jules and Gwen Knapp Charitable Foundation.

References

1. Weksler BB (1988) Roles for human platelets in inflammation. Prog Clin Biol Res 283: 611–638
2. Worner P (1981) Arachidonic acid-induced chemiluminescence of human platelets: contribution of the prostaglandin and lipoxygenase pathways. Thromb Haemost 46:584–589
3. Joseph M, Capron A, Ameisen J-C, Capron M, Vorng H, Pancre V, Kusnierz J-P, Auriault C (1986) The receptor for IgE on blood platelets. Eur J Immunol 16:306–312
4. Larsen T, Sorensen MB, Olsen R, Jorgensen L (1989) Effect of scavengers of active oxygen species and pretreatment with acetyl-salicylic acid on the injury to cultured endothelial cells by thrombin-stimulated platelets. In Vitro Cell Devel Biol 25:276–282
5. Houle JJ, Leddy JP, Rosenfeld SI (1989) Secretion of the terminal complement proteins, C5-C9, by human platelets. Clin Immunol Immunopath 50:385–393

6. George JN, Saucerman S, Levine SP, Knieriem LK, Bainton DF (1985) Immunoglobulin G is a platelet alpha granule-secreted protein. J Clin Invest 76:2020–2025

7. Johnson RJ, Guggenheim SJ, Klebanoff SJ, Ochi RF, Wass A, Baker P, Schulze M, Couser WG (1988) Morphologic correlates of glomerular oxidant injury induced by the myeloperoxidase-hydrogen peroxide-halide system of the neutrophil. Lab Invest 58:294–301

8. Johnson RJ, Alpers CE, Pruchno C, Schulze M, Baker PJ, Pritzl P, Couser WG (1989) Mechanisms and kinetics for platelet and neutrophil localization in immune complex nephritis. Kidney Int 36:780–789

9. Cattell V (1979) Focal mesangial proliferative glomerulonephritis in the rat caused by habu snake venom: the role of platelets. Br J Exp Pathol 60:201–208

10. Johnson RJ, Pritzl P, Iida H, Alpers CE. Platelet-complement interactions in mesangial proliferative nephritis in the rat. Amer J Path (in press)

11. Duffus P, Parbtani A, Frampton G, Cameron JS (1982) Intraglomerular localization of platelet related antigens, platelet factor 4 and β-thromboglobulin in glomerulonephritis. Clin Nephrol 17:288–297

12. George CRP, Slichter SJ, Quadracci LJ, Striker GE, Harker L (1974) A kinetic evaluation of hemostasis in renal disease. N Engl J Med 29:1111–1115

13. Parbtania A, Frampton G, Cameron JS (1980) Platelet and plasma serotonin concentrations in glomerulonephritis, II. Clin Nephrol 14:112–123

14. Lowenhaupt RW (1982) Human platelet chemotaxis can be induced by low molecular substance(s) derived from the interaction of plasma and collagen. In: Jamieson GA, Scipio AR (eds) Interaction of platelets and tumor cells. Alan R. Liss, New York, pp 269–280

15. Ito S, Camussi G, Tetta C, Milgrom F, Andres G (1984) Hyperacute renal allograft rejection in the rabbit. Lab Invest 51:148–161

16. Poelstra K, Hardonk MJ, Koudstaal J, Bakker WW (1990) Intraglomerular platelet aggregation and experimental glomerulonephritis. Kidney Int 37:1500–1508

17. Yamamoto T, Wilson CB (1987) Complement dependence of antibody-induced mesangial cell injury in the rat. J Immunol 138:3758–3765

18. Meuer S, Ecker U, Hadding U, Bitter-Suermann D (1981) Platelet-serotonin release by C3a and C5a: Two independent pathways of activation. J Immunol 126:1506–1509

19. Kniker WT, Cochrane CG (1968) The localization of circulating immune complexes in experimental serum sickness. J Exp Med 127:119–135

20. Camussi G (1986) Potential role of platelet-activating factor in renal pathophysiology (editorial review). Kidney Int 29:469–477

21. Barnes JL, Venkatachalam MA (1985) The role of platelets and polycationic mediators in glomerular vascular injury. Semin Nephrol 5:57–68

22. Kincaid-Smith P (1972) Coagulation and renal disease. Kidney Int 2:183–190

23. Walsh PN (1985) Platelet-mediated coagulant protein interactions in hemostasis. Semin Hematol 22:178–186

24. Johnsen ULH, Lyberg T, Galdal KS, Prydz H (1983) Platelets stimulate thromboplastin synthesis in human endothelial cells. Thromb Haemost 49:69–72

25. Niemetz J, Marcus AJ (1974) The stimulatory effect of platelets and platelet membranes on the procoagulant activity of leukocytes. J Clin Invest 54:1437–1443

26. Tipping PG, Worthington LA, Holdsworth SR (1987) Quantitation and characterization of glomerular procoagulant activity in experimental glomerulonephritis. Lab Invest 56:155–159

27. Johnson RJ, Alpers CE, Pritzl P, Schulze M, Baker P, Pruchno C, Couser WG (1988) Platelets mediate neutrophil-dependent immune complex nephritis in the rat. J Clin Invest 82:1225–1235

28. Schlondorff D (1987) The glomerular mesangial cell: an expanding role for a specialized pericyte. FASEB J 1:272–281

29. Jorgensen L, Glynn MF, Hovig T, Murphy EA, Buchanan MR, Mustard JF (1970) Renal lesions and rise in blood pressure caused by adenosine diphosphate-induced platelet aggregations in rabbits. Lab Invest 23:347–357
30. Gabbiani G, Badonnel M-C, Vassalli P (1975) Experimental focal glomerular lesions elicited by insoluble immune complexes. Lab Invest 32:33–45
31. Kant KS, Pollak VE, Weiss MA, Glueck HI, Miller MA, Hess EV (1981) Glomerular thrombosis in systemic lupus erythematosus: Prevalence and significance. Medicine (Baltimore) 60:71–86
32. Purkerson ML, Heinrich-Joist J, Yates J, Valdes A, Morrison A, Klahr S (1985) Inhibition of thromboxane synthesis ameliorates the progressive kidney disease of rats with subtotal renal ablation. Proc Natl Acad Sci USA 82:193–197
33. Zoja C, Perico N, Bergamelli A, Pasini M, Morigi M, Dadan J, Belloni A, Bertani T, Remuzzi G (1990) Ticlopidine prevents renal disease progression in rats with reduced renal mass. Kidney Int 37:934–942
34. MacKay K, Striker LJ, Stauffer JW, Doi T, Agodoa LY, Striker GE (1989) Transforming growth factor-β. Murine glomerular receptors and responses of isolated glomerular cells. J Clin Invest 83:1160–1167
35. Border WA, Okuda S, Languino LR, Ruoslahti E (1990) Transforming growth factor-β regulates production of proteoglycans by mesangial cells. Kidney Int 37:689–695
36. Henson PM, Cochrane CG (1969) Immunological induction of increased vascular permeability. I. A rabbit passive cutaneous anaphylactic reaction requiring complement, platelets, and neutrophils. J Exp Med 129:153–164
37. Ward PA, Macconi D, Sulavik MC, Till GO, Warren JS, Johnson KJ, Powell J (1988) Rat neutrophil-platelet interactions in oxygen radical-mediated lung injury. UCLA symposium on molecular and cellular biology, new series, 82:83–98
38. Yahalom J, Eldor A, Fuks Z, Vlodavsky I (1984) Degradation of sulfated proteoglycans in the subendothelial extracellular matrix by human platelet heparitinase. J Clin Invest 74:1842–1849
39. Kanwar YS, Linker A, Farquhar MG (1980) Increased permeability of the glomerular basement membrane to ferritin after removal of glycosaminoglycans (heparan sulfate) by enzyme digestion. J Cell Biol 86:688–693
40. Shigematsu H, Niwa Y, Takizawa J, Akikusa B (1979) Arthus-type nephritis I. Characterization of glomerular lesions induced by insoluble and poorly soluble immune complexes. Lab Invest 40:492–502
41. Johnson RJ, Garcia RL, Pritzl P, Alpers CE (1990) Platelets mediate glomerular cell proliferation in immune complex nephritis induced by anti-mesangial cell antibodies in the rat. Am J Pathol 136:369–374
42. Kurki P, Vanderlaan M, Dolbeare F, Gray J, Tan EM (1986) Expression of proliferating cell nuclear antigen (PCNA)/cyclin during the cell cycle. Exp Cell Res 166:209–219
43. Hawrylowicz CM, Santoro SA, Platt FM, Unanue ER (1989) Activated platelets express IL-1 activity. J Immunol 143:4015–4018
44. Shultz PJ, Dicorleto PE, Silver BJ, Abboud HE (1988) Mesangial cells express PDGF mRNAs and proliferate in response to PDGF. Am J Physiol 255:F674–F684
45. Silver BJ, Jaffer FE, Abboud HE (1989) Platelet-derived growth factor synthesis in mesangial cells: Induction by multiple peptide mitogens. Proc Natl Acad Sci USA 86:1056–1060
46. Gesualdo L, Abboud HE, Pinzani M, Floriano J, Lamm ME, Emancipator SN (1990) Platelet-derived growth factor (PDGF) expression in increased in murine IgA nephropathy (IgAN). Kidney Int 37:414
47. Kartha S, Bradham DM, Grotendorst GR, Toback FFG (1988) Kidney epithelial cells express c-sis protooncogene and secrete PDGF-like protein. Am J Physiol 255:F800–F806
48. Iida H, Alpers CE, Seifert R, Gown A, Ross R, Bowen-Pope D, Johnson R. (1990) Platelet-derived growth factor (PDGF) and PDGF receptor (PDGF-R) expression in mesangial

proliferative nephritis. J Amer Soc Neph 1:526 (abstr)
49. Fellstrom B, Klareskog L, Heldin CH, Larsson E, Ronnstrand L, Terracio L, Tufveson G, Wahlberg J, Rubin K (1989) Platelet-derived growth factor receptors in the kidney—upregulated expression in inflammation. Kidney Int 36:1099–1102
50. Johnson RJ, Iida H, Alpers CE, Majesky MW, Schwartz SM, Pritzl P, Gordon K, Gown AM (1991) Expression of smooth muscle cell phenotype by rat mesangial cells in immune complex nephritis. J Clin Invest (in press)

The Role of Eicosanoids in Glomerular Immune Injury

ROLF A.K. STAHL[1]

Introduction

The characteristic features of several models of experimental glomerular immune injuries are reduction of the glomerular filtration rate and loss of the permselectivity of the glomerular filtration barrier, with the appearance of proteinuria [1]. These alterations are, in most cases, the consequence of glomerular antibody binding, immune complex formation, activation of mediator systems, and the glomerular infiltration of inflammatory cells (polymorphonuclear neutrophils (PMNs), monocytes, and platelets) [2]. In this initial process of experimental glomerular injuries, formation of eicosanoids in whole isolated glomeruli is enhanced [3–6].

Eicosanoids are oxygenic products of 20 carbon polyunsaturated fatty acids. In the enzymatic pathway of arachidonic acid the cyclooxygenase forms prostanoids (prostaglandins (PGE_2, PGI_2, $PGF_{2\alpha}$) and thromboxane A_2, the lipoxygenase converts polyunsaturated fatty acids in hydroxyeicosatetraenoic acids (HETEs) and leukotrienes ($LTBC_4$, LTB_4) (see Fig. 1). Eicosanoids exert their functional effects as local hormones and represent a group of autacoids.

Recent studies have addressed the question of which mechanisms lead to increased glomerular eicosanoid formation in experimental glomerular injury and which cellular components in whole nephritic glomeruli are the sources of increased eicosanoid formation. There is good evidence that prostanoids and thromboxane A_2 (TxA_2) are produced by resident glomerular cells and infiltrating monocytes [5–7], whereas HETE and leukotrienes derive from glomerular resident cells and PMNs [8,9]. It has also become clear that the intraglomerular activation of the complement system plays an important role in the release of eicosanoids in glomerular immune injury [6,7,9]. Even though the mechanisms of the release, and the cellular sources of eicosanoids

---

[1]University of Frankfurt, Department of Medicine, Division of Nephrology, Theodor-Stern-Kai 7, 6000 Frankfurt 70, Federal Republic of Germany

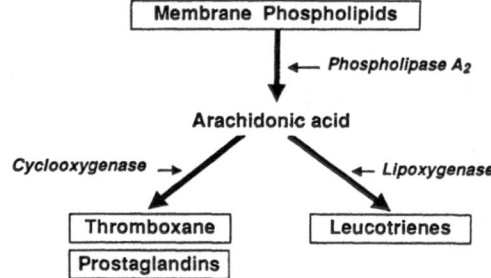

Fig. 1. Eicosanoids are products of arachidonic acid, which is converted by cyclooxygenase to thromboxane and prostaglandins and by lipoxygenase to leukotrienes

in nephritic glomeruli have been reasonably well characterized, their possible role in experimental glomerular injury is still being debated. There is now sufficient evidence to support the view that eicosanoids participate in the regulation of renal hemodynamics in glomerular disease. In most animal models studied, the reduction of glomerular filtration rate can be ameliorated by inhibition of the synthesis of TxA_2 or by its blockade [3,10]. On the other hand, increased formation of PGE_2 and PGI_2 in glomerular injury maintains impaired hemodynamic renal function [4,11]. Besides these hemodynamic functions, which are at least partially attributable to changes in the contractility of mesangial cells [12], there is still little information on whether eicosanoids are actively involved in other processes which appear in glomerular diseases, i.e., the attraction of inflammatory cells, growth of resident glomerular cells, formation of matrix components, or effects on the permselectivity of the glomerular filtration barrier.

This short review will therefore focus on information which deals with the role of eicosanoids, other than their vasoactive effects on the glomerulus. This review includes data from animal experiments; however, the majority of the information is derived from cell culture studies.

The Effect of Prostaglandins of the E Series on Experimental Glomerular Immune Injuries

The first evidence that prostaglandins of the E series might effect glomerular immune injury is derived from Zurier et al. [13]. NZB/NZW mice treated with prostaglandin E_1 had a decrease of immune complexes deposited in the glomeruli and a reduction of glomerular hypercellularity. PGE treatment also increased survival of these animals.

Similar data on different animal models of glomerular immune injury were collected by other investigators [14–17].

Most investigators observed beneficial effects on glomerular morphology and function. The beneficial effects, however, were attributed to different mechanisms by different investigators. These included influences of PGE_1 on immune complex formation [14], antibody synthesis [15], recruitment of PMNs [16], or recruitment of monocytes [17,18].

These experiments demonstrate that exogenous prostaglandins of the E series uniformly improve morphology and function of different models of glomerular immune diseases. The mechanisms by which PGs of the E series exert their beneficial effects, however, seem to be different and might involve immune complex formation, antibody synthesis, inflammatory cell recruitment, and more or less undefined effects. The influences of exogenous PGs might thus be systemic or could also appear on the glomerular level. The question therefore arises, whether prostaglandins formed locally, either by glomerular resident cells or by blood borne inflammatory cells during glomerular injury, participate in disease mechanisms.

There is currently no evidence from animal experiments, besides the hemodynamic function, which would clearly demonstrate that endogenous PGE_2 has such effects. There is, however, some information, obtained from recent studies in cell cultures of glomerular mesangial cells, which suggests that PGs can be involved in the growth of resident glomerular cells, and that PGs might be involved in the release of cytokines and in the formation of matrix components.

Prostanoids and Mesangial Cell Function

The mesangial cell, due to its ability to regulate perfusion, produce matrix components, express antigens of the MHC II class, proliferate and release several inflammatory mediators, has a central role in the pathophysiology of glomerular disease [19]. The mesangial cell is also a source of prostanoid formation in the glomerulus, $PGF_{2\alpha}$, PGE_2, and PGI_2 being the major products. In inflammatory processes, several mediators, including cytokines and growth factors, complement components, free oxygen radicals, bacterial toxins, and antibody binding stimulate mesangial cell prostanoid formation (for review see [20]).

Since increased formation of prostanoids and enhanced mesangial cell proliferation are characteristic features of several entities of glomerular immune injury, we addressed the question whether endogenous prostanoids formed by mesangial cells might be involved in the growth of mesangial cells. For this purpose rat mesangial cells were exposed to the cytokines interleukin-1β (IL-1β), tumor necrosis factor (TNF), and granulocyte macrophage colony stimulating factor (GMCSF), all inflammatory mediators which are supposed to be released during the process of inflammation on the glomerular level [19].

Without exception, all cytokines increased mesangial cell PGE_2 formation (see Fig. 2). On a molar basis TNF was the most potent stimulator of mesangial cell PGE_2 formation, whereas the effect of IL-1β was comparatively mild.

With regard to the effects on mesangial cell DNA synthesis there were, however, differences between the cytokines studied (see Fig. 3). IL-1β induced a small but significant increase of mesangial cell growth (evaluated by ^{3}H-thymidine uptake), whereas TNF and GMCSF reduced ^{3}H-thymidine incorporation in mesangial cells (see Fig. 3). The decrease in mesangial cell growth with TNF and GMCSF was paralleled by an increase in mesangial cell PGE_2 formation. The growth promoting activity of IL-1β was not dose-dependent, but rather showed a decrease when the concentration of the cytokine was increased.

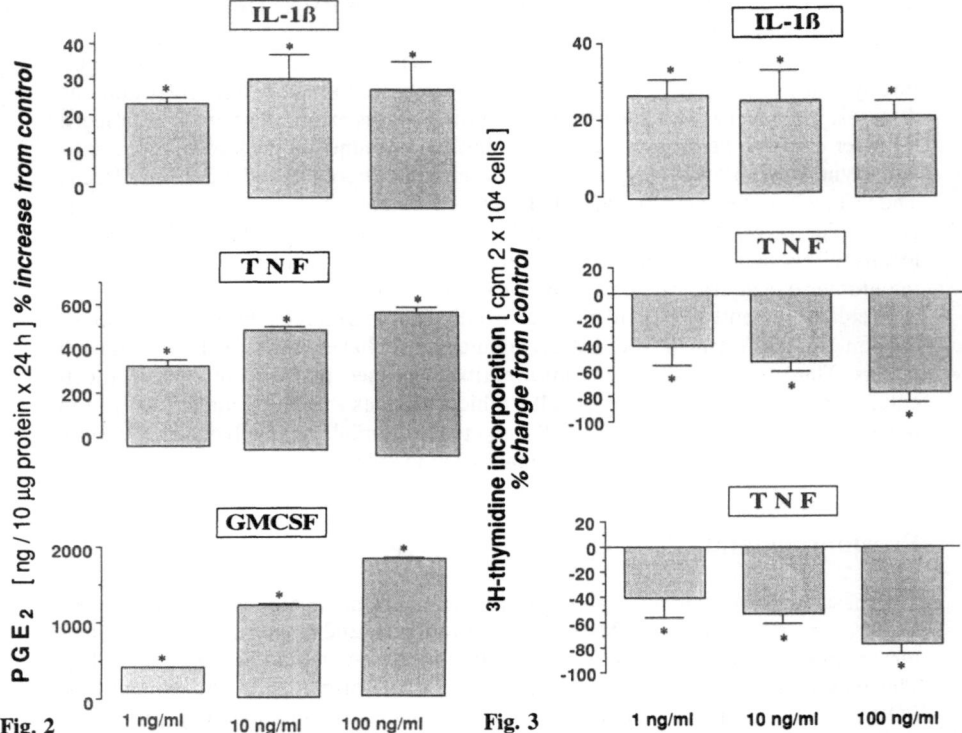

Fig. 2. To study the effect of recombinant Interleukin-1β (IL-1β) (rat), Tumor Necrosis Factor (*TNF*) (human), and Granulocyte Macrophage Colony Stimulating Factor (*GMCSF*) (murine) on proliferating mesangial cell prostaglandin E_2 production, rat mesangial cells (2nd subculture) were grown in 24 well dishes in 5% fetal calf serum (*FCS*) and were incubated for 24 hours with increasing concentrations (1,10,100 ng/ml) of the cytokines. Prostaglandin E_2 (*PGE₂*) formation was analyzed in the supernatants by radioimmunoassay. Compared to control levels (5% FCS alone) all cytokines significantly increased PGE_2 production. The relative responses, however, were different. The most potent stimulator on a molar basis was TNF, whereas the stimulatory influence of IL-1β was relatively mild. The data (*n*=6, each variable) are given as means ± S.E. in % change from control. *P values < 0.05 were considered significant

Fig. 3. To assess the influence of IL-1β, TNF, and GMCSF (see Fig. 2 for definitions) on cell growth, mesangial cells (2nd subculture) were incubated in 96 well dishes (2×10^4 cells) either with 5% FCS or with 5% FCS and increasing concentrations of the cytokines (1,10,100 ng/ml). Prior to the experiments, cells were kept for 48 h on 0.5% FCS. Growth effects were evaluated over 48 h. ³H-thymidine incorporation (last 6 h of the experimental period) and cell counts were applied to study growth.

Interleukin-1β induced a small, but significant increase of ³H-thymidine uptake which was independent of the increasing concentration of the cytokine. TNF and GMCSF, however, significantly inhibited mesangial cell growth with increasing concentrations. The data (*n*=12, each variable) are given in % changes from control (5% FCS alone). *P values < 0.05 were considered significant

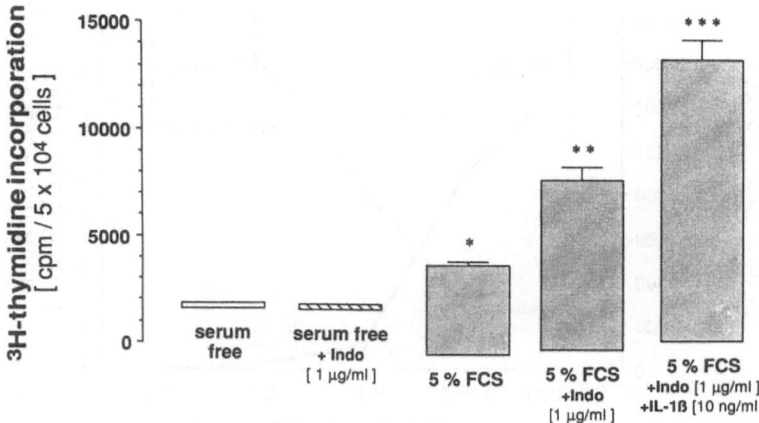

Fig. 4. To study the role of endogenous cyclooxygenase products of mesangial cells on growth, cells were incubated with endomethacin (*Indo*) in the presence and absence of serum. Indomethacin significantly increased ³H-thymidine uptake by mesangial cells, however, only when serum was present. When IL-1β was added to the cyclooxygenase inhibitor, the growth promoting activity of FCS and indomethacin was further enhanced. Data ($n=12$, each variable) are given as means ± S.E. P values < 0.05 were considered significant.[a] FCS vs serum free; [b]FCS + Indo vs FCS; [c]FCS + Indo + IL-1β vs FCS + Indo

To study the possible role which endogenous cyclooxygenase products have in this growth promoting activity of IL-1β and fetal calf serum (FCS), mesangial cells were incubated with the cyclooxygenase inhibitor indomethacin (see Fig. 4).

Incubation with indomethacin significantly enhanced the ³H-thymidine uptake in rat mesangial cells; however, the effect required the presence of FCS. In the absence of serum the cyclooxygenase inhibitor did not influence DNA synthesis.

The growth stimulatory effect of IL-1β increased with the degree of the reduction of mesangial cell PGE₂ formation, which appeared in a dose-dependent manner with increasing indomethacin concentrations (see Fig. 5).

These data demonstrate that endogenous formation of cyclooxygenase products might inhibit serum or cytokine (IL-1β) stimulated mesangial cell growth in culture. This growth inhibitory effect is unmasked when cyclooxygenase is inhibited. It appears from our experiment that TNF and GMCSF significantly stimulate mesangial cell prostaglandin formation and thereby might enhance growth inhibitory effects. These cytokines, however, do not further stimulate mesangial cell growth in mesangial cells incubated with a cyclooxygenase inhibitor (data not shown). It is unclear which cyclooxygenase metabolite derived from mesangial cells is responsible for the antiproliferative effect. When exogenous eicosanoids (PGE₂, PGF₂ₐ, AA), however, are added to mesangial cells in the presence of cyclooxygenase, only PGE₂ exerts antiproliferative effects [20]. It might therefore be possible that PGE₂ produced on the glomerular level, either by resident glomerular cells or by infiltrating inflammatory cells (i.e., monocytes), might inhibit mesangial cell growth in glomerular diseases.

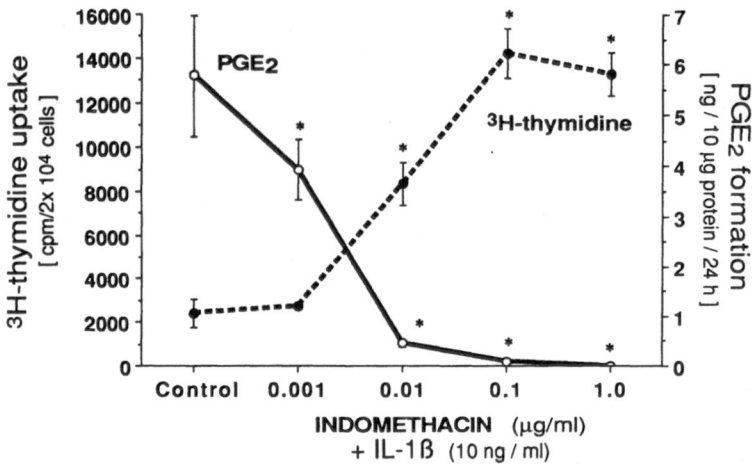

Fig. 5. Rat mesangial cells were incubated with increasing concentrations of indomethacin in the presence of interleukin 1-β and FCS 5% in order to evaluate the effect of endogenous cyclooxygenase products on mesangial cell growth. With the stepwise increase of indomethacin (0.001 to 1.0 μg/ml) PGE$_2$ formation decreased and was almost completely inhibited with 0.1 μg/ml indomethacin. Corresponding with the reduction of mesangial cell PGE$_2$ formation, ^{3}H-thymidine uptake increased significantly and reached a maximum at an indomethacin concentration of 0.1 μ/ml, when PGE$_2$ formation was completely inhibited. PGE$_2$, Prostaglandin E$_2$. The data ($n = 12$, each variable) are given as means ± S.E. *P values < 0.05 were considered significant

There is also evidence, however, that endogenously added cyclooxygenase products can enhance mesangial cell growth in culture. Mene and Dunn [22] found that prostaglandin F$_{2\alpha}$, a compound which is present in significant amounts in isolated glomeruli, can induce rat mesangial cell proliferation in culture and, further, this compound enhances growth factor-induced proliferation. In a way similar to the stimulatory effect of the cyclooxygenase inhibitors (as mentioned), PGF$_{2\alpha}$ did not exert its effect without additional cofactors or serum.

In addition to the effects of eicosanoids on mesangial cell proliferation, endogenous cyclooxygenase products are probably involved in the release of cytokines and matrix components of resident glomerular cells.

Baud et al. [23] studied the mechanism of lipopolysaccharide (LPS)-induced release of TNF by rat mesangial cells in culture. In their studies LPS caused an increase in TNF secretion which was paralleled by stimulated mesangial cell PGE$_2$ formation. Treatment of mesangial cells with indomethacin promoted an increase in TNF synthesis, an effect which could be suppressed by the addition of PGE$_2$ and a cyclic AMP analogue. These observations strongly suggest that PGE$_2$ might regulate the release of TNF on a feedback mechanism.

There is also some evidence that cyclooxygenase products might be involved in the formation of basement membrane proteins and matrix components of the glomerulus.

In diabetic mice with progression of the disease, Ledbetter et al. [24] found an increase in mRNA expression of the α-1 chain of type IV collagen in the kidneys, which was paralleled by an increase in albuminuria. When the diabetic mice were treated with an inhibitor of thromboxane synthesis over a period of 1 month, albuminuria was reduced and mRNA expression of type IV collagen was not different from that of non-diabetic control mice. The authors conclude from their studies that thromboxane might play a role in progressive renal disease in diabetic mice and that thromboxane might be a mediator of increased collagen type IV production in diabetic mice.

Preliminary evidence, derived from studies by Ardaillou et al. [25], suggests that prostaglandin E_2 inhibits mesangial cell uptake of proline, probably due to the activation of cAMP, and that prostaglandin E_2 might be of significance in the production of matrix components, suggestions which have also been made earlier by others [26].

In summary, these recently obtained data suggest that endogenous eicosanoids are involved in the process of glomerular resident cell growth, cytokine release, and possibly, in glomerular matrix formation. Prostaglandin E_2 in this context might exert a "protective" effect by inhibiting cell growth, cytokine release, and matrix component formation. On the other hand $PGF_{2\alpha}$ and TxA_2 seem to exert effects which might be interpreted as "propagating" glomerular disease. One has to consider, however, that most of this information is obtained from tissue culture experiments and has yet to be confirmed in disease states.

References

1. Wilson CB, Blantz RC (1985) Nephroimmunopathology and pathophysiology (editorial review). Am J Physiol 248:F319–327
2. Couser WG, Baker PJ, Adler S (1985) Complement and the direct mediation of immune glomerular injury: A new perspective. Kidney Int 28:879–886
3. Lianos EA, Andres GA, Dunn MJ (1983) Glomerular prostaglandin and thromboxane synthesis in rat nephrotoxic nephritis. J Clin Invest 72:1439–1448
4. Stork JE, Dunn MJ (1985) Hemodynamic roles of thromboxane A_2 and prostaglandin E_2 in glomerulonephritis. J Pharmacol Exp Ther 233:672–678
5. Kelley VE, Sneve S (1986) Increased renal thromboxane production in murine lupus nephritis. J Clin Invest 77:252–259
6. Stahl RAK, Adler S, Baker PJ, Chen YP, Pritzl PM, Couser WG (1987) Enhanced glomerular prostaglandin formation in experimental membranous nephropathy. Kidney Int 31:1126–1131
7. Stahl RAK, Thaiss F, Kahf S, Schoeppe W, Helmchen UM (to be published) Immune mediated mesangial cell injury: biosynthesis and function of prostanoids. Kidney Int
8. Lianos EA (1988) Synthesis of hydroxyeicosatetraenoic acids and leukotrienes in rat nephrotoxic serum glomerulonephritis. J Clin Invest 82:427–435
9. Lianos EA, Noble B, Hucke B (1989) Glomerular leukotriene synthesis in Heymann nephritis. Kidney Int 36:998–1002
10. Thaiss F, Germann PJ, Kahf S, Schoeppe W, Helmchen U, Stahl RAK (1989) Effect of thromboxane synthesis inhibition in a model of membranous nephropathy. Kidney Int 35:76–83
11. Stahl RAK, Kudelka S, Paravicini M, Schollmeyer P (1986) Prostaglandin and thromboxane formation in glomeruli from rats with reduced renal mass. Nephron 42:252–257

12. Mene P, Dunn MJ (1988) Eicosanoids and control of mesangial cell contraction. Circ Res 62:916–925
13. Zurier RB, Damjanov I, Syadoff M, Rothfield NF (1977) Prostaglandin E₁ treatment of NZB/NZW F₁ hybrid mice. II. Prevention of glomerulonephritis. Arthritis Rheum 20:1449–1456
14. McLeish KR, Gohara AF, Gunning III WT, Senitzer D (1980) Prostaglandin E₁ therapy of murine chronic serum sickness. J Lab Clin Med 96:470–479
15. McLeish KR, Gohara AF, Gunning III WT (1982) Suppression of antibody synthesis by prostaglandin E as a mechanism for preventing murine immune complex glomerulonephritis. Lab Invest 47:147–152
16. Kunkel SL, Thrall RS, Kunkel RG, McCormick JR, Ward PA, Zurier RB (1979) Suppression of immune complex vasculitis in rats by prostaglandin. J Clin Invest 64:1525–1529
17. Kelley VE, Winkelstein A, Izui S (1979) Effect of prostaglandin E on immune complex nephritis in NZB/W mice. Lab Invest 41:531–537
18. Cattell V, Smith J, Cook HT (1990) Prostaglandin E₁ suppresses macrophage infiltration and ameliorates injury in an experimental model of macrophage-dependent glomerulonephritis. Clin Exp Immunol 79:260–265
19. Sterzel RB, Lovett DH (1988) Interactions of inflammatory and glomerular cells in the response to glomerular injury. In: Brenner BM, Stein JH (eds) Immunopathology of renal disease. Churchill Livingstone, pp 18:137–173
20. Stahl RAK, Thaiss F: Eicosanoids (1987) biosynthesis and function in the glomerulus. Renal Physiol 10:1–13
21. Stahl RAK, Thaiss F, Haberstroh U, Kahf S, Shaw A, Schoeppe W (to be published) Cyclooxygenase inhibition enhances rat II-1β induced proliferation of mesangial cells. Am J Physiol
22. Mene P, Dunn MJ (1990) Prostaglandins and rat glomerular mesangial cell proliferation. Kidney Int 37:1256–1262
23. Baud L, Oudinet J-P, Bens M, Noe L, Peraldi M-N, Rondeau E, Etienne J, Ardaillou R (1989) production of tumor necrosis factor by rat mesangial cells in response to bacterial lipopolysaccharide. Kidney Int 35:1111–1118
24. Ledbetter S, Copeland EJ, Noonan D, Vogeli G, Hassell JR (1990) Altered steady state mRNA levels of basement membrane proteins in diabetic mouse kidneys and thromboxane synthase inhibition. Diabetics 39:196–203
25. Ardaillou N, Nivez PM, Ardaillou R (1990) Effect of prostaglandin E2 on proline uptake and collagen synthesis by cultured human mesangial cells (abstract). Kidney Int 37:344
26. Homma T, Ichikawa I, Hoover RL (1988) Prostaglandins of mesangium origin inhibit mesangial cell (MC) proliferation and matrix synthesis (abstract). Kidney Int 33:268

Mechanisms of Glomerular Fibrin Deposition in Glomerulonephritis

S. R. HOLDSWORTH and P. G. TIPPING[1]

SUMMARY. Evidence points to glomerular fibrin deposition (GFD) as an important mediator of renal injury and crescent formation. GFD appears to be initiated by intraglomerular stimuli related to local immune inflammatory events. Macrophages expressing augmented procoagulant activity (PCA) are likely to be important initiators of GFD. Antibody Fc direction or delayed type hypersensitivity (DTH) mechanisms may be the primary initiating event. Other factors, including contact activation of coagulation and inhibition of fibrinolytic clearance, may act in concert to exacerbate fibrin accumulation, especially in Bowman's space. The importance of GFD in human GN is highlighted by evidence that it may be prevented or reversed by therapeutic intervention, thereby offering the potential for limiting the progression of injury in these forms of GN.

Introduction

Glomerular deposition of fibrin is observed in the most severe forms of glomerulonephritis (GN), in which the outcome for renal function is often poor. Paradoxically however, it is these forms of GN which offer the greatest potential for treatment. Defibrination studies in experimental GN demonstrate that prevention of fibrin deposition preserves renal function and abrogates crescent formation. Fibrin deposition in GN is restricted to the glomerulus, and is deposited in response to local immunologically initiated inflammatory events.

Fibrin Deposition in GN

Glomerular fibrin deposition (GFD) is observed in many histological types of GN but is most prominent in association with proliferative GN, and particularly with crescent formation [1,2]. Similar observations have been made in experimental GN. It is

---

[1]Department of Medicine, Prince Henry's Hospital, St. Kilda Road, Melbourne 3004, Australia

those forms of injury which are associated with severe proliferation, renal failure, and crescent formation where GFD is also most abundant. This occurs regardless of the nature of the immune initiating events. GFD occurs in GN initiated by anti-glomerular basement membrane (GBM) antibodies, immune complexes, and planted antigens and is common to a variety of species, including rabbit, mouse, rat, and sheep. Recent studies also suggest a close association between GFD and macrophage accumulation in human and experimental GN.

Pathological Effects of Glomerular Fibrin Deposition

Observations of human GN confirm the association of prominent GFD with loss of glomerular filtration, crescent formation, and a poor prognosis. In experimental GN, specific depletion of fibrin can be induced without altering other immune initiating events, allowing studies of the specific consequences of GFD. Ancrod is a component of cobra venom which converts fibrinogen to soluble fibrin monomer which cannot crosslink and is rapidly cleared from the circulation, resulting in severe hypofibrinogenemia. When employed in models of experimental GN with prominent GFD, immunofluorescence studies demonstrate complete abrogation of GFD with the use of this agent [3–5]. Similar results can be obtained with the fibrinolytic agent streptokinase [6,7]. Blocking GFD maintains urine output and preserves glomerular filtration, suggesting that fibrin deposition may result in a physical barrier limiting filtration. The second striking consequence of preventing GFD is the reduction in crescent formation. Early in experimental GN, fibrin collects in Bowman's space, forming an acellular proteinaceous crescent. Accumulation of monocytes and prolif-eration of epithelial cells leads to cellular crescent formation. Prevention of crescent formation by defibrination suggests a pivotal role for fibrin in the pathogenesis of these events. Fibrin is chemotactic for macrophages [8] and may induce macrophage localization in Bowman's space, but is also likely to act as an extracellular substratum facilitating cellular proliferation and organization. Studies in vitro demonstrate that fibrin degradation products may be toxic to mesangial cells [9], however, the obser-vation of prominent mesangial proliferation in fibrin related GN in man clearly demonstrates that this potential toxicity is not a limiting feature in vivo.

Systemic Coagulation Changes in GN

A variety of alterations in systemic coagulation have been reported in patients with GN. These are largely due to the consequences of the nephrotic syndrome or the effects of systemic inflammation in diseases where GN is secondary to disease pro-cesses such as sepsis, vasculitis, or connective tissues diseases (principally SLE). In these inflammatory diseases, disturbance of coagulation may include thrombocyto-sis, hyperfibrinogenemia, and increased levels of acute phase proteins with anti-fibrinolytic activity [10–12], including C4 binding protein and $\alpha 2$ antiplasmin. Reduction in levels of anti-thrombin III may occur as a result of the nephrotic syn-drome [13,14]. All of these changes in circulating coagulation factors shift the balance of procoagulant and anti-coagulant pathways in favor of clotting. Increased

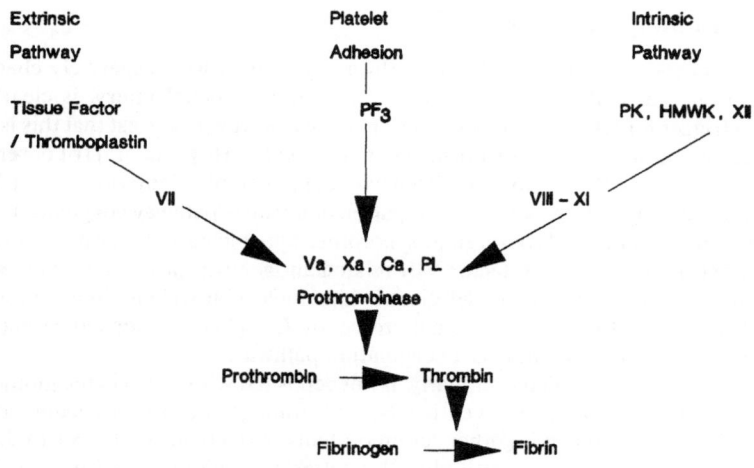

Fig. 1. Potential pathways for initiation of fibrin deposition in GN

levels of activated Factor VIII have been reported in some patients with GN [10,11]. Despite these reports, the majority of patients with GFD in association with GN have no systemic disturbance in coagulation. Similarly, experimental animal studies strongly support the view that GFD occurs as the result of local procoagulant stimuli rather than systemic coagulation changes.

Local Events Initiating Coagulation

The occurrence of GFD in glomeruli with evidence of capillary wall injury (manifested by histological changes and proteinuria) naturally led to the view that GFD was initiated by contact coagulation activation. Fibrin deposition is not a universal feature of all histological types of GN. In human GN, it is usually associated with proliferative and crescentic disease. However, in some types of GN associated with significant GBM injury, significant glomerular fibrin deposition is absent. These observations suggest that GFD is not a consequence of GBM injury alone.

Support for this hypothesis is provided by studies of experimental models of anti-GBM antibody initiated GN in rabbits [15]. Comparing the heterologous and autologous phases of this disease, similar levels of proteinuria and histological evidence of glomerular injury were observed. However, significant GFD was seen only in the autologous phase, indicating that capillary wall damage per se was not sufficient to initiate GFD. The mechanisms responsible for GFD have recently been explored in some detail.

Coagulation may be initiated by a number of different mechanisms, as demonstrated in Fig. 1.

Intrinsic Pathway Activation

Activation of the intrinsic coagulation pathway by contact with negatively charged molecules such as collagen, exposed as a result of endothelial injury, is clearly a potential trigger for GFD. A number of observations, however, suggest that this is not a significant initiating factor for fibrin deposition in GN. Hoyer et al. [16] observed that GFD in human GN was not associated with demonstrable glomerular factor VIII related antigen, suggesting lack of participation of intrinsic pathway coagulation factors. In contrast, in hemolytic-uremic syndrome, hyperacute homograft rejection, and post partum renal failure, factor VIII related antigen was prominent in association with GFD. Rats congenitally deficient in high molecular weight kininogen show no impairment of GFD in experimental crescentic GN [17], further indicating the lack of participation of the intrinsic coagulation pathway.

Hageman Factor (factor XII), similarly, is not deposited with fibrin in the glomerular tufts in rabbits developing crescentic GN, [18] although late passive accumulation in Bowman's space, along with other serum proteins, was noted. Factor VIII related antigen deposition also occurs well after the initiation of glomerular fibrin deposition and is restricted to Bowman's space in crescentic GN in rabbits [19]. These studies together provide consistent evidence for the lack of participation of intrinsic coagulation pathway factors in glomerular fibrin deposition.

Platelets and GFD

Platelets are a major component of intravascular thrombus although they are not essential for coagulation in vitro. Platelet phospholipid membrane provides an important co-factor for activation of coagulation proteins, and platelets themselves are a source of coagulation factors, including thrombin. Therefore it would seem difficult to entirely discount a role for platelets in GFD. However, available evidence does not suggest an important role for platelets in GFD associated with GN. Platelets are infrequently observed in proliferative forms of human GN [20], although they have been identified in experimental anti-GBM GN [21] and immune complex GN [22]. Induction of profound thrombocytopenia or use of anti-platelet drugs in experimental GN, however, did not reduce GFD [23,24].

Extrinsic Pathway Activation

The lack of involvement of intrinsic pathway factors and platelets in GFD in GN, raises the potential of a pivotal role for extrinsic pathway activation. The extrinsic pathway is triggered by activation of factor VII by tissue thromboplastin (tissue factor). Tissue factor is a membrane bound phospholipid expressed constitutively by many cells and may be upregulated in inflammation. Monocytes and macrophages in particular are an abundant source of tissue factor. The recognition of the close association between macrophages and GFD, both in human [25-28] and in experimental GN [1,5,7,15], suggested that monocytes may be responsible for glomerular fibrin deposition via tissue factor induced activation of the extrinsic coagulation pathway. We assessed the capacity of monocytes to induce glomerular fibrin deposition by studying the effects of monocyte depletion and selective repletion in a model of anti-GBM GN with prominent fibrin deposition in rabbits [15] (Fig. 2). These studies

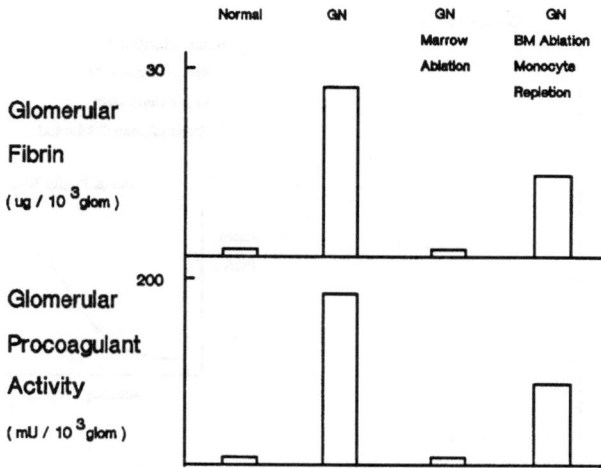

Fig. 2. The effect of macrophage depletion and repletion on glomerular fibrin deposition and procoagulant activity in anti-GBM GN

clearly indicated that GFD was dependent on monocyte infiltration in this model. Fibrin deposition was associated with monocyte induced GN, but not with neutrophil induced glomerular injury, indicating that the capacity of these leukocytes to induce glomerular injury was unrelated to their capacity to initiate GFD. Although both neutrophils and monocytes have the capacity to induce glomerular injury, only macrophages express procoagulant activity enabling them to initiate fibrin deposition by activation of the extrinsic pathway. To assess extrinsic pathway activation during development of GN, expression of procoagulant activity by nephritic glomeruli was measured. When compared to normal glomeruli and glomeruli from rabbits with heterologous phase injury, monocyte infiltrated nephritic glomeruli had greatly augmented levels of PCA. Depletion and repletion studies confirmed that glomerular monocyte influx accounted for the augmented expression of PCA [15] (Fig. 2).

The functional characteristics of glomerular PCA indicate it activates the extrinsic pathway and is tissue factor. Its activity is dependent on coagulation factors VIII and V and independent of factors VIII and XII. It is inhibited by phospholipase C and concanavalin A and by antibodies to tissue factor [29] (Fig. 3). Expression of PCA by macrophages isolated from nephritic glomeruli was compared with PCA expression by blood monocytes and pulmonary alveolar macrophages in the same animals. These studies indicated that infiltrating glomerular macrophages express vastly augmented levels of procoagulant activity (PCA) compared to other macrophage populations during the development of GN, indicating that they are locally activated, further suggesting a pivotal role for macrophages in the initiation of fibrin deposition in GN [30].

Macrophage Mechanisms for Promoting Coagulation (Fig. 4)

Activated monocytes are capable of influencing coagulation directly, by their expression of procoagulant and anti-coagulant molecules and indirectly, by their production

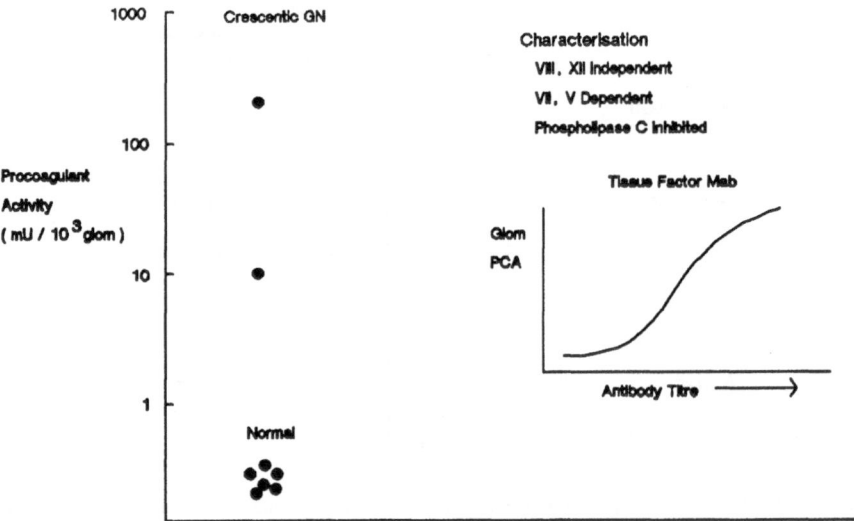

Fig. 3. Procoagulant activity in glomeruli from 2 patients with crescentic GN, and in normal glomeruli. Functional characteristics of glomerular procoagulant activity and its inhibition by a monoclonal anti-tissue factor antibody

of proinflammatory cytokines, principally interleukin 1 (IL1) and tumor necrosis factor (TNF), which alter the expression of procoagulant and anti-coagulant molecules by endothelial cells [31–33]. Endothelial cells normally exhibit a number of functions which result in a net anti-coagulant effect [12]. These include thrombomodulin, heparin-like proteoglycans that facilitate anti-thrombin III activity, plasminogen activator, and PGI_2 (prostacycline) which inhibits platelet aggregation. Macrophage cytokines have been shown both to downregulate these functions and to upregulate procoagulant endothelial function including plasminogen activator inhibitor, procoagulant activity, and Von Willebrand factor activity [31] (Fig. 4).

Mechanisms of Activation of Macrophage Procoagulant Functions

There are a number of mechanisms, of potential relevance to GN, by which macrophages may be stimulated to augment their PCA expression and thereby initiate GFD.

Complement

Glomerular complement deposition is prominent in many types of human and experimental GN and is often present in association with GFD. In experimental GN, depletion studies have demonstrated that complement is a pivotal chemoattractant

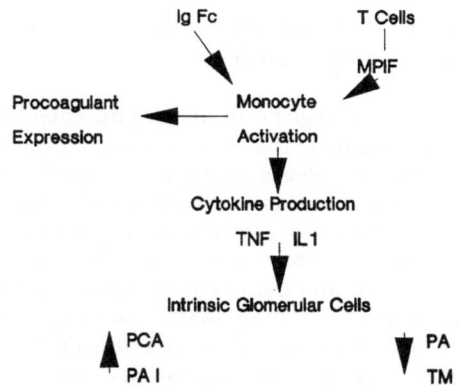

Fig. 4. Potential mechanisms for macrophage initiation of fibrin deposition. MPIF, macrophage procoagulant inducing factor; PA, plasminogen activator; PA1, plasminogen activator inhibitor; TM, thrombomodulin.

for neutrophils, but is not essential for glomerular monocyte accumulation. Complement fragments can activate macrophages and then augment monocyte PCA expression [33], however, in experimental GN, complement depletion does not alter glomerular PCA expression. (Lowe, Tipping and Holdsworth, unpublished observations)

Immunoglobulin

Immunoglobulin Fc is an important stimulus for macrophage localization in GN. Immunoglobulin and immune complexes are potent stimuli for augmentation of macrophage PCA expression [34–35], however the contribution of these to the augmented glomerular PCA in GN is unknown.

T Lymphocytes

T lymphocytes have recently been demonstrated in proliferative forms of human and experimental GN. They are particularly abundant in human GN, with prominent glomerular fibrin deposition macrophage accumulation and tissue factor expression. T lymphocytes are potent activators of macrophages [26–28], and have the capacity to augment macrophage PCA expression via release of the lymphokine macrophage procoagulant inducing factor (MPIF). T cell directed macrophage induced fibrin deposition is a characteristic feature of delayed type hypersensitivity (DTH) reactions occurring in the skin in response to a locally represented antigen. In both human and experimental GN there is now good evidence for the participation of these same mediators of injury, T cells [39–41], macrophages expressing tissue factor, and fibrin deposition [42], suggesting the potential for T cell augmentation of glomerular fibrin deposition via mechanisms akin to DTH.

The Role of Intrinsic Glomerular Cells
in Glomerular Fibrin Deposition

Epithelial, endothelial, and mesangial cells all have the potential to interact in the coagulation process. However, there is a scarcity of studies addressing their contribution to GFD in GN. Indirect evidence comes from demonstration of the potential of intrinsic glomerular cells to release products which interact with various elements of the coagulation cascade, particularly via effects on endothelial cell procoagulant and anti-coagulant molecules. Isolated glomeruli can produce both thromboxane and PGI_2 in response to oxygen radicals [43]. Isolated glomeruli and mesangial cells can synthesize platelet aggregation factor (PAF) [43] and mesangial cells have the potential to express augmented PCA activity following TNF stimulation [44]. Mesangial cells have the potential to produce proinflammatory cytokines [45] which may modulate endothelial cell functions.

Both endothelial and mesangial cells synthesize tissue type plasminogen activator (t-PA) [46] and glomerular endothelial cells express thrombomodulin, and important anticoagulant molecule expressed by endothelial cells elsewhere [47]. Human glomeruli contain t-PA and a minor component of urokinase type plasminogen activator (u-PA). It is reported that mesangial cells release t-PA and plasminogen activator (PA) inhibitor type 1 while epithelial cells release an inactive form of u-PA [48].

Macrophage Modulation of Intrinsic
Glomerular Cell Coagulant Functions

Endothelial cell expression of PCA is augmented by soluble products released from monocyte infiltrated isolated nephritic glomeruli [30]. This effect is not observed with culture supernatants of normal glomeruli or with nephritic glomeruli from macrophage depleted animals, suggesting that macrophage products (possibly proinflammatory cytokines) are responsible for this endothelial cell PCA augmentation. Monocytes in experimental models of GN with prominent GFD have been shown to express augmented levels of IL-1 and TNF [49] and these cytokines have the capacity to augment endothelial cell PCA in vitro. While these data confirm the potential for intrinsic cells to contribute to the augmented PCA in GN there is no direct evidence of a significant contribution to glomerular PCA by this mechanism in vivo, as nephritic glomerular supernatants capable of enhancing endothelial cell PCA failed to measurably enhance the PCA of intact glomeruli in vitro. Intrinsic glomerular cells and cytokine activated endothelial cells express 100–1000-fold less PCA than glomerular macrophages. This suggests that the contribution of intrinsic cells to the augmented PCA in GN with prominent macrophage infiltration may be insignificant, and that macrophages themselves are likely to account for most of the augmented procoagulant activity observed in nephritic glomeruli with prominent GFD.

Alterations in other coagulant functions of intrinsic cells may be relevant to GFD in GN. Glomerular fibrinolytic activity and t-PA activity has been assessed in models of GN with prominent fibrin depositions. In rabbits with chronic serum sickness, glomerular fibrinolytic activity was reduced in association with glomerular deposition of fibrin [50]. In anti-GBM antibody induced GN in rats, glomerular fibrinolytic activity and t-PA expression were enhanced [51] while procoagulant activity was reduced [52]. This is consistent with the observation that rats appear resistant to the development of crescentic GN and develop only sparse GFD. Blockade of fibrinolytic activity enhances crescent formation [53] in this model. In mercuric chloride induced GN in rats, enhanced glomerular PCA is associated with prominent GFD [54].

Mechanisms of Fibrin Deposition in Human Glomerulonephritis

In human GN, fibrin deposition is associated with the severe proliferative crescentic forms of GN. This has been demonstrated by immunohistochemical staining for fibrin in renal biopsies [1,2] and measurement of urinary fibrin degradation products [55,56]. The cellular mechanisms of GFD in human GN can only be studied indirectly, however there are now a number of histological studies of the participation of coagulation factors in renal tissue of patients with GN.

Absence of Factor VIII in glomeruli of patients with prominent GFD mitigates against a major role for intrinsic pathway initiation of fibrin deposition in human GN. Aggregation of platelets in glomeruli is not a prominent feature in human GN [20].

Recent evidence suggests that mechanisms similar to those observed in experimental GN may be operative in man. Glomerular macrophage influx is observed in forms of GN accompanied by prominent GFD [25–28]. Studies of the expression of procoagulant activity in human GN have recently been performed. Two patients who died with acute crescentic GN with prominent fibrin deposition and without substantial immunosuppression therapy provided renal tissue soon after death [57]. Isolated glomeruli from these patients showed vast augmentation of procoagulant activity when compared to levels expressed by non-nephritic human glomeruli. The procoagulant had the functional characteristics of tissue factor, being factor VII and V dependent and factor VIII and XII independent, and being inhibitable by phospholipase C and by a monoclonal antibody specific for human tissue factor. Nonspecific esterase staining demonstrated a significant macrophage presence in these glomeruli, indicating the potential for macrophages to be responsible for the augmented glomerular PCA in these patients.

The recent demonstration of the participation of T lymphocytes, particularly in proliferative forms of GN where fibrin deposition is associated with prominent macrophage infiltration, raises the possible involvement of delayed type hypersensitivity mechanisms in GFD. In a study of 62 renal biopsies, all those showing GN with fibrin deposition and random biopsies showing fibrin negative GN were studied for the presence of the essential elements of DTH; T lymphocytes, macrophages, and tissue factor [42]. Fibrin negative biopsies did not have substantial lymphocyte, monocyte, or tissue factor presence and, in general, exhibited features of less aggressive forms of GN. Fibrin positive biopsies, however, had marked tissue factor expression together with evidence of lymphocyte and macrophage accumulation, indicating the simultaneous deposition of the essential components of DTH in association with fibrin in human GN (Table 1).

Glomerular fibrin deposition occurs in experimental anti-GBM GN in association with macrophages and augmented PCA when injury is induced passively by antibody, without involvement of sensitized T lymphocytes. In this passive model of anti-

218 Immunological and Cellular Mechanisms of Glomerulonephritis

Table 1. The association of mediators of delayed type hypersensitivity, (*DTH*) and fibrin deposition in human GN

DTH Reactant	Fibrin negative biopsies $n = 19$	Fibrin positive biopsies $n = 10$
Macrophages	0.6 ± 0.02	18.9 ± 6.2
T Cells	0.2 ± 0.002	9.9 ± 0.6
Tissue Factor	−	++/+++

GBM GN, GFD, assessed quantitatively by ^{125}I fibrinogen accumulation, was substantially less than in the active form of this disease which is associated with glomerular T lymphocyte accumulation. A greater augmentation of glomerular PCA is also seen in the active model in association with T cells. Thus, in experimental GN, although T lymphocytes may have an important role in augmenting GFD, glomerular injury, initiated by immunoglobulin and mediated by macrophages in the absence of T cells, has the capacity to induce GFD.

On the other hand, GFD in human GN has been observed in the absence of any immunoglobulin deposition. In these patients with so called "immune negative" GN, fibrin deposition occurs in the presence of T cells and macrophages [42], providing strong evidence for the capacity of DTH, in the absence of antibody induced mechanisms, to induce GFD.

Alterations in the glomerular fibrinolytic system have been assessed in human GN. In the large study of human biopsies by Bergstein and Michael [56] no overall change in glomerular fibrinolytic or t-PA activity was observed. Recent studies have reported increased expression of PA inhibitor in crescentic GN with fibrin deposition [59]. Increased expression of PA inhibitor, synthesized by glomerular epithelial cells, may represent a further mechanism for preventing the clearance of deposited fibrin [48].

References

1. Kincaid-Smith P (1972) Coagulation and renal disease. Kidney Int 2:183–190
2. McCluskey RT, Vassalli P, Gallo G, Baldwin DS (1966) An immunofluorescent study of pathogenic mechanisms in glomerular diseases. N Engl J Med 274:695–701
3. Naish P, Penn GB, Evans DJ, Peters, DK (1972). The effect of defibrination on nephrotoxic serum nephritis in rabbits. Clin Sci 42:643–646
4. Naish PF, Evans DJ, Peters DK (1975) The effects of defibrination with ancrod in experimental allergic glomerular injuries. Clin Exp Immunol 20:303–309
5. Thomson NM, Simpson IJ, Evans DJ, Peters, DK (1975) Defibrination with ancrod in experimental chronic immune complex nephritis. Clin Exp Immunol 20:527–535
6. Tipping PG, Holdsworth SR (1986) Fibrinolytic therapy with streptokinase in established experimental glomerulonephritis. Nephron 43:258–264
7. Tipping PG, Thomson NM, Holdsworth SR (1986) A comparison of fibrinolytic and defibrinating agents in established experimental glomerulonephritis. Brit J Exp Pathol 67:481–491
8. Humair L, Kwann HC, Potter E (1969) The role of fibrinogen in renal disease II. Effects of anticoagulants and urokinase on experimental lesions in mice. J Lab Clin Med 74:72–78
9. Tsumagari T, Tanaka K (1984) Effects of fibrinogen degradation products on glomerular mesangial cells in culture. Kidney Int 26:712–718

10. Salem HH, Whitworth JA, Koutts J (1981) Hypercoagulation in glomerulonephritis. Br Med J 282:2083–2086
11. Adhikari M, Coovadia HM, Greig HBW, Christensen S (1978) Factor VIII procoagulant activity in children with nephrotic syndrome and post-streptococcal glomerulonephritis. Nephron 22:301–305
12. Esmon CT (1987) The regulations of natural anticoagulant pathways. Science 235: 1348–1352
13. Kendall AG, Lohmann RC, Dossetor JB Nephrotic syndrome a hypercoagulable state. Ann Intern Med 127:1021–1031
14. Vaziri ND (1983) Nephrotic syndrome and coagulation and fibrinolytic abnormalities. Am J Nephrol 3:1
15. Holdsworth SR, Tipping PG (1985) Macrophage induced fibrin deposition in experimental glomerulonephritis in the rabbit. J Clin Invest 76:1367–1374
16. Hoyer JR, Michael AF, Hoyer LW (1974) Immunofluorescent localization of antihemophiliac factor antigen and fibrinogen in human renal disease. J Clin Invest 53:1375–1384
17. Villaro J, Errasti P, Goni M, Monzo A, Purroy A, Sanchez-Ibarrola A (1984) Pathogenesis of glomerular fibrin deposition: Role of the contact system (abstract). Kidney Int 26:219
18. Wiggins RG (1985) Hageman factor in experimental nephrotoxic nephritis in the rabbit. Lab Invest 53:335–348
19. Tipping PG, Holdsworth SR (1986) The participation of macrophages, glomerular procoagulant activity and factor VIII in glomerular fibrin deposition. Studies in anti-glomerulonephritis basement membrane antibody induced glomerulonephritis in rabbits. Am J Pathol 124:10–17
20. George CPR, Clark WF, Cameron JS (1975) The role of platelets in glomerulonephritis. Adv Nephrol 5:19–65
21. Vassali P, McCluskey RT (1964) The pathogenic role of the coagulation process in rabbit Masugi nephritis. Am J Path 45:653–677
22. Gabbiani G, Boadonnel MC, Vassoli P (1975) Experimental focal glomerular lesion elicited by insoluble immune complexes: ultrastructural and immunofluorescent studies. Lab Invest 32:33–45
23. Ogawa S, Naruse T (1982) Effects of various antiplatelet drugs and a defibrinating agent on experimental glomerulonephritis in rats. J Lab Clin Med 99:428–435
24. Sindrey M, Marshall TI, Naish P (1979) Quantitative assessment of the effects of platelet depletion in the autologous phase of nephrotoxic serum nephritis. Clin Exp Immunol 36:90–96
25. Atkins RC, Holdsworth SR, Glasgow EF, Matthews FE (1976) The macrophage in human rapidly progressive glomerulonephritis. Lancet I:830–832
26. Monga G, Mazzucco G, Barbiano di Belgiojoso GB, Busnach G (1979) The presence and possible role of monocyte infiltration in human chronic proliferative glomerulonephritides. Light microscopic, immunofluorescence and histochemical correlation. Am J Pathol 94:271–284
27. Ferrario F, Castiglione A, Colasanti G, Barbiano di Belgiojoso G, Bertoli S, D'Amico G (1985) The detection of monocytes in human glomerulonephritis. Kidney Int 28:513–519
28. Magil AB, Wadsworth AB (1981) Monocytes in human glomerulonephritis. An electromicroscopic study. Lab Invest 34:77–81
29. Tipping PG, Worthington LA, Holdsworth SR (1987) The quantitation and characterization of glomerular procoagulant activity in experimental glomerulonephritis. Lab Invest 56:155–159
30. Tipping PG, Lowe MG, Holdsworth SR (1988) Glomerular macrophages express augmented procoagulant activity in experimental glomerulonephritis in rabbits. J Clin Invest 82:1253–1259
31. Cotran RS (1987) New roles for the endothelium in inflammation and immunity. Am J Pathol 129:407–413

32. Bevilacqua MP, Schleef RR, Gimbrone MA, Loskutoff DJ (1986) Regulation of the fibrinolytic system of cultured human vascular endothelium by interleukin 1. J Clin Invest 78:581–591
33. Mulfelder TW, Niemetz J, Kreutzer D, Beebe D, Ward PA, Rosenfeld SI (1979) C5 chemo-tactic fragment induces leukocyte production of tissue factor activity: A link between com-plement and coagulation. J Clin Invest 63:147–150
34. Rothberger H, Zimmerman TS, Spiegleberg HL, Vaughan JH (1977) Leukocyte pro-coagulant activity. Enhancement of production "in vitro" by IgG and antigen-antibody complexes. J Clin Invest 59:549–557
35. Schwartz BS, Edgington TS (1981) Immune complex-induced human monocyte procoagulant activity. I. A rapid unidirectional lymphocyte instructed pathway. J Exp Med 154:892–906
36. Edwards RL, Rickles FR, Bolorove AM (1979) Mononuclear cell tissue factor. Cell of ori-gin and requirements for activation. Blood 54:359–370
37. Helin H, Edgington TS (1983) Allogenic induction of the human T cell instructed mono-cyte procoagulant response is rapid and is elicited by HLA-DR. J Exp Med 58:962–975
38. Gregory SM, Edgington TS (1985) Tissue factor induction in human monocytes. Two dis-tinct mechanisms displayed by different alloantigen-responsive T cell clones. J Clin Invest 76:2440–2445
39. Tipping PG, Neale TJ, Holdsworth SR (1985) T-lymphocyte participation in antibody induced experimental glomerulonephritis. Kidney Int 27:530–537
40. Stachura I, Si L, Whiteside TL (1984) Mononuclear cell subsets in human idiopathic crescentic glomerulonephritis: Analysis in tissue sections with monoclonal antibodies. J Clin Immunol 4:203–208
41. Nolasco FEB, Cameron JS, Hartley B, Coelho A, Hildreth G, Reuben R (1987) Intra-glomerular T cells and monocytes in nephritis: Study with monoclonal antibodies. Kidney Int 31:1160–1166
42. Neale TJ, Tipping PG, Carson S, Holdsworth SR (1988) Evidence for the participation of cell mediated immunity in the deposition of fibrin in glomerulonephritis. Lancet II:421–424
43. Baud L, Sraer J, Delarue F, Bens M, Balavoine F, Schlondorff D, Ardaillou R, Sraer JD (1985) Lipoxygenase products mediate the attachment of rat macrophages to glomeruli in vitro. Kidney Int 27:855–863
44. Wiggins RC, Njoku N, Sedor JR (1990) Tissue factor production by cultured rat mesangial cells. Stimulation by TNFα and lipopolysaccharide. Kidney Int 37:1281–1285
45. Boswell JM, Tui MA, Burt DW, Kelly VE (1988) Increased tumor necrosis factor and IL1-β gene expression in the kidneys of mice with lupus nephritis. J Immunol 141:3052–3054
46. Angles Cano E, Balaton A, Le Bonniec B, Genot E, Elion J, Sultan Y (1985) Production and immunolocalization of monoclonal antibodies to the high fibrin affinity tissue type plasminogen activator of human plasma: Demonstration of its endothelial origin by immunolocalization. Blood. 66:913–920
47. Hancock WW (1990) IL1 and TNF depress glomerular endothelial thrombomodulin expression in vitro and in vivo (abstract). Kidney Int 38:557.
48. Sraer JD, Kanfer A, Rondeau E, Lacaux R (1988) Glomerular hemostasis in normal and pathologic conditions. Adv Nephrol 17:27–56
49. Tipping PG, Lowe MG, Holdsworth SR (1991) Glomerular interleukin 1 production is dependent on macrophage infiltration in anti-GBM glomerulonephritis. Kidney Int (in press)
50. Stark H, Miller K, Michael AF (1979) Renal cortical fibrinolytic activity in rabbits with chronic immune complex nephritis. Isr J Med Sci 14:610–612
51. Giroux L, Verroust P, Morel-Maroger L, Delarue F, Delauche M, Sraer JD (1979) Glomerular fibrinolytic activity during nephrotoxic nephritis. Lab Invest 40:415–422

52. Kanfer A, De Prost D, Le Floch V (1985) Procoagulant activity in isolated glomeruli from normal and glomerulonephritic rats (abstract). Eur J Clin Invest 15:A43.
53. Clark BE, Ham KN, Tange JD, Ryan GB (1983) Macrophages and glomerular crescent formation: Studies with rat nephrotoxic nephritis. Pathology 15:75–81
54. Kanfer A, de Prost D, Guettier C, Nochy D, Le Floch V, Hinglais N, Druet P (1987) Enhanced glomerular procoagulant activity and fibrin deposition in rats with mercuric chloride-induced autoimmune nephritis. Lab Invest 57:138–143
55. Ekberg M, Pandolli M (1975) Origin of urinary fibrin fibrinogen degradation products in glomerulonephritis. Br Med J [Clin Res] 2:17–21
56. Clarkson AR, McDonald MK, Petrie JJB, Cash JD, Robson JS (1971) Serum and urine fibrin/fibrinogen degradation products in glomerulonephritis. Br Med J [Clin Res] 3:447–451
57. Tipping PG, Dowling JP, Holdsworth SR (1988) Glomerular procoagulant activity in human proliferative glomerulonephritis. J Clin Invest 81:119–125
58. Bergstein JM, Michael AF (1972) Cortical fibrinolytic activity in normal and diseased human kidneys. J Lab Clin Med 79:701–709
59. Mougenot B, Rondeau E, Kruithof B, Sraer JD (1988) Presence of type 1 plasminogen activator inhibitor (PA1-1) in renal fibrin deposits in human pathological conditions (abstract) Kidney Int 33:330

Hapten-Specific Cellular Immune Response Producing Glomerular Injury

Takashi Oite[1]

SUMMARY. A new model of experimental glomerulonephritis (GN), in which a cell-mediated reaction predominated, was established. Attachment of the haptens trinitrophenol (TNP) and fluorescein isothiocyanate (FITC) to a cationic carrier protein (bovine serum albumin:BSA) enabled their plantation in the glomerular capillary wall. Epicutaneous sensitization of the TNP without carrier protein induced a TNP-specific cell-mediated immunity. When we perfused the left kidneys of these sensitized rats with cationized TNP-BSA, proliferative glomerulonephritis with proteinuria could be induced without deposition of any autologous immunoglobulins and complement. Here, we will focus on the involvement of the cellular immune response in this experimental glomerulonephritis (GN) model.

Materials and Methods

Rats

All experiments were performed on male Wistar rats of body weight 160–180 g (Doken Japan).

Preparation of Hapten-Carrier Proteins and Their Cationization

2,4,6-trinitrobenzene-1-sulfonic acid sodium salt (TNBS), and fluorescein isothiocyanate (FITC) were conjugated to bovine serum albumin (BSA) by the method previously described [1]. Then TNP-BSA and FITC-BSA preparations were cationized as described previously [2]. Isoelectric points of the antigenic materials

[1]Department of Immunology, Institute of Nephrology, Niigata University School of Medicine, Asahimachi-dori 1, Niigata, 951 Japan

used in this study were determined by isoelectric focusing. The average degree of conjugation of haptens to BSA was determined spectrophotometrically.

Estimation of Serum Anti-TNP Antibody

Rat anti-TNP antibody was determined by enzyme-linked immunosorbent assay (ELISA), described previously [3].

Contact Hypersensitivity to the Haptenic Groups

Wistar rats were sensitized by applying 0.1 ml of 4% TNP or 4% FITC in absolute ethanol intradermally to the abdominal wall. Seven days later, 0.02 ml of 1% TNP or 1% FITC in olive oil was supplied to each side of the ear from a 25 gauge needle. Ear thickness was measured using a Peacock G1 dial thickness gauge (Ozaki Co., Tokyo). The results were expressed as the mean increment of ear thickness (10^{-2} mm).

Glomerular Labeling

Isolated glomeruli were incubated with monoclonal antibodies according to a modification of the method described by Schreiner et al. [4]. After washing, each preparation was incubated with FITC-conjugated rabbit anti-mouse immunoglobulins. The number of labeled cells per glomerulus was determined by focusing through whole glomerulus and counting.

Histological Examination

For light microscopy, renal tissue was fixed in buffered formalin and embedded in paraffin; 4 µm sections were stained with hematoxylin-eosin, periodic acid-Schiff, or periodic acid silver hematoxylin. For immunofluorescence, the material was snap-frozen in hexane cooled to -70 C.

Experimental Schedule

Unilateral renal perfusion was carried out to examine the nephritogenic potential of the test materials. Four groups of experiments were performed according to Table 1 in the Result section.

Results and Discussion

Characterization of Antigen Preparation

Table 1 shows the experimental schedule and characterization of the hapten-carrier protein used in each group. Native or cationized hapten-carrier protein, 500 µg, was injected intrarenally.

Table 1. Experimental design

Group	Sensitization	Renal perfusion
Group A	TNP	TNP.cat-BSA ($P\,I \geq 9.3$)
Group B	TNP	FITC.cat-BSA ($P\,I = 6.5 - 7.5$)
Group C	FITC	TNP.cat-BSA ($P\,I \geq 9.3$)
Group D	–	TNP.nat-BSA ($P\,I = 4.6$)

TNP, trinitrophenol; BSA, bovine serum albumin; FITC, fluorescein isothiocyanate

Contact Hypersensitivity to the TNP Haptenic Group

In TNP-sensitized group A, the standard ear-reaction when challenged with TNP showed an enhancement significantly greater than that of the FITC-sensitized group (Table 2).

Histological Changes

Light microscopically, there were no significant abnormalities in the right, unperfused kidneys from rats in TNP-sensitized group A and in bilateral kidneys from control groups B, C, and D. In the perfused kidneys from group A, there were prominent histological changes, such as endocapillary cell proliferation and adhesion of the glomerular capillary wall to Bowman's capsule, as described previously [1]. Figure 1 shows localization of immune reactants in the left kidney from group A. Hapten-specific binding to the glomerular capillary was found, as shown in Fig. 1a (1 hour after injection). The TNP bound to the glomerular capillary wall decreased rapidly with time, leading to moderate staining in a focal pattern within the first 24 hours (Fig. 1b). An interesting finding was that there was no deposition of rat IgG and C3, even in the TNP-sensitized group A, during the examination period (Fig. 1c and d). Immunofluorescent examination revealed a similar distribution and disappearance of TNP in both groups A and C. This finding is consistent with similar disappearance kinetics of ^{125}I-labeled cationized TNP-BSA from the perfused, left kidneys in both groups A and B, as described previously [1]. We have already reported that the presence of cationized antigen in the glomeruli, especially in the glomerular capillary walls, is markedly prolonged when complexed with antibody [2,5]. Since the elimination of the cationized TNP-BSA was not prolonged in sensitized animals, it is unlikely that, in group A, enough antibody was present to produce abnormal lesions with proteinuria.

Table 2. Contact hypersensitivity to TNP

Group	Sensitization	Challenge	Increment of ear thickness (10^{-2} mm)		
			Day 1	Day 2	Day 3
A	TNP	TNP	0.68 ± 0.07	0.85 ± 0.15	0.59 ± 0.14
B	FITC	TNP	0.30 ± 0.03	0.30 ± 0.14	0.18 ± 0.005

TNP, trinitrophenol; FITC, fluorescein isothiocyanate

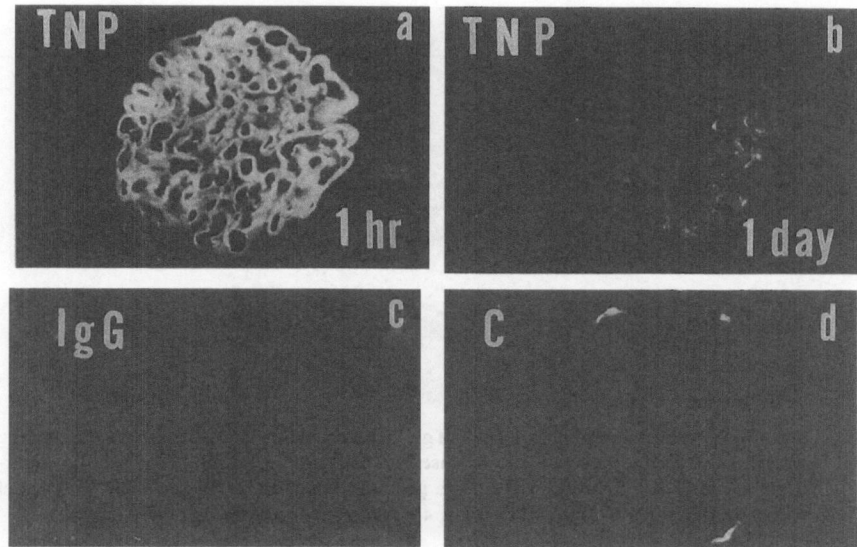

Fig. 1a-c. Cryostat sections of rat glomeruli from group A rats, **a** staining with FITC-anti-TNP-human IgG. At 1 h after renal perfusion with cationized TNP-BSA, **b** Staining with FITC-anti-TNP-human IgG. At 24 h after renal perfusion with cationized TNP-BSA, **c** and **d** Staining for rat IgG (Fig. 2c), and for rat C3 (Fig. 2d), at 1 h. FITC, fluorescein isothiocyanate; TNP, trinitrophenol; BSA, bovine serum albumin

Urinary Protein Analysis

Abnormal urinary protein excretion was seen on day 1 in all rats of the TNP-sensitized group A. The mean was 95 mg per day, but the level varied individually from rat to rat within a range of 35–170 mg per day. The amount of urinary protein in group A decreased rapidly to the point when, by day 2, it was already 13 mg per day. In groups B, C, and D there was no abnormal urinary protein excretion.

Labeled Cells Present in Isolated Glomeruli in this Experimental Glomerulonephritis

We quantified the number of cells bearing the rat leukocyte common antigen, and the Ia antigen, detected by mouse monoclonal antibodies. Many cells were significantly positive for leukocyte common antigen and Ia antigen in the glomerulus from the diseased left kidney (Fig. 2a). In contrast, fewer cells with these markers could be seen in the unperfused right kidney (Fig. 2b). As a control, the monoclonal antibody, RVG1, of the same subclass, IgG1, was substituted for the primary antibody (Fig. 2c).

In general, exudates induced by inflammatory, nonimmunological stimuli, such as thioglycollate broth or mineral oil were enriched for Ia-negative cells. Only 1%–4% of circulating monocyte-macrophages were Ia-positive. On the other hand, it is well

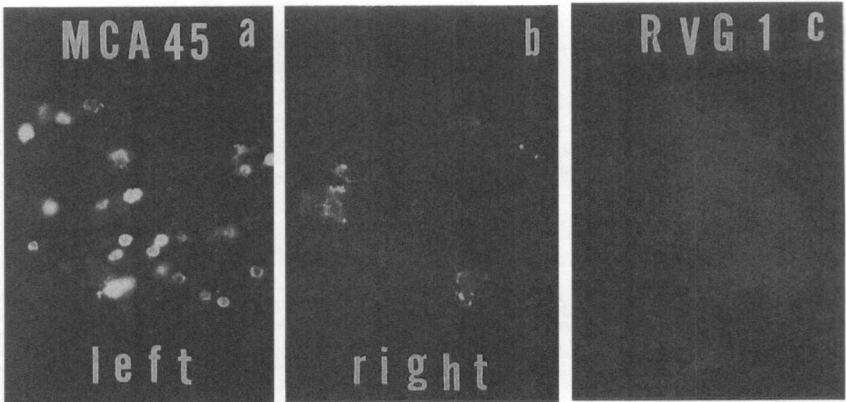

Fig. 2a-c. Fluorescent micrographs of isolated glomeruli on day 1, stained for cells bearing the rat Ia antigen, **a** A glomerulus from the perfused left kidney, **b** A glomerulus from the unperfused right kidney, **c** A glomerulus from the perfused left kidney, reacted with the control monoclonal antibody RVG1, instead of MCA 45, as a primary antibody

known that Ia-positive macrophages predominate in the exudates induced by the interaction of antigen-stimulated T cells and macrophages.

We have reported here that the development of proliferative glomerulonephritis with transient, but significant, proteinuria resulted from sensitization with a hapten, TNP. A cellular influx, including Ia-positive cells, was seen without deposition of any autologous antibody. We believe that the glomerular injury produced in this model is induced solely by cell-mediated immune reaction.

Acknowledgment. This work was supported by research grants (59570145, 60570153, 63570155) from The Ministry of Education, Science and Culture, Japan.

References

1. Oite T, Shimizu F, Kagami S, Morioka T (1989) Hapten-specific cellular immune response producing glomerular injury. Clin Exp Immunol 76:463–468
2. Oite T, Batsford SR, Mihatsch MJ, Takamiya H, Vogt A (1982) Quantitative studies of in situ immune complex glomerulonephritis in the rat induced by planted, cationized antigen. J Exp Med 155:460–474
3. Kagami S, Miyao M, Shimizu F, Oite T (1988) An active in situ immune complex glomerulonephritis using the hapten-carrier system: role of epitope density in cationic antigens. Clin Exp Immunol 74:121–125
4. Schreiner GF, Kiely J-M, Cotran RS, Unanue ER (1981) Characterization of resident glomerular cells in the rat expressing Ia determinants and manifesting genetically restricted interactions with lymphocytes. J Clin Invest 68:920–931
5. Oite T, Shimizu F, Kihara I, Batsford SR, Vogt A (1983) An active model of immune complex glomerulonephritis in the rat employing cationized antigen. Am J Pathol 112:185–194

Role of Potassium
in Acid-Base Disturbances

Chair: F. John Gennari (USA)
Yasushi Asano (Japan)

Acid-Base Implications of the K-NH$_4$ Interactions

RICHARD L. TANNEN[1]

SUMMARY. Observations in animals and humans in vivo, as well as direct investigation of kidney tissue in vitro, indicate that alterations in potassium have a profound effect on renal ammonia production. Potassium depletion results in an adaptive increase in ammonia production by the kidney similar to the changes produced by chronic metabolic acidosis, suggesting that altered ammoniagenesis in both conditions may be initiated by a decrease in proximal tubular intracellular pH. Hyperkalemia inhibits ammonia production directly, but does not appear to induce an adaptive down regulation in the renal capacity to produce ammonia. The direct effects of a low potassium concentration on ammonia production are not definitively resolved.

Potassium-induced alterations in ammonia homeostasis appear to play an important role in the pathogenesis of metabolic alkalosis induced by potassium depletion and in the hyperchloremic metabolic acidosis found in patients with Type IV renal tubular acidosis (RTA).

Introduction

Ammonia production and excretion are crucial components of the kidney's capacity to excrete acid. It is now well established that potassium as well as on acid-base status can exert profound effects on ammonia metabolism. This review will address the physiologic observations relevant to this relationship in animals and humans, the biochemical studies focused on the impact of potassium on the regulation of ammonia production, and the role played by the interaction between potassium and ammonia in the production of the acid-base abnormalities which accompany states of potassium depletion and excess.

---

[1]LA County/USC Medical Center, 2025 Zonal Ave., Rm. 7900, Los Angeles, CA 90033, USA

Physiologic Observations

Studies, dating back to the 1950s, of potassium depletion induced experimentally or produced clinically by several conditions, including laxative abuse, primary hyperaldosteronism, and fasting, have suggested that urinary pH and ammonium excretion were perturbed. Increased ammonium excretion, a high urine pH with normal ammonium excretion, and a high rate of ammonium excretion relative to urine pH, were all described (See [1] for a listing of these publications).

In order to investigate the relationship between potassium depletion and ammonia in more detail, I carried out a study of urine acidification in normal men, who were subjected to mild, experimentally-induced potassium depletion [2]. After ingestion of a standard acute ammonium chloride load, urine pH was found to be higher in the potassium depleted state in comparison with paired observations obtained under conditions of normal potassium balance. The increase in urine pH was accompanied by an increase in ammonium and net acid excretion; calculated urinary free ammonia concentration was also higher during potassium depletion. These changes were demonstrable with deficits of potassium as modest as approximately 200 mEq.

This combination of findings, i.e., a concurrent increase in both urine pH and ammonium excretion, seemed to be best explained by an enhanced rate of ammonia diffusion into the urine as a result of a primary increase in renal ammonia production. Alternatively, a decrease in renal blood flow could, theoretically, result in urinary elimination of a higher percentage of the ammonia produced by the kidney, with a concurrent reduction of ammonia release into the renal venous effluent.

Similar studies of urine acidification were also performed in normal men who had had a high potassium intake (3.0 − 6.0 mmoles/kg per day) for five days [3]. As found in studies of potassium depletion, chronic potassium loading produced no detectable effects on blood acid-base parameters, on urinary flow rate, or on nonvolatile buffer excretion (i.e., phosphate, creatinine, and organic acids). Urine pH in the potassium loaded state was lower than during control conditions by a mean of 0.21 U. Furthermore, the largest decrements in urine pH were accompanied by decreased excretion rates of both ammonium and net acid.

These findings suggested that a potassium surfeit diminished renal ammonia production. However, the possibility that an increase in renal blood flow accounted for the primary decrease in ammonia diffusion into the urine could not be excluded [4].

In the aggregate, these studies with potassium depletion and loading indicated that an important relationship existed between potassium homeostasis and renal ammonia production. Furthermore, the ability to detect alterations in ammonia metabolism with a modest potassium depletion of only 200 mmoles (i.e., approximately 5% of total body stores) and an equally modest potassium retention, which approximated 219 mmoles, suggested that this relationship might be a physiologic, rather than a pathologic, phenomenon. A variety of experimental approaches have been utilized to more precisely delineate the biochemical mechanisms underlying the influence of potassium on ammonia metabolism.

Biochemical Studies

The impact of potassium depletion on ammoniagenesis has been subjected to intense scrutiny. Increased renal ammonia production, with potassium depletion, has been documented in intact humans and rats by the simultaneous measurement of urinary and renal venous ammonia content [5-8]. Furthermore, studies utilizing renal cortical tissue and isolated mitochondria from both rats and dogs have shown that an adaptive increase in the capacity to produce ammonia is induced by potassium depletion [9-14].

The adaptive alterations produced by potassium depletion in the rat are virtually identical, for the most part, with those manifested during the adaptation of ammoniagenesis to chronic metabolic acidosis (see [1]). Both these conditions increase the activity of the cytosolic enzymes of the glutaminase II pathway and purine nucleotide cycle, and decrease the conversion of glutamate to glutamine, suggesting an inhibition of glutamine synthetase activity. They also similarly affect the intramitochondrial ammoniagenic pathway, which is currently believed to be the primary regulator of renal ammoniagenesis. The activity of phosphate dependent glutaminase (PDG) is increased with specific localization to the proximal tubule [15]; mitochondrial entry of glutamine is enhanced; ammonia production by rotenone-inhibited mitochondria is increased, providing a functional correlate of increased glutamine transport and/or PDG activity; flux through glutamate dehydrogenase is accelerated; the activity of phosphoenolpyruvate carboxykinase (PEPCK) and the production of glucose is increased; the generation of 14 CO_2 from U-14C glutamine is modified, suggesting alterations in metabolism of the glutamine carbon skeleton by the tricarboxylic acid (TCA) cycle; and the rate of citrate decarboxylation is increased.

The controversy regarding which metabolic alteration is primarily responsible for the increase in ammoniagenesis in potassium depletion is as equally unresolved as the controversy over metabolic acidosis. The data suggest that alterations, in either the mitochondrial glutamine transporter and/or the activity of PDG, are essential components of the adaptive response, but the precise importance of alterations in flux through glutamate dehydrogenase and through PEPCK to glucose are still unclear.

In view of the similarities, it is tempting to suggest that a similar mechanism might account for the development of an adaptive increase in the capacity to produce ammonia with both potassium depletion and chronic metabolic acidosis. Supporting this view, the production of metabolic alkalosis by the ingestion of sodium bicarbonate suppresses renal ammonia production in rats with potassium deficiency [7]. The most attractive unifying hypothesis is that both conditions are accompanied by a similar decrease in intracellular pH of the proximal tubular cells. This concept is supported, indirectly, by the changes in citrate metabolism produced by both conditions [16]. Direct measurements of renal intracellular pH using nuclear magnetic resonance (NMR) are also consistent with this hypothesis [17].

The direct effect of a low potassium concentration, per se, on renal ammonia production is not resolved definitively. Studies employing renal cortical slices bathed in a potassium free medium have reported an increase in ammonia production [18]. However, experiments in our laboratory did not detect increased ammoniagenesis by isolated renal cortical mitochondria exposed to a low potassium concentration; nor did we detect increased ammoniagenesis by either isolated cortical tubules or the isolated perfused rat kidney subjected to a reduction of ambient potassium concentration to 2.0 mM [13,19]. A recent preliminary report, in which isolated microperfused proximal tubules from the mouse were used, found that when the bath potassium was reduced to 2.0 mM there was a 20% increase in ammonia production [20].

There has been considerably less investigation of the effects of a potassium surfeit, as compared with a deficit, on ammonia production. To date, despite a variety of observations in humans, rats, and dogs, that a high potassium diet decreases urine pH and ammonium excretion, no direct measurements of the effects of high potassium on renal ammoniagenesis in vivo have been reported.

Furthermore, studies of isolated tissues in vitro have not yielded any convincing evidence that a potassium surfeit results in an adaptive down regulation of the ammoniagenic capacity of the kidney. Ingestion of a high potassium diet had no discernible effect on ammonia production by either isolated renal cortical mitochondria or by the isolated perfused kidney [13,19]. An earlier report from our laboratory found that ingestion of a high potassium diet produced a 5% decline in ammoniagenesis, seen in slices from the renal cortex, and a more impressive 36% decline, seen in slices from the outer medulla, but the implications of this finding are currently unclear [14]. However, it is important to emphasize that all these studies examined only the effects of a high potassium diet and not the potential effects of sustained hyperkalemia on adaptive changes in ammoniagenesis.

The direct effect of a high potassium concentration on renal ammonia production has also not undergone extensive investigation; but the results reported are quite uniform. Studies utilizing the isolated perfused kidney, renal cortical tubules, renal cortical slices, and isolated microperfused mouse proximal tubules, all indicate that a high potassium concentration directly inhibits ammonia production [18–20]. The suppressive effect has been demonstrated with potassium concentrations in the range of 7.5–10.4 mM. While it is tempting to speculate that this direct effect of potassium concentration accounts for the apparent inhibition of ammonia production by a potassium surfeit in vivo, it is important to recognize that some studies have reported urinary changes consistent with diminished ammoniagenesis in the absence of detectable changes in plasma potassium concentration [3,21].

The precise metabolic step at which hyperkalemia influences ammoniagenesis is also unresolved. Some data point to inhibition of glutamate deamination, while other information suggests an inhibition of glutamine deamidation [18,19]. More direct methods of investigating the pathways of ammoniagenesis are required to resolve this issue.

In addition to its effects on ammonia production, hyperkalemia may also directly inhibit the excretion of ammonium into the urine. Recent studies have shown that an increase in bath potassium concentration reduces ammonium absorption by isolated perfused thick ascending limbs of Henle [22,23]. Since ultimate elimination of the ammonium produced and secreted by the proximal tubule is dependent upon reabsorption by the ascending limb, hyperkalemia might directly impair urinary secretion, as well as production, of ammonium.

Acid-Base Abnormalities

As discussed in detail in another contribution to this symposium, (see List of Contents) there is now convincing evidence that potassium depletion can play a role in the development and maintenance of metabolic alkalosis. It seems highly likely that, when an increase in acid excretion is a central part of the pathophysiology, the potassium depletion-induced increase in ammonia production contributes to the generation of alkalosis. Furthermore, potassium depletion-induced increase in ammonia production may also play an important role in the maintenance of metabolic alkalosis by sustaining ammonium, and thereby acid excretion, in the face of the suppressive effects of metabolic alkalosis.

Although ingestion of a high potassium diet in normal humans appears to have no effect on systemic acid-base homeostasis [3], the hyperkalemic effect on ammonia production appears to play a crucial role in the metabolic acidosis associated with two important clinical hyperkalemic syndromes. It is now widely recognized that hyperkalemia, often in association with hyperchloremic metabolic acidosis, is a manifestation of the renal disease which is associated with either hyporeninemic hypoaldosteronism or with aldosterone independent defects in tubular potassium secretion.

The seminal study in humans, done by Szylman and co-workers [24], and subsequent detailed investigations by Sebastian, Schambelan, and their co-workers [25,26], demonstrated that correction of hyperkalemia by the use of cation exchange resins, mineralocorticoids, or dietary potassium restriction, produced a concomitant correction of metabolic acidosis. Furthermore, the improvement in acid-base status was accompanied by changes in urinary pH and ammonium excretion consistent with an increase in renal ammonia production.

In contrast to the findings in humans, correction of hyperkalemia in mineralocorticoid-deficient dogs does not improve metabolic acidosis, despite the anticipated changes in urine pH and ammonium excretion [27]. However, additional studies from this same laboratory have elegantly shown that adrenalectomized, steroid-replaced dogs maintained on a phosphate restricted diet develop hyperkalemia and metabolic acidosis when challenged with a high KCl intake [28]. In response to KCl, these animals exhibited a reduction in urinary net acid excretion, accompanied by a decrease in urine pH and ammonium excretion, which was consistent with a reduction in ammonia production. Thus, it seems clear that in certain circumstances in animals, as well as in humans, hyperkalemia can result in metabolic acidosis. Furthermore, the acid-base abnormality appears to result, at least in part, from an effect of potassium on ammonia metabolism.

References

1. Tannen RL (1977) Relationship of renal production and potassium homeostasis. Kidney Int 11:453–465
2. Tannen RL (1970) The effect of uncomplicated potassium depletion on urine acidification. J Clin Invest 49:813–827
3. Tannen RL, Wedell E, Moore R (1973) Renal adaptation to a high potassium intake: The role of hydrogen ion. J Clin Invest 52:2089–2101
4. Hollenberg NK, Williams G, Burger B, Hooshmand I (1975) The influence of potassium on the renal vasculature and the adrenal gland, and their responsiveness to angiotensin II in normal man. Clin Sci 48:527–534
5. Baertl JM, Sancetta SM, Gabuzda GH (1963) Relation of acute potassium depletion to renal ammonium metabolism in patients with cirrhosis. J Clin Invest 42:696–706
6. Gabuzda GJ, Hall PW III (1966) Relation of potassium depletion to renal ammonium metabolism and hepatic coma. Medicine (Baltimore) 45:481–490

7. Tollins JP, Hostetter MK, Hostetter MK, Hostetter TH (1987) Hypokalemic nephropathy in the rat: The role of ammonia in chronic tubular injury. J Clin Invest 79:1447–1458

8. Yablon S, Relman AS (1977) Excretion and total renal production of ammonia in K$^+$-depleted rats. Clin Res 25:452A

9. Adam WR, Simpson DP (1975) Renal mitochondrial glutamine metabolism and dietary potassium and protein content. Kidney 7:325–330

10. Kamm DE, Strope GL (1973) Glutamine and glutamate metabolism in renal cortex from potassium-depleted rats. Am J Physiol 224:1241–1248

11. Pagliara AS, Goodman AD (1970) Relation of renal cortical gluconeogenesis, glutamate content, and production of ammonia. J Clin Invest 49:1967–1974

12. Sastrasinh S, Sastrasinh M (1986) Renal mitochondrial glutamine metabolism during K$^+$ depletion. Am J Physiol 250:F667–F673

13. Tannen RL, Kunin AS (1976) Effect of potassium on ammoniagenesis by renal mitochondria. Am J Physiol 231:44–51

14. Tannen RL, McGill J (1976) The influence of potassium on renal ammonia production. Am J Physiol 231:1178–1184

15. Nonoguchi H, Takehara Y, Endou H (1986) Intra- and inter-nephron heterogeneity of ammoniagenesis in rats: effects of chronic metabolic acidosis and potassium depletion. Pflugers Arch 407:245–251

16. Adler S, Zett B, Anderson B (1974) Renal citrate in the potassium deficient rat: Role of potassium and chloride ions. J Lab Clin Med 84:307–316

17. Adam WR, Koretsky AP, Weiner MW (1986) ^{31}P-NMR in vivo measurement of renal intracellular pH: Effects of acidosis and K$^+$ depletion in rats. Am J Physiol 251:F904–F910

18. Sleeper RS, Belanger P, Lemieux G, Preuss HG (1982) Effects of in vitro potassium on ammoniagenesis in rat and canine kidney tissue. Kidney Int 21:345–353

19. Sastrasinh S, Tannen RL (1983) Effect of potassium on renal NH$_3$ production. Am J Physiol 244:F383–F391

20. Nagami GT, Lee P (1987) Ammonia production by isolated perfused mouse proximal tubules. Effect of bath and luminal potassium concentration. Abstr Am Soc Nephrol 20:258A

21. Kamm DE (1971) Dissociation of urine pH and NH$_3$ excretion during KCl and NaCl loading. Abstr Am Soc Nephrol 5:36

22. Good DW (Nov 1987) Effects of potassium on ammonia transport by medullary thick ascending limb of the rat. J Clin Invest 80:1358–1365

23. Good DW (1988) Active absorption of NH$^+_4$ by rat medullary thick ascending limb: inhibition by potassium. Am J Physiol 255 (Renal Fluid Electrolyte Physiol 24):F78–F87

24. Szylman P, Better OS, Chaimowitz C, Rosler A (1976) Role of hyperkalemia in the metabolic acidosis of isolated hypoaldosteronism. New Engl J Med 294:361–365

25. Sabastian A, Schambelan M, Lindenfeld S, Morris RC Jr (1977) Amelioration of metabolic acidosis with fluorocortisone therapy in hyporeninemic hypoaldosteronism. New Engl J Med 297:576–583

26. Maher T, Schambelan M, Kurtz I, Hulter HN, Jones JW, Sebastian A (1984) Amelioration of metabolic acidosis by dietary potassium restriction in hyperkalemic patients with chronic renal insufficiency. J Lab Clin Med 103:432–445

27. Hulter HN, Licht JH, Glynn RD, Sebastian A (1979) Renal acidosis in mineralocorticoid deficiency is not dependent on NaCl depletion or hyperkalemia. Am J Physiol 236:F283–F294

28. Hulter HN, Toto RD, Iinicki LP, Sebastian A (1983) Chronic hyperkalemic renal tubular acidosis induced by KCl loading. Am J Physiol 244:F255–F264

Reabsorption of Bicarbonate Along the Nephron: Importance of Potassium

Giovambattista Capasso[1], Robert Unwin[2], and Gerhard Giebisch[3]

SUMMARY. In order to assess the relationship between potassium and renal bicarbonate transport, micropuncture studies were carried out on superficial rat nephrons. The microcalorimetric method was used to quantitate bicarbonate reabsorption ($JHCO_3$). Two segments were studied: 1) the loop of Henle and 2) the distal tubule. In the first set of experiments, superficial loops of Henle were microperfused in vivo from late proximal to early distal tubule. Three groups of rats were investigated: 1) control rats 2) rats maintained either on 2) low or 3) high potassium diets. The loops were perfused with solutions containing 2 or 4 mM K^+. In control conditions $JHCO_3$ was 150.3 ± 5.0 pmol/min. This value was not affected by low or high potassium diet. In the second set of experiments free-flow micropuncture studies were carried out on superficial rat distal tubules. Experiments were performed in a) control conditions and b) during dietary potassium withdrawal. In normal conditions we observed highly significant, load dependent, net $JHCO_3$. Distal bicarbonate reabsorption persisted in hypokalemic alkalosis and, at comparable early distal loads, hypokalemia exerted a powerful stimulation on distal $JHCO_3$. These data demonstrate that along the loop of Henle, $JHCO_3$ is unaffected by changes in potassium intake, while in the distal tubule $JHCO_3$ is stimulated by potassium depletion.

Introduction

It is well established that, between potassium and hydrogen ions, there is a very close interaction at the cellular level that can lead to a mutual interplay of acid-base and potassium regulation. For example, changes in whole acid-base balance have been shown to influence the level of intracellular potassium activity [1], while alterations

---

[1]Chair of Nephrology, University of Naples, 80100 Naples, Italy

[2]Department of Cellular and Molecular Physiology, Yale Medical School, USA

[3]Department of Clinical Pharmacology, Hammersmith Hospital, London, UK

in potassium balance exert important effects on intracellular pH [2]. With respect to the kidney function it has been found that acidosis inhibits K^+ secretion in the distal tubule [2], while changes in body potassium distribution may influence acid-base transport along the nephron [3].

Although the proximal tubule is thought to be the major site of renal acidification [4], recent studies have shown that the distal nephron can make a significant contribution to the final urine pH. Our interest has been focused on two nephron segments: the loop of Henle and the cortical distal tubule. As opposed to the so-called proximal nephron, these segments have a much more pronounced heterogeneity, both from a morphological and from a functional point of view [5]. The loop of Henle comprises: a part of the late proximal convoluted tubule and the straight portion of the proximal tubule, the thin descending and ascending limbs, the thick ascending limb, and a small portion of the early distal tubule. The distal tubule is considered to be the segment starting at the macula densa and ending at the first junction with another distal tubule to form the collecting duct. It is certainly the most heterogeneous segment of the nephron; it contains at least three distinct sub-segments. The first of these is the distal convoluted tubule; the following segment is the connecting tubule which is lined by connecting tubule cells and by intercalated cells in relatively low density. The last segment is the initial cortical collecting duct, composed of a majority of principal cells and containing, in addition, intercalated cells (alfa and beta forms).

In the present study we have pursued two objectives: first, to assess the contribution and to elucidate the mechanisms involved in acid-base transport along these two heterogeneous segments. Second, to evaluate, in the same segments, the relationship between serum potassium level and bicarbonate transport. This last issue was studied by modulating the potassium intake through diets of different potassium content.

Methods

Preparation of Animals

Male rats were anesthetized with Inactin (Promonta, West Germany) using a dose of 120 mg/kg body weight, intraperitoneally; they were then tracheostomized and placed on a thermoregulated table designed to hold body temperature at 37°C. The right carotid artery was catheterized for blood pressure monitoring and periodic blood sampling for measurements of hematocrit, radioactive inulin, pH and total CO_2 concentration. The left jugular vein was cannulated with PE-50 tubing and used for infusion via a syringe pump. The left kidney was exposed through a flank incision, made free of perirenal fat, decapsulated and immobilized in a lucite chamber. The left ureter was catheterized for collection of urine. Three groups of rats were studied: (1) control rats maintained on a diet of standard Purina laboratory chow; (2) low potassium rats, maintained on a low potassium diet for at least three weeks; and (3) rats maintained on 10% potassium diet (potassium adapted animals).

Microperfusion of the loop of Henle

A perfusion pipette was inserted in the last surface loop of the proximal tubule and a castor oil block was placed upstream of the perfusion pipette. Microperfusion was

Table 1. Summary of baseline data (mean $\pm$ SEM) of rats fed with diet at different K content (*$p < 0.005$ vs control)

Rats	Blood K+ (nEq/lt)	Blood pH	Blood HCO3 (mM)
Control	4.1 $\pm$ 0.1	7.348 $\pm$ 0.04	29.3 $\pm$ 0.3
Low K	2.5 $\pm$ 0.1*	7.532 $\pm$ 0.1*	36.0 $\pm$ 1.3*
K adapted	4.0 $\pm$ 0.2	7.372 $\pm$ 0.05	29.1 $\pm$ 0.7

started at 20 nl/min with a thermally shielded microperfusion pump. The perfusion solution was an end-proximal solution containing, in addition, 0.07% FD&C blue dye and ^{14}C-insulin.

Free-flow collections

After completion of surgery, methoxy-^{3}H-inulin (110 µCi/h following a priming injection of 90 µCi) was infused i.v. Collections of tubule fluid samples were begun after a 1 h equilibration period. Early and late distal segments were identified by the i.v. injection of 20 µl FDC solution. Puncture sites were recognized by filling the tubule with a microfil silicone rubber compound. The kidneys were then macerated overnight in 25% NaOH and the puncture sites determined by microdissection.

Analytical methods

Tubule fluid total CO_2 concentration was determined by microcalorimetry. The blood acid-base status of each animal was measured with a blood-gas analyzer. Radioactivity was measured by a liquid scintillation counter and plasma electrolytes were measured by flame photometry.

Results

Table 1 summarizes data on blood electrolytes and systemic acid-base parameters in control, potassium depleted, and potassium adapted animals. As expected, plasma potassium was markedly depressed in group (2), whereas blood pH and bicarbonate were significantly increased. In potassium adapted rats (group 3) no changes were detected.

Loop of Henle

Figure 1 shows the effects of various inhibitors on fractional bicarbonate transport (FRHCO$_3$) along the loop of Henle. In the presence of the carbonic anhydrase inhibitor methazolamide (2.10^{-4} M) FRHCO$_3$ was reduced by 73% (P < 0.01); the Na+-H+ exchange inhibitor ethylisopropylamiloride (2.10^{-4} M) reduced FRHCO$_3$ by 39% (P < 0.01); and the H+-ATPase inhibitor bafilomycin A$_1$ reduced FRHCO$_3$ by 26% (P < 0.01). The Cl$^-$ channel blocker NPPB (5-nitro-2'-(3-phenylpropylamino)-benzoate) (2.10^{-4} M) and the anion exchange inhibitor DIDS (diidothiocyanato-2,2'-stilbenedisulfonate) (5.10^{-5} M) had no effect on FRHCO$_3$.

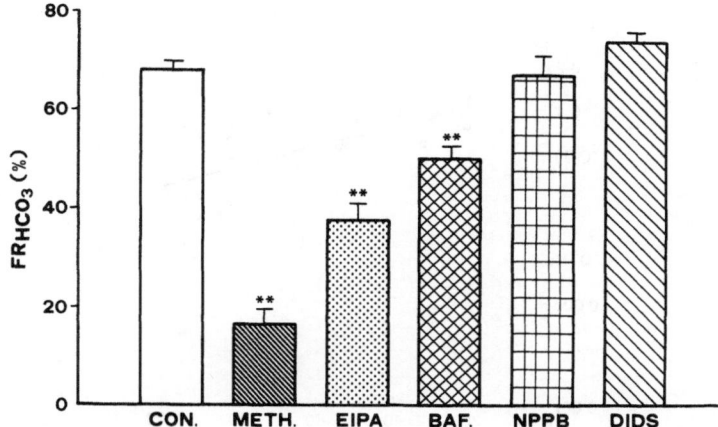

Fig. 1. Effect of several transport inhibitors on fractional bicarbonate reabsorption (*FRHCO₃*) along the loop of Henle (**P<0.01 vs CON). CON, control; METH, methazolamide; EIPA, ethylisopropylamiloride; BAF, bafilomycin A_1; NPPB, 5-nitro-(-3-phenylpropylamino) benzoate; DIDS, diisothiocyanato-2-2′-stilben edisulfonate

In hypokalemic rats, $JHCO_3$ in the loop was 150.9 ± 8.6 pmol/min (n=19); this value was not different from that obtained in control rats perfused with the same solution containing 2 mM K^+ (152.3 ± 11.2 pmol/min, n=17).

In potassium adapted animals, loop $JHCO_3$ was 152.1 ± 6.3; this value was similar to that found in control animals.

Distal tubule

Figure 2 shows fractional bicarbonate delivery in the control group plotted as function of distal tubular length. Between 20% and 95% distal tubular length, a mean of some 6% of the filtered bicarbonate was reabsorbed. Accordingly, significant bicarbonate reabsorption takes place along the superficial distal tubule.

Figure 3 shows the data on the fractional reabsorption of bicarbonate along the distal tubule during hypokalemia. The figure clearly indicates that significant net bicarbonate reabsorption was uniformly observed along the distal tubule in hypokalemic rats.

Figure 4 provides a schematic overview of absolute bicarbonate reabsorption rates along the distal tubule, with and without bicarbonate loading, in control and hypokalemic conditions. It is important to note that in the presence of closely similar early distal bicarbonate loads in control and in K depletion, distal $JHCO_3$ was significantly higher in low-K rats compared with control rats. Moreover, both values are several-fold higher than corresponding values for bicarbonate reabsorption in the non-bicarbonate-loaded conditions. Thus, distal $JHCO_3$ in bicarbonate loaded control rats was 3.6 times higher than in non loaded rats, whereas in low-K rats, bicarbonate loading resulted in 5.4-fold stimulation of $JHCO_3$.

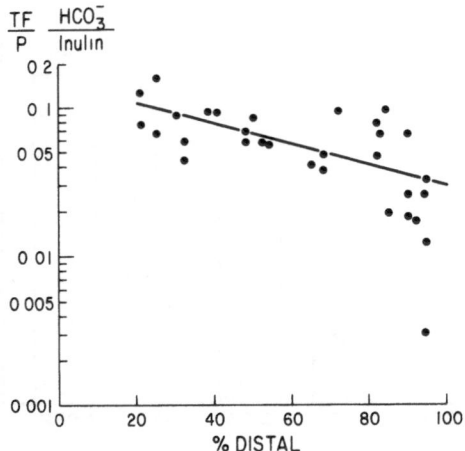

Fig. 2. Summary of fractional bicarbonate concentration ratios as function of distal tubular length of control rats. (From [10] with permission)

Discussion

Bicarbonate transport along the loop of Henle

The data presented show that about 15% of filtered bicarbonate is reabsorbed along the loop of Henle. Such transport is sensitive to inhibition by carbonic anhydrase, but there appears to be a carbonic anhydrase insensitive component. There was no major

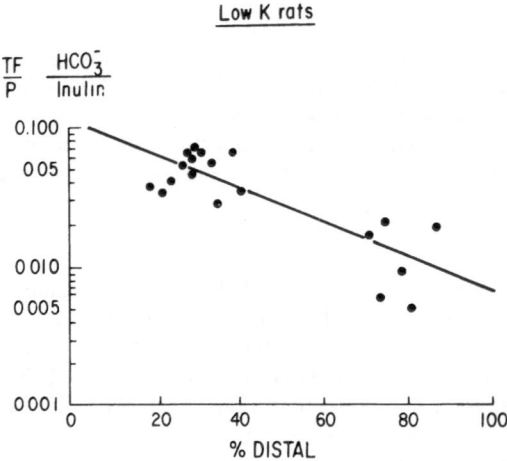

Fig. 3. Summary of fractional bicarbonate concentration ratios as function of distal tubular length of hypokalemic rats. (From [10] with permission)

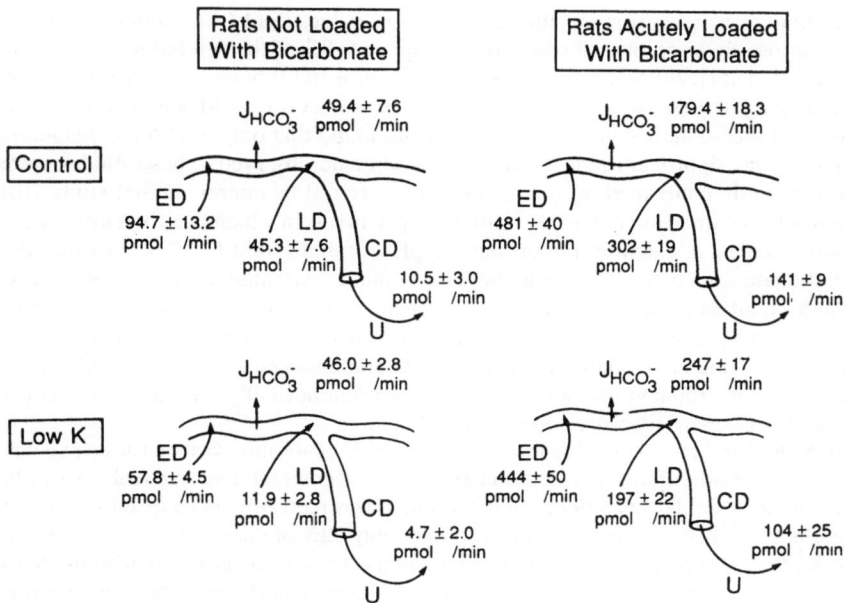

Fig. 4. Schematic summary of bicarbonate reabsorption along the superficial distal tubule of the rat. (From [14] with permission).

contribution to net bicarbonate transport by the Cl-HCO₃ exchanger. The bulk of loop of Henle bicarbonate transport is dependent on the presence of Na⁺-H⁺ exchanger and the proton pump. The data on the effect of potassium depletion on JHCO₃ are interesting. In contrast with the distal tubule, where in low K rats we found an increase in JHCO₃, we measured no difference in JHCO₃ between control and low K rats, when the loops were perfused with the same potassium concentration. One possible explanation could be related to the higher back-flux of bicarbonate. This effect would be facilitated by the steeper bicarbonate gradient and the relatively high bicarbonate permeability of the various segments that make up the loop of Henle. Such an interpretation is consistent with the data of Byers et al. [6], who found an accumulation of 6 mM bicarbonate in loops of Henle perfused with bicarbonate free solutions; and consistent with our observations that even in the presence of a potent carbonic anhydrase inhibitor, like methazolamide, we did not measure a bicarbonate concentration of less than 4 mM in collected fluid. Therefore it is entirely possible that in low potassium rats there could be an increase in bicarbonate transport, but this is offset by the larger bicarbonate back flux. With respect to JHCO₃ along the loop in potassium adapted animals the data presented seem to indicate that such a maneuver has no significant influence on loop bicarbonate handling.

Bicarbonate transport in the distal tubule

Studies in which luminal pH was used to estimate bicarbonate concentrations showed that bicarbonate remained approximately constant along the distal tubule. Distal bicarbonate reabsorption calculated from these values, and from inulin concentration ratios, yields an overall reabsorption rate of 5–8% of the filtered load along the distal tubule [7]. Pump-perfusion experiments in distal tubules have cast doubts on the capacity of these segments to acidify the urine. Lucci et al. [8] perfused these tubules with bicarbonate containing solutions and found that only in chronic metabolic acidosis was significant reabsorption of bicarbonate observed. These studies were more recently confirmed by Levine [9]. In our free-flow micropuncture study [10] the results obtained did not differ from the experiments in which bicarbonate concentrations were evaluated by measuring the pH of tubule fluid [7]. The fact that the bicarbonate concentration along the distal tubule was maintained at low levels, despite significant fluid reabsorption, demonstrates significant net bicarbonate reabsorption along the distal tubule in conditions of normal acid-base balance. Very recently, Levine et al. found that overnight fasting induced significant, load dependent distal bicarbonate reabsorption, whereas when normally fed rats were studied no net bicarbonate reabsorption was found [11].

In K-depleted rats, a distal reabsorption rate of 46 pmol/min was measured at a distal load of 58 pmol/min, that is, about 80% of the segmental load was reabsorbed. In control rats a similar net amount of bicarbonate was reabsorbed at a distal load of 95 pmol/min, corresponding to a reabsorption of only 52% of the segmental load. When low K rats were compared with control rats subject to acute bicarbonate loading, both groups having a similar distal bicarbonate load, significantly more bicarbonate was reabsorbed along the distal tubule in low K rats. Although direct cell pH measurements have not yet been done in cells of the distal tubule, it is possible that cell acidification, postulated to occur in tubule cells during hypokalemia, may be responsible for enhanced bicarbonate transport. Furthermore, the observation that during potassium depletion there is an activation along the distal tubule of a K/H-ATPase [12], would be consistent with our findings. Such an interpretation would be strengthened by the observation that the intercalated cells of the rat medullary collecting duct exhibit an increase in luminal membrane surface area under conditions of K$^+$ depletion [13]. Finally we would like to emphasize that the changes in bicarbonate transport could not have been due to alteration in circulating aldosterone, since hypokalemia depressed aldosterone secretion.

References

1. Kubota TK, Biagi BA, Giebisch G (1983) Effects of acid base disturbances on basolateral membrane potential and intracellular potassium activity in the proximal tubule of Necturus. J Membr Biol 73:61–68
2. Stanton BA, Giebisch G (1982) Effects of pH on K$^+$ transport by renal distal tubule. Am J Physiol 241:F544–F551
3. Chan YL, Biagi B, Giebisch G (1982) Control mechanisms of bicarbonate transport across the rat proximal convoluted tubule. Am J Physiol 242:F532–F543
4. Cogan MG, Alpern RJ (1984) Regulation of proximal bicarbonate reabsorption. Am J Physiol 247:F387–F395
5. Madsen KM, Tisher CC (1986) Structural-functional relationship along the distal nephron. Am J Physiol 250:F1–F15
6. Byers MK, Levine DZ, McLeod RA, Luisello JA (1979) Loop of Henle bicarbonate accumulation in vivo in the rat. J Clin Invest 63:59–66

7. Malnic G, De Mello, Aires M, Giebisch G (1972) Micropuncture study of renal tubular hydrogen ion transport in the rat. Am J Physiol 222:147–158
8. Lucci MS, Pucacco LR, Carter NW, Dubose TD (1982) Evaluation of bicarbonate transport in rat distal tubule: effects of acid-base status. Am J Physiol 243:F335–F341
9. Levine DZ (1985) An in vivo microperfusion study of distal tubule bicarbonate absorption in normal and ammonium chloride rats. J Clin Invest 75:588–595
10. Capasso G, Kinne R, Malnic G, Giebisch G (1986) Renal bicarbonate reabsorption in the rat. I, Effects of hypokalemia and carbonic anhydrase. J Clin Invest 78:1558–1567
11. Levine DZ, Iacovitti M, Nash L, Vandorpe D (1988) Secretion of bicarbonate by rat distal tubules in vivo. J Clin Invest 81:1873–1878
12. Doucet A, Marsy S (1987) Characterization of K-ATPase activity in distal nephron: stimulation by potassium depletion. Am J Physiol 253:F418–F423
13. Stetson DL, Wade JB, Giebisch G (1980) Morphologic alteration in the rat medullary collecting duct following potassium depletion. Kidney Int 17:4556
14. Capasso G et al. (1987) Renal bicarbonate reabsorption in the rat -II. Distal tubule load dependence and the effect of hypokalemia. J Clin Invest 80:409–414

Role of Acid-Base Disturbance on Potassium Transport Along the Nephron

KAORU TABEI, SHIGEAKI MUTO, HIROAKI FURUYA, YASUNORI SAKAIRI, YASUHIRO ANDO, and YASUSHI ASANO[1]

SUMMARY. We evaluated the role of acidosis on the regulation of transepithelial potassium transport in rabbit early proximal convoluted tubules (PCT) and cortical collecting ducts (CCD) by using in vitro microperfusion and conventional microelectrode methods. In PCT, when the bath medium pH declined from 7.4 to 6.8, transepithelial voltage (Vt) and net potassium flux (JK) increased; however, in CCD, Vt and JK decreased significantly without changing net Na flux. In CCD, basolateral acidosis decreased basolateral membrane voltage and increased transepithelial resistance, with an increment of calculated fractional resistance of apical membrane in principal cells. Inhibition of JK by basolateral acidosis remained significant in the presence of 2mM luminal $BaCl_2$. Elimination of ambient bicarbonate (Hepes buffer solution) did not affect the inhibitory effect of basolateral acidosis on JK. Basolateral 1 mM amiloride diminished the inhibitory effect of basolateral acidosis on JK. The ^{86}Rb and ^{22}Na efflux coefficients were not significantly affected by basolateral acidosis.

In conclusion, the present study demonstrates that basolateral acidosis affects JK in both PCT and CCD, but it does so in opposite directions. In CCD, basolateral pH is indeed an important modulator of epithelial K transport. Mechanistically, basolateral acidosis appears to inhibit apical K conductance independently of Na conductance or ambient bicarbonate in rabbit CCD.

Introduction

The maintenance of potassium balance is vital in several respects; in particular, a high intracellular potassium concentration is essential for operating cell functions and for keeping the normal electrical gradients across the cell membranes, which is essential for various forms of electrolyte transport. Since the maintenance of potas-

[1]Div. of Nephrology, Dept. of Medicine, Jichi Medical School, 3311-1 Minamikawachi-machi, Kawachi-gun, Tochigi, 329-04 Japan

sium balance is critical for the maintenance of cellular metabolism, potassium homeostasis should be efficiently regulated in a narrow range by several mechanisms. The acid-base balance is also critical for cell viability, therefore, several buffering systems should be necessary. It has long been known that changes in acid-base balance have significant effects on both renal and extrarenal potassium homeostasis [1]. It has been generally accepted that acidosis increases, while alkalosis decreases, plasma potassium concentration [2]. A common rule of thumb states that for every 0.1 unit change in blood pH the potassium concentration will change in the opposite direction by approximately 0.1–1.2 mEq/l [3,4]. Whether the acidosis is respiratory or metabolic in origin has an important effect on the magnitude of the hyperkalemic response. Respiratory acidosis causes little increase in the plasma potassium concentration; for every 0.1 unit change in blood pH the plasma potassium concentration increases by only 0.1–0.3 mEq/l [5]. Recent studies have indicated that the relationship between changes of blood pH and plasma potassium concentration is quite complex, and is influenced by several factors, including the origin of the acid-base disturbance, the nature of the anion accompanying the increase in hydrogen ion, change in plasma bicarbonate concentration, per se, duration of acidosis, and extent of intracellular buffering. Extrarenal potassium homeostasis is very important in keeping plasma potassium levels within a narrow range, especially in a rapid potassium loaded condition such as occurs just after meals. Several factors, such as insulin, catecholamines, aldosterone, and maybe other peptides, by controlling renal and/or extrarenal potassium regulatory systems, may contribute to keeping plasma potassium levels constant [1].

We have examined the relationship between acid-base disturbance and potassium transport in hemodialyzed patients [6]. In hemodialyzed patients, erythrocyte potassium concentration increased in patients with severe metabolic acidosis, and the amount of potassium removed into the dialysate was significantly smaller than that in patients without metabolic acidosis. These findings clearly showed the shift of potassium into the cells when metabolic acidosis was corrected by hemodialysis. To confirm this finding, in vitro ^{86}Rb uptake was examined in erythrocytes of control subjects and uremic patients. ^{86}Rb uptake was performed by incubation of cell suspensions of erythrocytes for 60 min with Hepes buffer. Acidification of the incubation medium, from 7.4 to 6.8, diminished Rb uptake significantly, by 15% [7]. In the presence of 10^{-5}M ouabain, Rb uptake was markedly inhibited, and the pH-dependent suppression of Rb uptake was also abolished. In the presence of 10^{-5} M amiloride and furosemide, acidification of the incubation medium failed to suppress Rb uptake in control subjects; however, in uremic patients, furosemide did not affect the pH-dependent suppression of Rb uptake. These data suggested that 1) in extrarenal potassium regulatory mechanisms, erythrocytes also play an important role in regulating plasma potassium level, 2) metabolic acidosis depletes erythrocyte potassium contents, and rapid correction of metabolic acidosis during hemodialysis shifts potassium into erythrocytes, and 3) metabolic acidosis, directly or indirectly, suppresses ouabain-sensitive Na-K ATPase activity. In renal potassium homeostasis, a number of clearance studies have demonstrated that both metabolic and respiratory acidosis decrease urinary potassium excretion; in contrast, both metabolic and respiratory alkalosis increase urinary potassium excretion [8–11]. In renal potassium regulatory mechanisms, increased plasma potassium concentration, itself, stimulates urinary potassium secretion [12,13]; however, both metabolic and respiratory acidosis depress urinary potassium excretion independent of changes in plasma potassium concentration [14].

The role of acidosis in potassium transport along the nephron has been examined only in distal tubules. In the proximal tubules, several microelectrode and patch clamp studies suggest the possibility that metabolic acidosis affects potassium transport in these segments [15–20]; however, up to the present, no direct data is available. Nephron segments responsible for the alteration of potassium secretion in acid-base disturbance have been examined by the use of the free flow micropuncture method. Malnic et al. [21] and Stanton et al. [22] demonstrated that both metabolic and respiratory acidosis decreased potassium secretion in distal tubules. They also demonstrated that both metabolic and respiratory alkalosis stimulated potassium secretion in distal tubules. However, by using the micropuncture method, the nephron segments really responsible were not identified, because the distal tubules included distal convoluted tubules, connecting tubules, and cortical collecting ducts. So far, the nephron segments most responsible for final urinary potassium excretion have not yet been determined. Using isolated tubular microperfusion, Boudry et al. [23] reported the effect of luminal acidosis on potassium secretion in rabbit cortical collecting ducts. They demonstrated that luminal acidification, from 7.4 to 6.8, depolarized transepithelial voltage and decreased bath to lumen ^{86}Rb flux, without changing lumen to bath ^{22}Na flux. O'Neil et al. [24] demonstrated that luminal acidification, from 7.4 to 4.0, markedly inhibited luminal potassium conductance, by 70%, in rabbit cortical collecting ducts with microelectrode techniques. However, the effect of basolateral acidosis on potassium transport has not been examined. Using the in vitro microperfusion method, we examined the effect of metabolic acidosis on potassium transport in rabbit proximal convoluted tubules and cortical collecting ducts.

Methods

Protocol 1. The Effect of Metabolic Acidosis on Potassium Transport in Rabbit Proximal Convoluted Tubules

Proximal convoluted tubules, dissected from New Zealand white rabbits anesthetized with pentobarbital (50 mg/kg body weight), were placed in Euro Collins solution (mM): $NaHCO_3$ 10, K_2HPO_4 42.5, KH_2PO_4 15.0, KCl 15.0, and Glucose 3.5 g/dl; osmolarity was adjusted to 375 mOsm/kg.H_2O, at 4°C. Isolated tubular microperfusion was performed by the method of Burg et al. [25] with minor modifications [26]. Artificial solution was used as perfusate; the composition was (mM): NaCl 105, $NaHCO_3$ 25, KCl 5, NaH_2PO_4 1.6, Na_2HPO_4 0.4, $CaCl_2$ 1.8, Na acetate 10, d-glucose 8.3, and l-alanine 5.0; pH was adjusted to 7.4 after bubbling with 95% O_2/5% CO_2 gas mixture; osmolarity was adjusted to 298 mOsm/kg H_2O. For the bathing medium, bovine serum albumin 6.0 g/dl was added instead of d-glucose and l-alanine. The pH and osmolarity were identical with those of the perfusate. Metabolic acidosis was carried out by reducing the $NaHCO_3$ concentration from 25 to 5 mM/l and replacing the amount removed with 20 mmol Na cyclamate. pH was adjusted to 6.8, and osmolarity was identical with the control solution. The perfusate contained methoxy ^{3}H Inulin for a volume marker, and FD and C Green dye was used for the detection of damaged cells. Potassium transport was examined as a net flux by measuring the potassium concentration of the perfusate and collected fluid. Potassium concentration was measured with an ultramicroflamephotometer (Apel Co. Japan). Sample collections were performed, one by one, for measurement of water flux and potassium flux. After dissection, PCT were transferred to a Lucite bath chamber and were perfused in vitro. After a 20 min equilibrium period, control collections were performed: three for measuring water flux and three for measuring potassium flux. The bathing medium was then changed to an acidic solution, and the same samplings were performed, followed by consecutive changes of perfusate to acidic solution, change of bathing medium to 7.4 solution and, lastly, perfusate and bathing medium were returned to 7.4 solution.

Protocol 2. The Effect of Metabolic Acidosis on Potassium Transport in Rabbit Cortical Collecting Ducts

Rabbit cortical collecting ducts were perfused by the in vitro microperfusion method, as described above. In addition to measuring the net potassium flux under various conditions, ^{86}Rb flux and ^{22}Na flux were also examined. Either ^{86}Rb or ^{22}Na was added to the perfusate for measuring the unidirectional efflux coefficient. The isotope count was measured by the Chelencof method in ^{86}Rb and by gamma counter in ^{22}Na. In order to clarify the detailed mechanisms of the effect of acid-base disturbance on potassium transport, several maneuvers were performed: 2 mM BaCl$_2$ was added to the perfusate; 1 mM amiloride was added to the bathing medium. In order to examine the effect of bicarbonate on K transport, Hepes buffer was used instead of NaHCO$_3$ in both the 7.4 solution and the 6.8 solution. Conventional microelectrodes were used to impale the principal cells of rabbit cortical collecting ducts, in order to measure the basolateral membrane voltage by the method reported previously [27]. The electrolyte composition of the perfusate and the bath solution was identical to that used in the in vitro microperfusion experiments, except that the perfusate did not contain d-glucose and l-alanine, and the bath solution did not contain bovine serum albumin. Also, a constant current was passed through the perfusate and the bath solution, so that the transepithelial and fractional apical membrane resistances could be calculated.

Statistical analysis was performed by Student's t-test. A P value less than 5% was considered as significant.

Results

Protocol 1. The Effect of Metabolic Acidosis on K Transport in Rabbit Proximal Convoluted Tubules

Basolateral acidosis achieved by changing the bathing medium pH from 7.4 to 6.8 solution decreased transepithelial voltage by -2.36 ± 1.4 to -1.48 ± 0.85 mV ($P < 0.05$); however, water transport did not significantly change. On the other hand, basolateral acidosis enhanced potassium secretion from -5.08 ± 1.76 to -11.97 ± 2.14 pmol/min per mm ($P < 0.05$) without any change of sodium flux. Additional luminal acidosis depressed potassium secretion to -2.84 ± 3.04 pmol/min

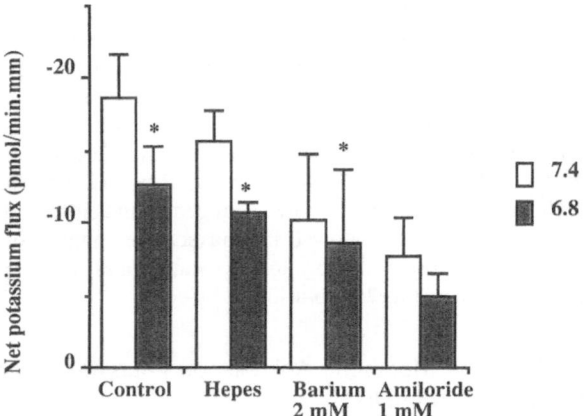

Fig. 1. Basolateral acidosis suppressed potassium secretion in rabbit cortical collecting duct. This effect was studied in isolated microperfused tubules in vitro. The inhibitory effect of basolateral acidosis on potassium transport was not affected by the elimination of bicarbonate, but was diminished in the presence of either luminal 2 mM barium or basolateral 1 mM amiloride

per mm; however, transepithelial voltage did not change. The change of bath solution to pH 7.4 did not affect potassium transport, water transport, and transepithelial voltage.

Protocol 2. The Effect of Metabolic Acidosis on Potassium Transport in Rabbit Cortical Collecting Ducts

When the pH of the bathing medium was changed from 7.4 to 6.8, transepithelial voltage was depolarized from -9.62 ± 2.18 to -3.84 ± 2.70 mV ($P < 0.005$), without significant recovery. Net potassium flux also decreased from -18.69 ± 3.00 to -10.98 ± 2.16 pmol/min per mm ($P < 0.025$), however, net sodium flux did not significantly change. In the presence of 2 mM barium chloride, a potent potassium channel blocker in the perfusate, the inhibitory effect of basolateral acidosis on potassium secretion and transepithelial voltage was diminished, but still remained significant (Fig. 1). Basolaterally, a high dose of amiloride, (1 mM), which is thought to inhibit both sodium channel and sodium-proton exchanger, diminished the inhibitory effect of basolateral acidosis on potassium flux and transepithelial voltage. When Hepes buffer solution was used as perfusate and bathing medium instead of bicarbonate, the inhibitory effect of basolateral acidosis remained unchanged. Neither the ^{86}Rb efflux coefficient nor the [22]Na efflux coefficient was significantly affected by the basolateral acidosis. Electrophysiological studies also revealed that basolateral acidosis depolarized transepithelial voltage and a simultaneous record of basolateral membrane voltage also showed deporalization in the principal cells, from -83.5 ± 2.3 to -74.75 ± 3.07 mV ($P < 0.001$). Basolateral acidosis also significantly increased transepithelial resistance, from 81.7 ± 7.08 to 93.4 ± 9.7 ohm.cm²

(P < 0.001), and significantly increased the calculated fractional resistance of apical membrane, from 0.47 ± 0.07 to 0.57 ± 0.08 (P < 0.001).

Discussion

A high intracellular potassium concentration, essential for operating cell functions, is kept by sodium-potassium ATPase on the various epithelial membranes. Potassium ions can be shifted out of the extracellular space and taken up by body cells so that only a small fraction of any potassium added remains in the extracellular fluid compartment. Conversely, extracellular losses can be mitigated by transfer of potassium ions from the cell pool to the extracellular fluid. Since potassium imbalance, whether manifested as hypokalemia or hyperkalemia, leads to lethal disorders, plasma potassium levels should be regulated within a strictly narrow range. Clinically, it is a well-known phenomenon that acidosis induces hyperkalemia and that alkalosis induces hypokalemia. The real mechanisms of these interactions between acid-base disturbance and potassium homeostasis has remained uncertain [1].

Both metabolic and respiratory acidosis decrease urinary potassium excretion and, in contrast, both metabolic and respiratory alkalosis increase urinary potassium excretion, independently of extrarenal potassium regulatory systems [14]. In the renal potassium regulatory mechanisms, increased plasma potassium concentration, itself, stimulates urinary potassium secretion [12,13]; however, both metabolic and respiratory acidosis depress urinary potassium excretion, independently of changes in plasma potassium concentration.

Bulk reabsorption of electrolytes and water in the kidney occurs mainly in the proximal tubules and in Henle's loop, but the site of the final regulation of renal water and electrolyte excretion is the distal nephron segment, particularly the collecting duct system.

In the proximal tubules, there are no data available which would allow us to assume the effect of metabolic acidosis on net potassium transport. We demonstrated previously that potassium was secreted in rabbit proximal convoluted tubules in vitro when studied by isolated tubular microperfusion [28]; however, micropuncture studies have found that potassium is reabsorbed in the proximal tubules, to the extent of about 50%–80% of the filtered load. Similar findings were reported from Wasserstein [29] and Work [30] in proximal straight tubules. We further examined the effect of basolateral barium on potassium secretion in proximal convoluted tubules. Basolateral barium stimulated potassium secretion, perhaps due to the inhibition of basolateral barium-sensitive potassium channel [28], resulting in reduced potassium leaking out from basolateral membrane and an increment of luminal potassium extrusion. Intracellular recordings with conventional microelectrodes have demonstrated that changes in extracellular pH greatly affect the basolateral membrane potential in renal proximal tubules [15–18]. This fact may suggest that the basolateral potassium conductance is sensitive to external pH. As a change in extracellular pH is known to give rise to a change in intracellular pH [19], the potassium conductance might be regulated by intracellular pH [20]. Recent patch clamp studies in opossum kidney proximal tubular cells revealed that apical membrane potassium channel was calcium sensitive and basolateral membrane potassium channel was barium sensitive [20]. As we have shown in this paper, in the proximal convoluted tubules, basolateral acidosis enhanced potassium channels, contrary to our expectations. Although the detailed mechanisms have not yet been clarified, it is suggested that basolateral acidosis may enhance potassium secretion by the inhibition of basolateral barium sensitive potassium channel. Unless sodium and water reabsorption is reduced, proximal potassium transport is thought to be less important in the regulation of final urinary potassium excretion. However, the fact should be mentioned that basolateral acidosis stimulates potassium secretion in proximal convoluted tubules, although the physiological significance of this phenomenon has not yet been clarified.

In the loop nephron, the interaction of metabolic acidosis and potassium transport has not been examined; however, the upper portion of long-loop nephron segments is highly cation selective [31] and potassium permeability is very much higher here than that in other nephron segments [32]. A mathematical model of the transport profiles along the descending loop clearly demonstrated that potassium loading from the proximal tubules does not affect potassium transport in the long-loop nephron [33].

Thus, the cortical collecting duct has been identified as a major site of potassium secretion; it is also at this nephron site that hormones exert their typical sodium and potassium effects. The original potassium secretion model in cortical collecting ducts consists of a two-step process. The first step includes active, ATP-dependent sodium extrusion and active potassium uptake across the basolateral membrane, resulting in a high cell potassium concentration and an appropriate potassium gradient. The second step consists of potassium extrusion from cell to lumen, via potassium conductance of apical membrane [34].

Segments responsible for the interaction of acid-base disturbance and potassium transport along the nephron were examined by in vivo micropuncture and microperfusion [21,22] and in vitro microperfusion [23]. Luminal acidification depolarized transepithelial voltage and depressed bath to lumen ^{86}Rb flux, without changing lumen to bath ^{22}Na flux. However, the detailed mechanisms of the relationship between acid-base disturbance and potassium secretion in distal tubules remained unclear. We examined the effect of basolateral acidosis on potassium transport in the rabbit cortical collecting ducts. Our data clearly showed the inhibitory effect of basolateral acidosis on potassium secretion. Basolateral acidosis suppressed potassium secretion and depolarized transepithelial voltage, as seen in the luminal acidosis reported previously [23]. However, sodium flux did not change as a result of the acidification of the bathing medium.

It is well established that two distinct cell types constitute the cortical collecting duct; principal cells and intercalated cells. Several kinds of evidence suggest that principal cells are involved in sodium reabsorption and potassium secretion. As mentioned before, sodium is extruded and potassium is taken up by sodium-potassium ATPase pump in the basolateral membrane of the principal cell, and potassium diffuses and sodium enters across the apical membrane. These transporters of the apical membrane are mediated by amiloride-sensitive sodium channels and barium-sensitive potassium channels [35]. However, recent patch clamp studies clearly demonstrated the existence of at least three types of potassium channels; a so-called Maxi K channel, a small conductance channel, and a calcium-activated K channel [35–38]. The Maxi K channel is identified in the apical membrane of rat cortical collecting duct; this channel has a high conductance, is barium sensitive, and may be involved in potassium secretion; the pH sensitive conductance change is still controversial. The small conductance K channel is located in both apical and basolateral membranes; however, its role in potassium secretion is much different. The apical small conductance K channel is involved in potassium secretion in cortical collecting duct; this channel is pH-sensitive, barium-insensitive, and voltage independent. The calcium-activated K channel exists in basolateral membrane, although the physiological role of this channel is limited to that of cell volume regulation, and it has almost no significant role in the potassium secretory mechanism. That is, in hypotonic shock, membrane stretch activates this calcium-sensitive K channel.

Regarding the inhibitory effect of basolateral acidosis on potassium secretion, we showed that in the presence of luminal barium, the inhibitory effect of basolateral acidosis diminished, but still remained significant. However, the question remains whether 2 mM barium is enough to block luminal potassium channel, since recent microelectrode studies have suggested that more than 5 mM barium is required to completely block the potassium channel [24]. Thus, although it is indirect evidence, intracellular acidosis might inhibit barium-sensitive and, probably, barium-insensitive, pH-dependent K channels in the apical membrane, the so-called small K conductance channels.

However, problems remained in the interpretation of our data. We showed that basolateral acidosis inhibited potassium secretion via barium-sensitive and -insensitive pathways and that basolateral acidosis also deporalized transepithelial voltage. If pH-sensitive potassium channel blockade is the primary event in the inhibitory effect in cortical collecting ducts, the decrement of potassium secretion should result primarily in transepithelial voltage hyperporalization, because basolateral acidosis did not affect either net sodium reabsorption or unidirectional sodium efflux. This means that neither the change of sodium channel activity nor the change of sodium-proton ATPase activity might be involved in the effect of basolateral acidosis. How basolateral acidosis depolarizes transepithelial voltage remained to be resolved. There are two possibilities. One is that basolateral acidosis affects conductances other than sodium or potassium, such as sodium-proton exchanger, potassium-chloride cotransporter, and chloride-bicarbonate exchanger, in depolarizing transepithelial voltage. Another possibility is that basolateral acidosis affected intercalated cells, in which proton secretion might be stimulated in basolateral acidosis, resulting in deporalization of transepithelial voltage, independent of changes in sodium and potassium conductance. Indirect evidence suggested that this latter thesis better explained the facts. The addition of ouabain to the bathing medium induced marked depolarization, from negative transepithelial voltage to markedly positive voltage. This finding suggests that the complete block of principal cell function by ouabain revealed the voltage generation of intercalated cells. That is, the stimulation of proton secretion in the intercalated cells can deporalize transcellular voltage, resulting in the reduction of voltage-dependent potassium secretion. However, our electrophysiological data suggested that principal cells are the cells responsible, at least in part, for the inhibitory effect of basolateral acidosis on potassium secretion. The fact that addition of high dose amiloride from the basolateral side diminished the inhibitory effect of basolateral acidosis also suggested an effect of the sodium-proton exchanger system on the basolateral membrane of either principal cells or intercalated cells.

We summarized the data as follows: 1) Basolateral acidosis inhibited potassium secretion without changing sodium reabsorption in rabbit cortical collecting ducts, 2) basolateral amiloride diminished the effect of basolateral acidosis on potassium secretion, 3) luminal barium diminished the inhibitory effect of basolateral acidosis on potassium secretion, 4) ambient bicarbonate ion was not essential for the inhibitory effect of basolateral acidosis on potassium secretion, and 5) basolateral acidosis depolarized both transepithelial voltage and basolateral membrane voltage by increasing relative luminal resistance.

The present study further confirmed the previous assumption, based on clearance studies and in vivo micropuncture data, that the cortical collecting duct is involved in an reduced renal potassium secretion in acidosis. The mechanism of basolateral acidosis-induced inhibition of potassium secretion appears to involve: the inhibition of luminal barium-sensitive and barium-insensitive potassium channels and the basolateral amiloride-sensitive Na-H exchanger system, but not bicarbonate ion on either side of the epithelium in the principal cells.

References

1. De Fronzo RA, Bia M (1985) Extrarenal potassium homeostasis. In: Seldin DW, Giebisch G (eds) The kidney; physiology and pathophysiology. Raven, New York, pp 1179–1206
2. Simmons DH, Avedon M (1959) Acid base alterations and plasma potassium concentration. Am J Physiol 197:319–326
3. Burnell JM, Villamil MF, Uyeno BT, Scribner BH (1956) Effect in humans of extracellular pH change in relationship betwen serum potassium concentration and intracellular potassium. J Clin Invest 35:935–939
4. Adrogue HJ, Madias NE (1981) Changes in plasma potassium concentration during acute acid-base disturbances. Am J Med 71:456–467
5. Schwartz WB, Brackett N, Cohen JJ (1965) The response of extracellular hydrogen ion concentration to graded degrees of chronic hypercapnia. The physiologic limits of the defense of pH. J Clin Invest 44:291–301
6. Tabei K, Furuya H, Shimanaka K, Shindo Y, Hosoi H, Asano (1986) Changes of erythrocyte K concentration and K removal by hemodialysis. J Japn Soc Dial Ther 19:793–802
7. Sakairi Y, Tabei K, Furuya H, Ando H, Asano Y (1990) Regulation of extrarenal potassium (K) homeostasis in chronically hemodialyzed patients (pts) (abstract). Proceedings of the XIth international congress of nephrology, July 15–20, 1990. Tokyo, Japan
8. Berliner RW, Kennedy TJ, Orloff J (1951) Relationship between acidification of the urine and potassium metabolism. Am J Med 11:274
9. Berliner RW (1952) Renal secretion of potassium and hydrogen ions. Fed Proc 11:695
10. Schwartz WB, Cohen JJ (1978) The nature of the renal response to disorders of acid-base equilibrium. Am J Med 64:417
11. Seldin DW, Rector FC Jr (1972) The generation and maintenance of metabolic alkalosis. Kidney Int 1:306
12. Khuri RN, Windderholt M, Strieder N, Giebisch G (1975) Effects of flow rate and potassium intake on distal tubular potassium transfer. Am J Physiol 228:1249
13. Muto S, Giebisch G, Sanson S (1988) An acute increase of peritubular K stimulates K transport through cell pathways of CCT. Am J Physiol 255:F108–F114
14. Toussaint C, Vereerstraeten P (1962) Effect of blood pH changes on potassium excretion in the dog. Am J Physiol 202:768
15. Biagi B, Kubota T, Sohtell M, Giebsch G (1981) Intracellular potentials in rabbit proximal tubules perfused in vitro. Am J Physiol 240:F200–F210
16. Boron WF, Boulpaep EL (1983) Intracellular pH regulation in the renal proximal tubules of the salamander. J Gen Physiol 81:53–94

17. Kubota T, Biagi BA, Giebisch G (1983) Effects of acid base disturbances on basolateral membrane potential and intracellular potassium activity in the proximal tubule of Necturus. J Membr Biol 73:61–68

18. Steels PS, Boulpaep EL (1987) pH-dependent electrical properties and buffer permeability of the Necturus renal proximal tubule cell. J Membr Biol 100:165–182

19. Burckhardt BC, Fromter E (1987) Evidence for OH^-/H^+ permeation across the peritubular cell membrane of rat renal proximal tubule in HCO_3^--free solution. Pflügers Arch 409:132–137

20. Ohno-Shosaku T, Kubota T, Yamaguchi J, Fujimoto M (1990) Regulation of inwardly rectifying K^+ channels by intracellular pH in opossum kidney cells. Pflügers Arch 416:138–143

21. Malnic G, deMello-Aires M, Giebisch G (1971) Potassium transport across renal tubules during acid-base disturbance. Am J Physiol 211:1192

22. Stanton BA, Giebisch G (1982) Effect of pH on potassium transport by renal distal tubules. Am J Physiol 242:F544

23. Boudry JF, Stoner LC, Burg MB (1976) The effect of luminal pH on potassium transport in renal cortical collecting tubules. Am J Physiol 230:239

24. O'Neil RG, Sansom SC (1984) Characterization of apical cell membrane Na^+ and K^+ conductances of cortical collecting duct using microelectrode techniques. Am J Physiol 247:F14–F24

25. Burg MB, Grantham J, Abramow M, Orloff J (1966) Preparation and study of fragments of rabbit nephron. Am J Physiol 210:1293–1298

26. Ando Y, Tabei K, Furuya H, Asano Y (1989) Glucagon stimulates chloride transport independently of cyclic AMP in the rat medullary TAL. Kidney Int 31:760–767

27. Muto S, Sansom S, Giebisch G (1988) Effects of a high potassium diet on electrical properties of cortical collecting ducts from adrenalectomized rabbits. J Clin Invest 81:376–380

28. Tabei K, Furuya H, Muto S, Asano, Y (1988) Potassium (K) is secreted in rabbit proximal convoluted tubules (PCT) in vitro. Kidney Int 35:489

29. Wasserstein AG, Agus ZS (1983) Potassium secretion in the rabbit proximal straight tubule. Am J Physiol 245:F167–F174

30. Work J, Troutman L, Schafer JA (1982) Transport of potassium in the rabbit pars recta. Am J Physiol 242:F226–F237

31. Tabei K, Imai M (1986) Permselectivity for cations over anions in the upper portion of the descending limb of the long-loop nephron (LDLu) of hamsters. Pflügers Arch 406:279–284

32. Tabei K, Imai M (1987) K transport in upper portion of descending limb of long-loop nephron from hamsters. Am J Physiol 252:F387–F392

33. Taniguchi J, Tabei K, Imai M (1987) Profile of water and solute transport along long-loop descending limb: analysis by a mathematical model. Am J Physiol 252:F393–F402

34. Giebisch G, Malnic G, Berliner RW (1986) Renal transport and control of potassium excretion. In: Brenner BM, Rector FC Jr (eds) The kidney. Saunders, Philadelphia, pp 177–205

35. Giebel J, Zweifach A, White S, Wang W, Giebisch G (1990) K^+ channels of the mammalian collecting duct. Renal Physiol Biochem 13:5969

36. Koeppen B, Biagi BA, Giebisch G (1983) Electrophysiology of mammalian renal tubule: influences from intracellular microelectrode studies, Annu Rev Physiol 45:497–517

37. Wang W, Giebisch G (1989) The regulation of the small conductance K^+ channel in the apical membrane of rat cortical collecting tubule (abstract). Proc Am Soc Nephrol 21:386A

38. Frint G, Palmer IG (1987) Ca-activated K channels in apical membrane of mammalian CCT, and their role in K secretion. Am J Physiol 252:F458–F467

Mechanisms of Transcellular Potassium Shifts in Acid-Base Disorders

HORACIO J. ADROGUÉ[1]

Introduction

A substantial improvement in our understanding of the determinants of internal potassium balance, the regulation of acidity within body fluids, and the relationship between potassium transport and pH levels has been accomplished in the last forty years [1–4]. Yet, a number of fundamental questions on the linkage between acid-base and potassium transport at the cellular level remain unanswered. I will attempt to summarize our view of this puzzling relationship with the understanding that alternative explanations have been or might be offered at this time. Our analysis of the internal K^+ exchanges in acid-base disorders will be performed considering the existence of basic determinants of the K^+-H^+ relationship as well as modulators of this relationship. The wide range of $\Delta [K^+]/\Delta$ pH values in the extracellular fluid observed among the various acid-base disorders [5] may be largely explained by the differential effects of the basic determinants of the K^+-H^+ relationship on each disorder. The modulators of the K^+-H^+ relationship might either ameliorate or exaggerate the translocation of potassium under a variety of pathophysiological conditions.

A. Basic Determinants

All cells contain a cytosolic fluid rich in proteins and phosphate compounds, which are polyvalent macromolecules essential for normal cell function. These macromolecules have, at normal cell pH, a net negative charge that accounts for more than two thirds of the anionic equivalency of the intracellular fluid. Furthermore, these cell-restricted anions are responsible for the peculiar distribution of the diffusable anions and cations on both sides of the cell membrane, as dictated by the physical

---

[1]Chief, Renal Section (151-B), Veterans Affairs Medical Center, 2002 Holcombe Blvd., Houston, TX 77030, USA

chemical principles of equilibrium in aqueous solutions, theoretically conceived by Gibbs and experimentally verified by Donnan. In most cells potassium and chloride are the dominant conductive species across the cell membrane and, in accordance with Gibbs-Donnan postulates, these permeant ions must be in electrochemical equilibrium. The negative charge of the cell-restricted anions is predominantly carried by the amino-acid residues of proteins, by ATP, and by other organic phosphate compounds. This charge is balanced by the positive charge of potassium, the exclusively permeant cation. Although sodium is not strictly impermeant, its rapid extrusion upon entering the cell makes this cation effectively impermeant. As a consequence a K^+-rich cytosolic fluid is created; the cell-restricted anions produce a much higher concentration of this diffusable cation within the cell compared to the extracellular fluid. In addition, the cell-restricted anions force an unequal distribution of chloride, the permeant anion, which largely accumulates in the extracellular fluid. Obviously, another cation must balance the negative charge of chloride outside the cells; the cation that fills this function is sodium.

The cellular accumulation of K^+ and exclusion of Cl^- generates an electrical potential across the membrane where the cytosol is negative with respect to the extracellular fluid. The polarized cell membrane, which repels anions and attracts cations, develops an electrical potential difference that satisfies the electrochemical equilibrium of the permeant ions potassium and chloride. The experimental verification of these assumptions required the measurement of ion permeabilities, intracellular voltage, and the chemical composition of the cytosolic fluid. Since several ions are permeant under steady-state conditions in most cells (i.e., K^+, Cl^- and to some extent Na^+) the membrane potential may be estimated by the Goldman-Hodgkin-Katz (GHK) constant field equation, that is a modification of the Nernst equation:

$$E_m = \frac{RT}{F} \ln \frac{P_K[K]_e + P_{Na}[Na]_e + P_{Cl}[Cl]_i}{P_K[K]_i + P_{Na}[Na]_i + P_{Cl}[Cl]_e}$$

which takes into account the main permeant (P = permeability) ions at rest which are Na^+, K^+ and Cl^-. Most cells have resting cell membrane potentials of -60 mV to -90 mV and these values are close to E_K (equilibrium potential for potassium) since their highest permeability at rest is to potassium ions. The cell membrane also has a relatively high resting permeability to Cl^- and low permeability to Na^+ which accounts for the proximity of the resting cell membrane potential to the equilibrium potential for potassium and chloride ions, but not to sodium. An examination of the Nernst potentials at $37\,°C$, calculated according to the extracellular and intracellular concentrations of the different ions in mammalian cells, depicted below, helps to better recognize these phenomena.

Nernst Equilibrium
Potential (mV)   Concentration (mmol/l)

Na^+	$+71$	(i = 10; e = 142)
Ca^{2+}	$+150$	(i = <0.0001; e = 2.5)
K^+	-98	(i = 155; e = 4)
Cl^-	-29 to -90	(i = 5-30; e = 101)

The application of the Gibbs-Donnan rules to the cellular membrane satisfactorily explains a large fraction of the available data on the peculiar distribution of electro-

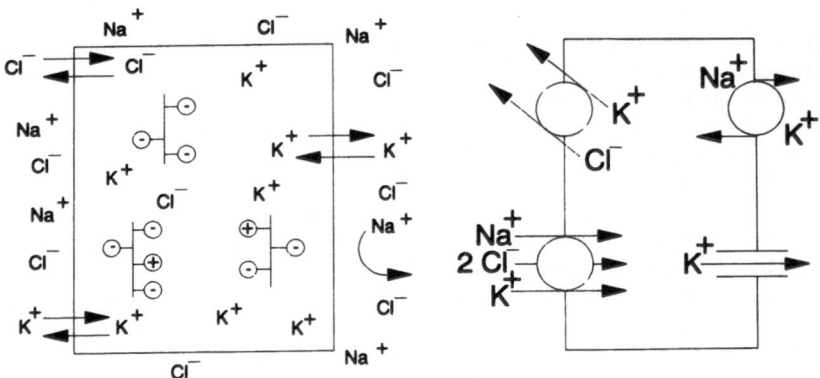

Fig. 1. The Gibbs-Donnan theory (*left panel*) and Pump/Leak hypothesis (*right panel*) properly account for the distribution of major electrolytes across the cell membrane (Modified from [6])

lytes in the cytosolic and extracellular fluids [6]. We believe that additional information, collectively described as the Pump/Leak hypothesis, completes the Gibbs-Donnan rules, resulting in a coherent overall account of the distribution of electrolytes in cells and extracellular fluid (Fig. 1). The exclusion of Na^+ from cells, for example, is not simply the result of a nonpermeant condition of this ion but is best explained by active pumping of sodium from cells by the Na^+, K^+ ATPase. Since this pump moves 3 Na^+ out in association with 2 K^+ into the cell, it generates an electrical potential. The Na^+-K^+ pump maintains the steady-state intracellular levels of high potassium and low sodium by creating a flux of ions that counterbalance the passive cellular loss of potassium and the influx of sodium. The action of the pump also accounts for the presence in some cells of K^+ levels that are above its electrochemical equilibrium.

The combination of ionic gradients of K^+, Cl^-, and Na^+ across the cell membrane, the permeability of the membrane to these ions, and the contribution from electrogenic pumping (i.e., Na^+-K^+ pump) determine the resting membrane potential. In most cells the resting membrane potential is largely generated by the potassium diffusion potential.

Effect of Cell pH on the Interaction Between Intracellular Proteins and Potassium

Intracellular proteins interact with potassium almost exclusively by electrostatic binding, that is in a salt-type manner, and the approximately 55 mEq/l of anionic proteins within skeletal muscle are balanced by equal amounts of potassium ions. Since proteins in an electrolyte solution contribute to both the anionic and the cationic properties of the solution, the 55 mEq/l of anionic proteins referred to above, are also known as the *net cationic equivalency* or *net negative charge* of the proteins. It has been estimated that the minimum acid/base buffer value of cell proteins in muscle is about 15 mmol/l per unit pH change (slyke), and this value agrees with data obtained in vivo in muscle from intact animals [7]. The ion-binding sites of proteins appear to

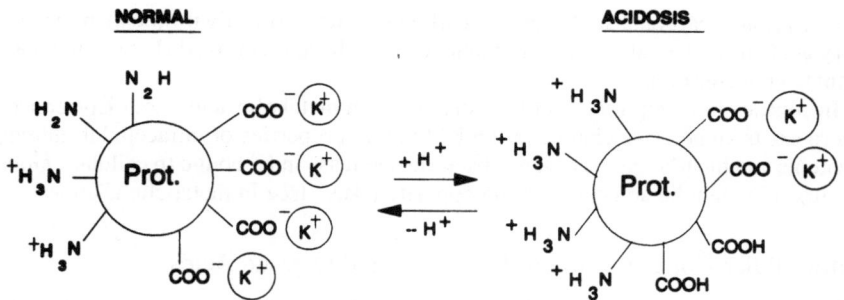

Fig. 2. Schematic representation of the decreased potassium-binding capacity of intracellular proteins in acidosis (Modified from [1])

have preference for H^+ ions so that other cations can compete only if their concentration is considerably higher than that of the H^+-ions [8]. This requisite is amply satisfied in the cytosolic fluid by K^+-ions because their concentration is six orders of magnitude higher than that of H^+-ions ($[K^+] = 10^{-1}M$; $[H^+] = 10^{-7}M$). Thus, as cell pH falls, the electrostatic binding of K^+-ions to cytosolic proteins decreases and H^+ ions displace K^+ ions from the proteins (Fig. 2); the opposite process occurs when pH increases. The magnitude of the change in K^+-binding capability is similar to the change in the net cation equivalency of intracellular proteins, which is a function of the deviation in cell pH multiplied by the buffer value of the proteins. The nature of the phenomenon that takes place in the cytosolic fluid is similar to the pH-related effect on plasma proteins, which partially accounts for the alteration in the plasma anion gap in the course of acid-base disturbances [9].

The diminished binding of K^+ by proteins within the cell in acidosis will alter the electrochemical equilibrium for this ion, favoring the cellular exit of potassium. By contrast, an increased intracellular pH will have the opposite effect which will favor the uptake of potassium by cells.

Intracellular Concentration of Bicarbonate

The intracellular level of bicarbonate of about 12 mEq/l in skeletal muscle balances an equal concentration of cations, most of which are potassium ions. Thus, increases and decreases in cytosolic bicarbonate concentration should be accompanied by parallel alterations in the levels of potassium bound to this anion within the cell. Respiratory acidosis and metabolic alkalosis are characterized by elevated levels of intracellular bicarbonate and consequently they have increased levels of anionic sites for K^+-binding. The opposite occurs in respiratory alkalosis and metabolic acidosis. The magnitude of the alteration in the concentration of bicarbonate is dependent on the severity of the acid-base disorder.

Increases and decreases of about 4 mEq/l in the cellular bicarbonate concentration have been described in skeletal muscle in moderately severe respiratory acidosis and respiratory alkalosis, respectively [10]. Yet, the changes in K^+-binding by cytosolic bicarbonate in each respiratory acid-base disorder occur in association with an opposite change in the K^+-binding properties of intracellular proteins. In fact, the titration of carbonic acid by non-bicarbonate buffers (mostly proteins) in respiratory acidosis and alkalosis fully accounts for the above mentioned changes in bicarbonate concentration.

In contrast to respiratory acid-base disorders, in metabolic acid-base disturbances there exists an additive change in the K^+-binding properties of intracellular anions, proteins and bicarbonate. Thus, a substantial decrease in K^+ bound to cellular anions occurs in metabolic acidosis and the opposite takes place in metabolic alkalosis.

Intracellular Concentration of Phosphate and Organic Acids

The concentration of organic and inorganic phosphate in skeletal muscle is high, with levels between 40 and 70 millimols per liter. The pK′ of all these phosphate compounds is about 6.5 and the resulting aggregate buffer value amounts to approximately 18 slykes [7]. By contrast, creatine phosphate has a very low pK′ of about 4.5, so that its buffer value is negligible.

The substantial acid/base buffer value of cell phosphates should result in a significant decrement in potassium-binding capability in acidosis and the opposite effect in alkalosis. However, changes in the levels of organic and inorganic phosphates in the cytosol, due to alterations in energy requirements, metabolic pathways, or other processes may substantially alter the predicted change in K^+-binding by phosphate moieties in acidosis and alkalosis.

Organic acid acidosis results in abnormally high cellular levels of protons and organic anions. Proton accumulation will displace potassium ions that were electrostatically bound to proteins, phosphate, and bicarbonate. Yet the organic anion may act as a sink for the displaced potassium ions, counterbalancing the effects of the protons released by the organic acid. The effect of changes in cell pH on organic acid production and disposal further complicates the basic interaction just mentioned.

In contrast to organic acid-acidosis, the cellular retention of protons, due to an impairment in renal acid excretion or to infusion of mineral acids, will not only diminish the K^+ binding by proteins, phosphate, and bicarbonate but also fails to offer a cellular anion to help with the disposal of the displaced potassium ions.

B. Modulators of the K^+-H^+ Relationship

The effect of changes in the cytosolic levels of hydrogen ions and sodium, and the role of insulin will be summarized below, since these are the dominant modulators of the K^+-H^+ relationship. Other influences of less importance [11], that include the effects of catecholamines, mineralocorticoids, and osmolality, will not be reviewed due to space limitation. A brief overview of the transport pathways of H^+ and K^+ will precede our evaluation of the interplay of these ions at the cell membrane.

A lipid bilayer that prevents the translocation of most ions is a basic component of the cell membrane. Yet, the exchange of potassium and other ions between cells and the interstitial fluid is allowed to occur through proteins that span the lipid bilayer of the cell membrane. Four distinct pathways are involved in the traffic of potassium.

Potassium may exit the cytosol satisfying the electrochemical gradient, either through K^+-channels or by a K^+/Cl^- cotransport, given that chloride is also accumulated above its electrochemical equilibrium in at least some cells.

The most important and best studied potassium influx mechanism occurs via the Na$^+$-K$^+$ pump, also known as Na$^+$-K$^+$ ATPase. This pump, which is present in all animal cells, is an ATP-dependent enzyme that catalyzes the movement of both Na$^+$ and K$^+$ in opposite directions. ATP hydrolysis acts as the energy source. A second K$^+$-influx pathway has been described in several cell types and involves the obligatory cotransport of one K$^+$, one Na$^+$ and two Cl$^-$ ions across the cell membrane. This pathway is electroneutral and from an energetic point of view is a secondary active transport process. The uphill movement of K$^+$ and Cl$^-$ into the cell is driven by the downhill movement of Na$^+$ toward the cells. The sodium gradient is in turn established by the Na$^+$-K$^+$ pump, which is the primary active transport mechanism.

The development of accurate measurements of intracellular pH and voltage has demonstrated that H$^+$ activity inside cells is lower than would be predicted if protons were simply distributed to satisfy electrochemical equilibrium. Thus, the cells are faced with a passive influx of protons which must be counterbalanced by active pumping of H$^+$ toward the extracellular fluid. An exception to this rule occurs in red cells and possibly hepatocytes, where H$^+$ efflux is passive. Since cell metabolism is also a significant source of intracellular acidification, cells have developed effective acid-extruding mechanisms. The Na$^+$/H$^+$ exchange system is the most important mechanism that protects cells against intracellular acidosis by the countertransport of external Na$^+$ for internal H$^+$. This system extrudes H$^+$ from the cells because the net thermodynamic driving force on the Na$^+$-H$^+$ exchangers in the plasma membrane favors this process. The higher ratio of [Na$^+$]e/[Na$^+$]$_i$ in comparison with the [H$^+$]e/[H$^+$]$_i$ accounts for the direction of the ion fluxes mentioned above. This countertransport process is not directly dependent upon ATP hydrolysis, but the energy for the uphill extrusion of H$^+$ derives from the downhill inwardly directed Na$^+$ gradient. The primary active extrusion of Na$^+$ mediated by the Na$^+$-K$^+$ ATPase is responsible for the sodium gradient between interstitial and cytosolic fluid.

The Na$^+$/H$^+$ countertransport mechanism appears to play an important role in the control of cell pH, protecting cells against intracellular acidosis. A second system involved in cell pH regulation is an electroneutral Cl$^-$/HCO$_3$-exchanger that, under physiological conditions, protects cells against intracellular alkalosis. The latter mechanism exchanges external Cl$^-$ for internal HCO$_3$. The pH-dependence of the two systems is quite different. The Na$^+$/H$^+$ exchanger predominates at acidic cell pH values and the defense of cell acidosis takes place at the expense of the transmembrane sodium gradient. By contrast, at alkaline cell pH levels the Cl$^-$/HCO$_3$ exchanger is activated, extruding cytosolic bicarbonate, which is driven by the transmembrane chloride gradient in the opposite direction.

Changes in cell and extracellular acidity alter the acid-loading and/or the acid-extruding mechanisms previously described, which in turn regulate the absolute values of pH in all the body compartments. In addition, the interdependence of intracellular and extracellular pH results from passive fluxes of H$^+$, HCO$_3$ and other weak acids and bases.

Intracellular Ion Levels

Changes in intracellular pH may alter K$^+$ transport across the cell membrane, acting on the Na$^+$-K$^+$ pump and on the conductance of K$^+$ channels [4,6]. Cell acidosis has been shown to depress both the activity of the pump and K$^+$-conductance through the cell membrane in some cell-types. Conversely, an alkaline cell pH stimulates the Na^+/K^+ pump and activates K^+ channels. The magnitude of this effect as well as the significance in overall extrarenal K^+ homeostasis is yet undefined.

The cytosolic concentration of sodium may also modulate the activity of the Na^+-K^+ pump as well as the activity of some K^+ channels. The effects of $[Na^+]_i$ on the pump have been previously discussed. The physiologic importance of the effects of intracellular sodium levels on the conductance of cell membrane K^+ channels remains unknown.

Insulin

Insulin is a major modulator of extrarenal potassium homeostasis and promotes potassium uptake in many cell types, including those from skeletal muscle and liver. The hypokalemic action occurs at very low concentrations of insulin and is independent from the effect of insulin on glucose uptake. The precise mechanism of action remains to be defined but appears to involve the activation of several transport proteins. Stimulation of Na^+-H^+ countertransport, resulting in cytosolic alkalinization, has been demonstrated in response to insulin in the skeletal muscle. The rise of cell pH caused by insulin is inhibited by lowering the extracellular Na^+ level and by amiloride. The insulin-induced cell alkalosis increases the K^+-binding capacity of intracellular anions and also stimulates the Na^+-K^+ pump, therefore favoring cellular K^+-loading. The increased cellular Na^+ concentration secondary to enhanced Na^+ entry via Na^+-H^+ exchange is also a stimulus for the action of the Na^+-K^+ pump to enhance potassium influx. This is the case because the Na^+ concentration for half-maximal activity of this pump is between 10 and 50 mM and the cellular concentration of sodium in most cells is 10–20 mM.

A direct stimulatory effect of insulin on the Na^+, K^+-ATPase in skeletal muscle and adipose tissue has been described. This stimulatory action is blocked by ouabain, a specific inhibitor of the pump. The mechanisms involved are an increase in the turnover rate of the pump or an unmasking of latent pump sites. In contrast with the action of thyroid hormones and adrenal steroids on the Na^+-K^+ pump, insulin does not appear to promote the synthesis of new pump units. The extent to which the activation by insulin of other transport mechanisms, including the Na^+-H^+ exchange, is important in the K^+ uptake by the pump remains undefined.

The hypokalemic action of insulin might also involve a direct effect on potassium channels [12]. One type of K^+ channel of significant relevance in the skeletal muscle is the inward rectifier channel, which accounts for most of the K^+ conductance in the resting state. This channel allows potassium to flow into cells much more easily than to exit cells. Thus, when the cell membrane is hyperpolarized the high inward conductance facilitates K^+ entry to cells. When the cell membrane is depolarized the low outward conductance reduces potassium exit from cells. The effect of insulin on the conductance of the inward rectifying potassium channels of skeletal muscle has been examined in potassium-depleted rats. Under these conditions a large K^+ conductance, defined by the presence of a steep slope in the current-voltage relationship, was found when the membrane was hyperpolarized. Insulin had no effects on this K^+ conductance. Preservation of the high conductance coupled to the hyperpolarization of the cell membrane due to stimulation of the Na^+-K^+ pump by insulin, would enhance cell potassium stores. By contrast to the lack of effect of insulin on K^+ conductance when

Table 1. Insulin-mediated cellular K^+ loading mechanisms

Primary action	Immediate result	Secondary effect
Stimulation of Na^+-H^+ exchanger	Cytosolic alkalinization	Increased K^+ binding capacity Stimulation of Na^+-K^+ ATPase
	Increased cell $[Na^+]$	Stimulation of Na^+-K^+ ATPase
Stimulation of Na^+-K^+ ATPase	Hyperpolarization of cell membrane	New electrical gradient favors K^+ entry Deactivation of K^+ channels turned on by depolarization prevents K^+ exit
K^+ Channels (inward rectifier)	Depressed K^+ conductance when membrane is depolarized	Exaggeration of the inward rectifying properties

the cell was hyperpolarized, a major depression of K^+ conductance occurred when the cell membrane was depolarized. This latter effect of insulin is in fact an exaggeration of the inward rectifying properties of this class of potassium channels. Thus insulin action on the inward rectifier K^+ channels may facilitate the accumulation of potassium by a dual effect of stimulation of K^+ entry and depression of K^+ exit.

Insulin produces hyperpolarization of the cell membrane in a number of tissues, including the skeletal muscle. The hyperpolarization might result from stimulation of the sodium-potassium pump or, less likely, might be the result of an increased K^+ conductance. Since the effect on membrane potential precedes cellular potassium accumulation, a primary effect on the pump is presumed. Yet the specific inhibitor of the Na^+-K^+ pump, ouabain, does not consistently block this insulin action.

The effect of insulin on the cell membrane potential might be of great relevance to the hypokalemic effect by a different mechanism that involves the modulation of K^+ currents in voltage-gated K^+ channels. Many potassium channels are activated by depolarization of the membrane (i.e., Ca^{2+}-activated K^+ channels, classic Hodgkin-Huxley/delayed rectifier K^+ channels) which increases the fraction of time that the channel is in the open state. In this circumstance K^+ is lost from the cell into the extracellular fluid. An example of this situation occurs in uremia, in which the depressed skeletal muscle potential may facilitate the cellular exit of potassium. The administration of insulin will hyperpolarize the cell membrane, which will in turn deactivate K^+ channels preventing the exit of cellular potassium. In some cells, such as those in the renal proximal tubule, gating of K^+ channels has the opposite voltage dependence so that when the membrane is hyperpolarized more channels are open. Thus, insulin action will enhance the potassium stores in these and other cells which have channels activated at hyperpolarized potentials.

Insulin action on glucose metabolism is pH-dependent and known to be impaired in acidosis [13]. Whether changes in pH have a similar effect on the kalemic effect of insulin remains unknown. It should be also recognized that increased insulin levels in the course of an acid-base disorder, as in the case of exogenous ketoacidosis, might substantially alter the K^+-H^+ relationship [14,15]. Table 1 summarizes the various insulin-mediated potassium loading mechanisms.

In summary, we envision the existence of basic determinants, as well as modulators, of the K^+-H^+ relationship. The action of the basic determinants is the result of changes in the anionic binding sites for K^+ in the cytosol, which in turn alter the electrochemical equilibrium for this ion, favoring either the cellular exit or the uptake of potassium. Intracellular proteins and phosphate interact with K^+ by electrostatic binding and their net anionic change is balanced with K^+ ions. As cell pH falls, H^+ ions displace K^+ ions from these compounds, while the opposite process occurs when cell pH increases. The intracellular level of bicarbonate also balances an equal concentration of cations, most of which are potassium ions. Thus, elevated levels of intracellular bicarbonate (respiratory acidosis and metabolic alkalosis) should be accompanied by parallel alterations in the levels of potassium bound to this anion within the cell. The opposite occurs in respiratory alkalosis and metabolic acidosis. Consequently, the changes in K^+ binding by cytosolic bicarbonate in each respiratory acid-base disorder occur in association with an opposite change in the K^+-binding properties of intracellular proteins. In contrast to the respiratory type, in metabolic acid-base disturbances there exists an additive change in the K^+-binding properties of intracellular anions, proteins and bicarbonate. The net result is the development of a substantial decrease in K^+ bound to cellular anions in metabolic acidosis; the opposite occurs in metabolic alkalosis. Organic acid acidosis is a special situation which results in abnormally high cellular levels of protons and anions of organic acids; the latter act as a sink for the displaced K^+, counterbalancing the effects of cell acidosis on the K^+-H^+ relationship. The most significant modulators of the K^+-H^+ relationship include the effects of cell pH and cytosolic $[Na^+]$ on K^+ pathways and the action of insulin on the transport of H^+ and K^+ across the cell membrane. The importance of the modulators is modest in comparison to that of the basic determinants with respect to the $\Delta [K^+] \Delta$ pH in the various acid-base disorders.

Acknowledgments. I am indebted to Debby S. Verrett for skillful assistance in preparing the manuscript. This study was supported in part by the Medical Research Service of the Veterans Affairs Medical Center in Houston and by the American Heart Association, Texas Affiliate.

References

1. Davenport HW (1974) The ABC of acid-base chemistry. The University of Chicago Press, Chicago, pp 3–53
2. Pitts RF (1976) Volume and composition of the body fluids. In: Pitts RF (ed) Physiology of the Kidney and Body Fluids. Year Book Medical Publishers, Chicago, pp 11–35
3. Boron WF (1989) Cellular buffering and intracellular pH. In: Seldin DW, Giebisch G (eds) The regulation of acid-base balance. Raven, New York, pp 33–56
4. Williams ME, Epstein FH (1989) Internal exchanges of potassium. In: Seldin DW, Giebisch G (eds) The regulation of potassium balance. Raven, New York, pp 3–29
5. Adrogué HJ, Madias NE (1981) Changes in plasma potassium concentration during acute acid-base disturbances. Am J Med 71:456–467
6. Palmer LG (1989) The regulation of intracellular potassium. In: Seldin DW, Giebisch G (eds) The regulation of potassium balance. Raven, New York, pp 89–119
7. Woodbury JW (1974) Regulation of pH. In: Ruch TC, Patton HD (eds) Physiology and Biophysics. WB Saunders, Philadelphia, pp 901–933

8. Van Leeuwen AM (1964) Net cation equivalency ("base binding power") of the plasma proteins. Acta Med Scand [Suppl] 422:1–212
9. Adrogué HJ, Brensilver J, Madias NE (1978) Changes in the plasma anion gap during chronic metabolic acid-base disturbances. Am J Physiol 235:F291–F297
10. Brown EB Jr (1965) Blood and tissue buffers. Arch Intern Med 116:665–669
11. Susuki H, Hishida A, Ohishi K, Kimura M, Honda N (1990) Role of hormonal factors in plasma K alterations in acute respiratory and metabolic alkalosis in dogs. Am J Physiol 258:F305–F310
12. Ruff RL (1989) Periodic paralysis. In: Seldin DW, Giebisch G (eds) The regulation of potassium balance. Raven, New York, pp 303–323
13. Adrogué HJ, Chap Z, Okuda Y, Michael L, Hartley C, Entman M, Field JB (1988) Acidosis-induced glucose intolerance is not prevented by adrenergic blockade. Am J Physiol 255:E812–E823
14. Adrogué HJ, Chap Z, Ishida T, Field JB (1985) Role of the endocrine pancreas in the kalemic response to acute metabolic acidosis in conscious dogs. J Clin Invest 75:798–808
15. Adrogué HJ, Lederer ED, Suki WN, Eknoyan G (1986) Determinants of plasma potassium levels in diabetic ketoacidosis. Medicine Baltimore 65:163–172

Hypokalemia in Metabolic Alkalosis: A New Look at an Old Controversy

F. John Gennari[1]

SUMMARY. Metabolic alkalosis can be induced in humans either by potassium, or by chloride depletion, but the selective removal of one of these ions is almost invariably associated with losses of the other. As a result, a controversy persists concerning which of these ions is critical for the development of this common acid-base disorder. In the last decade, epithelial membrane ion transporters, identified in the loop and distal nephron, have provided new insights into the close linkage between K^+ and Cl^- transport in this part of the nephron. These transporters can also explain how each of these ions influences H^+ and HCO_3^- transport. Results from membrane transport studies provide the basis for explaining the effect of K^+ depletion on stimulating NH_4^+ excretion, impeding Cl^- reabsorption, and on stimulating H^+ secretion. The membrane transport studies also show how Cl^- depletion promotes K^+ excretion and inhibits HCO_3^- excretion. Review of human and animal studies reveals a coherent story, which indicates that both K^+ and Cl^- depletion contribute to the pathogenesis and maintenance of metabolic alkalosis.

Introduction

Metabolic alkalosis is invariably associated with potassium depletion and hypokalemia. However, the role of potassium depletion, per se, in the pathogenesis and maintenance of this acid-base disturbance has been a matter of controversy for over 30 years. The extreme positions in this controversy are: 1) potassium depletion is an essential feature, causing the changes in renal bicarbonate reabsorption and acid excretion responsible for maintaining metabolic alkalosis, and 2) potassium depletion is simply an epiphenomenon, playing no role whatever in maintaining the disorder in the most common forms of metabolic alkalosis. The latter position maintains that chloride depletion, rather than K^+ depletion, is the responsible factor for induc-

---

[1]University of Vermont, Burlington, VT 05405, USA

ing and maintaining the most common form of sustained metabolic alkalosis. The controversy has persisted, because in whole animal studies, it is difficult to separate K^+ depletion from Cl^- depletion. Despite this experimental problem, it is now clear that both Cl^- and K^+ depletion can play contributory roles in maintaining metabolic alkalosis, and that their respective roles vary depending on the pathogenetic mechanism involved. Most exciting has been the identification of apical membrane transport proteins which specifically link K^+, Cl^-, HCO_3^-, H^+ and NH_4^+ transport in the loop of Henle and distal nephron. From our new knowledge of these membrane transporters, a logical story is emerging which can explain the pathogenesis and maintenance of metabolic alkalosis. This story illustrates the interdependence of K^+ and Cl^- transport in the renal response to metabolic alkalosis.

Discussion

Metabolic alkalosis can be induced in a variety of ways (Table 1). To undertake a discussion of the role of K^+ and Cl^- in the pathogenesis of this disorder, one first needs to define what type or types of metabolic alkalosis one is discussing. Although metabolic alkalosis can be induced by acute bicarbonate loading, this model has little relevance to the clinical disorder. From a clinical perspective, two types of metabolic alkalosis are of interest. The first type is initiated primarily by selective loss of chloride from either the gastrointestinal tract (vomiting, nasogastric drainage) or kidney (after administration of certain diuretics). This type accounts for over 90% of the metabolic alkalosis seen in clinical settings and is termed "chloride-responsive." The second type is initiated by a primary increase in distal nephron hydrogen ion secretion, in most cases induced by increased mineralocorticoid activity (due either to endogenous secretion or exogenous administration). This type is termed "chloride-resistant."

The first issue to be addressed is whether the maintenance of the alkalosis in these two subtypes is due to different factors. In both types, K^+ depletion and hypokalemia occur. In both types, in addition, chloride loss occurs, although the loss may be

Table 1. Experimental models of metabolic alkalosis

1. Acute alkali administration
2. Chloride depletion
    - gastric drainage
    - peritoneal dialysis with $NaHCO_3$
    - hemofiltration and replacement with $NaHCO_3$
    - Furosemide
    - Furosemide + $NaHCO_3$
    - recovery from respiratory acidosis
3. Potassium depletion
    - low K^+ diet
    - low K^+ diet + $NaHCO_3$
    - low K^+ diet + DOCA
    - Aldosterone administration
    - DOCA + $NaHCO_3$

DOCA, desoxycorticosterone acetate

minimal in some models of chloride-resistant alkalosis. In clinical medicine, management of the two types of metabolic alkalosis differs, and thus it is useful to subdivide them. From a pathophysiologic perspective, however, it is less clear that a major difference exists. This point is illustrated below in reviewing the experimental studies directed at gaining insight into the pathophysiology of this disorder.

Role of Potassium Depletion

The best experiment to determine whether K^+ depletion plays a specific role in the production and maintenance of metabolic alkalosis is to induce negative K^+ balance by means of dietary K^+ restriction. This type of experiment has been carried out in rats [1–8], dogs [2,9,10], and humans [11,12]. Although at first glance, the results appear to differ in all three species, on further analysis it appears that the rat and human are quite similar in their response to this maneuver.

In the rat, dietary K^+ restriction for 3 weeks or longer leads to marked and sustained metabolic alkalosis ($HCO_3^- > 35mEq/l$) [2,3]. Shorter term K^+ restriction, which presumably produces less severe K^+ depletion, fails to produce alkalosis [4,5]. The increase in bicarbonate concentration that occurs with K^+ depletion in the rat is modulated by the concurrent Cl^- intake [2,6]. In rats given NaCl in their drinking water, the increase in bicarbonate concentration is less than one-third as great as that in animals drinking tap water [2]. In addition, renal Cl^- wasting and Cl^- depletion occur in severely K^+ depleted rats, in association with metabolic alkalosis [7,8]. These same features are found in human K^+ depletion. In humans fed a normal salt intake (1.8mEq/kg body weight), dietary K^+ restriction produces a small but significant increase in serum bicarbonate concentration (2mEq/l) [11]. When chloride as well as K^+ is restricted, the accompanying K^+ depletion induces an increment in bicarbonate concentration that is nearly four times as great as that in the K^+ only restricted cases [12]. Although the increase in bicarbonate in humans is smaller in magnitude than that in the rat, it should be noted that the K^+ depletion is much less severe in these human studies than in the rat. In severely K^+ depleted humans, the alkalosis is quite severe, and in addition, renal Cl^- wasting has been documented to occur, just as it does in the rat [13].

The response in the dog to dietary K^+ restriction is strikingly different. In this species, K^+ depletion produces a mild metabolic acidosis rather than metabolic alkalosis [2,9,10]. Thus, K^+ depletion stimulates renal H^+ secretion in the human and rat kidney, but inhibits it in the dog. The reason for this striking species difference is unclear, but suggests that the dog may not be a useful model for studying this type of metabolic alkalosis. In contrast to its response to dietary K^+ depletion, the dog responds in the same fashion as do humans and rats to mineralocorticoid administration. In all 3 species, mineralocorticoids induce metabolic alkalosis, if sufficient sodium is present in the diet [1,7,14–19]. The effect is enhanced, moreover, if mineralocorticoids are given together with sodium bicarbonate [1,15,18]. In addition, prior K^+ depletion, or concomitant K^+ restriction, worsens the resultant alkalosis [1,16]. In humans, there is no direct experimental evidence for this last observation, but a clear correlation exists between the severity of the hypokalemia and the steady-state bicarbonate concentration in primary hyperaldosteronism [19].

Although the response in humans and animals to mineralocorticoid administration clearly indicates that K^+ depletion is a contributory factor in the development and maintenance of metabolic alkalosis, it should be pointed out that mineralocorticoids also produce chloride depletion by increasing renal chloride excretion [15]. Moreover, to the extent that chloride losses exceed dietary intake, chloride administration is required for full correlation of the alkalosis [15]. To summarize, K^+ depletion produces alkalosis in humans and rats, but not in dogs. In all species tested, chloride is a modulating factor and is necessary for full repair of the acid-base disorder when chloride depletion is also present.

Role of Chloride Depletion

Experiments designed to isolate a specific role for chloride depletion in the generation and maintenance of metabolic alkalosis have been carried out in rats [20,21], dogs [15,22], and humans [23] as well. In all 3 species, chloride depletion produces metabolic alkalosis. Unfortunately, it is virtually impossible to avoid producing simultaneous K^+ depletion in experimental Cl^- depletion alkalosis. To get around this problem, Kassirer and Schwartz tested whether the alkalosis induced by chloride depletion could be fully corrected by Cl^- administration without repair of the accompanying K^+ deficit [23]. They induced metabolic alkalosis by gastric drainage in subjects on a low electrolyte diet. After stable metabolic alkalosis was present (and K^+ stores were depleted by some 300mEq), they administered 120mEq/day of NaCl and demonstrated full correction of the alkalosis with no change in body K^+ stores [23]. This experiment has often been cited as evidence that K^+ depletion is not a contributory factor in maintaining chloride-depletion metabolic alkalosis in man. However, correction of metabolic alkalosis in these K^+ depleted subjects did not occur until 400–500 mEq of chloride was retained above and beyond the chloride originally lost during induction of the alkalosis [23]. An alternative explanation of Kassirer and Schwartz's experiment is that chloride retention and extracellular fluid (ECF) volume expansion markedly increased distal Cl^- delivery, overcoming the effect of K^+ depletion on distal nephron acid and bicarbonate transport (see later for proposed mechanism) [12].

Galla and co-workers produced chloride depletion alkalosis in the rat by a single peritoneal dialysis against 150mM $NaHCO_3$ [20]. This maneuver results in selective chloride loss and alkalosis which is sustained by dietary chloride restriction. In this model, as in other forms of chloride-depletion alkalosis, significant K^+ depletion develops over time [20,21]. These investigators showed that chloride-depletion alkalosis in the rat could be corrected by chloride administration, without repleting K^+ losses, or indeed, without even administering Na^+ (using choline chloride) [20,21]. This experiment provides evidence for a specific role for chloride in the maintenance of this type of metabolic alkalosis. Even in this experiment, however, some K^+ retention occurred during the correction phase. Thus, a contributing role for potassium cannot be excluded.

The most striking experiment constructed to try and separate K^+ depletion from metabolic alkalosis was carried out in the dog by Bleich and co-workers [22]. They induced metabolic alkalosis by gastric drainage in animals fed a low electrolyte diet, and then completely corrected the alkalosis by HCl administration. After a new steady-state was achieved, they administered either potassium sulfate or potassium phosphate to these K^+ depleted, sodium-avid animals. This maneuver produced a dramatic increase in serum bicarbonate concentration (metabolic alkalosis) while at

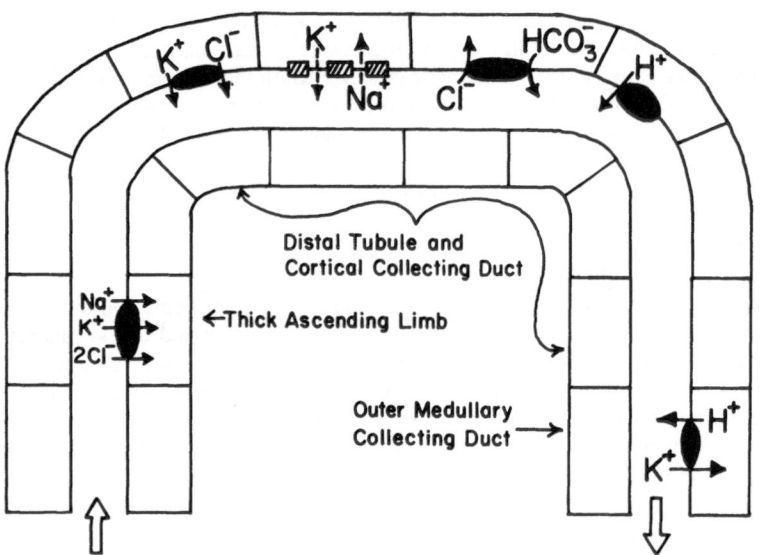

Fig. 1. Membrane ion transporters and channels linking potassium and chloride with hydrogen and bicarbonate secretion in the loop of Henle and the distal nephron

the same time completely replacing the K^+ lost as a result of the original gastric alkalosis. Bleich and co-workers concluded that as K^+ was retained, sodium was released from cells and delivered to the distal nephron with phosphate or sulfate rather than with chloride. Delivery of sodium without chloride to this site in the nephron in these sodium-avid animals stimulated hydrogen ion secretion, inducing metabolic alkalosis again. Although these ingenious experimental manipulations would seem to exclude a causal role for K^+ depletion in metabolic alkalosis, one must be cautious in extrapolating these findings to metabolic alkalosis in man. Firstly, as noted earlier, K^+ depletion in dogs does not produce metabolic alkalosis as it does in man. Secondly, it is possible that HCl administration conditioned the nephron to respond to sodium delivery by secreting hydrogen ions. These chloride-depletion studies in dogs, rats, and humans demonstrate a key role for chloride in the pathogenesis and maintenance of metabolic alkalosis, but they do not exclude a contributory role for K^+ depletion.

Linkage Between K^+, Cl^-, and H^+ Transport

The difficulty of separating the roles of K^+ and Cl^- in producing and maintaining metabolic alkalosis may well be due to the linked transport pathways of these two ions along the nephron. Potassium and chloride reabsorption and secretion are not only linked with one another by specific transporters, but also are linked with H^+, HCO_3^- and NH_4^+ transport in the loop and distal nephron [24–28]. Figure 1 illustrates the apical transporters where such interaction occurs. The primary cation reabsorptive site in the thick ascending limb of Henle's loop requires 2 Cl^- ions and one K^+ ion for each Na^+ ion which enters the apical membrane of the epithelial cell. Thus, severe K^+ depletion could impair Na^+ and Cl^- reabsorption in the loop. In fact, early distal Cl^- concentration is increased significantly in rats with K^+ depletion [29]. On this transporter, NH_4^+ can substitute for K^+ [28], and thus K^+ depletion could also enhance NH_4^+ entry, leading to more delivery of NH_4^+ to the papillary interstitium. This effect probably accounts for the stimulation of NH_4^+ excretion by K^+ depletion [30]. In the distal tubule and cortical collecting duct, a K^+/Cl^- cotransporter has been identified [31,32]. A low chloride concentration in the tubular fluid in this segment of the nephron promotes K^+ secretion by this mechanism, and a high chloride concentration inhibits it [31,32]. This could be one mechanism whereby chloride depletion promotes K^+ loss. A K^+ conductive channel is also present, and Cl^- depletion coupled with a driving force for Na^+ reabsorption creates a favorable electrochemical gradient for K^+ secretion via this channel [24]. The same luminal factors also create a favorable environment for H^+ secretion via the apical H^+-ATPase transporter.

Two additional transporters link K^+ and Cl^- directly with acid and alkali secretion. A K^+/H^+ exchanger, which reabsorbs K^+ in exchange for H^+ by an ATP driven mechanism, has been identified in the outer medullary collecting duct [25]. In K^+ depletion this transporter could be activated, promoting H^+ secretion (and thereby, bicarbonate reabsorption). Luminal chloride concentration is independently linked to bicarbonate transport through an apical transporter, the Cl^-/HCO_3^- exchanger, in the cortical collecting duct. The presence of chloride in the lumen promotes HCO_3 secretion (and excretion); the absence of chloride inhibits this process [26,27]. Microperfusion studies in the rat distal tubule have shown that the addition of chloride to the perfusate can convert a bicarbonate reabsorptive epithelium into a bicarbonate secreting epithelium [27]. This transporter could be the mechanism by which chloride ions modulate the alkalosis induced by K^+ depletion; it could also be the mechanism by which chloride depletion prevents recovery from alkalosis.

Conclusions

Thus, the presence of these newly identified membrane ion transporters can, in theory, account for 1) the effect of K^+ depletion to stimulate NH_4^+ excretion and to enhance distal H^+ secretion, 2) the effect of chloride intake to modulate the alkalosis-producing potential of K^+ depletion, 3) the effect of severe K^+ depletion to produce renal chloride wasting, 4) the effect of chloride depletion to promote renal K^+ excretion, and 5) the effect of chloride depletion to sustain alkalosis by inhibiting distal nephron bicarbonate secretion. The relative roles of each of these transporters in producing and maintaining metabolic alkalosis remains to be determined. Nonetheless, they provide a logical framework for understanding how K^+ and Cl^- interact to regulate bicarbonate reabsorption and NH_4^+ excretion by the kidney. Given this new information, further studies aimed at determining which ion is the "critical" one for maintaining metabolic alkalosis are not likely to be useful. It is clear that loss of either potassium or chloride can lead to a loss of the other ion, and that relatively normal stores of each of these ions are necessary for the kidney to regulate acid-base homeostasis in a normal fashion.

References

1. Seldin DW, Welt LG, Cort JH (1956) The role of sodium salts and adrenal steroids in the production of hypokalemic alkalosis. Yale J Biol Med 29:229–247
2. Garella S, Chang B, Kahn SI (1979) Alterations of hydrogen ion homeostasis in pure potassium depletion: Studies in rats and dogs during the recovery phase. J Lab Clin Med 93:321–331
3. Capasso G, Kinne R, Malnic G, Giebisch G (1986) Renal bicarbonate reabsorption in the rat. I. Effects of hypokalemia and carbonic anhydrase. J Clin Invest 78:1558–1567
4. Levine DZ, Walker T, Nash LA (1973) Effects of KCl infusions on proximal tubular function in normal and potassium-depleted rats. Kidney Int 4:318–325
5. Adam WR, Simpson DP (1975) Renal mitochondrial glutamine metabolism and dietary potassium and protein content. Kidney Int 7:325–330
6. Cooke RE, Segar WE, Reed C, Etzwiler DD, Vita M, Brusilow S, Darrow DC (1954) The role of potassium in the prevention of alkalosis. Am J Med 17:180–195
7. Luke RG, Levitin H (1967) Impaired renal conservation of chloride and the acid-base changes associated with potassium depletion in the rat. Clin Sci 32:511–526
8. Luke RG, Wright FS, Fowler N, Kashgarian M, Giebisch GH (1978) Effects of potassium depletion on renal tubular chloride transport in the rat. Kidney Int 14:414–427
9. Burnell JM, Teubner EJ, Simpson DP (1974) Metabolic acidosis accompanying potassium depletion. Am J Physiol 227:329–333
10. Hulter HN, Sebastian A, Sigala JF, Licht JH, Glynn RD, Schambelan M, Biglieri EG (1980) Pathogenesis of renal hyperchloremic acidosis resulting from dietary potassium restriction in the dog: Role of aldosterone. Am J Physiol 238:F79–F91
11. Jones JW, Sebastian A, Hulter HN, Schambelan M, Sutton JM, Biglieri EG (1982) Systemic and renal acid-base effects of chronic dietary potassium depletion in humans. Kidney Int 21:402–410
12. Hernandez RE, Schambelan M, Cogan MG, Colman J, Morris RC Jr, Sebastian A (1987) Dietary NaCl determines severity of potassium depletion-induced metabolic alkalosis. Kidney Int 31:1356–1367
13. Garella S, Chazan JA, Cohen JJ (1970) Saline-resistant metabolic alkalosis or "chloride-wasting nephropathy." Ann Intern Med 73:31–38
14. Orloff J, Kennedy TJ Jr, Berliner RW (1953) The effect of potassium in nephrectomized rats with hypokalemic alkalosis. J Clin Invest 32:538–542
15. Atkins EL, Schwartz WB (1962) Factors governing correction of the alkalosis associated with potassium deficiency; the critical role of chloride in the recovery process. J Clin Invest 41:218–229
16. Hulter HN, Sigala JF, Sebastian A (1978) K$^+$ deprivation potentiates the renal alkalosis-producing effect of mineralocorticoid. Am J Physiol 235:F298–F309
17. Relman AS, Schwartz WB (1952) The effect of DOCA on electrolyte balance in normal man and its relation to sodium chloride intake. Yale J Biol Med 24:540–558
18. Kassirer JP, Appleton FM, Chazan JA, Schwartz WB (1967) Aldosterone in metabolic alkalosis. J Clin Invest 46:1558–1571
19. Kassirer JP, London AM, Goldman DM, Schwartz WB (1970) On the pathogenesis of metabolic alkalosis in hyperaldosteronism. Am J Med 49:306–315
20. Galla JH, Bonduris DN, Luke RG (1983) Correction of acute chloride-depletion alkalosis in the rat without volume expansion. Am J Physiol 244:F217–F221
21. Wall BM, Byrum GV, Galla JH, Luke RG (1987) Importance of chloride for the correction of chronic metabolic alkalosis in the rat. Am J Physiol 253:F1031–F1039
22. Bleich HL, Tannen RL, Schwartz WB (1966) The induction of metabolic alkalosis by correction of potassium deficiency. J Clin Invest 45:573–579
23. Kassirer JP, Schwartz WB (1966) Correction of metabolic alkalosis in man without

repair of potassium deficiency. A reevaluation of the role of potassium. Am J Med 40:19–26

24. Field MJ, Giebisch G (1989) Mechanisms of segmental potassium reabsorption and secretion. In: Seldin DW, Giebisch G (eds) The regulation of potassium balance. Raven, New York, pp 139–155

25. Wingo CS (1989) Active proton secretion and potassium absorption in the rabbit outer medullary collecting duct. J Clin Invest 84:361–365

26. Star RA, Burg MB, Knepper MA (1985) Bicarbonate secretion and chloride absorption by rabbit cortical collecting ducts. Role of chloride/bicarbonate exchange. J Clin Invest 76:1123–1130

27. Levine DZ, Vandorpe D, Iacovitti M (1990) Luminal chloride modulates rat distal tubule bidirectional bicarbonate flux in vivo. J Clin Invest 85:1793–1798

28. Knepper MA, Packer R, Good DW (1989) Ammonium transport in the kidney. Physiol Rev 69:179–249

29. Luke RG, Booker BB, Galla JH (1985) Effect of potassium depletion on chloride transport in the loop of Henle in the rat. Am J Physiol 248:F682–F687

30. Tannen RL (1987) Effect of potassium on renal acidification and acid-base homeostasis. Semin Nephrol 7:263–273

31. Ellison DH, Velazquez H, Wright FS (1986) Unidirectional potassium fluxes in renal distal tubule: Effects of chloride and barium. Am J Physiol 250:F885–F894

32. Wingo CS (1989) Reversible chloride-dependent potassium flux across the rabbit cortical collecting tubule. Am J Physiol 256:F697–F704

Role of Kidney in the Pathogenesis of Hypertension

Chair: Maarten ADH Schalekamp
(The Netherlands)
Takao Saruto (Japan)

The Renin Angiotensin System, the Kidney, and the Pathogenesis of Hypertension

Norman K. Hollenberg[1] and Gordon H. Williams[2]

SUMMARY. Some individuals enjoy a high salt diet with impunity: others, on the other hand, raise their blood pressure and suffer the consequences. Multiple observations suggest that familial, probably genetic, factors are involved and that the abnormality resides in the kidney. We have identified a group of patients, called "non-modulators," in whom impaired responsiveness of the kidney and adrenal to Angiotension II (AII) with shifts in salt intake, is associated with failure of renal blood flow to change as salt intake changes, impaired ability to handle a salt load, and sodium-sensitive hypertension. The abnormality is familial and probably inherited. Angiotensin converting enzyme (ACE) inhibition corrects many of the associated abnormalities, increases renal blood flow, and enhances the ability of the kidney to handle a salt load—an important contribution, we believe, to the antihypertensive effect. The renal abnormality may also predispose to progressive renal injury if an additional abnormality, such as diabetes mellitus, is superimposed.

Introduction

Recognition of a crucial contribution of genetics to the pathogenesis of hypertension is longstanding, but precisely what is inherited as the predisposing abnormality has remained remarkably elusive. Interest in the kidney has recently been renewed by recognition of the fact that hypertension follows the kidney after transplantation in animals and in humans [1–5]. A series of abnormalities, potentially involving the kidney and sodium homeostasis, has been recognized over the years, including familial factors in renal sodium handling [6] and in the control of the renal circulation [7,8]. Relevant abnormalities in angiotensin-mediated control of the renal circulation and adrenal aldosterone release have been documented worldwide, in the relatively homogeneous populations of Japan [8] and Switzerland [9], and the relatively heterogeneous population of the United States [10].

---

[1]Departments of Medicine[1] and Radiology[2], Harvard Medical School and Brigham and Women's Hospital, Boston, MA 02115, USA

The thrust of this essay will be to organize a growing body of evidence which indicates that an abnormality of the kidney, and the adrenal, involving disordered regulation through the renin-angiotensin system, is responsible for the pathogenesis in about 45% of patients—a discrete subgroup that may be the most common cause of hypertension. That fundamental abnormality leads to disordered renal sodium handling and sodium-sensitive hypertension, abnormalities in the renal vascular response to changes in sodium intake and to angiotensin II, blunted decrements of renin release in response to saline or angiotensin II, and an accentuated renal vasodilator response to angiotensin converting enzyme (ACE) inhibition. ACE inhibition increases renal blood flow substantially more in these patients than it does in normal subjects or other essential hypertensives. ACE inhibition also restores to normal the renal vascular and adrenal response to angiotensin II, renin release in response to angiotensin II, renal sodium handling, and, ultimately, blood pressure. Finally, and perhaps most intriguing, similar abnormalities have been found in 50% of the normotensive offspring of patients with essential hypertension; evidence is accruing to indicate that the abnormality is inherited, perhaps via a major gene.

Sodium and Renal Vascular Responses to Angiotensin II

Dahl, in a 1963 review of metabolism in hypertension, was puzzled by five then recent publications, which described a paradoxical, natriuretic response to angiotensin II associated with a blunted or absent renal vascular response in some patients with essential hypertension [11]. He noted the parallel with hepatic cirrhosis. Since then, the mechanism in cirrhosis has become clear [12]. The paradoxical natriuresis reflects the effects on renal sodium handling of the pressor response, when the renal vascular bed can no longer respond to angiotensin II because of angiotensin-mediated renal vasoconstriction.

During the time since Dahl's review, two separate lines of investigation on disordered control of the renal blood supply [13] and the adrenal [14] with shifts in state of sodium balance led to the recognition that both abnormalities occur in the same patient [15]. This followed recognition of a highly predictable shift in renal vascular and adrenal responses to angiotensin II with changes in sodium intake: the renal vasculature is more sensitive to angiotensin II on a high salt diet, and adrenal aldosterone release is more sensitive with restriction of sodium intake [16]. Because the term "modulation" had been employed to describe such shifts in responsiveness in other endocrine systems, the inability of these individuals to change renal vascular and adrenal responsiveness to angiotensin II [17] was called "non-modulation" [10,18].

Several lines of evidence indicate that "non-modulation" is not part of a continuum, but rather represents a discrete subgroup present in about 45% of patients with normal renin and high renin essential hypertension [10,18].

Sodium Sensitive Hypertension

The frequent sensitivity of hypertension to sodium intake has long been recognized. In 1904, within a few years of the first recognition that hypertension represents a clinical disorder, Ambard and Baujard proposed that the increase in blood pressure reflected a failure to adapt to an excess of salt in the diet [19]. Not long thereafter, Allen, in the United States, demonstrated that a severe reduction of salt in the diet was effective in reducing blood pressure in about 60% of patients with hypertension [20]. Both the French group and Allen believed that hypertension reflected an unknown renal defect that limited the individual's ability to handle salt. Since that time, confirmation of the frequency of sodium sensitive hypertension has come from estimates based on sodium intake as therapy [21], the frequency of response to diuretics [22], and from careful metabolic balance studies [23,24], which have confirmed a frequency of about 50%–60%. The metabolic balance studies failed to identify a mechanism responsible for the blood pressure rise, but did demonstrate that individuals with salt-sensitive hypertension showed more positive sodium balance and gained more weight as their blood pressure rose [23,24].

An abnormality involving the renal blood supply and adrenal aldosterone release, both crucial for sodium handling, raised the possibility, intriguing to us, that the unidentified patients in the metabolic balance studies were the non-modulators. Indeed, that has turned out to be the case. Whether the pattern by which external sodium balance is achieved when sodium intake is restricted [25] or the acute response to a saline load [26] is employed as the index, non-modulators show a clear inability to handle sodium. When the earlier metabolic balance study was replicated in a study in which external balance was first achieved on a restricted and then on a high salt intake, the non-modulators showed more positive sodium balance, as they gained more weight [25]; all of the sodium-sensitive hypertension that was identified occurred in that group [27].

Control of the Renal Circulation

In addition to blunted renal vascular responses to angiotensin II, two other abnormalities in the control of the renal circulation, that are germane both to renal vascular responses to angiotensin II and to renal sodium handling, occur in non-modulators. Normal individuals display parallel changes in renal blood flow as they change salt intake: in a shift from a high sodium to a low sodium intake renal blood flow falls, and rises with an increase in salt intake [10,13,17]. Patients with essential hypertension who have intact modulation show similar changes, but renal blood flow is fixed with shifts in sodium intake in non-modulators [10,13,17,15–17]. Again, this abnormality is not part of a continuum, but rather reflects a discrete limitation reflected in a bimodal distribution [25]. To the extent that intrarenal physical forces and filtration fraction contribute to the ability of the kidney to handle sodium, the limited renal vascular response to changes in sodium intake could account for the limited capacity of the kidney to handle sodium (described above).

A fixed renal blood supply in response to a physiological stimulus could reflect fixed, organic disease so common as a byproduct of hypertension. On the other hand, multiple lines of evidence suggest that in some patients there is a functional abnormality of the renal blood supply, vasoconstriction, that contributes to the reduced renal blood flow [10]. ACE inhibition, long recognized as inducing a potentiated renal vasodilatation in essential hypertension [28,29], is now recognized as producing preferential renal vasodilatation in the non-modulator. Indeed, only non-modulators display renal vasodilatation when an ACE inhibitor is administered on a high salt diet, when the renin system is suppressed [27].

ACE inhibition also restores renal vascular responsiveness to angiotensin II [27] and restores the capacity of the kidney to handle a sodium load [26]. We believe that the restoration of the ability of the kidney to handle a sodium load represents a major factor by which ACE inhibitors are effective at achieving goal blood pressure in patients with essential hypertension who enjoy a typical high salt diet, and thus have a suppressed circulating renin-angiotensin system.

The restoration of the renal vascular response to angiotensin II following ACE inhibition also provides insight into mechanisms. If the renal vasodilatation reflected the accumulation of bradykinin because of reduced degradation, or because of prostaglandin release, the renal vasodilator response to ACE inhibition should have been associated with further blunting of renal vascular responsiveness to angiotensin II, since both prostaglandins and kinins share this characteristic [30].

Renin Release and Non-Modulation

Patients with non-modulation at the steady state have either a normal or increased level of plasma renin activity [10,15–17], but two abnormalities of renin release have been identified in non-modulators. In normal subjects on a low salt diet, intravenous infusion of saline rapidly reduces plasma renin activity and plasma aldosterone concentration, but only about 50% of the patients with essential hypertension show this rapid fall [31]. The same patients that had a blunted renin response also had a reduced rate of sodium excretion, and a transient pressor response to the saline infusion. These observations suggested the possibility that non-modulation was involved. Indeed, subsequent studies showed that it was the non-modulator that showed the delayed response to saline [32].

Saline induced suppression of the renin-angiotensin system in the normal subjects did not involve simple plasma volume expansion, since the infusion of dextran in a volume to produce similar or more plasma volume expansion aldosterone concentration [31]. This observation made it possible to divide the stimulus into "sodium sensitive" and "volume sensitive" elements. The rate of fall of plasma renin activity in response to saline in non-modulators is identical to the normal response to dextran, the volume-sensitive signal. One attractive, but speculative, interpretation of these data is that non-modulators have a normal volume-sensing system, but lack the ability to respond to the specific signal emitted by sodium.

A second evidence of disregulation of renin release involves the so-called "short feedback loop," by which angiotensin II reduces renin release. The response occurs within minutes, as opposed to the "long feedback loop," which involves aldosterone release and sodium retention. Patients with essential hypertension frequently do not show renin suppression with angiotensin II infusion [33], an abnormality once again corrected by converting enzyme inhibition [34]. Again, after identification of the non-modulating group, this abnormality was found to occur only in the non-modulator [35].

Genetic Factors

A contribution of heredity to hypertension in many patients has long been recognized, but the precise factors inherited have been remarkably elusive. Information from renal transplantation, both in inbred animal models [1–3] and in man [4,5], has suggested that the genetic information, at least some of the time, is coded in the kidney. Four lines of investigation have suggested that non-modulation is inherited.

The first clue came from the frequency of a family history of hypertension in the parents of non-modulators [25]. In the neighborhood of 90% of the non-modulators in two studies have a parent with hypertension, where the family history could be evaluated, as opposed to a rate of about 30% in essential hypertensives in whom modulation was intact. The second line of investigation involves the identification of features identical to non-modulation, involving both the adrenal gland and the kidney, in the offspring of hypertensives. In the adrenal, plasma aldosterone concentration in the offspring of hypertensives studied on a low salt diet was substantially lower than the concentration in the offspring of normotensive parents, despite a similar level of plasma renin activity and plasma angiotensin II concentration [7]. In an elegant study on aldosterone release in response to angiotensin II infusion, performed by Beretta-Piccoli and his co-workers, aldosterone release was shown to be blunted in the offspring of hypertensives [9], but not normotensive, parents. In Japan, ACE inhibition increased renal blood flow, not only in essential hypertensives with a family history of hypertension, but also in their normotensive offspring [8]. This study was especially impressive because it was performed in Japan, where an ad libitum intake is especially rich in sodium chloride. We have confirmed that observation retrospectively in data for our earlier studies, and prospectively, the calcium channel blocking agent, diltiazem, increased renal blood flow, preferentially in 50% of the offspring of hypertensives, but not in the control group made up of the normotensive offspring of normotensive parents [37]. Diltiazem blocked the action of angiotensin II on the renal blood supply in that study. The specificity of that response was confirmed by the observation that no difference could be identified, in the renal vascular response to the vasodilator acetylcholine, as a function of family history.

A third line of evidence involves red blood cell sodium:lithium countertransport. Lithium countertransport is increased not only in many hypertensives, but also in their normotensive offspring [36–38]. There is a striking increase in the frequency with which increased lithium countertransport occurs in non-modulation [39]. Unfortunately, because of the number of confounding variables that influence lithium countertransport, that determination will be useful in identifying non-modulators only at the extremes of countertransport.

In a study still in progress, involving multiple family members, renal plasma flow and its response to angiotensin have been found in aggregate significantly in the non-modulator [40,41]. There is evidence that sodium handling also is influenced by heredity, and is modified by a family history of hypertension [6]. It will be intriguing to ascertain whether that genetic influence reflects non-modulation and its influence on the renal circulation and aldosterone, or abnormalities in other systems identified in these patients [39,40].

Equally speculative, and equally intriguing, is the possibility that non-modulation has implications for the pathogenesis of renal disease. About one-third of patients with type I diabetes mellitus will develop nephropathy, and two thirds will not, despite an apparently identical severity and duration of disease. Studies in animal models have suggested a powerful role for renal hemodynamic factors, but have not provided an explanation for the fact that 100% of rats but only 33% of people will progress to nephropathy. The information to indicate that the control of the renal circulation is altered not only in non-modulators, but also in their normotensive offspring, may be relevant. Patients with diabetes mellitus at risk of nephropathy display elevated red blood cell sodium: lithium countertransport and a striking family history of hypertension [41,42], features that they share with non-modulators. To the extent that non-modulators and their normotensive offspring act as though they have elevated intrarenal angiotensin II concentration – reflected in a blunted renal vascular response to angiotensin II, blunted renin release in response to saline and angiotensin II, and a potentiated renal vascular response to converting enzyme inhibition – the metabolic disarray of diabetes mellitus superimposed on a disordered control of the renal circulation could lead to glomerular hypertension and its consequences.

That speculation is most sweet when it leads to a testable hypothesis. The speculation that we have indulged in passes that test.

References

1. Bianchi G, Fox U, DiFrancesco GF, et al (1974) Blood pressure changes produced by kidney cross transplantation between spontaneously hypertensive rats (SHR) and normotensive rats (NR). Clin Sci 47:435–448
2. Dahl LK, Heine M (1975) Primary role of renal hemografts in setting blood pressure levels in rats. Circ Res 36:692–696
3. Kawabe K, Watanabe TX, Shiono K, et al (1978) Influence of blood pressure of renal isografts between spontaneously hypertensive and normotensive rats utilizing the F1 hybrids. Jpn Heart J 19:886–894
4. Guidi E, Bianchi G, Dallosia V, et al (1982) Influence of familial hypertension of the donor on the blood pressure and antihypertensive therapy of kidney grafat recipients. Nephron 30:318–323
5. Curtiss JJ, Luke RG, Dustan HP, et al (1983) Remission of essential hypertension after renal transplantation. N Engl J Med 309:1009–1015
6. Luft FC, Rankin LI, Bkloch R, et al (1979) Cardiovascular and humoral responses to extremes of sodium intake in normal black and white men. Circulation 60:697–703
7. Blackshear JL, TGarnic D, Williams GH, et al (1987) Exaggerated renal vascular response to calcium entry blockade in first degree relatives of essential hypertensives: Possible role of intrarenal angiotensin II. Hypertension 9:384–389
8. Uneda S, Fukishima S, Fujika Y, et al (1986) Renal hemodynamics and renin angiotensin system in adolescents genetically predisposed to essential hypertension. J Hypertens 2(Suppl 3):437–439
9. Beretta-Picolli C, Pusterla C, Stadler P, et al (1988) Blunted aldosterone responsiveness to AII in normotensive subjects with familial predisposition to essential hypertension. J Hypertens 61:57–61
10. Hollenberg NK, Williams GH (1986) Sensitivity to sodium and nonmodulation of renal and adrenal responsiveness to angiotensin II. Implications for the pathogenesis of hypertension. In: Zanchetti A, Tarazi RC (eds) Handbook of hypertension, vol 8. Elsevier, New York, pp 520–522
11. Dahl LK (1963) Metabolic aspects of hypertension. Annu Rev Med 14:69–98
12. Gutman RA, Forrey AW, Flet WP, et al (1973) Vasopressor-induced natriuresis and altered intrarenal hemodynamics in cirrhotic man. Clin Sci 45:19–34
13. Hollenberg NK, Merrill JP (1970) Intrarenal perfusion in the young essential hypertensive: A subpopulation resistant to sodium restriction. Trans Assoc Am Physicians 83:93–101
14. Williams GH, Rose LI, Dluhy RG, et al (1970) Abnormal responsiveness of the renin aldosterone system to acute stimulation in patients with essential hypertension. Ann Intern Med 72:317–326

15. Williams GH, Tuck ML, Sullivan JM, et al (1982) Parallel adrenal and renal abnormalities in the young patient with essential hypertension. Am J Med 72:907–914

16. Hollenberg NK, Chenitz WR, Adams DF, et al (1974) Reciprocal influence of salt intake on adrenal glomerulosa and renal vascular responses to angiotensin II in normal man. J Clin Invest 54:34–42

17. Shoback DM, Williams GH, Hollenberg NK, et al (1983) Endogenous angiotensin II as a determinant of sodium modulated changes in tissue responsiveness to angiotensin II in normal man. J Clin Endocrinol Metab 57:764–770

18. Williams GH, Hollenberg NK (1985) Abnormal adrenal and renal responses to angiotensin II in essential hypertension: Implications for pathogenesis. In: Carey RM (ed) Clinical endocrinology: is essential hypertension an endocrine disease?, vol 7. Butterworth, London, pp 184–211

19. Ambard L, Beaujard E (1904) Causes de l'hypertension arterielle. Arch Intern Med 1:520–533

20. Allen FM (1925) Treatment of kidney disease and high blood pressure. The Psychiatric Institute, Morristown, p 206

21. Chapman B (1951) Some effects of the rice-fruit diet in patients with essential hypertension. In: Bell ET (ed) Hypertension: A symposium. Minneapolis, pp 504–516

22. Freis E (1979) Comparative effects of tierynafen and hydrochlorothiazide in the treatment of hypertension (Veterans Administration Cooperative Study Group on Antihypertensive Agents). N Engl J Med 301:293–297

23. Kawasaki T, Delea CS, Bartter FC, et al (1978) The effect of high sodium and low sodium intakes on blood pressure and other related variables in human subjects with idiopathic hypertension. Am J Med 64:193–198

24. Fujita T, Henry WL, Bartter FC, et al (1980) Factors influencing blood pressure in salt sensitive patients with hypertension. Am J Med 69:334–344

25. Hollenberg NK, Williams GH (1986) Abnormal renal sodium handling in essential hypertension: Relation to failure to renal and adrenal modulation of responses to angiotensin II. Am J Med 81:412–418

26. Rystedt LL, Williams GH, Hollenberg NK (1986) The renal and endocrine response to saline infusion in essential hypertension. Hypertension 8:217–222

27. Redgrave JE, Rabinowe SL, Hollenberg NK, et al (1985) Correction of abnormal renal blood flow response to angiotensin II by converting enzyme inhibition in essential hypertensives. J Clin Invest 75:1285–1290

28. Williams GH, Hollenberg NK (1977) Accentuated vascular and endocrine responses to SQ 20881 in hypertension. N Engl J Med 297:184–188

29. Hollenberg NK, Meggs LG, Williams GH, et al (1981) Sodium intake and renal responses to captopril in normal man and in essential hypertension. Kidney 20:240–245

30. Meggs LG, Katzberg RW, DeLeeuw P, et al (1985) Specific desensitization of the canine renal vasculature to angiotensin II despite cycloxygenase inhibition. Yale J Biol Med 58:453–458

31. Tuck ML, Williams GH, Dluhy RG, et al (1976) A delayed suppression of the renin aldosterone axis following saline infusion in human hypertension. Circ Res 39:711–716

32. Rabinowe SL, Redgrave JE, Rysedt LL, et al (1987) Renin-suppression by saline is blunted in non-modulating essential hypertension. Hypertension 10:404–408

33. Dluhy RG, Bavli SZ, Leung FK, et al (1979) Abnormal adrenal responsiveness and angiotensin II dependency in high renin essential hypertension. J Clin Invest 64:1270–1276

34. LeBoff MS, Dluhy RG, Hollenberg NK, et al (1982) Abnormal renin short feedback loop in essential hypertension is reversible with converting enzyme inhibition. J Clin Invest 70:335–341

35. Seely EW, Moore TJ, Rogacz S, Gordon M, Gleason RE, Hollenberg NK, Williams GH

(1989) Angiotensin-mediated renin suppression is alterd in non-modulating hypertension. Hypertension 13:31–37

36. Redgrave JE, Canessa M, Gleason R, Hollenberg NK, Williams GH (1989) Red blood cell Na-Li countertransport in non-modulating essential hypertensives. Hypertension 13:721–726

37. Dluhy RG, Hopkins P, Hollenberg NK, Williams GH, Williams RR (1988) Heritable abnormalities of the renin-angiotensin-aldosterone system in essential hypertension. J Cardiovasc Pharmacol 12(3):149–154

38. Lifton RP, Hopkins PN, Williams RR, Hollenberg NK, Williams GH, Dluhy RG (1989) Evidence for heritability of non-modulating essential hypertension. Hypertension 13:884–889

39. Gordon MS, Steunkel CA, Conlin PR, Hollenberg NK, Williams GH (1989) The role of dopamine in nonmodulating hypertension. J Clin Endocrinol Metab 69(2):426–432

40. Conlin PR, Gleason RE, Hollenberg NK, Williams GH (1989) Altered aldosterone and norepinephrine responses to upright posture in nonmodulating hypertension (abstract No. 61). Hypertension 14:346

41. Krolewski AS, Canessa M, Warram JH, et al (1988) Predisposition to hypertension and susceptibility to renal disease in insulin-dependent diabetes mellitus. N Engl J Med 318:140–145

42. Mangill R, Bending JJ, Scott G, et al. Increased sodium-lithium countertransport activity in red cells of patients with insulin-dependent diabetes and nephropathy. N Engl J Med 318:146–150

Renal Microcirculation in Essential Hypertension

KOICHI HAYASHI, MURRAY EPSTEIN[1,2], and RODGER D. LOUTZENHISER[1,2]

SUMMARY. The past several years have witnessed important advances in characterizing the renal microvascular response to pressure as a determinant of renal autoregulation. Utilizing diverse in vitro models, including the juxtamedullary nephron preparation and the isolated perfused hydronephrotic kidney, several investigators have demonstrated that pressure-dependent alterations of the renal microvessels are mediated, in part, independent of signals from the macula densa. Furthermore, recent evidence indicates that the afferent arterioles of normotensive and genetically hypertensive animals respond differently to changes of renal arterial pressure (RAP). Thus, hypertension is associated with a compensatory shift in the pressure response of the afferent arteriole, such that higher RAPs are required to elicit vasoconstriction in this vessel. Calcium antagonists attenuate pressure-induced afferent arteriolar vasoconstriction, suggesting the participation of dihydropyridine-sensitive calcium channels in mediating pressure-induced vasoconstriction of this microvessel.

Introduction

The rediscovery, by Goldblatt and his co-workers [1], that partial ligation of the renal artery induces hypertension raised the possibility that essential hypertension could be renal in origin due to abnormalities of renal perfusion. Subsequently, a large body of evidence has accumulated, recognizing the important role of structural and functional changes in the renal microcirculation in the initiation and maintenance of hypertension in animals, as well as in humans [2–4]. In this brief survey, we review recent studies which further characterize the renal microvascular response to pressure elevation utilizing diverse in vitro models.

[1]Nephrology Section, Veterans Administration Medical Center, Miami, FL 33125, USA
[2]Nephrology Division, Department of Medicine, University of Miami School of Medicine, Miami, FL 33125, USA
(Address correspondence to: Dr. Murray Epstein, at above address.)

Sustained hypertension markedly alters the renal response to elevations in renal perfusion pressure; shifting the threshold pressure of autoregulation of renal blood flow [5] and pressure-induced natriuresis [6,7] to higher pressures. This resetting of the renal response to pressure represents a renal adaptation to hypertension. Pressure-induced vasoconstriction of renal microvessels constitutes an important determinant of renal autoregulation [8,9]. It is extremely difficult, however, to assess directly the renal microvascular response to pressure in situ. The ability to directly observe microvascular responses would obviously facilitate the characterization of the determinants of the autoregulatory response. Unfortunately, the vascular pole of the glomerulus is not accessible to direct intravital microscopic observation. An early attempt to circumvent this problem involved transplantation of glomeruli into the hamster cheek pouch and subsequent observation following revascularization [10]. Using this approach, Click et al. demonstrated differences in the responsiveness of renal microvessels to various hormones in normotensive and hypertensive animals [10]. The effects of hypertension on renal microvascular responsiveness during acute changes of perfusion pressure have, until recently, not been directly ascertained.

Finally, it is apparent that when arterial pressure is altered in vivo, concomitant changes in the neural and humoral determinants of renal microvascular tone tend to counter the induced changes, thereby confounding the interpretation of results [11,12]. Recently, a number of investigators have succeeded in characterizing the determinants of the renal autoregulatory response to pressure, utilizing diverse in vitro models.

Role of TGF and Myogenic Vasoconstriction in Autoregulation

Sanchez-Ferrer et al. [13] utilized the in vitro perfused juxtamedullary nephron preparation perfused with cell-free artificial media to directly assess the determinants of the microvascular response to elevated pressure. Their studies demonstrated an afferent arteriolar vasoconstriction in response to elevated renal arterial pressure (120–180 mm Hg). When the tubuloglomerular feedback mechanism was blocked, either with furosemide administration, or by removal of the renal papilla (by interrupting the delivery of fluid to the macula densa), pressure-induced afferent arteriolar vasoconstriction was eliminated. Based on these observations, the authors concluded that pressure-induced pre-glomerular vasoconstriction is mediated entirely by feedback signals from the macula densa without any remaining, i.e., myogenic, component.

In contrast, Moore [14] has advocated that an important tubuloglomerular feedback (TGF)-independent component contributes to the renal microvascular response to pressure. Carmines et al. [15] demonstrated myogenic pressure-dependent contractions of interlobular arteries in the blood-perfused juxtamedullary nephron preparation.

Recently our laboratory has investigated, in a quantitative manner, the role of pre-glomerular microvessels, i.e., the interlobular artery and the afferent arteriole, in mediating the vasoconstrictor response to changes in perfusion pressure [16]. We have utilized the isolated perfused hydronephrotic kidney model to delineate the renal microvascular response to changes in perfusion pressure. This model is uniquely

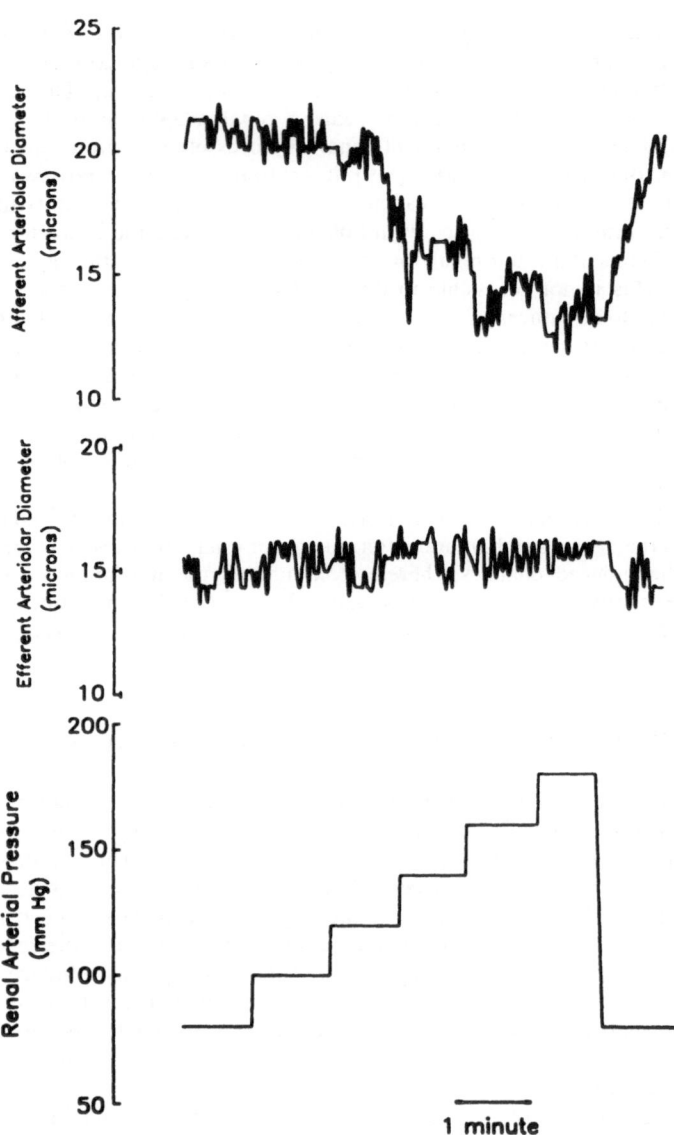

Fig. 1. Representative tracings depicting the response of afferent and efferent arterioles of an isolated perfused hydronephrotic kidney to alterations in renal arterial pressure. Increasing pressure in the renal artery (*bottom*) elicited a vasoconstriction of the afferent arteriole (*top*), but not of the efferent arteriole (*center*). (Reproduced from [11] with permission)

suited for the study of renal microvascular responsiveness to alterations in perfusion pressure [11]. The renal microvessels can be visualized in an intact in situ setting, but under in vitro conditions in which RAP is under direct experimental control. Extrarenal neural and humoral influences on renal vascular tone are eliminated. Furthermore, as detailed previously [11], because hydronephrosis induces tubular atrophy [17], tubulo-glomerular feedback is absent in this model. Thus, pressure-dependent alterations of the renal microvessels must occur independent of signals from the macula densa. As demonstrated by the original tracing in Fig. 1, the afferent arteriole constricted markedly as renal arterial pressure was elevated, whereas the efferent arteriole was unresponsive to this manipulation.

Recent studies by Hayashi et al. [16] utilizing the isolated perfused hydronephrotic kidney have delineated the marked segmental heterogeneity in the response of the afferent arteriole to pressure. These findings are summarized in Fig. 2. Both SHR and WKY manifested a blunted response to elevated perfusion pressure at the segment near the glomerulus. Thus, this segment of the afferent arteriole vasoconstricted only modestly in response to elevating RAP from 80 mm Hg to 180 mm Hg (i.e., $7.4 \pm 2.5\%$ and $8.1 \pm 2.0\%$ decreases in vessel diameters in WKY and SHR, respectively). In contrast, the same change in RAP resulted in marked decreases in the diameters of the segments of the afferent arteriole near the interlobular artery ($-22.3 \pm 1.6\%$ and $-19.9 \pm 1.6\%$ in WKY and SHR, respectively and at the mid-portion ($-20.2 \pm 1.6\%$ and $-18.5 \pm 2.7\%$ in WKY and SHR, respectively). These findings are in accord with the observation by Steinhausen et al. [18] that reducing renal arterial pressure in vivo causes less vasodilation in the afferent arteriolar segment near the glomerulus than in the more proximal portions of this vessel. In contrast to these observations in both in vivo and in vitro hydronephrotic kidneys, Carmines [19] reported that in the perfused juxtamedullary nephron preparation the portion of the afferent arteriole nearest the glomerulus manifests the major resistance adjustment to alterations in RAP. These divergent findings may be attributable to differences in the role of TGF in these two models. In the juxtamedullary nephron, TGF is intact, whereas the tubular atrophy associated with chronic hydronephrosis disrupts this mechanism [11,17]. In concert, these observations suggest that the portion of the afferent arteriole near the glomerulus may be under predominant control by TGF [20], whereas more proximal segments exhibit an intrinsic, e.g., myogenic, vasoconstrictor response to elevated pressure.

As discussed above, Sanchez-Ferrer et al. have recently reported that the pressure-induced decrement in arteriolar diameter and regulation of glomerular pressure in juxtamedullary nephrons were completely abolished by pharmacologic or surgical disruption of TGF [13]. Based on these findings, the authors concluded that TGF-induced vasoconstriction represented the sole mechanism whereby afferent arteriolar tone is modulated by elevated pressure. Our demonstration that the afferent arteriole of the hydronephrotic kidney constricts in response to pressure elevation, despite the absence of TGF mechanism, clearly indicates an important contribution of non-TGF mediated vasoconstriction in the pressure response of the renal microvasculature.

One possible explanation for these apparent discrepancies relates to the region of the afferent arteriole under observation. As detailed above, the segment of the affer-

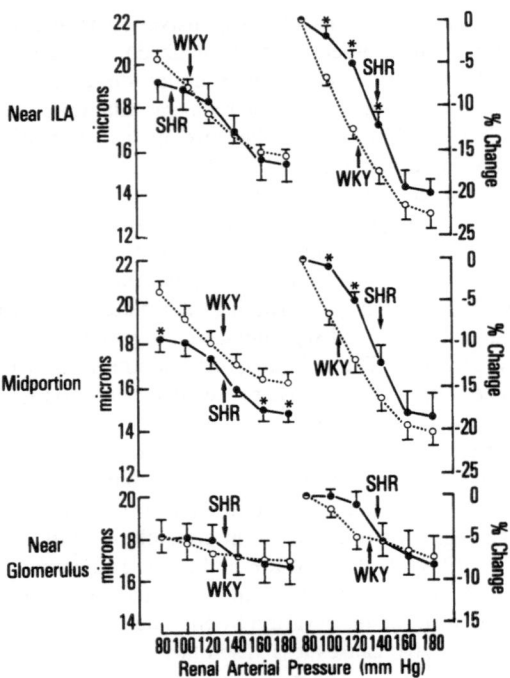

Fig. 2. Effects of renal arterial pressure on the diameters of afferent arterioles in kidneys from WKY (*open circle*) and SHR (*closed circle*). Regions of afferent arterioles observed were classified as segments near the interlobular artery (*ILA, top*), of midportion (*center*), and near the glomerulus (*bottom*). In the lower range of renal arterial pressure, pressure-induced afferent arteriolar vasoconstriction was blunted in SHR as compared with that in WKY (*left panel*). Plotting the data as the percent change in vessel diameter revealed a marked shift of the response of afferent arterioles in SHR kidneys (*right panel*). Note the diminished response of segments near the glomerulus to an increase in renal arterial pressure as compared with other segments. Results are mean±SE; *P<0.05 vs. WKY. (Reproduced from [16] by permission of the American Heart Association, Inc.)

ent arteriole near the glomerulus does not respond directly to elevated pressure (Fig. 2), whereas this site is the major region affected by TGF [20]. In contrast, more proximal portions of the afferent arteriole respond markedly to pressure, but are not likely to be influenced by the macula densa signal. Finally, it should be noted that we studied vessels arising from small caliber (ca. 30 µm) interlobular arteries, suggesting an origin in the superficial cortex. These afferent arterioles had a mean basal diameter of approximately 20 µm. In contrast, the afferent arterioles observed in the juxtamedullary nephron preparation arise primarily from the arcuate artery and have basal diameters of 32 µm. Thus, differences in myogenic responsiveness may be related to regional factors and may be influenced by vessel diameter.

Sites of Preglomerular Vasoconstriction

Although pre-glomerular vessels are thought to be primarily responsible for the autoregulatory response [21,22], controversy remains concerning the relative role of the afferent arteriole and the interlobular artery. Tønder et al. [23] demonstrated that the pressure within the interlobular artery in the outer cortex was substantially lower than that of the aorta. Furthermore, Källskog et al. [24] demonstrated that within the autoregulatory range, the pressure in the superficial interlobular artery was maintained relatively unchanged. These observations indicate that the interlobular artery contributes importantly to renal autoregulation. In contrast, Carmines and colleagues [15] reported that in juxtamedullary nephrons, afferent arteriolar pressure was variably regulated, whereas interlobular arterial pressure was not. Thus, these observations suggest a predominant contribution of the afferent arteriole to renal autoregulation, at least in the juxtamedullary portion of the renal microcirculation. Of interest, Carmines et al. demonstrated the presence of pressure-induced vasoconstriction in both afferent and interlobular artery [15]. Thus, the lack of pressure regulation within this segment of the interlobular artery may simply reflect the larger diameter of this vessel near the arcuate artery (ca. 50 µm).

We have recently demonstrated that the intralobular artery of the isolated perfused hydronephrotic kidney responds markedly to elevated pressure. More importantly, the responsiveness of this vessel to pressure is dependent on the basal diameter, with the smaller diameter, i.e., distal, segments demonstrating a much more marked response than the larger, i.e., proximal, segments [25]. Since vascular resistance is inversely related to the fourth power of the radius, it follows that a pressure-induced vasoconstriction of the smaller caliber segments of this vessel, i.e., in the outer cortex, may contribute more to autoregulation than the larger segments, i.e. in the juxtamedullary region. Taken together, these findings are consistent with the postulate that the segments of the interlobular artery in the superficial cortex contribute importantly to the regulation of renal hemodynamics.

Altered Autoregulation in Hypertension

Sustained hypertension influences several aspects of the renal response to elevated renal perfusion pressure. Autoregulation of renal blood flow and the pressure-natriuresis relationship are both reset toward higher pressure level in hypertensive animals [5–7]. In a recent study [16], we have demonstrated that the RAP at which a significant increase in total renal vascular resistance is attained is higher in kidneys isolated from SHR (180 mm Hg) than in those from WKY (140 mm Hg). This observation indicates a resetting of the relationship between RAP and total renal vascular resistance in our experimental model.

There is little information on the functional modification of the responsiveness of microvessels to changes of perfusion pressure in hypertensive animals. Previous investigations have demonstrated that arterioles from the gracilis muscle in SHR exhibited a higher threshold for pressure-induced vasoconstriction than in WKY, indicating the shift of pressure-diameter relationship at arteriolar levels in the microcirculatory bed of skeletal muscle [26].

We recently characterized for the first time, in a controlled in vitro setting, the responsiveness of the renal microvessels to changes of RAP in kidneys from normotensive and hypertensive rats. Direct assessment of the microvascular response to elevated RAP suggests that the renal hemodynamic adaptation in hypertension involves an alteration in the responsiveness of the afferent arteriole. Thus, we observed a shift to the right in the pressure response curves of afferent arterioles in kidneys from SHR (Fig. 2). The threshold RAP that elicited a significant afferent arteriolar vasoconstriction was 20 mm Hg higher in SHR than in WKY. Furthermore, the pressure at which half maximum vasoconstrictor response was elicited was also shifted to a higher pressure level in SHR at every segment of the afferent arteriole (Fig. 2). In contrast, interlobular arteries exhibited no shift of pressure-diameter relationship in kidneys from hypertensive animals. Thus, our study indicates that the adaptive changes in the responsiveness of renal microvessels to changes of RAP in hypertensive animals is restricted to the afferent arteriole. To our knowledge, this finding constitutes the first direct demonstration that renal arteriolar behavior adapts to a higher pressure level in hypertensive animals.

Although our recent study clearly demonstrates a shift in the relationship between RAP and pressure-induced afferent arteriolar tone, an influence of pre-afferent arteriolar resistance cannot be ruled out. Sustained hypertension causes structural changes which could decrease vessel diameters and thus increase passive resistance of larger vessels [27]. Thus, a greater pressure drop in pre-afferent arteries may be responsible for the observed shift in the relationship between RAP and afferent arteriolar vasoconstriction in kidneys from SHR. However, as detailed elsewhere in this volume [25], we observed that hypertension alters the responsiveness of the interlobular artery in an entirely different manner, potentiating the response of the intermediate segment. The distal portions of the interlobular arteries that we examined exhibited no shift in pressure-induced response. Furthermore, the basal (i.e., at 80 mm Hg) vessel diameters of the interlobular artery were identical (WKY; 28.4 ± 1.6 vs. SHR; 27.3 ± 2.0 μm, $P > 0.5$). This latter observation tends to militate against a difference in luminal pressure in WKY and SHR arterioles.

Effects of Calcium Antagonists

Calcium antagonists have been demonstrated to abolish autoregulation both in isolated kidney preparations [28,29] and in intact animals [30,31]. In isolated renal interlobular arteries from the dog, Harder et al. have demonstrated that verapamil abolishes pressure-induced vascular tone [32]. In an attempt to directly characterize the effects of calcium antagonists on the renal microvascular response to pressure, we have examined the actions of nifedipine on pressure-induced afferent arteriolar vasoconstriction in WKY and SHR in isolated perfused hydronephrotic kidneys.

The effects of nifedipine on pressure-induced afferent arteriolar vasoconstriction in kidneys from WKY and SHR are depicted in Figs. 3 and 4. As depicted in Fig. 3, before administration of nifedipine, the afferent arteriole constricted in response to graded increases in RAP. In the presence of nifedipine (10^{-6} M), the pressure-induced afferent arteriolar vasoconstriction was completely abolished.

Figures 4a and 4b depict the effects of nifedipine on pressure-induced afferent arteriolar vasoconstriction in WKY (n=7) and SHR kidneys (n=6). As detailed

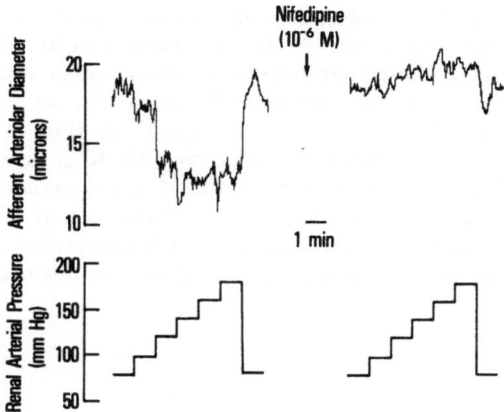

Fig. 3. Representative tracings depicting the effects of nifedipine on the pressure-induced vasoconstrictor response of an afferent arteriole in an isolated perfused kidney from SHR. In the absence of nifedipine, an increase in renal arterial pressure induced a pressure-dependent vasoconstriction (*left*). The addition of 10^{-6} M nifedipine to the perfusate abolished this response (*right*). (Reproduced from [16] by permission of the American Heart Association, Inc.)

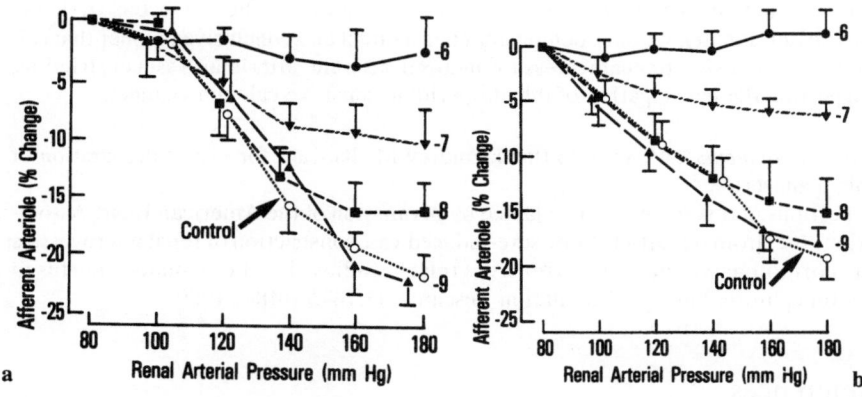

Fig. 4a,b. Effects of nifedipine on pressure-induced afferent arteriolar vasoconstriction in kidneys from Wistar Kyoto control (*WKY*) **a,** n=7 and Spontaneously hypertensive rat (*SHR*) **b,** n=6. In the absence of nifedipine (control, *open circle*), an increase in perfusion pressure induced a decrease in afferent arteriolar diameter. The addition of nifedipine to the perfusate inhibited the afferent arteriolar vasoconstriction in a dose-dependent manner (nifedipine concentrations depicted on *right* as log M). At 10^{-6} M, nifedipine completely abolished the response in both WKY (P>0.5) and SHR (P>0.1). Results are mean±SE. (Reproduced from [16] by permission of the American Heart Association Inc.)

above, in the absence of nifedipine, afferent arteriolar diameters decreased in both WKY and WHR as RAP was increased. The administration of 10^{-9} M–10^6 M of nifedipine did not alter basal afferent arteriolar diameters in either strain. Nevertheless, nifedipine markedly inhibited pressure-induced afferent arteriolar vasoconstriction in a dose dependent manner in both WKY (Fig. 4a) and SHR (Fig. 4b). The concentrations at which half maximal inhibition was observed, i.e. IC_{50}, were identical (WKY; 63 ± 27 nM vs. SHR; 60 ± 32 nM, $P > 0.5$). At 10^{-6} M, nifedipine completely abolished the pressure-induced afferent arteriolar vasoconstriction in both strains. In concert, these observations suggest the participation of dihydropyridine-sensitive calcium channels in mediating pressure-induced vasoconstriction of this microvessel.

Conclusions

It is evident that major strides have been made in characterizing the renal microvascular response to pressure. Utilizing diverse in vitro models, including the juxtamedullary nephron preparation and the isolated perfused hydronephrotic kidney, investigators have demonstrated that elevated pressure elicits afferent arteriolar vasoconstriction directly by a pressure-dependent (i.e., myogenic) mechanism, and indirectly by signals originating from the macula densa (i.e., TGF). Therefore, the available evidence suggest that both TGF-induced and myogenic vasoconstriction act in concert to mediate renal autoregulation. Furthermore, recent evidence indicates that hypertension is associated with a compensatory shift in the pressure response of the afferent arteriole, such that higher RAPs are required to elicit vasoconstriction in this vessel. Finally, we have demonstrated in a direct and conclusive manner that calcium antagonists attenuate pressure-induced afferent arteriolar vasoconstriction, suggesting the participation of dihydropyridine-sensitive calcium channels.

Acknowledgments. We wish to thank Audrey M. Kincaid for expert preparation of this manuscript.

Portions of this review were adapted by permission of the American Heart Association, Inc. from our article "Pressure-induced vasoconstriction of renal microvessels in normotensive and hypertensive rats: Studies in the isolated perfused hydronephrotic kidney", Circulation Research 65:1475–1484, 1989.

References

1. Goldblatt H, Lynch J, Hanzal RF, Sommerville WW (1934) Studies in experimental hypertension. The production of a persistent elevation of systolic blood pressure by means of renal ischemia. J Exp Med 59:347–379
2. Folkow B, Hallback M, Lundgred Y, Sivertson R, Weiss L (1973) Importance of adaptive changes in vascular design for establishment of primary hypertension, studied in man and in spontaneously hypertensive rats. Circ Res 32:2–16
3. Mulvany MJ, Hansen PK, Aalkjaer C (1978) Direct evidence that the greater contractility of resistance vessels in spontaneously hypertensive rats is associated with a narrowed lumen, a thickened media, and an increased number of smooth muscle cell layers. Circ Res 43:854–864

4. MacKay A, Brown JJ, Lever AF (1983) Unilateral renal disease in hypertension. In: Roberson JIS (ed) Handbook of hypertension, vol 2: Clinical aspects of secondary hypertension. Elsevier, Amsterdam, pp 33–78
5. Iversen BM, Sekse I, Ofstad J (1987) Resetting of renal blood flow autoregulation in spontaneously hypertensive rats. Am J Physiol 252:F480–F486
6. Roman RJ, Cowley AW Jr (1985) Abnormal pressure-diuresis-natriuresis response in spontaneously hypertensive rats. Am J Physiol 248:F199–F205
7. Roman RJ (1987) Altered pressure-natriuresis relationship in young spontaneously hypertensive rats. Hypertension 9 (Suppl III):130–136
8. Aukland K, Øien AH (1987) Renal autoregulation:models combining tubuloglomerular feedback and myogenic response. Am J Physiol 252:F768–F783
9. Lush DJ, Fray JCS (1984) Steady-state autoregulation of renal blood flow: a myogenic model. Am J Physiol 247:R89–R99
10. Click RL, Joyner WL, Gilmore JP (1979) Reactivity of glomerular afferent and efferent arterioles in renal hypertension. Kidney Int 15:109–115
11. Loutzenhiser R, Epstein M (1990) Renal hemodynamic effects of calcium antagonists. In: Epstein M, Loutzenhiser R (eds) Calcium antagonists and the kidney. Hanley and Belfus, Philadelphia, pp 33–75
12. Epstein M, Flamenbaum W, Loutzenhiser R (1980) Characterization of the renin-angiotensin system in the isolated perfused rat kidney. Renal Physiol 2:244–256
13. Sanchez-Ferrer CF, Roman RJ, Harder DR (1989) Pressure-dependent contraction of rat juxtamedullary afferent arterioles. Circ Res 64:790–798
14. Moore LC (1984) Tubuloglomerular feedback and SNGFR autoregulation in the rat. Am J Physiol 247:F267–F276
15. Carmines PK, Inscho EW, Gensure RC (1990) Arterial pressure effects on preglomerular microvasculature of juxtamedullary nephrons. Am J Physiol 258:F94–F102
16. Hayashi K, Epstein M, Loutzenhiser R (1989) Pressure-induced vasoconstriction of renal microvessels in normotensive and hypertensive rats: Studies in the isolated perfused hydronephrotic kidney. Circ Res 65:1475–1484
17. Fleming JT, Garthoff B, Mayer D, Rosen B, Steinhausen M (1987) Comparison of the effects of antihypertensive drugs on pre- and postglomerular vessels of the hydronephrotic kidney. J Cardiovasc Pharmacol 10(Suppl 10):S149–S153
18. Steinhausen M, Fleming JT, Holz FG, Parekh N (1987) Nitrendipine and the pressure-dependent vasodilation of vessels in the hydronephrotic kidney. J Cardiovasc Pharmacol 9(Suppl 1):S39–S43
19. Carmines PK (1989) Responses of the renal microvasculature to changes in renal arterial pressure (abstract). FASEB J M19:A1381
20. Schnermann J, Briggs J (1985) Function of the juxtaglomerular apparatus; local control of glomerular hemodynamics. In: Seldin DW, Giebisch G (eds) The kidney: physiology and pathology, vol 1. Raven, New York, pp 669–697
21. Navar LG, Marsh DL, Blantz RC, Hall J, Ploth DW, Nasjletti A (1982) Intrinsic control of renal hemodynamics. Fed Proc 41:3022–3030
22. Øien AH, Aukland K (1983) A mathematical analysis of the myogenic hypothesis with special reference to autoregulation of renal blood flow. Circ Res 52:241–252
23. Tønder KJH, Aukland K (1979) Interlobular arterial pressure in the rat kidney. Renal Physiol 80;2:214–221
24. Källskog Ö, Lindbom LO, Ulfendahl HR, Wolgast M (1976) Hydrostatic pressure within the vascular structures of the rat kidney. Pflügers Arch 363:205–210
25. Hayashi K, Epstein M, Loutzenhiser R (1991) Role of the interlobular (ILA) in protection against glomerular barotrauma in hypertension (abstract). Proceedings of the XIth International Congress of Nephrology, July 15–20 1990. Tokyo, Japan
26. Alson RL, Dusseau JW, Hutchins PM (1985) Arteriolar and systemic autoregulatory

responses during the development of hypertension in the spontaneously hypertensive rats. Proc Soc Exp Biol Med 180:62–71

27. Heptinstall RH (1983) Pathology of the kidney, vol 1, 3rd edn. Little, Brown, Boston, pp 181–246

28. Ono H, Kokubun H, Hashimoto K (1974) Abolition by calcium antagonists of the autoregulation of renal blood flow. Naunyn Schmiedebergs Arch Pharmacol 285:201–207

29. Cohen AJ, Fray JCS (1982) Calcium ion dependence of myogenic renal plasma flow autoregulation: evidence from the isolated perfused rat kidney. J Physiol 330:449–460

30. Lin H, Young DB (1988) Verapamil alters the relationship between renal perfusion pressure and glomerular filtration rate and renin release: The mechanism of the antihypertensive effect. J Cardiovasc Pharmacacol 12(Suppl 6):S57–S59

31. Navar LG, Champion WJ, Thomas CE (1986) Effects of calcium channel blockade on renal vascular resistance responses to changes in perfusion pressure and angiotensin-converting enzyme inhibition in dogs. Circ Res 58:874–881

32. Harder DR, Gilbert R, Lombard JH (1987) Vascular muscle cell depolarization and activation in renal arteries on elevation of transmural pressure. Am J Physiol 253:F778–F781

The Pathogenesis of Salt-Sensitive Hypertension

TOSHIRO FUJITA[1]

SUMMARY. Patients with normal plasma renin and essential hypertension can be divided into two groups according to blood pressure response to salt loading; salt-sensitive (SS) and non-salt-sensitive (NSS). With a high-sodium diet SS patients retained more sodium, and had a greater increase in cardiac output, as compared to NSS patients. Despite the markedly increased cardiac output, systemic vascular resistance did not change with sodium loads in the SS patients, suggesting inappropriately elevated systemic vascular resistance. The greater increase in blood pressure with sodium loads seems to be characterized by a very inhomogeneous distribution of local flow and resistance in SS patients; renal and hepatic blood flow remains essentially unchanged and skeletal muscle blood flow receives almost all of the increase in cardiac output. Moreover, systemic vascular resistance changes did not reflect the resistance of individual beds because vasoconstriction appeared in the kidney and in the splanchnic area but was masked by prominent vasodilation in the skeletal muscle. Because this hemodynamic pattern is similar to the pattern evoked during defense reaction, it is suggested that sympathetic overactivity on a selective basis might be involved in the impaired renal function for sodium excretion and the increase in blood pressure with sodium loads in SS patients.

Introduction

It is widely believed that excessive sodium intake plays a role in the development of hypertension in man. Epidemiological studies have shown that the prevalence of hypertension in a population increases with the usual sodium intake of that population. Even in populations habitually consuming large amounts of sodium, however, 60% of the population remains free of hypertension, suggesting that some individuals are susceptible to the pressor effects of sodium while others are resistant.

[1]The Fourth Department of Internal Medicine, University of Tokyo School of Medicine, 3-28-6 Mejirodai, Bunkyo-ku, Tokyo, 112 Japan

In our previous studies [1–6], we found that patients with essential hypertension could be divided into two groups according to the blood-pressure response to salt load; salt-sensitive (SS) and non-salt-sensitive (NSS). On a high-salt diet, the salt-sensitive hypertensive patients retained more sodium and gained more weight, with greater increase in blood pressure, as compared to the non-salt-sensitive patients [1]. It seems that human hypertensive subjects show heterogeneous responses to sodium loading.

Systemic Hemodynamics in Patients with Salt-Sensitive Hypertension

In partially nephrectomized dogs, salt loading increases blood pressure, possibly by causing sodium retention. During the early period of salt loading, cardiac output increases, but later, systemic vascular resistance increases in association with the restoration of cardiac output. Although the precise mechanism for the increased vascular resistance with salt loading is still unknown, Guyton et al. [7] postulated that total body autoregulation might contribute to an increase in vascular resistance during exposure to salt and water in excess.

Cardiac output increased with salt loading in all patients, but the extent of the increase was significantly greater in the salt-sensitive patients than in the non-salt-sensitive ones. The elevation of blood pressure with salt loading in the salt-sensitive patients may be partly due to the increased cardiac output, possibly caused by sodium retention [1,6].

With increased cardiac output, the non-salt-sensitive patients had significantly decreased systemic vascular resistance with salt loading. In contrast, systemic vascular resistance remained unchanged with salt loading in the salt-sensitive patients, in spite of the pronounced increase in cardiac output. In the salt-sensitive patients, the fall in peripheral resistance was not adequate to maintain pressure hemeostasis when the magnitude of the increase in cardiac output with salt loading was relatively greater than in the non-salt-sensitive patients.

In another study [5], we investigated sodium susceptibility and hemeodynamics in young patients with borderline hypertension, since young borderline hypertensives are at least three times more likely to develop established essential hypertension than are age-matched normotensive subjects. After a period of sodium depletion with a diuretic, short-term sodium loading caused blood pressure to increase significantly in a group of young subjects with borderline hypertension but not in a group of normal subjects of comparable age, sex, and body weight.

Hemodynamic responses of borderline hypertensives to sodium loads after sodium depletion showed increased cardiac output, while in the normal subjects cardiac output did not change significantly. Calculated systemic vascular resistance did not change in either group. The blood pressure of borderline hypertensives was associated with an apparent increase in cardiac output and with inappropriately elevated systemic vascular resistance. Further, we divided thirty-four borderline hypertensives into two groups, according to blood-pressure responses to salt loads. Of the 34 borderline hypertensives 14 salt-sensitive patients had greater increases in cardiac output with salt loading than did the 20 non-salt-sensitive patients. With increased cardiac output, the non-salt-sensitive patients had significantly decreased

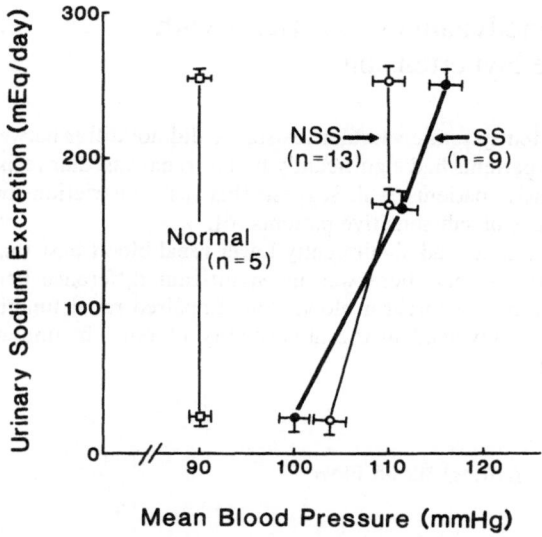

Fig. 1. Renal function curve in salt-sensitive (*SS*) and non-salt-sensitive (*NSS*) patients

systemic vascular resistance with salt loading. In contrast, systemic vascular resistance remained unchanged with salt loading in the salt-sensitive patients, which is consistent with the hemodynamic pattern in salt-sensitive essential hypertensive patients. Salt-induced elevation of blood pressure in the salt-sensitive patients with both borderline and established hypertension might be due to a disproportionate increase in cardiac output and inadequate fall in systemic vascular resistance.

Impaired Renal Function in Patients with Salt-Sensitive Hypertension

During salt loading, the salt-sensitive patients excreted less sodium in the urine than did the non-salt-sensitive patients. The salt-sensitive patients retained more sodium than did the other patients. In fact, the extent of the increases in plasma volume and body weight was significantly greater in the salt-sensitive patients than in the non-salt-sensitive patients [1,6].

Guyton et al. postulated that the blood pressure/urinary sodium excretion curve for the kidney of hypertensive subjects is shifted to the right, with a decreased slope [7]. Renal function curves of both salt-sensitive and non-salt-sensitive patients were shifted to the right, as compared to those of normotensive subjects (Fig. 1). However, the slope of the renal function curve for the kidney of salt-sensitive patients apparently decreased as compared with that of the non-salt-sensitive patients.

There was no significant difference in blood pressure, nor in creatinine clearance, between the two groups. Salt-sensitive patients have impaired renal function for sodium excretion, despite having normal glomerular filtration rates.

Regional Hemodynamics in Patients with Salt-Sensitive Hypertension

Although calculated systemic vascular resistance did not differ between the groups, the salt-sensitive patients had significantly higher renal vascular resistance than did the non-salt-sensitive patients. This suggests that vasoconstriction appeared specifically in the kidneys of salt-sensitive patients [6].

Salt-sensitive patients had significantly lower renal blood flow than did the non-salt-sensitive patients, but there was no significant difference between the two groups in hepatic nor in forearm blood flow. Impaired renal function for sodium excretion might be involved in the abnormality of renal hemodynamics in salt-sensitive patients.

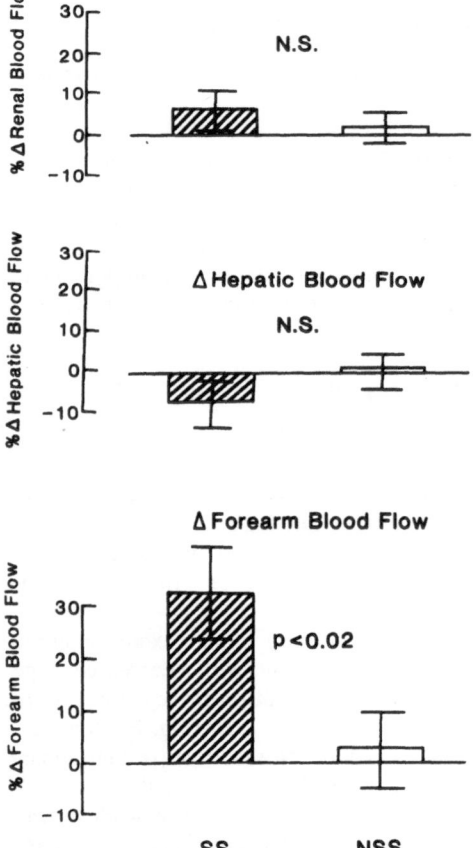

Fig. 2. Changes in renal, hepatic, and forearm blood flow with sodium loads in salt-sensitive (*SS*) and non-salt-sensitive (*NSS*) patients with hypertension. N.S., not significant

Although many extrarenal factors regulate renal vascular tone and change renal function in sodium excretion, neural mechanisms may play an important role in the control of renal sodium handling.

In our first study [1], we demonstrated that patients with salt-sensitive hypertension had inappropriately high levels of plasma norepinephrine during sodium loading, compared with the non-salt-sensitive hypertensive patients, thus suggesting that the persistence of autonomic "drive" in the sodium-loaded patients with salt-sensitive hypertension contributed to the relative sodium retention with sodium loads and to the increase in blood pressure.

In general, autonomic activation in essential hypertension is regional rather general, so that the measurement of total plasma norepinephrine and tests for generalized activation are inadequate. In our recent study [6], therefore, we measured regional blood flows in order to further assess changes in sympathetic nerve activity with salt loading in individual vascular beds.

We measured changes in renal, hepatic, and forearm blood flows with salt loading in the two groups [6]. Renal and hepatic blood flows remained essentially unchanged in both groups. In contrast, skeletal muscle blood flow increased profoundly in the salt-sensitive patients, and it received almost all of the increase in cardiac output (Fig. 2). Therefore, the greater increase in blood pressure with sodium loads seems to be characterized by a very inhomogeneous distribution of local flow and resistance in salt-sensitive patients.

Despite unchanged systemic vascular resistance, a high salt intake in salt-sensitive patients was associated with increases in hepatic and renal vascular resistances but with a decrease in forearm vascular resistance. This result suggests that analysis of systemic vascular resistance alone is inadequate for understanding the vascular changes that take place during elevation of blood pressure with sodium loading.

In this hemodynamic study, vasoconstriction appeared in the kidney and in the splanchnic area but, in salt-sensitive patients, vasoconstriction was masked by prominent vasodilation in skeletal muscle. Since this hemodynamic pattern is similar to the pattern evoked during defense reaction, in which sympathetic activity is selectively increased in the kidney and splanchnic area, this hemodynamic pattern might be involved in the impaired renal function for sodium excretion and blood pressure elevation which occurs with sodium loading in salt-sensitive patients [6].

The Antihypertensive Effect of Potassium in Salt-Sensitive Rats

A dietary potassium supplement is antihypertensive in animals and in humans, and protects against the hypertensinogenic effects of excessive dietary sodium. In our previous study [8], a high sodium diet for 4 weeks significantly increased blood pressure in salt-sensitive young spontaneously hypertensive rats (SHR). However, although potassium supplementation attenuated the elevation of blood pressure with the sodium loading, potassium had little effect on blood pressure in normal sodium-SHR.

The blood pressure/urinary sodium excretion curve for the kidneys of young SHR was shifted to the right and its slope apparently decreased as compared with that of Wistar Kyoto (WKY) control rats (Fig. 3). However, potassium supplements restored the slope toward normal, suggesting that potassium could normalize the increased salt-sensitivity of blood pressure in young SHR.

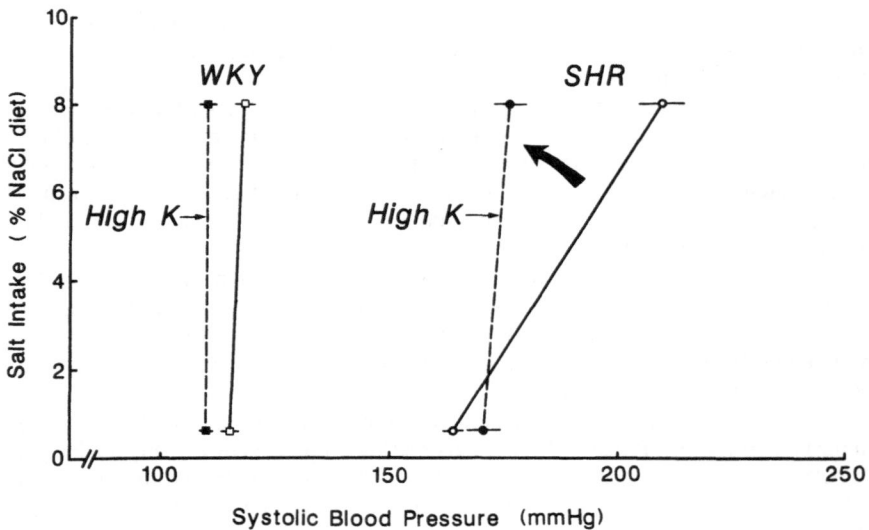

Fig. 3. Effects of potassium supplements on pressure-renal sodium excretion relationship in 5-week spontaneously hypertensive rats (*SHR*) and age-matched control Wistar-Kyoto rats (*WKY*) [8]

In the study of renal hemodynamics, sodium loads significantly increased renal vascular resistance in SHR, as was observed in salt-loaded patients with salt-sensitive hypertension. However, potassium supplementation attenuated the increased renal vascular resistance of salt-loaded SHR, although it did not affect renal vascular resistance in normal sodium-SHR. The salt-induced increase in renal vascular resistance, which might be intimately related to the impaired renal sodium handling, appears to be involved in the increased salt-sensitivity in young SHR.

Similar findings for potassium effects were observed in rats with desoxycorticosterone acetate (DOCA)-salt hypertension, another salt-sensitive model [9–11]. Salt loading increased blood pressure in DOCA-treated rats. However, the supplementation of potassium attenuated the development of hypertension in DOCA-salt rats.

From the data for cumulative sodium retention, it was found that potassium supplementation, as a result of natriuresis, attenuated the increase in the amount of sodium retained throughout the experimental period in DOCA-salt rats. We evaluated the effect of potassium supplementation on the blood pressure/urinary sodium excretion curve for the kidney of DOCA-salt rats. The slope of the renal function curve for DOCA-salt rats apparently decreased, with shifting, but potassium restored it toward normal (Fig. 4).

To further evaluate the role of renal sympathetic activity in the impaired sodium-excreting ability of the kidneys of DOCA-salt rats [11] and salt-sensitive SHR [12], the tissue norepinephrine turnover rate was measured in vivo by using alpha-methyl-p-tyrosine, an inhibitor of catecholamine synthesis. Norepinephrine turnover in the kidneys of DOCA-salt rats was significantly accelerated compared to that in control rats, but potassium supplement normalized this turnover [11,12]. According to

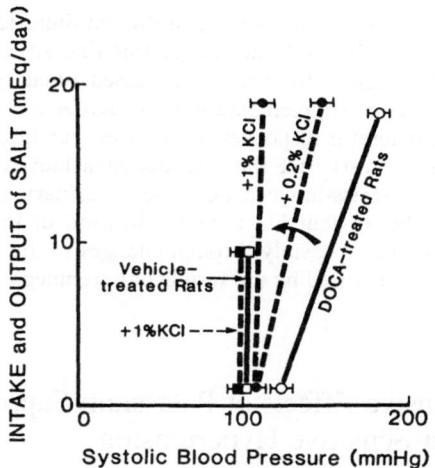

Fig. 4. Effects of potassium supplements on pressure-renal sodium excretion relationship in DOCA-salt treated rats. Potassium restored the decreased slope of the renal function curve toward normal but did not affect the curve in control vehicle-treated rats. DOCA, desoxycorticosterone acetate

changes in renal norepinephrine turnover, moreover, hypothalamic norepinephrine turnover, on exposure to cold, was markedly accelerated in salt-sensitive hypertensive animals, but the potassium supplement normalized this turnover [12]. The normalization of increased renal sympathetic activity, which is intimately related to central noradrenergic mechanisms, may be involved in the natriuretic and antihypertensive actions of potassium in salt-sensitive hypertensive animals [11,12].

Effects of Air Stress on Urinary Sodium Excretion in Salt-Sensitive Hypertensive Rats

Recently, Anderson reported that the combination of avoidance-conditioning tasks and saline infusion for 2 weeks could increase blood pressure in intact dogs, but blood pressure remained unchanged on an avoidance schedule or on saline infusion alone, indicating a significant interaction between environmental stress and dietary sodium in renal sodium handling and the development of hypertension [13]. We then studied the interaction of mental stress and dietary sodium and potassium in salt-sensitive hypertension.

To clarify the neural mechanisms for the antihypertensive and natriuretic actions of potassium in salt-sensitive hypertension, we studied the effects of potassium supplementation on urinary sodium excretion and renal function responses to a stressful environmental stimulus, air stress, in DOCA-salt rats (Y. Sato et al., manuscript in preparation).

In conscious DOCA-salt rats, air stress decreased urine flow rate and urinary sodium excretion, but in normotensive sham-operated rats air stress had no effects on these parameters. Renal denervation abolished the antidiuretic and antinatriuretic responses to air stress in DOCA-salt rats, suggesting that air stress decreased urinary sodium excretion, possibly by causing increased renal sympathetic activity. Correspondingly, potassium supplementation in DOCA-salt rats attenuated the antidiuretic and antinatriuretic responses to air stress, as in the renal-denervated DOCA-salt rats. This suggests that the attenuation achieved by potassium supplementation of the air stress-induced decrease in urinary sodium excretion in DOCA-salt rats might be attributable to normalization of the increased sympathetic activity in the kidney, possibly through changes in the central nervous system. This hypothesis is supported by the results of norepinephrine turnover studies [11,12].

The Antihypertensive Effects of Potassium Supplementation in Patients with Salt-Sensitive Hypertension

Salt loading after low sodium diets increased blood pressure in patients with essential hypertension. However, potassium supplementation during a high sodium diet period showed a lesser elevation of blood pressure with sodium loading than in the potassium-untreated group [14]. Potassium may counteract the pressor actions of dietary sodium in patients with salt-sensitive hypertension. In our previous studies [1,6], salt-sensitive patients had decreased urinary sodium excretion during high sodium diets, as compared to the non-salt-sensitive patients, but potassium supplementation promoted urinary sodium excretion in these hypertensive subjects with impaired renal sodium handling. Sodium retained during salt loading was attenuated by potassium supplementation. Correspondingly, potassium supplementation inhibited the increase in plasma volume with sodium loads. Moreover, potassium attenuated the salt-induced increase in cardiac output.

Further, we measured plasma norepinephrine in order to estimate sympathetic activity, since the sympathetic nervous system is known to control urinary sodium excretion. From the low sodium diet to Day 3 of the high sodium diet, plasma norepinephrine decreased significantly in the potassium-supplemented patients, but it remained unchanged in the non-potassium-supplemented patients. Concurrently, the heart rate of the potassium-supplemented patients decreased significantly in the early period of salt loading.

Concomitantly, in the potassium-supplemented group, as compared to the other group, urinary sodium excretion was significantly greater in the early period of salt loading. Moreover, there was a significant negative correlation between the degree of the decrease in plasma norepinephrine concentration from the end of the low sodium diet to the 3rd day of the high sodium diet and the amount of urinary sodium excretion in the early period of salt loading.

Taken together, these data suggest that potassium supplementation could shift the renal function curve toward normal, partly by inducing decreased sympathetic nerve activity in the kidney, which would result in natriuresis (Fig. 5).

Finally, we evaluated the antihypertensive effects of potassium when the potassium-supplemented patients were divided into two groups. The antihypertensive effect of potassium was greater in five salt-sensitive patients than in six non-salt-

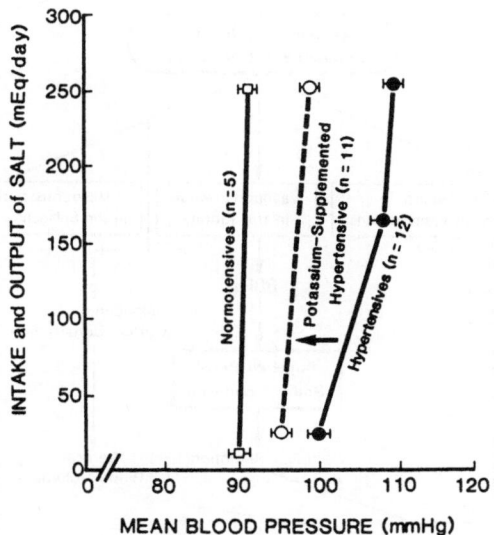

Fig. 5. Effects of potassium supplements on pressure-renal sodium excretion relationship in hypertensives

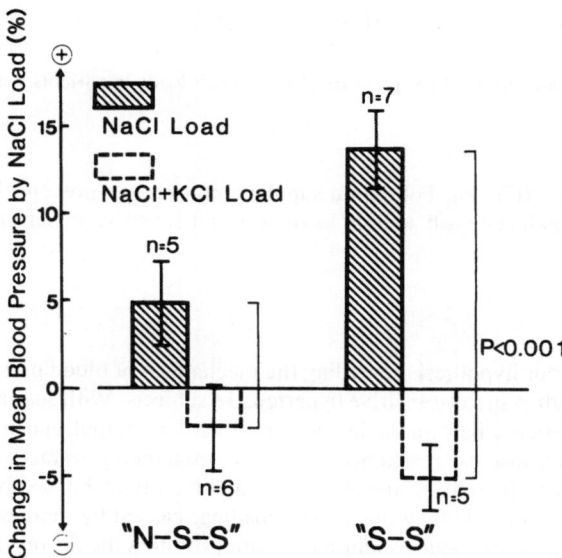

Fig. 6. Effects of potassium supplements on salt-loaded blood pressure increase in salt-sensitive (*SS*) and non-salt-sensitive (*NSS*) patients

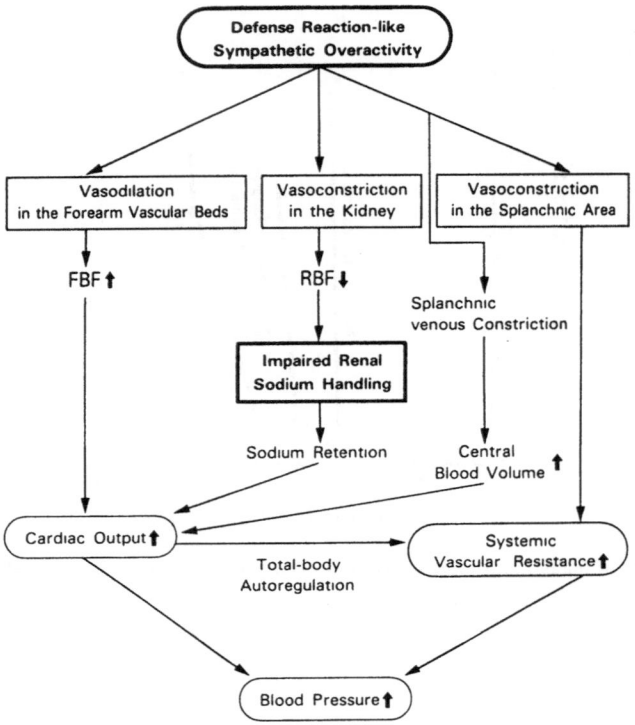

Fig. 7. The mechanism for blood-pressure rise with salt loads in patients with salt-sensitive hypertension

sensitive patients (Fig. 6). Potassium supplementation can prevent the increase in blood pressure induced with sodium loading in salt-sensitive hypertensive subjects.

Conclusion

Figure 7 shows our hypothesis regarding the mechanism of blood pressure elevation with sodium loading in salt-sensitive hypertensive subjects. With sodium loading, the salt-sensitive patients had markedly increased cardiac output and inappropriately elevated systemic vascular resistance, in which sympathetic overactivity on a selective basis, similar to that of the defense reaction, might be involved. Selective vasoconstriction in the kidney during salt loading, caused by increased renal sympathetic activity, may produce sodium retention, through the decreased slope of the renal function curve for sodium excretion, leading to increased cardiac output. In contrast, sympathetic nerve activity, which can readily be lowered by salt loading in the non-salt-sensitive patients, causes natriuresis through renal vasodilation. Vasoconstriction in the splanchnic bed during salt loading may contribute to the rise in blood pressure, not only by increased vascular resistance but also by increased cardiac output, through increased central blood volume via splanchnic venous constriction. In contrast to the renal and hepatic vasoconstriction, prominent vasodilation occurred in muscle blood flow in salt-loaded SS patients; this might contribute to the profound increase in cardiac output through a faster average venous return to the heart by means of the shorter time constant pathway, suggesting that, with sodium loading in the SS patients, skeletal muscle blood flow maintains high cardiac output. Not only this selective sympathetic overactivity, but also autoregulation in the setting might represent a response to the inappropriately high blood flow produced by increases in blood volume and cardiac output, resulting in increased vascular resistance during exposure to salt and water in excess. Because our study was a short-term one that did not include serial measurements of hemodynamic parameters, we could not examine the possibility of total body autoregulation as postulated by Guyton and his group [7].

Finally, an altered dietary sodium to potassium ratio may have possible significance in the development of hypertension. The high sodium-low potassium environment of civilized people, operating on a genetic substrate of susceptibility, is the cardinal factor in the genesis and perpetuation of 'essential hypertension'. Moreover, there is significant interaction between environmental stress and dietary sodium and potassium in renal sodium handling and the development of hypertension.

References

1. Fujita T, Henry WL, Bartter FC, Lake CR, Delea CS (1980) Factors influencing blood pressure in salt-sensitive patients with hypertension. Am J Med 69:334–344
2. Fujita T, Ando K, Noda H, Sato Y, Yamashita N, Yamashita K (1982) Hemodynamic and endocrine changes associated with captopril in diuretic-resistant hypertensive patients. Am J Med 73:341–347
3. Fujita T, Sato Y, Ando K (1983) Role of sympathetic nerve activity and natriuresis in the antihypertensive actions of potassium in NaCl hypertension. Jpn Circ J 47:1227–1231
4. Ando K, Fujita T, Ito Y, Noda H, Yamashita K (1986) The role of renal hemodynamics in the antihypertensive effects of captopril. Am Heart J 111:347–352
5. Fujita T, Noda H, Ando K (1984) Sodium susceptibility and potassium effects in young patients with borderline hypertension. Circulation 69:468–476
6. Fujita T, Ando K, Ogata E (1990) Systemic and regional hemodynamics in patients with salt-sensitive hypertension. Hypertension 16:235–244
7. Guyton AC, Coleman TG, Cowley AE, Scheeel KW, Manning RD, Norman RA (1972) Arterial pressure regulation: Overriding dominance of the kidneys in long-term regulation and in hypertension. 52:584–594
8. Sato Y, Ando K, Ogata E, Fujita T (to be published) High potassium diet attenuates salt-induced acceleration of hypertension in SHR. Am J Physiol
9. Fujita T, Sato Y (1983) Natriuretic and antihypertensive effects of potassium in DOCA-salt hypertensive rats. 24:731–739
10. Fujita T, Sato Y (1984) Changes in renal and central noradrenergic activity with potassium in DOCA-salt rats. 246:F670–F675
11. Sato Y, Fujita T (1984) Suppression of renal sympathetic activity with potassium supplement in DOCA-salt rats. Jpn Heart J 25:253–261
12. Sato Y, Ogata E, Fujita T (to be published) High potassium diet attenuates salt-induced acceleration of renal and hypothalamic norepinephrine turnover in young SHR. Hypertension

13. Anderson DE, Murphy P, Kearns WD (1983) Progressive hypertension via avoidance conditioning and saline infusion in the dog. Hypertension 5:286–293
14. Fujita T, Ando K (1984) Hemodynamic and endocrine changes associated with potassium supplementation in sodium-loaded hypertensives. Hypertension 6:184–192

Ion Transport Abnormalities in the Development of Hypertension

GIUSEPPE BIANCHI, DANIELE CUSI[1], PATRIZIA FERRARI,
MARIA GRAZIA TRIPODI, and BARRY BARBER[2]

During the last decade mechanisms of ion transport across the cell membrane have been studied by many investigators interested in arterial hypertension [1–4], because ion transport is fundamental in the regulation of body fluids, renal function, hormone secretion and activity, nerve activity, etc. So far, many abnormalities of various ion transport systems have been described in hypertensive rats and in men with "hereditary" forms of hypertension. Such abnormalities regarding Na-K cotransport [5–7], Na/Li countertransport [6,8–10], Na/H countertransport [11,12], Na-K pump [13], passive permeability or leak [14], Ca pump [15], Ca channels [16] etc. have been reported in the literature. Therefore, theoretically, an abnormality of ion transport might be involved in the pathogenesis of "hereditary" or "primary" forms of hypertension.

Instead of discussing all the experimental data so far collected on this issue, we would prefer to discuss in detail one of these ion transport abnormalities, namely the Na-K cotransport, in order to evaluate the problems to be solved before we can say whether or not a given ion transport abnormality is useful in the detection of the genes responsible for hereditary forms of hypertension. The reasons for this choice should be clear. In fact, in our present state of knowledge, we do not know whether abnormalities in ion transport are directly linked to the genetic causes of hereditary forms of hypertension, or whether they are just epiphenomena with no relevance to the genetic mechanisms of hypertension. This distinction is obviously crucial in establishing the role and the importance of these transport systems, which will lead toward understanding the pathogenesis of hypertension. The problems to be considered include:

1) Differences in the methodological approaches used to measure ion transport systems. For instance, some workers have measured outward ion transport and others

[1]University of Milan, Nephrology and Hypertension Unit, Department of Science and Biomedical Technology, Ospedale San Raffaele, Via Olgettina 60, Milan, Italy

[2]Prassis, Research Institute, Via Forlanini 1/3, Settimo Milanese, Milan, Italy

have measured inward ion transport, without considering that the same molecular mechanism may be involved, differently, in both modes of transport [17].

2) A variety of environmental or physiological variables can, per se, affect these ion transport systems; the influence of such variables has been considered in only very few publications [18,19].

3) In many of these studies, ion transport systems were measured in erythrocytes, on the assumption that the functional pattern is similar to that in the plasma membrane of the cells (renal, vascular, nervous) more directly involved in blood pressure regulation. However, for most of the ion transport systems, there is no real experimental basis for this assumption.

4) Differences may be found in opposite directions among different individual patients and different rat strains. For instance, the rate of Na-K cotransport in hypertensive patients or rat strains may be either similar to, lower than, or higher than that in their normotensive controls [6,20,21].

5) It is not clear whether the differences in ion transport are directly linked to the primary molecular genetic mechanisms, or whether these differences are just the expression of secondary efforts to re-establish a cellular ion homeostasis after cellular dysfunction that has been caused by another genetic-molecular mechanism far from those directly involved in the ion transport systems. Even though both possibilities may occur in nature, this distinction is crucial for establishing the usefulness of these ion transport system abnormalities for the detection of gene or gene product candidates for genetic forms of hypertension.

6) Even though there is general agreement about the multifactorial nature of human primary hypertension, there are no precise and accepted clinical or biochemical criteria for sub-classification of the overall population of patients into distinct clinical entities with distinct and specific pathogenetic mechanisms. Therefore, we do not know whether the variability of the different patients mentioned in point 4 is due to our inability to classify them correctly or whether it is just an expression of epiphenomena not closely related to the primary pathogenetic mechanisms.

All of this suggests to us that the most productive way to find a clear answer to these problems is to use animal models of primary hypertension in which the genetic and environmental backgrounds can be properly evaluated, in order to understand how abnormal cotransport is linked to both the primary genetic molecular mechanisms and to the other cellular or organic dysfunctions which we believe to be the cause of hypertension. Since the ion transport systems of the MHS and SHR strains of rats are the most widely studied, we shall consider these two strains first.

Na-K cotransport measured in washed MHS erythrocytes is faster than in MNS erythrocytes [21]. This has been confirmed by another group of investigators [22] using slightly different methods, but with rats supplied from our breeding colony. Kinetic studies showed that the Km for internal Na is lower for MHS than for MNS, while the Vmax is similar for both strains [23,24]. The MHS erythrocyte is smaller than the MNS erythrocyte [21]. In renal vesicles prepared from the luminal membrane of the ascending limb [25], or in cultured vascular smooth muscle cells [26], Na-K cotransport is faster in MHS than MNS. Therefore, the assumption that there is widespread abnormality of the same ion transport system in erythrocytes and in the cells more directly involved in blood pressure regulation may be considered as proven, at least for the MHS strain.

When the Na-K cotransport of SHR was compared with that of WKY, conflicting results were obtained. Rosati et al. [20] found decreased cotransport affinity for internal Na in the erythrocytes of SHR, with a consequent decrease in Na-K cotransport, measured as bumetanide sensitive sodium efflux within the physiological ranges of intracellular sodium. On the other hand, Orlov et al. [22] found increased Na-K cotransport, measured as furosemide-sensitive ^{86}Rb influx, in SHR erythrocytes. Others have also found more active Na-K cotransport in the erythrocytes of SHR than in those of WKY [27,28]. It is not possible to say whether these discrepancies are due to differences in the methodology or to the genetic heterogeneity of the WKY strains, which would affect comparisons of WKY and SHR rats carried out in different Institutions using different commercial rat suppliers [29]. Conflicting results were also obtained for cultured vascular smooth muscle cell Na-K cotransport from SHR and from WKY rats [30,31]. Therefore, at this time, it is not possible to know whether the abnormality of Na-K cotransport is the same in erythrocytes and in vascular or renal tubular cells of SHR, even though a more uniform picture seems to be demonstrable for other cell membrane abnormalities in Ca or Na handling [1]. However, the question of the genetic heterogeneity of the different WKY substrains casts serious doubt on the validity of comparing the results obtained in different Institutions [29]. For these reasons, we shall not consider the results in SHR and WKY rats in the present discussion, which is aimed at comparing abnormalities in different types of cells. In fact, to our knowledge, there are no published results generated in the same Institution, with the same WKY substrain, in which different ion transports across different cell types are compared. This is a rather sad conclusion, in view of the tremendous amount of work that has so far been published on the variety of biochemical abnormalities in SHR.

For man there have been studies aimed at correlating abnormal transport rates across erythrocyte cell membranes with renal functional abnormalities [32,33] and some correspondences have been found, although at a much lower degree of precision than for rats. We shall discuss the Na-K cotransport in the last paragraph.

How Can a Faster Rate of Na-K Cotransport be Linked to the Organ Dysfunctions Involved in the Pathogenesis of Hypertension?

We have tried to answer this question as follows: in MHS, hypertension can be transplanted with the kidney [34–36], therefore the genetic message responsible for it may be transmitted through modification of renal function. When studied in vitro, isolated kidneys of MHS showed faster Na reabsorption and greater O_2 consumption than MNS kidneys [37,38]. Na transport across the luminal membrane was also faster in vesicles from proximal [39,40] or ascending portions of the tubules [25]. For the luminal membrane of the proximal tubules, faster Na transport seems to be mediated, at least in part, by the Na-H exchange pathway, while in the luminal membrane of the ascending limb, it is Na-K cotransport that is responsible for faster sodium transport [25]. This last conclusion is also supported by the results of comparisons of the diuretic effects of bumetanide, hydrochlorothiazide and amiloride in kidneys isolated from MHS and MNS. Na excretion after bumetanide is higher in MHS than in

MNS kidneys or in MHS kidneys given the other two diuretics [41]. The key role of Na-K cotransport in the transmission of the signal into the macula densa cells for generation of the tubulo-glomerular feedback mechanism is supported by much experimental data [42]. When measured in MHS and MNS, the tubulo-glomerular feedback mechanism in MHS is depressed at the pre-hypertensive stage although it is more active during the development of hypertension [43,44]. This depression at the pre-hypertensive stage in MHS is very likely due to increased renal interstitial pressure, which disappears during the development of hypertension, thus unmasking the underlying greater sensitivity of the feedback in MHS. The Na-K ATPase activity of isolated proximal tubules is also higher in MHS than in MNS [45]. Taken together, these findings are consistent with the notion that faster Na transport across the tubular epithelial cells is an important cause of hypertension in MHS and that an abnormality of Na-K cotransport may well be linked to the primary defect responsible for renal dysfunction.

The Possible Link Between Faster Na-K Cotransport and the Primary Genetic Mechanisms of Hypertension

This is certainly most relevant to today's discussion. A biochemical abnormality on a plasma membrane may be due to three different causes: 1) genetic, 2) environmental, 3) secondary readjustment through extracellular mechanisms (for instance, hormonal or other humoral changes) or intracellular ones. In order to differentiate between some of these mechanisms we transplanted bone marrow from MHS or MNS into (MHS × MNS) F_1 hybrids that had been previously irradiated to destroy their own bone marrow [46]. Erythrocyte volume was measured three months after transplantation and was found to be smaller in recipients of MHS bone marrow than in those that received MNS bone marrow. Also, the rate of Na-K cotransport was faster in MHS recipients. This clearly demonstrates that the genetic message responsible for faster Na-K cotransport and for the smaller volume of MHS erythrocytes was present in the stem cells, and that environmental factors or secondary readjustments through extracellular mechanisms are not responsible for these differences between MHS and MNS. Moreover, in F_2 hybrids, obtained by crossing the (MHS × MNS) F_1 hybrids, the rate of erythrocyte Na-K cotransport and the erythrocyte cell volume were correlated with the level of blood pressure, suggesting a genetic association between these traits [46]. However, these experiments do not exclude the possibility that faster Na-K cotransport might result from a readjustment of the cellular biochemical machinery. This readjustment would be aimed at re-establishing a cell homeostasis compatible with life, after a given mutation of a gene whose product is quite distant from the proteins directly involved in controlling Na-K cotransport. To evaluate this possibility we carried out a series of experiments which we shall summarize as follows: first of all, we wanted to see whether Na-K cotransport was still faster in inside out vesicles (IOV) prepared from MHS erythrocytes [47]. In these vesicles the transmembrane proteins responsible for ion translocation across the cell membrane should remain, while all the cytoplasm and the membrane skeleton proteins are removed. Na-K cotransport was similar for IOV prepared from MHS and MNS, and the Km for the internal site of Na on the Na-K cotransport system became similar for the two strains, excluding the possibility that transmembrane protein, by itself, was a possible cause of the differences between the intact erythrocytes [24]. Moreover, for resealed ghosts, in which the membrane skeleton is still present without the cytoplasmic component of the cell, the difference in cell volume between MHS and MNS remained [48]. This suggests that the membrane skeleton component may be involved in causing the overall cell dysfunction of MHS. With the aim of discovering possible differences in structural protein between MHS and MNS, we then injected extracts of erythrocyte membranes or membrane skeletons from MNS into MHS and vice-versa. After two immunizations, MNS recipients treated with MHS extract selectively produced an antibody against 105 KDa membrane skeleton protein. This protein was subsequently characterized as adducin [49].

Using this antibody, a cDNA library was screened and a clone was isolated. The study of the structure of the adducin gene is still in progress. However, we know almost ⅓ of the nucleotide sequence; the determination of such sequences in the MHS and MNS genes revealed a point mutation which was responsible for the coding of a glutamine (GLN) in place of an arginine (ARG) [50]. We had already noticed some degree of polymorphism in the MNS strain, but not in the MHS, in the antibody responses of the two strains to injection of antigen [49]. Evaluation of the genotypes also confirmed this phenomenon. Namely, all the MHS rats studied were ARG/ARG, while there were three MNS genotypes, ARG/ARG, ARG/GLN and GLN/GLN, suggesting that, in spite of close inbreeding for more than 50 generations, something had prevented achievement of homozygosis for the adducin locus in the normotensive strain. It should be noted that 11 other loci of MNS were homozygotic (Barber BR, personal communication). Theoretically there are four possible reasons for this selective heterozygosis at the adducin locus in the MNS inbred strain of animals:

1) homozygosis is lethal
2) homozygosis reduces biological fitness
3) mutation
4) selection for lower pressure favours heterozygosis

The first two reasons are not likely because we have animals homozygotic at the adducin locus and they show no differences from heterozygotic animals in body growth. Possibility No. 3 is also unlikely, because the difference in the antibody response was detected for the first time 4 years ago, and since then more than 10 generations have been obtained, with the maintenance of heterozygosis throughout these generations. Therefore, if a point mutation occurred without any relationship to the process of selection, we would expect its disappearance in the following generations. We are left with possibility No. 4 as the most likely one; first, by exclusion of the other three, second, because the blood pressure of rats with the genotype ARG/GLN is significantly lower than that of the rats of genotype ARG/ARG (Tripodi G, Piscone A, Ferrari P, Torielli L, Baralle T, Bianchi G, 1990, unpublished work). Also, the GLN/GLN genotype has slightly lower BP than the ARG/GLN genotype, even though the difference is not statistically significant (Tripodi G et al., 1990, unpublished work). There are major differences in ion transport systems and in BP between MHS and MNS. The mutation within the adducin gene, detected in MNS, may account for only minor differences in BP within this strain, and we do not yet know whether it may also account for minor differences in ion transport systems. However, we do not know whether or not other differences between MHS and MNS in the adducin gene might generate other adducin alleles that could be responsible for differences in blood pressure and ion transport much greater than those caused by the mutation studied so far.

This series of experiments was one attempt to establish a cause/effect relationship between a given alteration of a gene, membrane ion transport, and renal dysfunction responsible for increase in blood pressure. In our opinion, this body of knowledge can be used to approach our stated problem No. 4, that is, the meaning of ion transport system abnormalities in human essential hypertension. In fact, we have already shown that a subgroup of patients with essential hypertension had increased erythrocytic outward Na-K cotransport, increased renal Na excretion after furosemide, increased proximal reabsorption of urate (an index of proximal tubular reabsorption) [33], and lower plasma renin, with a greater blood pressure fall with diuretic compared to ACE inhibitors or β blockers, than other hypertensive patients or normal controls [51]. This overall clinical picture may well delineate a new nosologic entity with its own pathogenetic mechanisms. However, to prove the existence of this new clinical entity, we need to demonstrate that such biochemical, cell or organ dysfunctions are accompanied by precise genetic-molecular abnormalities which might explain such dysfunctions. Only by measuring all these factors (or the most important of them), in individual patients or subjects within a family tree, can we evaluate the genetic mode of transmission of a given ion transport system abnormality and its relevance to the determination of the blood pressure level. Indeed, the complexity of the interaction between the variety of genetic and environmental factors that may determine the level of blood pressure hampers attempts to study the mode of genetic transmission of this variable in an individual member of a family tree [52]. We might reduce the complexity of these factors by studying the genetics of ion transport systems as an intermediate phenotype. A better understanding of such an intermediate phenotype might help to dissect such complexity into relatively simpler systems [52]. The recent studies, by mixture analysis, of erythrocyte Li-Na countertransport [9] and blood pressure, or recent studies of the differences in Li-Na countertransport between "modulators" and "non-modulators" [53] are very helpful for drawing our attention to the importance of a particular ion transport system abnormality, in understanding the genetic and physiological mechanisms of hypertension. However, we must recognize that we are only at the start of a new avenue of research. This will give us meaningful results only if we take into consideration all the requirements for the approaching clarification of the role of genetic-molecular mechanisms in understanding the pathogenesis of complex diseases like arterial hypertension. In our opinion, the most important of these requirements is genetic homogeneity of the strain of animals used for these experiments. Only when the sequence of events from a given genetic abnormality to arterial hypertension has been clarified in animal models of primary hypertension, will we have the theoretical background to approach the enormous complexity of the relationship, in man, between the ion transport system and both the primary genetic-molecular abnormality and the cell dysfunction responsible for arterial hypertension.

Acknowledgments. The studies reported in this paper were supported in part by grants from the Ministry of Public Institutions, 1985–1989, (2-GB+DC), and by Research Grant on Hypertension from the Cassa di Risparmio delle Province Lombarde, Milano.

References

1. Postnov YV (1990) An approach to the explanation of cell membrane alteration in primary hypertension. Hypertension 15:332–337
2. Ives HE (1989) Ion transport defects and hypertension: Where is the link? Hypertension 14:590–597
3. Aviv A, Lasker N (1990) Proposed defects in membrane transport and intracellular ions as pathogenic factors in essential hypertension. In: Laragh, Brenner (eds) Hypertension: Pathophysiology, Diagnosis, and Management, vol 1. Raven, pp 923–937
4. Bianchi G (1986) Ion transport across blood cell membrane in essential hypertension. Curr Opin Cardiol 1:634–639
5. Garay RP, Dagher G, Pernolett MG, Dewynck MA, Meyer P (1980) Inherited defect in Na$^+$,K$^+$-cotransport system in erythrocyte from essential hypertensive patients. Nature 284:281–283
6. Cusi D, Barlassina C, Ferrandi M, Lupi GP, Ferrari P, Bianchi (1981) Familial aggregation of cation transport abnormalities and essential hypertension. Clin Exp Hypertens [A] 3:871–884
7. Canessa M, Spalvins A, Adragna N, Falkner B (1984) Red cell sodium countertransport and cotransport in normotensive and hypertensive blacks. Hypertension 6:344–351
8. Canessa M, Adragna N, Solomon HS, Connolly TM, Torteson D (1980) Increased sodium-lithium countertransport in red cells of patients with essential hypertension. N Engl J Med 302:772–776
9. Weder AB, Schork NJ (1989) Mixture analysis of erythrocyte lithium-sodium countertransport and blood pressure. Hypertension 2:145–150
10. Woods JW, Falk RJ, Pittman AW, Klemmer PJ, Watson BS, Namboodiri K (1982) Increased red cell sodium-lithium counter-transport in normotensive sons of hypertensive patients. N Engl J Med 306:593–595
11. Livne A, Balfe JW, Veitch R, Marquez-Julio A, Grinstein S, Rothstein A (1987) Increased platelet Na$^+$-H$^+$ exchange rates in essential hypertension: Application of a novel test. Lancet I:533–536
12. Semplicini A, Canessa M, Mozzato MG, Ceolotto G, Marzola M, Buzzaccarini F, Casolino P, Pessina AC (1989) Red blood cell Na$^+$/H$^+$ and Li$^+$/Na$^+$ exchange in patients with essential hypertension. Am J Hypertens 2:903–908
13. Diez J, Hannaert P, Garay R (1987) Kinetic study of Na$^+$-K$^+$ pump in erythrocytes from essential hypertensive patients. Am J Physiol 252:H1–H6
14. Garay RP, Nazaret C (1985) Na$^+$ leak in erythrocytes from essential hypertensive patients. Clin Sci 69:613–624
15. de la Sierra A, Hannaert P, Ollivier JP, Senn N, Garay R (1990) Kinetic study of the Ca^{2+} pump in erythrocytes from essential hypertensive patients. J Hypertens 3:285–293
16. Hermsmeyer K, Rusch N (1989): Calcium channel alterations in genetic hypertension. Hypertension 4:453–456
17. Canessa M, Brugnara C, Tosteson DC, Cusi D (1986) Modes of operation and variable stoichiometry of furosemide-sensitive Na and K fluxes in human red cells. J Gen Physiol 87:113–147
18. Canessa M, Brugnara C, Escobales N (1987) The Li$^+$-Na$^+$ exchange and Na$^+$-K$^+$-Cl$^-$ cotransport systems in essential hypertension. Hypertension 10:4–10
19. Adragna NC, Chang JL, Morey MC, Williams R (1985) Effect of exercise on cation transport in human red cells. Hypertension 7:132–139
20. Rosati C, Meyer P, Garay R (1988) Sodium transport kinetics in erythrocytes from spontaneously hypertensive rats. Hypertension 1:41–48
21. Ferrari P, Ferrandi M, Torielli L, Canessa M, Bianchi G (1987) Relationship between erythrocyte volume and sodium transport in the Milan hypertensive rat and age-dependent changes. J Hypertens 5:199–206

22. Orlov SN, Postnov IY, Pokudin NI, Kukharenko VY, Postnov YV (1989) Na⁺-H⁺ exchange and other ion-transport systems in erythrocytes of essential hypertensives and spontaneously hypertensive rats: a comparative analysis. J Hypertens 7:781–788

23. Ferrari P, Torielli M, Ferrandi M, Bianchi G (1988) The role of membrane skeleton in the alteration of Na-K cotransport (CO) in Milan hypertensive rats (MHS) (abstract) 12th scientific meeting of the International Society of Hypertension, May 22–26 1988. Kyoto, Japan

24. Ferrari P, Torielli L, Cirillo M, Salardi S, Bianchi G (to be published) Sodium transport kinetics in erythrocytes and inside-out vesicles from Milan rats.

25. Ferrandi M, Salardi S, Parenti P, Ferrari P, Bianchi G, Braw R, Karlish SJD (1990) Na⁺/K⁺/Cl⁻-cotransporter mediated Rb⁺ fluxes in membrane vesicles from kidneys of normotensive and hypertensive rats. BBA Biomembranes 1021:13–20

26. Socorro L, Vallega G, Nunn A, Moore TJ, Canessa M (1990) Vascular smooth muscle cells from the Milan hypertensive rat exhibit decreased functional angiotensin II receptors. Hypertension 15(part 1)

27. Feig PU, Mitchel PP, Boylan JW (1985) Erythrocyte membrane transport in hypertensive humans and rats: Effect of sodium depletion and excess. Hypertension 7:423–429

28. Duhm J, Göbel BO, Beck FX (1983) Sodium potassium ion transport accelerations in erythrocytes of DOC, DOC-salt, two kidney, one clip, and spontaneously hypertensive rats: Role of hypokalemia and cell volume. Hypertension 5:642–652

29. Kurtz TW, Montano M, Chan L, Kabra P (1989) Molecular evidence of genetic heterogeneity in Wistar-Kyoto rats: Implications for research with spontaneously hypertensive rat. Hypertension 13:188–192

30. Tokushige A, Kino M, Tamura H, Hopp L, Searle BM, Aviv A (1986) Bumetide-sensitive sodium-22 transport in vascular smooth muscle cell of the spontaneously hypertensive rat. Hypertension 8:379–385

31. O'Donnel ME, Owen NE (1988) Reduced Na-K-Cl cotransport in vascular smooth muscle cells from spontaneously hypertensive rats. Am J Physiol 255 (Cell Physiol 24):C169–C180

32. Weder AB (1986) Red-cell lithium-sodium countertransport and renal lithium clearance in hypertension. N Engl J Med 314:198–201

33. Cusi D, Barlassina C, Tripodi G, Alberghini E, Pozzoli E, Stella P, Bianchi G (to be published) Mixture analysis of erythrocyte Na-K cotransport and Li-Na countertransport in essential hypertension. Am J Hypertens

34. Bianchi G, Fox U, Di Francesco G.F, Bardi U, Radice M (1973) The hypertensive role of the kidney in spontaneously hypertensive rats. Clin Sci Mol Med, 45(Suppl I):135S–139S

35. Bianchi G, Fox U, Di Francesco G.F, Giovanetti AM, Pagetti D (1974) Blood pressure changes produced by kidney cross-transplantation between spontaneously hypertensive rats and normotensive rats. Clin Sci Mol Med 47:435–448

36. Fox U, Bianchi G (1976) The primary role of the kidney in causing the blood pressure difference between the Milan Hypertensive strain (MHS) and the normotensive rats (MNS). Proceedings of the symposium on spontaneous genetic hypertension in rats, Dunedin, New Zealand, 4–6 March 1976. Clin Exp Pharmacol Physiol (Suppl 3):71–74

37. Salvati P, Pinciroli G.P, Bianchi G (1984) Renal function of isolated perfused kidneys from hypertensive (MHS) and normotensive (MNS) rats of the Milan strain at different ages. J Hypertens 2 (Suppl 3):351–353

38. Salvati P, Ferrario R.G, Parenti P, Bianchi G (1987) Renal function of isolated perfused kidneys from hypertensive (MHS) and normotensive (MNS) rats of the Milan strain: role of calcium. J Hypertens 5:31–38

39. Parenti P, Hanozet G, Bianchi G (1986) Sodium and glucose transport across renal brush-border membranes of Milan hypertensive rats. Hypertension 8:932–939

40. Hanozet GM, Parenti P, Salvati P (1985) Presence of potential-sensitive Na$^+$ transport across renal brush-border membrane vesicles from rats of the Milan hypertensive strain. BBA 819:179–186

41. Salvati P, Ferrario RG, Bianchi G (1990) Diuretic effect of bumetanide in isolated perfused kidneys of Milan hypertensive rats. Kidney Int 37:1084–1089

42. Lapointe JY, Bell PD, Cardinal J (1990) Direct evidence for apical Na$^+$:2Cl$^-$:K$^+$ cotransport in macula densa cells. Am J Physiol 258(Renal Fluid Electrolyte Physiol 27):F1466–F1469

43. Persson A.E, Bianchi G, Boberg U (1984) Evidence of defective tubuloglomerular feedback control in rats of the Milan hypertensive strain (MHS). Acta Physiol Scand 122: 215–217

44. Persson AE, Bianchi G, Boberg U (1985) Tubuloglomerular feedback in hypertensive rats of the Milan strain. Acta Physiol Scand 123:139–146

45. Melzi ML, Bertorello A, Fukuda Y, Muldin I, Sereni F, Aperia A (1989) Na, K-ATPase activity in renal tubule cells from Milan hypertensive rats. Am J Hypertens 2:563–566

46. Bianchi G, Ferrari P, Trizio D, Ferrandi M, Torielli L, Barber B.R, and Polli E (1985) Red blood cell abnormalities and spontaneous hypertension in the rat: A genetically determined link. Hypertension 7:319–325

47. Ferrari P, Torielli L, Ferrandi M, Cirillo M, Bianchi G (1986) Volumes and Na transports in intact red blood cells, resealed ghosts and inside-out vesicles of Milan hypertensive rats J Hypertens, 4(Suppl 6):S379–S381

48. Ferrari P, Torielli L, Ferrandi M, Bianchi G (1986) Volumes and Na transports in intact red blood cells, resealed ghosts and inside out vesicles of Milan hypertensive rats. In: Bianchi G, Carafoli E, Scarpa A (eds) Ann NY Acad Sci 488:561–563

49. Salardi S, Saccardo, Borsani, Modica, Ferrandi M, Tripodi G, Soria, Ferrari P, Barralle, Sidoli I, Bianchi G (1989) Erythrocyte Adducin Differential Properties in Normotensive and Hypertensive rats of the Milan Strain: Characterization of Spleen Adducin m-RNA. Am J Hypertens 2:229–237

50. Tripodi G, Borsani G, Piscone A, Tisminetzky S, Salardi S, Sidoli A, Baralle FE, Bianchi G (1990) Difference between MNS and MHS rats in the cDNA coding for adducin (abstract). 13th scientific meeting of the International Society of Hypertension, 24–29 June 1990. Montreal, Canada

51. Niutta E, Cusi D, Colombo R, Tripodi G, Pellizzoni M, Pati P, Cesana B, Alberghini E, Barlassina C, and Bianchi G (1988) Antihypertensive Effect of Captopril, Canreonate Potassium, and Atenolol; Relations with Red Blood Cell Sodium Transport and Renin. Am J Hypertens 1:364–371

52. Camussi A, Bianchi G (1988) Genetics of Essential Hypertension From the Unimodal-Bimodal Controversy to Molecular Technology. Hypertension 12:620–628

53. Redgrave J, Canessa M, Gleason R, Hollenberg NK, Williams GH (1989) Red blood cell lithium-sodium countertransport in non-modulating essential hypertension. Hypertension 13:721–726

Cellular and Integrative Functions of the Juxtaglomerular Apparatus

Chair: Jurgen B. Schnermann (USA)
Toshikazu Takabatake (Japan)

Cell Volume Regulation and Transport Characteristics of Macula Densa Cells

A. ERIK G. PERSSON, MAX SALOMONSSON, PER WESTERLUND[1],
RAINER GREGER, EBERHARD SCHLATTER[2], and ERNESTO GONZALEZ[3]

SUMMARY. To study the sensing step of the juxtaglomerular apparatus, we have performed studies using isolated perfused ascending limb of the loop of Henle with attached glomeruli and macula densa segments (c-TAL-MD). Both from measurement of macula densa cell volume and from measurements of the electrical potential of MD cells it can be proposed that a Na-K-2Cl cotransport mechanism is involved in the sensing step of the juxtaglomerular apparatus. To study this question further, measurements of MD cell chloride concentration have been made, using the fluorophore SPQ and a digital imaging system. A chloride concentration of 47 mM was found in the MD cells with 150 mM NaCl in both lumen and bath. The MD cell concentration was reduced to 6 mM when furosemide was added to the lumen solution and to 35 mM when lumen NaCl concentration was reduced to 30 mM. These results strongly support the view of a Na-K-2Cl cotransport mechanism in the entry step of the sensing mechanism. To study whether MD cell calcium concentration changes were involved in the activation of the MD cells, intracellular calcium was measured when changes in luminal NaCl were induced. NaCl was reduced from 150 to 30 mM and then there was an increase in macula densa cell calcium from 90 nM to 110 nM. However, we feel that this small change is not sufficient to explain activation of the cells. Other routes of activation could be involved and for the time being the exact mechanism for this activation is not clear.

Introduction

One way by which the kidney controls glomerular filtration is through the action of the tubuloglomerular feedback (TGF) control mechanism [1]. For the operation of this mechanism, the load to the distal nephron is sensed at the macula densa site,

---

[1]Department of Physiology and Biophysics, Sölvegatan 19, 223 62 Lund, Sweden
[2]Department of Physiology, University of Freiburg, Federal Republic of Germany
[3]Department of Physiology, University Central, Caracas, Venezuela

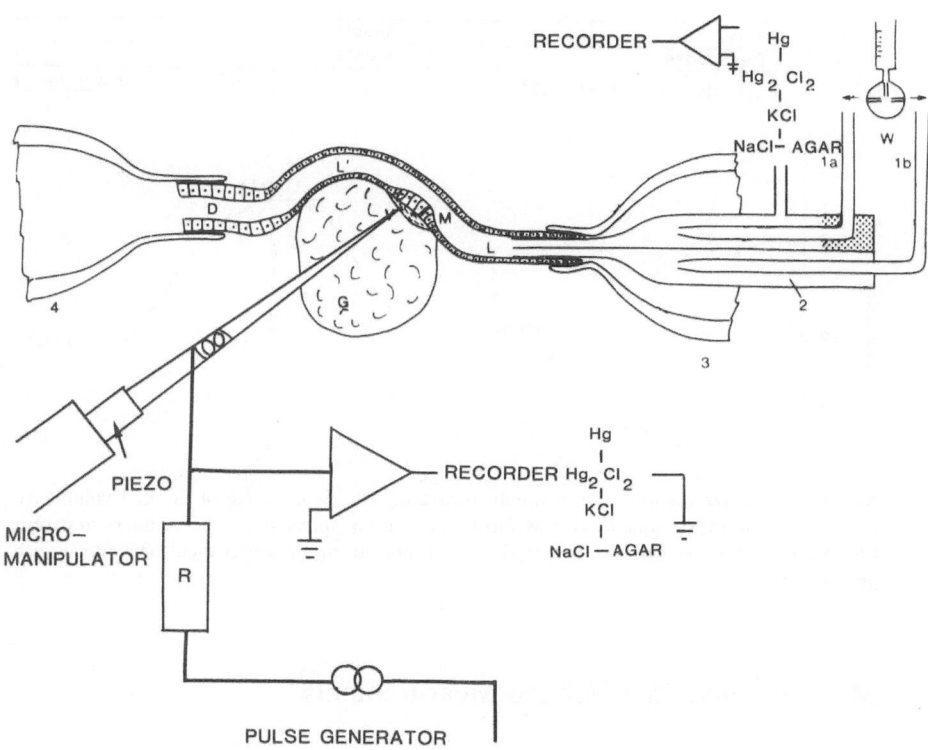

Fig. 1. Schematic view of the arrangement of the pipettes and the c-TAL and MD preparations. The tubular segment is perfused from right to left through a dual channel perfussion pipette. 2. The active channel is determined by the position of a pneumatic three-way valve *W*. The composition of the perfusate in the two channels of the perfusion pipette can be varied through two fluid exchange pipettes *1a* and *1b*. Two polyethylene catheters inserted through a lateral hole and sealed with epoxy resin serve as a fluid exchange pipette, *1a*. The tubular segment is held by the perfusion holding pipette *3* and by the collection holding pipette *4*, the latter coated with solid and liquid Sylgard 184. Note the cellular heterogeneity in the perfused tubular segment: the transition from the cortical ascending limb in front of (*L*) and behind (*L'*) and the macula densa (*M*) to the beginning of the distal convoluted tubule (*D*). The macula densa cells are interposed in the cortical ascending limb-macula densa (CAL-MD) only on the side that is in contact with the vascular pole of the juxtaglomerular apparatus (*V*). *G*, glomerulus. With another micromanipulator a microelectrode connected to a piezo stepper was used to puncture macula densa cells. A pulse generator was connected to the microelectrode to be able to continuously monitor electrical resistance

probably by the macula densa cells. Information about the load is then transferred to the effector site, the arterioles, via cells in the juxtaglomerular apparatus. The signal may become modulated during its transmission, possibly by the extraglomerular mesangial cells located between the sensing and effector sites.

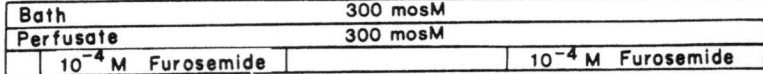

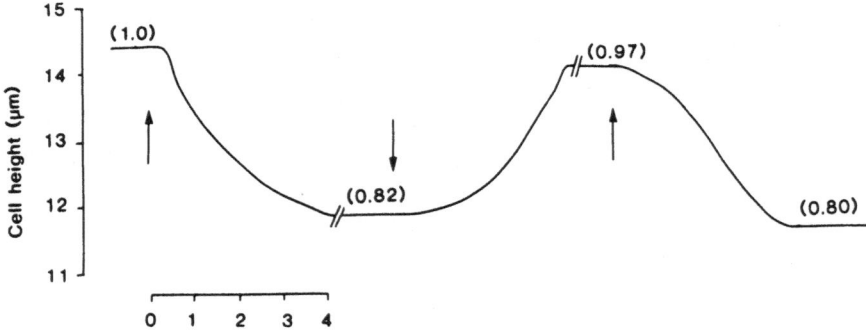

Fig. 2. Actual trace from an experiment illustrating the time course of the cell volume on exposure of the MD plaque to 10^{-4} M furosemide on the apical side. The numbers in parentheses are the relative cell volumes at different times during the experiment. (From [3] with permission)

Macula Densa Cell Volume Measurements

To study the sensing step, we performed the following sets of experiments [2–3]. The methods used were essentially the same as those described by Greger and Schlatter [4]. New Zealand white rabbits were used, and segments of cortical thick ascending limbs (c-TAL), 300–600 µm long, with attached glomeruli were isolated by manual dissection. Figure 1 shows how the tubules were mounted. The perfusion was carried out through a dual channel perfusion pipette which was put into the tubule and inserted into a holding pipette which kept the tubule in place. The tubule was mounted so that the macula densa (MD) cells were observed from the side. Experimental volume challenges caused no changes in the measured length or width of the MD cell plaque, but resulted in a change in its height [2]. The dimensions of these cells were measured with an image-splitting eyepiece to increase the resolution of the system. In the c-TAL segment the outer diameter was 25.2 µm, the inner tubular diameter was 7.1 µm, and the cell height was 4.8 µm. The height of the MD cell plaque was 13.3 µm, its length was 50 µm, and its width was 21.8 µm. Perfusion of furosemide rapidly reduced the cell volume to 0.82 compared with the control volume (see Fig. 2). This change was reversed on removal of the furosemide. When the luminal solution was modified by replacing most of the NaCl by mannitol, the cell volume decreased in the same way as with furosemide, resulting in an average cell volume of 0.83 compared with the control value. On calculation of the rate of cell volume decrease in the initial phase after removal of Na from the luminal fluid, a sodium flux of 0.28 nmol s^{-1} cm^{-2} was found. Since it is known from the work of Dr. Greger [5] that c-TAL segments reabsorb 5–10 nmol s^{-1} cm^{-2}, and from the work of Schnerman and Marver (in [1]) who found that the amount of Na-K-ATPase activity in MD cells was 1/37 of that in c-TAL cells, a sodium transport rate in MD cells of $0.14 - 0.27$ nmol s^{-1} cm^{-2} may be predicted. The measured value is in the same range as the calculated value. Thus, it seems clear that the rate of transport of the Na-K pump is only about 1/40 of that in the c-TAL cells, and that this rate is in good accordance with other data. The reduction in cell volume strongly suggested that furosemide inhibitable Na-K-2Cl co-transport was involved in the transport of Na and K into the MD cells.

We have also determined the osmotic water permeability of the basolateral and apical MD cell membranes [3]. Either the luminal or the basal side of tubules was perfused with oil, and an osmotic change of 150 mOsm was induced on the other side. The hydraulic conductance could then be calculated from the initial slope of the volume change curves. It was found that the water permeability of the apical cell membrane was much lower than on the basolateral side, and it was therefore concluded that the apical cell membrane constituted the primary barrier to water flow. The water permeability in c-TAL constituted about 10% of that in the MD cells. A greater membrane, due to a larger number of villi in the MD cells, might explain the higher water permeability in the MD cells, might explain the higher water permeability in the MD cells compared with the cells of the c-TAL. Nevertheless, the water permeability of the apical cell membrane was quite low. The high water permeability of the basolateral side, together with the low permeability of the luminal membrane, would mean that osmotic changes in the tubular lumen would give rise to only minor changes in cell volume, because of the rapid water movement across the basolateral cell membrane. When the luminal osmolarity was changed while the osmolarity of the outside bath was kept constant, only 10% of the expected volume change occurred, because of basolateral water flow. It was also found that when the luminal NaCl concentration was decreased from 60 mM to 15 mM without any compensation for a change in osmolarity, the steady state cell volume remained unaltered after the initial osmotic swelling and compensatory volume regulation. From these results it seems less likely to us that the lumen osmolarity, per se, is the factor involved in the sensing step.

Electrical Potential Measurements in Macula Densa Cell

The basolateral cell membrane potential in the macula densa cells has been measured [6]. The cortical thick ascending limbs were cannulated and perfused in vitro as described by Greger and Schlatter [4]. Both the transepithelial and the basolateral membrane voltages were measured with microelectrodes. The electrode tip was positioned next to macula densa cells by visual observation and was then advanced with the piezo stepper. Electrode resistances were constantly measured by injection of current pulses of 5 nA, 500 ms, and 1 Hz to detect any clogging of the pipette that might build up tip potentials in the order of -20 mV or more.

A concentration of 150 mM NaCl was usually used on both sides of the tubule. During the experiments of Schlatter et al. [6] on 166 perfused segments, some 3000 cell penetrations were attempted, and of these, eight impaled tubule cells showed stable recordings for up to 47 minutes. The mean PD_{bl} was -56 mV, and when furosemide was present in the lumen, PD_{bl} hyperpolarized by 27 mV, suggesting the

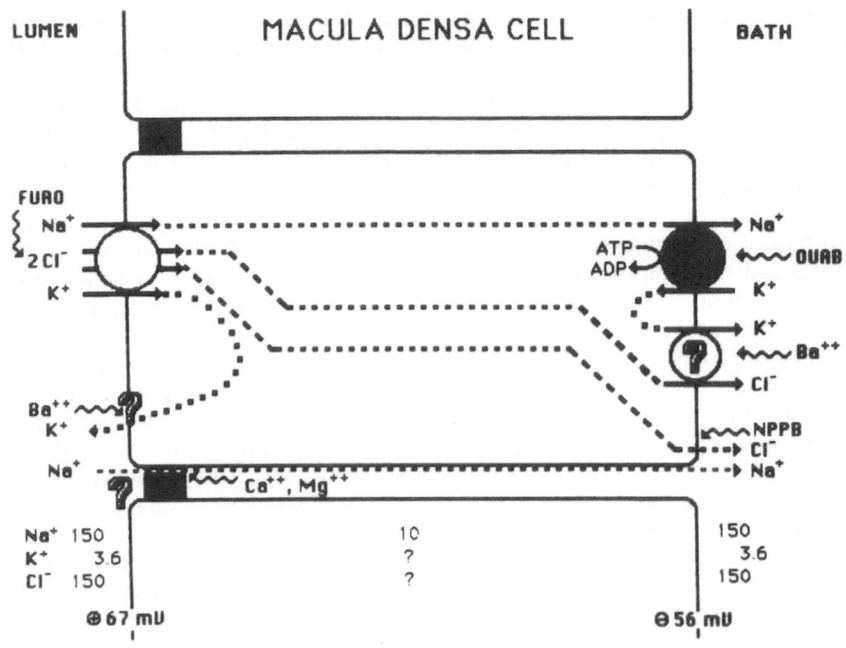

Fig. 3. Schematic diagram of ionic transport mechanisms in macula densa cells. Ouab, ouabain; Furo, furosemide. (From [16] with permission)

presence of a Na-K-2Cl co-transport system in the luminal cell membrane of the MD cells. This hyperpolarization dissipated when the furosemide was removed. It is possible that inhibition of Cl⁻ uptake hyperpolarized the cells, as the basolateral cell membrane was also Cl⁻ conductive. The Cl conductance of the basolateral cell membrane was also responsible for the increased depolarization of PD_{bl} when the bath Cl⁻ concentration was reduced from 150 to 30 mM.

The above results in the macula densa cells are compatible with the findings by Dr. Greger concerning the properties of c-TAL cells [5] (see Fig. 3). In the luminal membrane there is a Na-K-2Cl co-transport mechanism. When furosemide is added, the co-transport is blocked, the intracellular Cl concentration decreases, and the Cl conductance across the basolateral cell membrane is reduced, so that hyperpolarization of the basolateral cell membrane is reduced, so that hyperpolarization of the basolateral cell membrane takes place. The membrane potential then approaches the potassium equilibrium potential. Potassium recycling may also be suggested. The chloride conductance of the basolateral cell membrane is also supported by the finding of PD_{bl} depolarization when the bath concentration of Cl was reduced from 150 to 30 mM, as would be predicted for a Cl⁻ permeable membrane. In addition, the Cl channel blocker NPPB in the bath hyperpolarized PD_{bl}. Ouabain depolarized PD_{bl} from −68 to 12 mV, indicating the presence of Na-K pump activity.

Table 1.

Luminal perfusate	Macula densa cell (mM)	Thick ascending limb cell (mM)
150 mM NaCl	47	54
30 mM NaCl	35*	–
150 mM NaCl + 10^{-6} M furosemide	6*	5*

*$P < 0.06$

Macula Densa Cell Chloride Concentration

Recently, to test the hypothesis of Na-K-2Cl co-transport, we have performed direct measurements of chloride concentrations in cells of the cortical thick ascending limb and macula densa by use of the fluorophore SPQ, with a digital imaging system [7]. Chloride was measured in the macula densa and in the cortical thick ascending limb cells in the control states and after blockade with furosemide, or at a low sodium chloride concentration in the lumen perfusate. SPQ is quenched by a collisional mechanism without any change in the shape of its excitation or emission spectra [8]. SPQ follows a Stern-Volmer equation, and with knowledge of the Stern-Volmer constant K_{Cl^-}, the chloride concentration can be calculated;

$$F_o/F = 1 + K_{Cl}[Cl]$$

where F_o/F is the total fluorescence measured in the abscence of Cl divided by the fluorescence in the presence of Cl and K_{Cl} is the Stern-Volmer constant. The leakage of SPQ in the macula densa cells had a half-time of 197 minutes, which allowed sufficient time to perform the experimental protocol without losing too much SPQ. The chloride constant in the Stern-Volmer equation has to be determined for the macula densa cells, but it has been measured for proximal tubular cells [9] and for several types of fibroblasts [8] and does not seem to vary very much between the different cells. On the basis of the value for the proximal tubule, the concentration in the macula densa cells can be calculated. With this assumption the absolute value has to be considered with some caution. In the macula densa cells, as can be seen in Table 1, we found a chloride concentration of 47 mM at an NaCl concentration of 150 mM, both in the bath and in the lumen [7]. When furosemide was added to the luminal perfusion solution, the chloride concentration was reduced by 85% to 6 mM. The corresponding value in the cortical thick ascending limb cells was 54 mM, with a 90% reduction to 5 mM in the presence of furosemide. At a low NaCl of 30 mM in the tubular lumen, the chloride concentration in the macula densa cells was significantly reduced to 35 mM. The present results provide strong evidence that a Na-K-2Cl co-transport mechanism exists at the luminal cell membrane and that this mechanism allows NaCl to enter the macula densa cells and the cells of the cortical thick ascending limb at a fast rate, so that the chloride concentration is higher than that expected for passive distribution of chloride. When furosemide inhibits the Na-K-2Cl co-transport, the intracellular chloride concentration decreases to values close to the passive distribution of some 5 mM, calculated on theoretical grounds. On conversion of our furosemide values from ascending limb cells, the intracellular chloride activities were found not to be different from those obtained in rabbit cortical thick ascending limb cells by Dr. Greger and co-workers, using chloride selective microelectrodes [10].

Macula Densa Cell Calcium Concentration

It has been suggested that activation of macula densa cells may involve changes in the intracellular calcium concentration as one link in the chain of events leading to activation of TGF and release of renin. We therefore investigated the intracellular calcium concentration with fura-2, using a digital imaging system in macula densa cells, and compared it with the corresponding concentrations in the cells of the ascending limb of the loop of Henle. We found that our technique could be used to determine intracellular calcium. We found that the calibration curve for calcium and the K_d value of 228 nM was not different from that obtained by Grynkiewicz and co-workers [11]. An intracellular calcium concentration of about 90 nM was found both in the macula densa and in the cortical thick ascending limb cells, and the calcium concentration in the macula densa cells increased by about 20 nM when the tubular lumen was perfused with low Na and Cl concentrations. Addition of furosemide did not significantly increase the intracellular calcium concentration. We consider it less likely that this small change in the calcium concentration could be responsible for the full activation of renin release or the full inactivation of the TGF control mechanism. It would seem that the signal transmission from the macula densa cells could take routes other than through activation of intracellular calcium.

Sensing Step

Now, how can we envision the sensing step? Is it Na, Cl, NaCl, or osmolarity that is the flow dependent signal? On the basis of the present studies, it appears likely that MD cells have a Na-K-2Cl co-transport that carries Na-K and Cl into the cells. This can be concluded both from cell volume measurements and from the electrical measurements. An increase in the luminal NaCl concentration will increase the transport rate in the co-transport system, and a higher MD chloride will result, in association with a small increase in cell volume. The increase in conductive chloride flux across the basolateral cell membrane will depolarize the cell membrane potential. Since the Na-K-2Cl co-transport system has a higher affinity for Na than for Cl, as found in studies of the c-TAL segment [5], it is likely that the luminal Cl concentration is the most critical signal. The Na concentration will probably never fall so low as to limit the transport rate of the co-transporter.

Now, how is the signal from increased NaCl transport mediated across the macula densa cells to the effector site? For the time being there are several possibilities, of which we will briefly mention two. The first one is a metabolic control in which the intracellular formation of adenosine, and its leakage out of the cell, could transmit the response [12]. The formation of adenosine would increase on increased breakdown of ATP. These results are also particularly interesting in view of the findings of Bleich et al. [13], who demonstrated the existence of a luminal cell membrane K channel in the c-TAL cells that is inhibited by ATP. Thus, if a similar channel existed in the macula densa cells, increased NaCl transport through the macula densa cells would cause ATP breakdown. This would give rise to less inhibition of the K channel used for K recycling, thereby promoting this K recycling. At the same time more adenosine could leak out of the cell and mediate the response to the rest of the juxtaglomerular apparatus. One other possible explanation is that the NaCl concentration within the interstitial space of the extraglomerular mesangium is very high, and that this concentration is dependent on the NaCl transport in the macula densa. Dr. Bo Erik Persson and Dr. Marsh found that the Cl concentration within the renal interstitial space in the Amphiuma, as measured by chloride electrodes, was very high and was also flow-dependent [13]. It is possible that this high flow-dependent interstitial Cl concentration elicits the response from the arterioles or from the mesangial cells, as suggested by Dr. Kurokawa [14].

References

1. Schnermann J, Briggs J (1985) Function of the juxtaglomerular apparatus: local control of glomerular hemodynamics. In: Seldin DW, Giebisch G (eds) The kidney: physiology and pathophysiology. Raven, New York, pp 669–697
2. Gonzalez E, Salomonsson M, Müller-Suur C, Persson AEG (1988) Measurements of macula densa cell volume changes in isolated and perfused rabbit cortical thick ascending limb. I. Isosmotic and anisosmotic cell volume changes. Acta Physiol Scand 133: 149–157
3. Gonzalez E, Salomonsson M, Müller-Suur C, Persson AEG (1988) Measurements of macula densa cell volume changes in isolated and perfused rabbit cortical thick ascending limb. II. Apical and basolateral cell osmotic water permeabilities. Acta Physiol Scand 113:159–166
4. Greger R, Schlatter E (1983) Properties of the lumen membrane of the cortical thick ascending limb of Henle's loop of rabbit kidney. Pflugers Arch 396:315–324
5. Greger R (1985) Ion transport mechanisms in thick ascending limb of Henle's loop of mammalian nephron. Physiol Rev 65:760–797
6. Schlatter E, Salomonsson M, Persson AEG, Greger R (1989) Macula densa cells sense luminal NaCl concentration in furosemide sensitive $Na^+-2Cl^--K^+$ cotransport. Pflugers Arch 414:286–290
7. Salomonsson M, Gonzalez E, Westerlund P, Persson AEG (to be published) The effect of furosemide on chloride concentration in macula densa and in cortical thick ascending limb cells. Acta Physiol Scand
8. Chao AC, Dix JA, Sellers MC, Verkman AS (1989) Fluorescence measurement of chloride transport in nonlayer cultured cells. Biophys J 56:1071–1081
9. Krapf R, Berry CH, Verkman AS (1988) Estimation of intracellular chloride activity in isolated perfused rabbit proximal convoluted tubules using a fluorescent indicator. Biophys J 53:955–962
10. Greger R, Oberleitner H, Schlatter E, Cassola A, Weidtke C (1983) Chloride activity in cells of isolated perfused thick ascending limb of rabbit kidney. Pflugers Arch 399:29–34
11. Grynkiewicz G, Poenie M, Tsien RY (1985) A new generation of Ca^{2+} indicators with greatly improved fluorescence properties. J Biol Chem 260:3440–3450
12. Osswald H (1988) Metabolic control of organ function – does it apply to the kidney. In: Persson AEG, Boberg U (eds) The juxtaglomerular apparatus. Elsevier, Amsterdam, pp 155–166
13. Persson B-E, Marsh D (1988) The flow sensor of tubuloglomerular feedback in the early distal tubule of Amphiuma. In: Persson AEG, Boberg U (eds) The juxtaglomerular apparatus. Elsevier, Amsterdam, pp 121-128

14. Kurokawa K (1989) Biology of glomerular mesangial cells (abstract). Int Eup Physiol Sci Proc Int Union Physiol Sci XVII. Helsinki, p 130
15. Schnermann J, Ploth DW, Hermle M (1976) Activation of tubuloglomerular feedback by chloride transport. Pflugers Arch 362:229–240
16. Persson AEG, Salomonsson M, Westerlund P, Greger R, Schlatter R, Gonzalez E. Macula densa cell function. Kidney Int in press

Intracellular and Membrane Events in the Activation of Afferent Arteriolar and Granular Cells

ARMIN KURTZ[1]

SUMMARY. There is accumulating information about the existence of membrane-bound signal transduction systems in renal afferent arteriolar and granular cells. The second messenger generating systems, which include phospholipases, nucleotide cyclases, and ion channels, become activated upon ligand binding to cell surface receptors. Subsequently they exert influence on the cellular functions, which predominantly are contraction and renin secretion, in these cells.

It is the aim of this contribution to summarize what we know at present about the existence of signal transduction systems, about their way of activation, and about their possible intracellular effects in renal arteriolar and granular cells.

Introduction

The renal afferent arterioles fulfill two important physiological functions. Firstly, they regulate the rate of glomerular filtration by determining preglomerular resistance. Secondly, they secrete renin into the circulation and thus determine the activity of the systemic renin-angiotensin-aldosterone system. Regulation of renin secretion and regulation of afferent vascular tone share a number of similarities. Both functions are elaborated by the same cell type, namely vascular smooth muscle cells (VSMC), because renin producing granular juxtaglomerular (JG) cells develop from the neighboring VSMC by a reversible metaplastic transformation [1,2]. There exists moreover, a small but significant degree of electrical coupling between the VSMC and JG cells in the afferent arterioles [3]. In most instances, both functions are influenced by the same parameters. Those parameters, for instance, comprise blood pressure, a signal generated by the macula densa, sympathetic transmitters that are released from sympathetic nerve endings in the juxtaglomerular region, and a

[1]Physiologisches Institut der Universität Zürich, Winterthurerstrasse 190, CH-8057 Zürich, Switzerland

number of circulating or locally generated hormones. A superior principle in the regulation of preglomerular vascular tone and renin secretion even appears to exist. Factors causing a contraction of afferent arterioles usually lead to an inhibition of renin secretion, while stimulators of renin secretion most often cause a relaxation of afferent vessels. For instance, a rise of blood pressure, activation of the macula densa, and vasoconstrictive hormones such as angiotensin II cause a contraction of the VSMC in the afferent arterioles and inhibit renin secretion, cf [4]. A fall of blood pressure, β-adrenergic agonists, and other vasodilating hormones, on the other hand, lead to relaxation of VSMC and enhancement of renin secretion, cf [4]. From a physiological point of view, such a kind of interrelation between VSMC contraction and renin secretion appears ingenious. By its action renin generates the vasoconstrictor hormone angiotensin II (ANG II), which itself is an important determinant of blood pressure. Inhibition of renin secretion during states of contraction of the afferent arteriole therefore reflects a very powerful negative feedback control of renin release in particular, and of blood pressure in general.

The mechanism by which VSMC contraction and renin secretion are interrelated is still speculative. It is also not well understood how the blood pressure, the macula densa, and a number of hormones exert their effects on VSMC and JG cells located in afferent arterioles. A common feature of the parameters affecting afferent arteriolar function as alluded to above is that they exert their effects on cell contraction and exocytosis of renin via specific signal transduction systems.

The identification of such signal transduction systems in afferent arteriolar VSMC and in JG cells was hampered by the fact that these cells lie buried within the renal cortex and are not accessible for direct investigation. The development of new techniques, such as the split hydronephrotic kidney [5], isolation techniques for juxtaglomerular apparatuses [6] and JG cells [7], and the application of sophisticated techniques on these preparations have enabled investigators to get some first-hand insight into the intracellular and membrane events in VSMC and JG cells in afferent arterioles. In this contribution I shall summarize the knowledge which is presently available on those processes occurring in afferent vessels. In this context I will focus my considerations on classic signal transduction systems such as phospholipases, nucleotide cyclases, and ion channels as they occur in a variety of tissues.

Phospholipases

Phospholipase C

A phospholipase C (PLC) is a phosphodiesterase that splits a phospholipid into diacylglycerol and a phosphorester compound. As long as several decades ago it was recognized that phospholipases C and their substrates played a role in transmembrane signalling [8,9]. The hydrolysis of phosphatidylinositolbisphosphate (PIP$_2$) in particular, has attracted interest, because it provides two second messengers that cause release of calcium from intracellular stores (via inositoltrisphosphate) and that activate protein kinase C (via diacylglycerol) [10]. Today we know that this important reaction takes place in almost every eukaryotic cell, provided that the essential enzyme (PLC) is present in the cell membrane and is subject to regulated activation. The physiological relevance of PLC as a signal transduction system is made clear by the fact that PLC is coupled to cell surface receptors via coupling proteins that have been characterized as heterotrimer guanosine triphosphate GTP-binding proteins, cf. [11].

The first evidence that an activatable PLC also existed in JG cells was obtained in primary cultures of rat juxtaglomerular cells. Addition of angiotensin II (ANG II), arginine-vasopressin (AVP) and norepinephrine (NE) to those cells led to a significant breakdown of PIP_2 and simultaneous increase of diacylglycerol (DAG) [12]. Although a rise in IP_3 level was not demonstrated in that study it was considered likely that a receptor coupled PLC exists in JG cells and can be activated by ANG II, AVP, and to a lesser extent, by NE. This conclusion was recently supported by the observation that ANG II also causes the mobilization of calcium from intracellular stores in JG cells [3], an effect that is considered to be dependent on the generation of IP_3 [13]. Moreover, it was found that the calcium mobilizing effect of ANG II was dependent on the presence of intracellular GTP and could be mimicked by a stable GTP analogue, suggesting that the activation of PLC by ANG II in JG cells is also mediated by G-proteins [3]. Indirect evidence that the effect of ANG II on JG cells could be mediated by G proteins had already been provided by the findings that pertussis toxin, which functionally inactivates a number of GTP-binding proteins, attenuated the effect of ANG II on renin secretion from isolated kidneys and also attenuated the effect of ANG II on renal vascular resistance [14]. This was also the first indication that the signal transduction mechanisms for ANG II in renal VSMC and in JG are not principally different, a consideration that has been corroborated by two previous studies [3,15].

Summing up, there is good evidence for the existence of functional receptor -G-protein-PLC complexes in the membranes of VSMC and JG cells in afferent arterioles.

As already mentioned, activation of PLC, for instance by ANG II, leads to a rise of diacylglycerol (DAG) and subsequently to an activation of protein kinase C [16]. The subcellular effects of protein kinase C activation in afferent arteriolar and granular cells have so far been assessed in experiments with tumor promoting phorbol esters that are considered as artificial activators of C-kinase, as well as by the use of putative C-kinase inhibitors. It appears as if C-kinase activation is important for the contraction of renal VSMC induced by ANG II [17]. Phorbol esters in high concentrations were also found to enhance transmembrane calcium influx and to attenuate renin secretion from isolated JG cells [12]. Whether the latter effects are really due to C-kinase activation or to side effects of phorbol esters needs to be clarified. Recent findings, moreover, suggest that phorbol esters at concentrations typical for C-kinase activation cause an electrical decoupling of VSMC and JG cells in the afferent arterioles (A. Kurtz and R. Penner, unpublished work). Other effects of C-kinase activation that occur in cells and might be important in the future, but have so far not been proven for JG cells, are enhancement of phospholipase A_2 activity [18] and activation of sodium/proton exchange, cf [19]).

The partner messenger molecular arising simultaneously with DAG is inositol-trisphosphate (IP_3). The outstanding role of IP_3 as a second messenger causing intracellular calcium release is well established [10]. Recent evidence, moreover, suggests that IP_3 or its derivatives have — at least in some cell types — an important role in the regulation of transmembrane calcium influx [20]. The changes which take place in the intracellular concentration of calcium in JG cells and VSMC in afferent

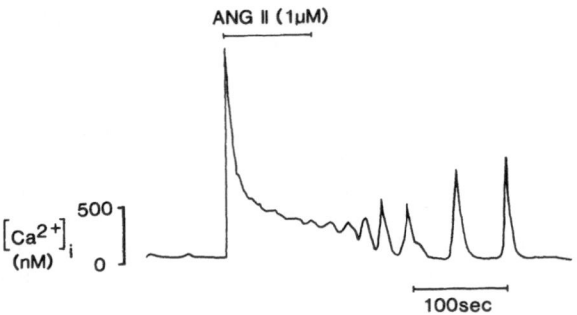

Fig. 1. Intracellular calcium concentration ($[Ca]_i$) in a juxtaglomerular cell from mouse kidney after addition of angiotensin II

arterioles upon activation of PLC by ANG II or by stable GTP-analogues are impressive (Fig. 1). Within a few seconds, cytosolic calcium rises transiently, as a result of calcium release from intracellular stores. This initial calcium transient, during which calcium levels rise from 90nM to 1μM or even higher, is then followed by an interval lasting 1–4 minutes, during which intracellular calcium stays constantly elevated at a level of about 200nM. When $[Ca^{2+}]_i$ declines to near resting levels, the cytosolic calcium concentration starts to oscillate. Such calcium oscillations after PLC-stimulation have already been observed in a number of cells, cf [21]. However, the pattern and the characteristics of the oscillations vary markedly between the cells. In JG cells the oscillations are very regular, with an average duration of 10 seconds and an average frequency of about 2 min^{-1} during continuous stimulation of PLC by stable GTP analogues [3]. The oscillatory calcium spikes result from intracellular calcium release. Their frequency, however, is strongly coupled to the extracellular concentration of calcium [3]. How extracellular calcium influences calcium release from internal stores in JG cells is not yet understood. Possible explanations could be that external calcium modulates PLC in a stimulatory fashion and/or that external calcium influences the refilling of internal calcium stores.

Another link between extra- and intracellular calcium concentrations is shown by the existence of calcium influx mechanisms, the activation of which causes the stable elevation of intracellular calcium after the initial calcium transient [3,12]. The mechanism activating the calcium influx in JG cells and in VSMC is not yet known. In analogy with other cell types, both receptor-operated or second messenger-operated calcium channels could be candidates. From the observation that not only ANG II, but also stable GTP analogues, can activate calcium influx in JG cells one could speculate that second messenger-operated channels rather than receptor-operated channels exist there. Whether IP_3 or one of its derivatives is the key activator of those channels still remains to be clarified.

What are the cellular events which follow a rise of calcium in renal afferent arteriolar VSMC and JG cells?

Doubtless, a rise of intracellular calcium is the key signal which activates myosin light chain kinase and it is thus the crucial event for the contraction of VSMC, the essential function of this cell type [22].

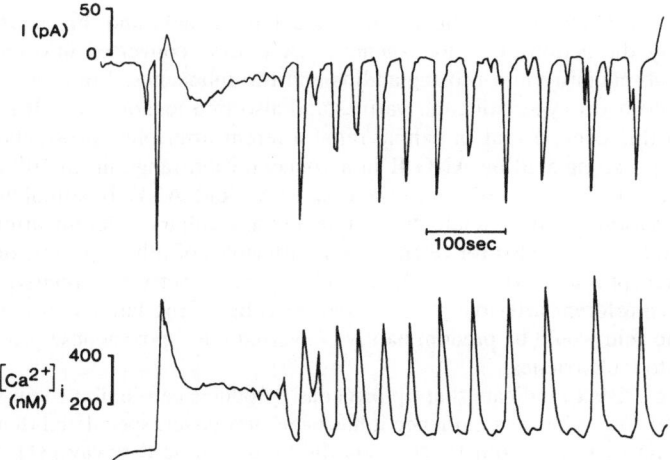

Fig. 2. Simultaneous recordings of membrane current and intracellular calcium concentration in a mouse JG cell during stimulation with GTP-γ-S (100μM). Voltage clamp potential was −60 mV

It is more difficult to find a clearcut answer for JG cells. Although it is generally assumed that a rise of calcium blocks the exocytosis of renin we still await unequivocal experimental proof of this hypothesis [23]. Therefore we should concentrate here on the cellular effects of calcium that have been measured in JG cells. In fact, so far, there is only one effect of calcium that has clearly been demonstrated in JG cells: the activation of calcium-dependent chloride channels (Fig. 2) that have been found to exist in high numbers in JG cells [3]. From the existence of these channels, a calcium-regulated cell volume control can be predicted for JG and VSMC cells in afferent arterioles [24]. A rise in internal calcium will lower the cell volume and, conversely, a drop in internal calcium will raise the cell volume. As outlined elsewhere, such a calcium-dependent volume control could, in fact, explain an inhibitory control function of calcium on renin secretion from JG cells [24].

Phospholipase A₂

Phospholipase A_2 (PLA$_2$) is a monoesterase that liberates fatty acids which are esterified in the 2 position of phospholipids. Since the bulk of arachidonic acid is bound in this position, activation of PLA$_2$ leads to a rise of the cytosolic level of arachidonic acid [25]. Arachidonic acid (AA) is the reaction limiting substrate for the AA-cascade leading to prostaglandins, thromboxanes, lipoxygenase products, and leukotriens. PLA$_2$-activity is highly calcium sensitive and it is not so surprising that it was at first thought that hormones activating PLC, and in consequence calcium release also led to an activation of PLA$_2$ [26,27]. This simpler view is now being expanded by recent findings that hormones can directly activate PLA$_2$, probably via GTP-binding proteins [28]. Regardless of the exact mechanisms of PLA$_2$ activation, it can be assumed that most hormones which stimulate PLC in JG cells and afferent arteriolar VSMC also lead to liberation of arachidonic acid and thus start the AA-cascade. By the action of cyclooxygenase AA is then converted into endoperoxides and subsequently into prostaglandins and thromboxanes. Lipoxygenases convert AA into hydroxyperoxide derivatives and also into leukotrienes. It is of some interest in this context that in canine renal afferent arterioles, prostaglandin formation is not stimulated by ANG II in a concentration range up to 100 nM [29]. Only at very high concentrations, such as 1 μM, did ANG II stimulate prostacyclin formation in superficial, but not in juxtamedullary afferent arterioles. If this observation holds also for renal afferent arterioles of other species, one would infer that receptor activation of PLA_2 or cyclooxygenase activity is relatively poorly expressed in afferent arteriolar VSMC and JG cells. If the latter is true then free arachidonic acid would be predominantly converted into lipoxygenase products and perhaps into leukotrienes.

Evidence exists to indicate that lipoxygenase products can inhibit renin secretion in vitro [30]. From indirect evidence it has been, moreover, speculated that ANG II inhibits renin secretion from JG cells via the lipoxygenase pathway [31]. Whether leukotrienes also affect renin secretion is not yet known. First evidence also suggests that lipoxygenase and epoxygenase products also affect the function of renal blood vessels [32].

Nucleotide Cyclases

Adenylate Cyclase

The adenylate cyclase (AC) generating cyclic AMP from ATP was the first among the, today, classic signal transduction systems whose existence was postulated for juxtaglomerular cells. Based on the observations that β-adrenergic agonists, as well as forskolin, exert profound stimulatory effects on renin secretion it was logical to assume first, the existence of AC and, secondly, the existence of a receptor coupling of AC in the membrane of JG cells, cf [4]. In experiments with isolated JG cells it has been confirmed that forskolin, isoproterenol, and also calcitonin gene related peptide (CGRP), increase the intracellular level of cAMP, cf [4]. The increase of cAMP caused by these agents is amplified when cAMP degradation is inhibited, thus suggesting strongly that they act, via cAMP formation, by stimulating adenylate cyclase. Forskolin causes receptor independent activation of AC, whereas, in contrast, receptor operated activation of AC, for instance, that caused by isoproterenol or by CGRP, only leads to a transient stimulation of AC (Fig. 3). This suggests that in JG cells, as in other cells, receptor mediated activation of AC is subject to desensitization, most likely to receptor downregulation. Irrespective of that fact, the effects of cAMP in JG cells appear to be longer lasting than the actual rise in cAMP (Fig. 3). This phenomenon is most likely due to phosphorylation processes that are performed by cAMP-dependent A-kinase and that last longer than the measurable rise of cAMP. It is generally agreed upon that a rise of cAMP enhances the exocytosis of renin from JG cells, cf [4]. The cellular mechanisms for this effect have not yet been identified. Recently it has been observed that the calcium mobilization induced by PLC activation is inhibited in JG cells if cAMP levels are elevated [3].

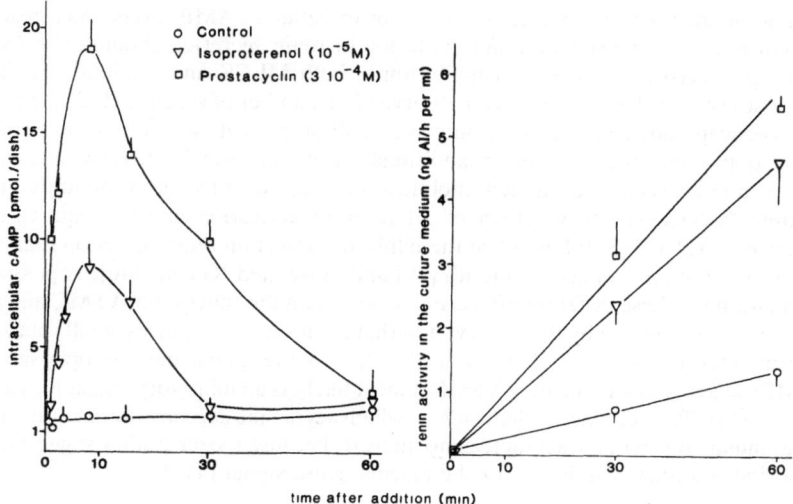

Fig. 3. Temporal change of intracellular cAMP levels (*left*) and renin secretion rates (*right*) from cultured rat juxtaglomerular cells after addition of prostacyclin and isoproterenol. (From [4])

Under the assumption that calcium is an inhibitory signal for renin secretion, the inhibition of calcium mobilization by cAMP could help us to understand, at least in part, the stimulatory effect of cAMP on renin secretion.

Cyclic AMP-dependent phosphorylation of the myosin light chain kinase has been recognized as a powerful negative regulatory element in the contraction of vascular smooth muscle cells [22]. If one assumes that receptor linked AC also exists in VSMC in afferent arterioles, then two potent vasorelaxant events can be postulated for these cells. First, inhibition of calcium mobilization, thus removing the key signal for smooth muscle cell contraction, and secondly, inhibition of myosin light chain kinase (MLCK), which is the key enzyme for the induction of smooth muscle cell contraction.

The juxtaglomerular region is well innervated with sympathetic nerve endings [1] and equipped with membrane bound β-adreno-receptors. Assuming continuous nerve activity, one can infer a steady activation of AC in VSMC and JG cells in the juxtaglomerular region.

This constellation provides a possible basis for another signal transduction system, namely for receptor mediated inhibition of cAMP formation. So far only a few hormones have been found to inhibit AC. Among these adenosine and α-adrenergic agonists are the best characterized ones, cf [33]. In several tissues, adenosine has been found to inhibit AC activity via A_1-subtype receptors, cf [33], while α-adrenergic agonists have been found to inhibit AC via α_2-subtype receptors, cf [33]. While the existence of α_2-receptors in afferent vessels is so far only speculative [34], there exists good evidence for the existence of adenosine A_1-receptors [35,36]. If they would negatively interfere with the steady state activation of AC in the juxtaglomerular region, then they should lower cellular cAMP levels. As a result, afferent arteriolar constriction and inhibition of renin secretion should arise from A_1-receptor activation, due to disinhibition of both MLCK and calcium mobilization. These effects have indeed been observed in a number of studies, cf [37]. Since, in this concept, adenosine appears only as a facilitator of calcium effects, one would expect that adenosine requires an additional agent that should directly stimulate PLC, and in consequence, calcium mobilization. Indeed, it has been found that the apparent "vasoconstrictory" effect of A1-receptor activation in vivo requires the presence of ANG II [38]; but not so the inhibitory effect on renin secretion that can also be observed in isolated glomeruli [39] and in isolated JG cells [40]. A possible explanation for these different effects of adenosine on the function of VSMC and JG cells could be provided by the observation that adenosine also causes small, but significant, elevations of cGMP in JG cells [40]. While guanosine monophosphate (cGMP) acts as a vasorelaxant in VSMC it most likely is an inhibitory signal for renin secretion [4]. The cellular mechanisms by which adenosine acts on afferent arteriolar and granular cells will attract increasing interest, because recent studies suggest that adenosine is a likely candidate for the macula densa signal [41,42].

Guanylate Cyclase

With the exception of the retina, a second messenger role of cyclic GMP in tissues has been speculated on for a long time. The discovery of atrial natriuretic peptide (ANP) as a physiologically important hormone has supported an important second messenger function of cGMP. The ANP-receptor that is anchored in the cell membrane has been identified as an intrinsic guanylate cyclase (GC), generating cyclic GMP from GTP [43].

Meanwhile several cGMP-mediated reactions have been characterized, cf [44], the most outstanding of which are, apart from light transduction, vasorelaxation and inhibition of renal sodium reabsorption.

The functional existence of ANP receptors has been shown for juxtaglomerular cells [7]. From that we may infer that JG cells and presumably also VSMC in the afferent arteriole are equipped with a membrane-bound guanylate cyclase.

There is good evidence that cGMP causes relaxation of VSMC in the afferent arterioles [45,46]. The precise mechanism leading to this effect is not yet known. It could be due to an increased calcium clearing from the cytosol, or could be due to a direct inhibitory action on myosin light chain kinase, cf [44].

The effect of ANP or cGMP on renin secretion from JG cells is less unequivocal. While the majority of the studies suggest an inhibitory effect of ANP and of cGMP on renin secretion, cf [4], there are also studies reporting no effect [47] and, in a single case, even a stimulatory effect of ANP/cGMP on renin secretion [48]. In my opinion these divergent results with ANP/cGMP result from the fact that cGMP has no direct effect on renin secretion, as cAMP has. In independent experiments, we have obtained evidence that ANP/cGMP requires calcium for its inhibitory effect on renin secretion [49] and that cGMP enhances the calcium sensitivity of the calcium-activated chloride channels in JG cells [3]. In consequence, ANP/cGMP requires at least normal calcium concentrations for its inhibitory effect on renin secretion. Given normal, or even elevated, calcium concentrations in JG cells an inhibitory effect of ANP/cGMP could be predicted for most experimental situations. Nevertheless, in some instances calcium levels could also drop below normal levels, and in these situations the inhibitory effect of ANP will be absent. An inhibitory effect of cGMP on renin secretion could gain importance in view of the fact that the recently discovered endothelial derived relaxing factor (EDRF) stimulates soluble guanylate cyclase activity and thus stimulates cGMP formation, cf [44]. Since there is evidence that JG cells contain a soluble guanylate cyclase [7], it is tempting to speculate about a possible endothelial control of renin secretion from JG cells via EDRF. First evidence in fact indicates that EDRF inhibits renin release in vitro [50]. Among the parameters stimulating EDRF formation by endothelial cells, the shear stress on the endothelial surface could play an important role, cf [51]. It will be interesting therefore, in future experiments, to test whether these mechanisms are involved in the process by which the blood pressure controls renin secretion from JG cells.

Ion Channels

Ion channels play an important role in signal transduction in excitable tissues. Since, in principle, vascular smooth muscle cells belong to the group of excitable cells it is obvious to question electrical events in JG cells upon activation and to consider the role of the membrane potential in the function of JG cells and VSMC in the afferent arterioles.

The first evidence for the occurrence of electrical events in JG cells was provided by microelectrode studies showing that the membrane potential of JG cells slightly hyperpolarized in response to β-adrenergic agonists [52]. More prominent, however, are changes of the membrane potential in response to vasoconstrictors. In elegant microelectrode investigations it was demonstrated that JG cells and VSMC in the afferent arterioles respond to ANG II and to other vasoconstrictors with a strong depolarization, with an amplitude ranging from 10 to 50mV [15]. In these studies no clear evidence for changes of electrical membrane resistance was found. Therefore it was not possible to attribute the observed depolarization to the opening or to the closing of certain types of ion channels. The resting membrane potential of VSMC and JG cells in afferent arterioles ranges between -70 to -80mV [3,15,52] and is thus close to the potassium equilibrium potential, suggesting that potassium conductances play a major role in the electrical properties of JG cells. In fact, a recent study has identified two types of potassium channels in JG cells and VSMC in afferent arterioles [3]. Both types are voltage activated but their activation potential differs markedly. One type of K^+-channel becomes activated upon depolarization of the cells to -10mV or more positive potentials. This type of K^+-channel is known in a variety of tissues; the sum current produced by these channels is named delayed (outward) rectifier for potassium. The second type of voltage gated K^+-channel present is inwardly rectifying and the channels become activated, upon hyperpolarization of the cells, to potential values lower than the resting membrane potential. This type of current, which also occurs in several other cell types, is named anomalous inward rectifier for potassium. So far no positive evidence has been produced for the existence of other potential activated ion channels, in particular sodium or calcium channels, in JG cells.

On the other hand there is good evidence for the existence of calcium-permeable channels which are activated by ANG II or by stable GTP analogues [3,53]. The question of whether these channels are directly coupled to receptors via GTP-binding proteins or whether they are activated by second messengers that result from G-protein mediated reactions, still has to be clarified.

Another type of second messenger operated ion channels has also been identified in JG cells and VSMC in afferent arterioles. These are calcium activated chloride channels, which have a small single channel conductance and which exist in high numbers in JG cells (Fig. 2) [3]. Together with the voltage gated K$^+$-channels the calcium activated chloride channels could manage an effective cell volume control, which in turn could govern renin secretion [24].

Having now considered the equipment of JG cells with ion channels we should recall the question of the mechanism by which ANG II leads to a depolarization of JG cells and VSMC in afferent arterioles.

As mentioned before, ANG II does cause calcium mobilization and calcium influx into JG cells. In parallel with the changes of calcium the chloride conductance of the cells will change and will therefore produce an electrical driving force toward the chloride equilibrium potential. The chloride equilibrium potential for JG cells has, so far, not been measured. If it is similar to that found in other smooth muscle cells it should be in the range of -20 to -30mV [54], a value that is far more positive than the resting membrane potential of -70 to -80mV in JG cells. In consequence, JG cells should depolarize upon a rise of intracellular calcium, and since the chloride conductance mirrors the intracellular calcium concentration, the time course of the membrane potential should mirror the time course of the intracellular calcium after stimulation of the cells by ANG II. In fact, the changes of membrane potential measured in microelectrode studies resemble the pattern of calcium changes in response to ANG II [15]. However, the depolarization usually lasts longer than the rise of calcium, suggesting that an additional depolarizing force is evoked by ANG II. This additional depolarizing force is most likely produced by a reversible inhibition of the anomalous inward rectifier for potassium caused by ANG II (Fig. 4), an event that removes a strong hyperpolarizing force. Interestingly, the inhibition of the inward rectifier can also be produced by stable GTP-analogues (Fig. 4), suggesting that it is mediated by a G-protein, or caused by a second messenger that is generated by G-protein mediated reaction. A third depolarizing force that is produced by the action of ANG II and also by stable GMP analogues is the increase of the calcium conductance of the cell membrane, which manifests itself as an increase of calcium influx [3,12,53]. Until recently, the depolarizing effect of ANG II in renal JG cells has been attributed mainly to the activation of potential operated calcium channels (POCC) [15]. However, a recent study failed to detect such channels in JG cells [53].

Summing up, the depolarization produced by ANG II in JG cells and VSMC in the afferent arterioles is probably a multifactorial event involving calcium activation of chloride conductance, increase of calcium conductance, and inhibition of potassium conductance.

Apart from the ion channels, ion exchange mechanisms could also gain importance for the regulation of function of JG cells. It has been observed that ANG II either directly, or indirectly via activation of protein kinase C, causes a stimulation of the sodium/proton exchange, cf [19]. This event leads to a transient alkalinization of the cytosol in response to ANG II. This effect could be of particular importance for JG cells, because recent studies on isolated JG cells have shown that inhibition of Na/H exchange leads to a marked stimulation of renin secretion (A. Kurtz et al., unpub-

Fig. 4. Block of inwardly rectifying potassium current in mouse JG cells by angiotensin II (*top*) and GTP-γ-S (*lower*). *Arrow* indicates establishment of whole cell configuration. Note that outward current is not blocked by GTP-γ-S

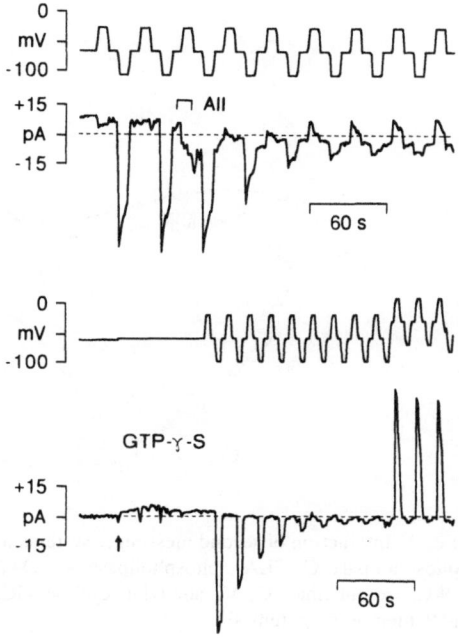

lished). If ANG II would activate Na/H exchange in JG cells also, then this action could causally contribute to the inhibitory effect of ANG II on renin secretion.

Cross-Talk Between Signal Transduction Systems

The accumulation of knowledge of intracellular events in JG cells has also revealed that the different signal transduction systems are not isolated units that produce specific cellular effects, but that the signal transduction systems communicate with each other (summarized in Fig. 5).

Receptor operated stimulation of PLC, for instance, causes activation of protein kinase C and the mobilization of calcium via IP_3 formation. C-kinase activation itself interferes with other second messenger systems in JG cells. First, it causes a negative feedback on PLC activation [55]. Secondly, presumably it activates Na/H exchange, cf [19], and could, as in neighboring mesangial cells, increase PLA_2 activity [18]. Calcium mobilization by IP_3 alters electrical behavior by influencing chloride channels [3]. Membrane depolarization, produced by calcium activation of chloride channels and by inhibition of potassium channels, has an inhibitory effect on the oscillatory calcium release [3].

A rise of cAMP produced by activation of adenylate cyclase impairs calcium mobilization in JG cells [3]. A rise of cGMP produced by activation of guanylate cyclase probably increases the calcium sensitivity of the chloride channels (A. Kurtz and R. Penner, unpublished work).

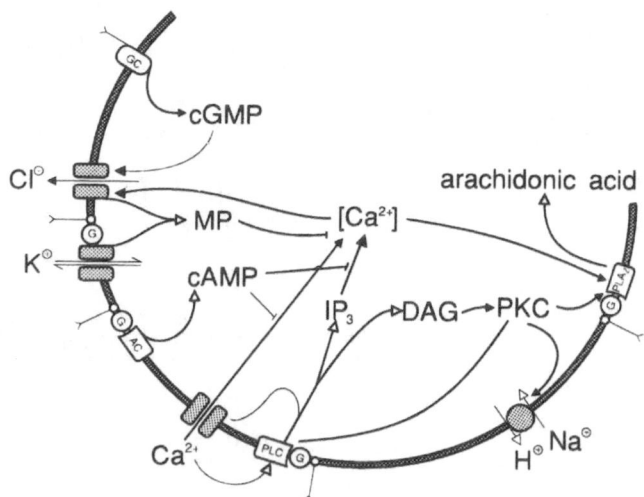

Fig. 5. Interaction of second messenger systems in afferent arteriolar and granular cells. PLC, phospholipase C; PLA$_2$, phospholipase A$_2$, DAG, diacyglycerol; IP$_3$, inositoltrisphosphate; PKC, protein kinase C; AC, adenylate cyclase; GC, guanylate cyclase; G, GTP-binding protein; MP, membrane potential

Acknowledgments. The author wishes to thank O. Stoupa for secretarial help and C. Gasser for doing the artwork. This work was financially supported by a grant from the Swiss National Science Foundation (31-26381.89)

References

1. Barajas L (1979) Anatomy of the juxtaglomerular apparatus. Am J Physiol 236:F333–F343
2. Taugner R, Bührle CP, Hackenthal E, Mannek E, Nobiling R (1984) Morphology of the juxtaglomerular apparatus and secretory mechanisms. In: Berlyne GM, Giovanetti S (eds) Contributions to nephrology, vol 43. Karger, Basel, pp 76–101
3. Kurtz A, Penner R (1989) Angiotensin II induces oscillations of intracellular calcium and inhibits anomalous inward rectifying potassium current in renal juxtaglomerular cells. Proc Natl Acad Sci USA 86:3423–3427
4. Kurtz A (1989) Cellular control of renin secretion. Rev Physiol Biochem Pharmacol 113:1–40
5. Steinhausen M, Snoei H, Parekh N, Baker R, Johnson PC (1983) Hydronephrosis: a new method to visualize vas afferens, efferens, and glomerular network. Kidney Int 23:794–806
6. Skott O, Briggs JP (1987) Direct demonstration of macula densa mediated renin release. Science 237:1618–1620
7. Kurtz A, Della Bruna R, Pfeilschifter J, Taugner R, Bauer C (1986) Atrial natriuretic peptide inhibits renin release from isolated renal juxtaglomerular cells by cGMP-mediated process. Proc Natl Acad Sci USA 83:4769–4773

8. Hokin MR, Hokin LE (1953) Enzyme secretion and the incorporation of ^{32}P into phospholipids of pancreas slices. J Biol Chem 203:967–977
9. Michell RH (1975) Inositol phospholipids and cell surface receptor function. Biochim Biophys Acta 415:81–147
10. Berridge MJ (1987) Inositoltriphosphate and diacylglycerol; two interactive second messengers. Annu Rev Biochem 56:159–193
11. Cockcroft S, Stutchfield (1988) G-proteins, the inositol lipid signalling pathway, and secretion. Philos Trans R Soc Lond [Biol] B320:247–265
12. Kurtz A, Pfeilschifter J, Hutter A, Bührle CP, Nobiling R, Taugner R, Hackenthal E, Bauer C (1986a) Role of protein kinase C in vasoconstrictor caused inhibition of renin release from isolated juxtaglomerular cells. Am J Physiol 250:C563–C571
13. Streb H, Irvine RF, Berridge MJ, Schulz I (1983) Release of Ca^{2+} from a nonmitochondrial store in pancreas acinar cells by inositol-1,4,5-triphosphate. Nature 306:67–68
14. Hackenthal E, Aktories K, Jakobs KH (1985) Pertussis toxin attenuates angiotensin II-induced vasoconstriction and inhibition of renin release. Mol Cell Endocrinol 42: 113–117
15. Bührle CP, Nobiling R, Taugner R (1985) Intracellular recordings from renin-positive cells of the afferent glomerular arteriole. Am J Physiol 249:F272–F281
16. Nishizuka Y (1984) Turnover of inositol phospholipids and signal transduction. Science 225:1365–1369
17. Scholz H, Kurtz A (1990) Role of protein kinase C in renal vasoconstriction caused by angiotensin II. Am J Physiol 259:C421–C426
18. Pfeilschifter J, Kurtz A, Bauer C (1986) Role of phospholipase C and protein kinase C in vasoconstrictor-induced prostaglandin synthesis in cultured rat renal mesangial cells. Biochem J 234:125–130
19. Smith JB (1986) Angiotensin receptor signalling in cultured vascular smooth muscle cells. Am J Physiol 250:F759–F769
20. Penner R, Matthews G, Neher E (1988) Second messenger control of calcium influx in rat peritoneal mast cells. Nature 334:499–504
21. Jacob R (1990) Calcium oscillations in electrically non-excitable cells. Biochim Biophys Acta 1052:427–438
22. Adelstein RS (1983) Regulation of contractile proteins by phosphorylation. J Clin Invest 72:1863–1866
23. Fray JCS (1990) Control of renin secretion by extracellular calcium. Cell Calcium 11:339–341
24. Kurtz A (1990) Do calcium-activated chloride channels control renin secretion? News Physiol Sci 5:43–46
25. Irvine RF (1982) How is the level of free arachidonic acid controlled in mammalian cells? Biochem J 204:3–16
26. Van den Bosch H (1980) Intracellular phospholipases A. Biochim Biophys Acta 604:191–246
27. Lapetina EG (1982) Regulation of arachidonic acid production: role of phospholipase C and A_2. Trends Pharmacol Sci 3:115–118
28. Axelrod J, Burch RM, Jelsema CL (1988) Receptor-mediated activation of phospholipase A_2 via GTP-binding proteins: arachidonic acid and its metabolites as second messengers. Trends Neurosci 11:117–123
29. Hura CE, Kunau RT (1988) Angiotensin II-stimulated prostaglandin production by canine renal afferent arterioles. Am J Physiol 254:F734–F738
30. Antonipillai I, Nadler JL, Robon EC, Horton R (1987) The inhibitory role of 12- and 15-lipoxygenase products on renin release. Hypertension 10:61–66
31. Antonipillai I, Nadler J, Horton R (1988) Angiotensin feedback inhibition on renin is expressed via the lipoxygenase pathway. Endocrinology 122:1277–1281

32. Takahashi K, Capdevila J, Karara A, Falck JR, Jacobson HR, Badr KF (1990) Cytochrome P-450 arachidonate metabolites in rat kidney: characterization and hemodynamic responses. Am J Physiol 258:F781–F789

33. Limbird LE (1988) Receptors linked to inhibition of adenylate cyclase: additional signalling mechanisms. FASEB J 2:2686–2695

34. Pettinger WA, Umemura S, Smyth DD, Jeffries WB (1987) Renal α_2-adrenoreceptors and the adenylate cyclase-cAMP system: biochemical and physiological interactions. Am J Physiol 252:F199–F208

35. Churchill PC, Churchill MC (1985) A1 and A2 adenosine receptor activation inhibits and stimulates renin secretion of rat renal cortical slices. J Pharmacol Exp Ther 232: 589–594

36. Holz FG, Steinhausen M (1987) Renovascular effects of adenosine receptor agonists. Renal Physiol 10:272–282

37. Spielman WS, Thompson CJ (1982) A proposed role for adenosine in the regulation of renal hemodynamics and renin release. Am J Physiol 242:F423–F435

38. Hall JE, Granger JP (1986) Adenosine alters glomerular filtration control by angiotensin II. Am J Physiol 250:F917–F923

39. Skott O, Baumbach L (1985) Effects of adenosine on renin release from isolated glomeruli and kidney slices. Pflugers Arch 404:232–237

40. Kurtz A, Della Bruna R, Pfeilschifter J, Bauer C (1988b) Role of cGMP as second messenger of adenosine in the inhibition of renin release. Kidney Int 33:798–803

41. Schnermann J, Weihprecht H, Briggs JP (1990) Inhibition of tubuloglomerular feedback during adenosine1 receptor blockade. Am J Physiol 258:F553–F561

42. Weihprecht H, Lorenz JN, Schnermann J, Skott O, Briggs JP (1990) Effect of adenosine 1-receptor blockade on renin release from rabbit isolated perfused juxtaglomerular apparatus. J Clin Invest 85:1622–1628

43. Chinkers M, Garbers DL, Chang MS, Lowe DG, Chin H, Goeddel DV, Schulz S (1989) A membrane form of guanylate cyclase is an atrial natriuretic peptide receptor. Nature 338:78–83

44. Walter U (1989) Physiological role of cGMP and cGMP-dependent protein kinase in the cardiovascular system. Rev Physiol Biochem Pharmacol 113:41–88

45. Marin-Grez M, Fleming JT, Steinhausen M (1986) Atrial natriuretic peptide causes preglomerular vasodilatation and post-glomerular vasoconstriction in rat kidney. Nature 324:473–476

46. Ohishi K, Hishida A, Honda N (1988) Direct vasodilatory action of atrial natriuretic factor on canine glomerular afferent arterioles. Am J Physiol 255:F415–F420

47. Takagi M, Franco-Saenz R, Mulrow PJ (1988) Effect of atrial natriuretic peptide on renin release in a superfusion system of kidney slices and dispersed juxtaglomerular cells. Endocrinology 122:1437–1442

48. Hiruma M, Ikemoto F, Yamamoto K (1986) Rat atrial natriuretic factor stimulates renin release from renal cortical slices. Eur J Pharmacol 125:151–153

49. Kurtz A, Della Bruna R, Pfeilschifter J, Bauer C (1986c) Effect of synthetic atrial natriuretic peptide on rat renal juxtaglomerular cells. J Hypertens 4:S57–S60

50. Vidal MJ, Romero JC, Vanhoutte PM (1988) Endothelium-derived relaxing factor inhibits renin release. Eur J Pharmacol 149:401–402

51. Daniel TO, Ives HE (1989) Endothelial control of vascular function. News Physiol Sci 4:139–142

52. Fishman MC (1976) Membrane potential of juxtaglomerular cells. Nature 260:542–544

53. Kurtz A, Skott O, Chegini S, Penner R (1990) Lack of direct evidence for a functional role of voltage gated calcium channels in renal juxtaglomerular cells. Pflugers Arch 416:281–287

54. Aickin CC, Brading AF (1985) Advances in the understanding of transmembrane ionic gradients and permeabilities in smooth muscle obtained by using ion-selective microelectrodes. Experientia 41:879–887
55. Kurtz A, Penner R (1990) Effects of angiotensin II on intracellular calcium and electrical function of mouse renal juxtaglomerular cells. Kidney Int 38:S-51–S-54

Macula Densa Control of Renin Secretion

JOSIE P. BRIGGS, JOHN N. LORENZ, HORST WEIHPRECHT, and
JÜRGEN SCHNERMANN[1]

SUMMARY. Macula densa (MD) controls on renin secretion have recently been
studied by examining the renin secretory response of the isolated perfused rabbit
juxtaglomerular apparatus (JGA). Single JGAs, consisting of a segment of distal
tubule including the macula densa, with adherent glomerulus and short vascular fragments, are dissected from rabbit kidney, and the tubule is perfused. Renin secretion
from this preparation shows an inverse dependency on NaCl concentration in the
tubular lumen. When perfused with a low NaCl solution, renin secretion is inhibited
by addition of NaCl, choline Cl, and RbCl, but not by addition of Na acetate or Na
isethionate. Renin secretion is stimulated by addition of 10^{-6}M bumetanide to the
tubular perfusate but not to the bathing solution. It is concluded that renin secretion
is inversely related to the rate of tubular transport, and that the pattern of ion specificity is consistent with participation of the Na-K-2Cl co-transporter. Other studies
examined possible stimulus-response coupling mechanisms. Renin secretion was
found to be stimulated by the adenosine1 analog CHA (N^6-cyclohexyladenosine), an
effect that was blocked by the specific adenosine 1 blocker, CPX(8-cyclopentyl-
1,3-dipropylxanthine). The inhibitory effect of a high luminal NaCl solution at the
MD was markedly blunted in the presence of the A1 blocker CPX, but CPX did not
significantly affect renin secretion when luminal NaCl was low, suggesting that
adenosine formation is dependent upon luminal NaCl concentration, and supporting
the hypothesis that variation in the local levels of adenosine may be at least partially
responsible for macula densa signal transmission.

Introduction

The terminal end of the thick ascending limb of Henle, the site of the macula densa
(MD), is a position uniquely suited for monitoring flow dependent changes of NaCl

[1]The University of Michigan, Department of Internal Medicine, Division of Nephrology, 1150
W. Medical Center Drive, 1560 MSRBII, Ann Arbor, MI 48109-0676, USA

338

concentration. Along the proximal tubule, flow is not a major determinant of salt concentration. In more distal nephron segments, Na and Cl concentrations are largely determined by the actions of aldosterone and vasopressin. At the macula densa, however, NaCl concentration is primarily dictated by tubular flow rate. The transport properties of the thick ascending limb of Henle (TALH), and active NaCl transport by a water impermeable epithelium, result in the transformation of a flow signal into a change in salt concentration.

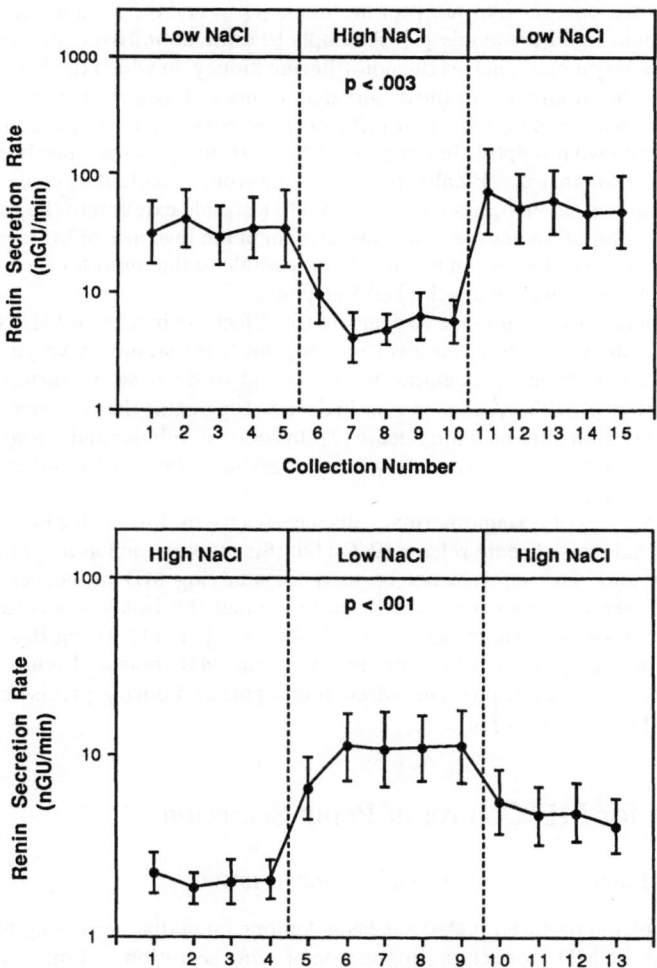

Fig. 1

An influence of tubular fluid composition on renin release was first proposed by Goormaghtigh [1]. In 1965 Vander summarized a substantial body of experimental evidence and concluded that a change in distal NaCl delivery induced inverse changes of renin secretion and that the input from the MD was the major control mechanism of renin secretion in states of salt depletion and excess [2]. Nevertheless, as judged from the continued controversy over existence and mechanisms of MD control of renin secretion, the experimental work in intact kidneys has remained remarkably inconclusive. Several problems have made limited progress in this area. First, the signal arriving at the MD often cannot be determined precisely, because the MD is located below the surface of the kidney. Secondly, renin secretion is also influenced by sympathetic tone, the baroreceptor mechanism [3], and the local levels of a number of hormones and autocoids [4]. Attempts to draw definitive conclusions from complex in vivo models, such as the non-filtering kidney, in which the MD influence is assumed to be eliminated, or the denervated, β-blocked, papaverine treated dog, in which sympathetic and baroreceptor influences are considered to be excluded [5,6], have been somewhat helpful, but in general these techniques have not been able to yield unequivocal answers. Finally, renin secreted from a single JGA cannot be sampled quantitatively in vivo, since it is secreted to a sizable extent into the renal interstitium. This limitation has prevented assessment of the response of MD secretion to single nephron perturbations in a manner comparable to that used for the evaluation of the tubuloglomerular feedback (TGF) response.

Two attempts have been made to evaluate the effect of changes in MD NaCl concentration at the single nephron level in vivo, but these studies have yielded contradictory results. Renin concentration was found to decrease in surface venules draining a group of oil-blocked nephrons in the cat, suggesting that a reduction in MD NaCl concentration inhibits renin release [7]. In contrast, tubular and postglomerular renin concentration varied inversely with changes in distal NaCl in micropuncture studies in the rat [8].

Isolated explants of juxtaglomerular cells have been a useful tool for in vitro evaluation of mechanisms of renin release [9,10] but this preparation has a disrupted JGA morphology and can therefore not be used for studying MD influences on renin secretion. Several laboratories have recently applied the isolated perfused tubule technique to studying various aspects of MD function [11–14]. Using this approach it has been possible, for the first time, to investigate MD control of renin secretion in the absence of baroreceptor and adrenergic inputs and during precise control of tubular fluid composition [14].

Evidence for MD Control of Renin Secretion

Effect of Changes in Luminal NaCl Concentration

Using the isolated perfused JGA it has been demonstrated that increasing NaCl concentration at the MD produces a suppression of renin secretion and that a reduction of NaCl concentration produces stimulation [14,15,16,17] (see Fig. 1). These results yield clear evidence for an inverse relationship between renin secretion and MD NaCl concentration. MD-dependent renin secretion is characterized by a rapid onset and offset following step changes in NaCl concentration and by reversibility of the induced changes [15,16]. Renin responses were independent of whether the tubule was perfused in an orthograde fashion from the TALH or in a retrograde fashion from the distal convoluted tubule [16]. Renin secretion was not altered when NaCl concentration was reduced from isotonicity to about 80 mM, but the full renin response was seen when NaCl concentrations were varied between 7 and 61 mM (Cl) and between 26 and 80 mM (Na)[17], that is, within the range that seems to be physiologically relevant. It is of note that this is the same concentration range in which the tubuloglomerular feedback response occurs.

These studies yield a quantitative estimate of the effect of MD NaCl concentration on renin secretion [16]. Assuming a linear relationship between the changes in NaCl concentration and renin release, the in vitro results predict that single JGA renin secretion increases by about 0.5 nGU/min per mM decrement of NaCl concentration. Using this approximation, one can estimate that plasma renin activity could increase approximately fivefold if NaCl concentration at the MD fell by 10 mM for ten minutes. Nonetheless, extrapolation from this in vitro system to the in vivo response must be made with caution. The assumption of a linear response of renin release over the concentration range studied may not be valid. Furthermore, in vitro, renin secretory responses are assessed in the absence of stabilizing feedback loops that may be important in vivo. For example, stimulation of renin secretion in vivo will increase angiotensin II levels and thereby depress steady-state renin secretion below that predicted for the prevailing MD NaCl concentration. Since renin is effectively removed in the in vitro preparation this negative feedback is eliminated. The TGF mechanism is another feedback system which would tend to minimize deviations in NaCl concentration at the MD and thereby dampen the signal for renin release.

NaCl Concentration vs NaCl Delivery

It has been an unresolved issue whether renin secretion responds to a reduction in NaCl concentration or in NaCl delivery (concentration times flow rate). When luminal NaCl load was reduced by 80% by decreasing perfusate flow at constant NaCl concentration, a small, approximately twofold increase in the rate of renin secretion was noted. In contrast, when NaCl load was reduced to a similar degree by decreasing perfusate NaCl concentration, renin secretion increased nearly eightfold [16]. These studies show clearly that, at least in the isolated perfused JGA, NaCl concentration is a more important determinant of renin release than NaCl delivery. The notion that NaCl load is of primary importance in MD-dependent renin secretion was derived from two observations. Stimulation of renin secretion by dietary Na restriction was associated with an increased distal NaCl concentration, but a reduced NaCl load [18], suggesting an inverse relationship between renin secretion and Na load, but not Na concentration. However, there is substantial evidence that NaCl measurements in the early distal tubule significantly overestimate NaCl concentrations at the MD when tubular flow rates are low, such as those observed in Na restricted animals [19,20]. It is therefore likely that NaCl at the level of the MD is in fact reduced during Na restriction. Another finding supporting load dependency of renin secretion was the observation that an osmotic diuresis produced by hypertonic mannitol infusions was associated with an inhibition of renin release, even though distal NaCl concentration was reduced [21-23]. A possible explanation is that the stimulatory signal exerted through the MD was overcome by other inputs. For example, the increase in plasma osmolality produced by mannitol may have suppressed renin release [24]. Studies with isolated superperfused glomeruli reveal marked sensitivity of renin release to the ambient osmolarity [25]. In contrast to the direct effects of osmolality on granular cells, stimulation of renin secretion by a reduction in luminal NaCl at the MD was also seen when perfusate osmolality was kept constant by the addition of mannitol [14]. Thus, changes in tubular fluid osmolality independent of NaCl variations do not seem to exert control over renin secretion. These findings attest to the specificity of compositional changes within the tubular compartment.

The Sensing Mechanism for MD-Mediated Renin Secretion

The Tubular Sensor

An important aspect of the use of the isolated JGA preparation is that it limits the possible sites of tubulo-vascular information transfer to cells present in the area of contact. Since only MD cells, and possibly a small number of surrounding TAL cells, are found in the area of contact, it is the cellular response of these cell types to luminal NaCl concentration which is probably the critical event in MD-regulated renin release.

It was suggested earlier that inhibition of MD Na transport is an early step in the stimulation of renin secretion [2,26]. This supposition was in part based on observations showing that increasing the delivery of NaCl to the MD prevented or reversed the stimulation of renin secretion produced by a fall in arterial pressure [26]. The subsequent finding that loop diuretics consistently stimulate renin secretion appeared to confirm transport dependency of MD-mediated renin secretion [4], but the in vivo effects of diuretics are complex, and alterations in the baroreceptor signal or in adrenergic input could also explain these effects. The first direct evidence for a MD mediated effect of furosemide on renin secretion came from experiments in which renin secretion from non-perfused afferent arterioles was measured; it was found to be lower when the MD segment was included in the dissected specimen, and higher in specimens which lacked a MD [27]. Addition of furosemide increased renin release in the presence of the MD, but not in its absence [27]. In the isolated perfused JGA preparation, luminal application of bumetanide in a concentration of 10^{-6} M stimulated renin secretion, while bath application had no effect [17]. Since bumetanide did not affect renin secretion when added to the bath it seems unlikely that it interacts directly with granular cells. In view of the low concentration required to observe this effect it seems likely that bumetanide interferes with the operation of the Na,K,2Cl-cotransporter and that the subsequent reduction in the rate of NaCl transport stimulates renin secretion. This proposal is consistent with the recent evidence in support of the presence of this transporter on MD cells [11,13,28].

Ion Specificity of Renin Secretory Responses

Renin secretion in intact animals has been shown to be suppressed by oral or intravenous administration of various Cl or Br salts, but not by Na salts including Na acetate [29,30]. An acute selective depletion of chloride by peritoneal dialysis increased plasma renin activity [31]. In addition, substitution of chloride by nitrate or thiocyanate in the perfusate of isolated kidneys has been shown to stimulate renin secretion [32]. In isolated perfused JGAs, ion selectivity has been examined by measuring the inhibitory effect of addition of various Na and Cl salts to a low NaCl perfusate. The inhibitory response was unchanged when most of the luminal Na was replaced by choline or rubidium. On the other hand, substituting chloride by isethionate or acetate virtually eliminated the response to increased Na concentration [17]. These results are similar to the pattern of ion specificity shown for TGF responses, and are compatible with the hypothesis that both mechanisms share a common sensing step. It has been outlined previously that the known binding affinities of the Na K 2Cl-cotransporter permit some predictions as to the efficacy of Na and Cl to affect MD-dependent processes. The expectation would be that changes in Cl concentration should have a more pronounced effect on renin secretion than changes in Na concentration, above a concentration of about 10 mM where Na binding sites are virtually saturated [33]. In summary, there is now good evidence in support of the hypothesis that the initiating signal for MD control of renin secretion is a change in NaCl transport rate, via a luminal Na K 2Cl-cotransporter whose physiological activity is determined by a change in luminal Cl concentration.

The Stimulus-Response Coupling Mechanism

Adenosine

In intact animals (rats or dogs) exogenous adenosine usually inhibits renin release [34–36]. Theophylline blocks the inhibitory effect of adenosine on renin secretion in dogs [37–40], and itself stimulates renin release [38]. Effects of adenosine analogs are generally dose dependent. At low concentrations, the adenosine1 analogs such as CHA (N^6-cyclohexyl adenosine) produce inhibition of release from intact kidneys [40,41], isolated cortical slices [42], and isolated perfused JGAs [43], but at higher concentrations these analogs may lose their specificity and stimulate renin secretion by interaction with adenosine 2 receptors [44].

In the isolated perfused JGA, addition of the adenosine1 analog CHA resulted in significant inhibition of renin release stimulated by low MD NaCl [43]. The selective adenosine$_1$-receptor blocker 8-cyclopentyl-1,3-dipropylxanthine (CPX) was noted to reverse the inhibiting effect of CHA [43]. Adenosine itself did not significantly inhibit renin secretion unless the adenosine deaminase inhibitor pentostatin (deoxycoformycin) was present in the bath (J. Briggs, H. Weihprecht, unpublished observations). These findings support the conclusion that receptors of the adenosine$_1$-subclass are present on renin-secreting cells at the glomerular vascular pole, and that their activation can initiate inhibition of renin secretion independent of changes in renal hemodynamics or sympathetic nerve activity.

Support for the hypothesis that transport-dependent alterations in local generation of adenosine serve as a paracrine mediator for renin release within the JGA comes from studies using agents which block adenosine receptors. Theophylline has been shown to stimulate renin secretion in isolated non-perfused arterioles that include a MD, but not in specimens lacking a MD [44]. Further evidence comes from experiments with perfused JGAs in which the MD signal was directly manipulated. The inhibitory effect of a high luminal NaCl solution at the MD was markedly blunted in the presence of the A1 blocker CPX, but CPX did not significantly affect renin secretion when luminal NaCl was low, suggesting that adenosine formation is dependent upon luminal NaCl concentration [43].

Prostaglandins

Alterations in renal prostaglandins are known to alter renin secretory responses to a variety of stimuli. For example, cyclooxygenase inhibition has been shown to reduce the stimulation of renin release by salt depletion [4], converting enzyme inhibitors [4], and adrenalectomy [45]. Infusion of arachidonic acid stimulates renin release from intact animals and isolated perfused kidneys; in most preparations administration of PGE_2 or PGI_2 is also stimulatory [4]. Indirect evidence supports PG participation in MD mediated effects on renin secretion. The acute stimulation of renin release produced by furosemide [4,46] and theophylline [38] is blunted by administration of indomethacin. Stimulation of renin secretion by supra-aortic constriction in denervated kidney of dogs treated with papaverine, a model of MD responses, is also blocked by indomethacin and meclofenamate [47].

Histochemical studies have provided evidence that cyclo-oxygenase, although abundant in renal endothelial cells, is low or absent in the MD [48]. This finding suggests that it is unlikely that a cyclo-oxygenase metabolite functions as a paracrine mediator transmitting a signal from the macula densa to the granular cell. However, cyclo-oxygenase products, particularly PGE_2 and PGI_2, appear to be produced by mesangial cells and isolated glomeruli [49,50]; a local autacoid or paracrine function of PGs within the JGA is possible. In cultured mesangial cells, medium Cl concentration has been shown to modify PGE_2 production, with reductions in Cl stimulating the formation of the measured prostaglandin [51].

Renin Secretion and Tubuloglomerular Feedback

Changes in NaCl concentration in the tubular fluid in the region of the MD exert two effects on cells of the afferent arteriole. They induce direct changes of the tone of contractile smooth muscle cells (the tubuloglomerular feedback response) and they inversely affect renin secretion from granular cells. Both responses have a number of similarities and it is possible that they are mediated through the same extracellular and intracellular mediators. One aspect of the MD-mediated control mechanisms which deserves some consideration is that they have the potential of influencing each other. Angiotensin has been shown to markedly enhance the contractile response of afferent arterioles to the MD signal [52,53]. An increase in NaCl at the MD will lead to an increase in afferent tone, which will tend to lower distal NaCl through its effect on GFR and proximal absorption. But since this compensation is likely to be incomplete, there will be a decrease in renin secretion simultaneously. The resulting change in plasma angiotensin concentration will decrease the sensitivity of the vascular response to NaCl and attenuate the dependency of GFR on the MD signal. These changes will relax control of NaCl at the MD and permit salt excretion to rise. The opposite sequence of events will occur when MD NaCl decreases.

This dual effect of MD NaCl may contribute to the adjustments in TGF responsiveness which are seen during alterations in extracellular volume. The reduction in TGF sensitivity, caused by volume expansion, is to a large extent explicable by reductions in angiotensin levels [52], suggesting that depression of renin secretion plays an important role in the adjustment of GFR during volume expansion, is predicted to uncouple GFR from MD control, because the simultaneous inhibition of renin secretion will, after a time, reduce TGF sensitivity. Since the resulting increase in GFR will further inhibit renin secretion, a positive feedback cycle is initiated which will allow filtrate formation to become independent of MD control. However, the fall in angiotensin levels will induce an increasing release of renin secretion from the inhibiting effects of angiotensin. Thus, resulting from a balance of these interconnected feedback loops, a new steady-state in salt excretion and in renin secretion will occur.

Acknowledgments. L.N. Lorenz is the recipient of an Individual National Research Service Award, DK-08411. H. Weihprecht is supported by a Fellowship from the Michigan Affiliate of the American Heart Association. Work performed in this laboratory is funded by the National Institutes of Health Grants DK-37448, DK-39255, and DK40042.

References

1. Goormaghtigh N (1939) Une glande endocrine dans la paroi des arterioles renales. Bruxelles-Med 19:1541–1549
2. Vander AJ (1967) Control of renin release. Physiol Rev 47:359–382
3. Bock HA, Hermle M, Fiallo A, Osgood RW, Fried TA (1990) Measurement of renin secretion in single perfused rabbit glomeruli. Am J Physiol 258:F1460–F1465
4. Keeton TK, Campbell WB (1980) The pharmacologic alteration of renin release. Pharmacol Rev 32:81–227
5. Blaine EH, Davis JO, Witty RT (1970) Renin release after hemorrhage and after suprarenal aortic constriction in dogs without sodium delivery to the macula densa. Circ Res 27:1081–1089
6. Witty RT, Davis JO, Johnson JA, Prewitt RL (1971) Effects of papaverine and hemorrhage on renin secretion in the non-filtering kidney. Am J Physiol 221:1666–1671
7. Morgan T, Gillies A (1977) Factors controlling the release of renin. A micropuncture study in the cat. Pflügers Arch 368:13–18
8. Leyssac PP (1986) Changes in single nephron renin release are mediated by tubular fluid flow rate. Kidney Int 30:332–339
9. Kurtz A (1989) Cellular control of renin secretion. Rev Physiol Biochem Pharmacol 113:1–40
10. Carey RM, Geary KM, Hunt MK, Ramos SP, Forbes MS, Inagami T, Peach MJ, Leong DA (1990) Identification of individual renocortical cells that secrete renin. Am J Physiol 258:F649–F659
11. Bell PD, Lapointe JY, Cardinal J (1989) Direct measurement of basolateral potentials from cells of the macula densa. Am J Physiol 257:F463–F468
12. Kirk KL, Bell PD, Barfuss D, Ribadeneira M (1985) Direct visualization of the isolated and perfused macula densa. Am J Physiol 248:F890–F894
13. Schlatter E, Salomonsson M, Persson AEG, Greger R (1989) Macula densa cells sense luminal NaCl concentration via furosemide sensitive $Na^+2Cl^-K^+$ cotransport. Pflügers Arch 414:286–290

14. Skøtt O, Briggs JP (1988) A method for superfusion of the isolated perfused tubule. Kidney Int 33:1009-1012
15. Skøtt O, Briggs JP (1987) Direct demonstration of macula densa-mediated renin secretion. Science 237:1618-1620
16. Lorenz JN, Weihprecht H, Schnermann J, Skøtt O, Briggs JP (to be published) Characterization of the macula densa stimulus for renin secretion. Am J Physiol
17. Lorenz JN, Weihprecht H, Schnermann J, Skøtt O, Briggs JP (to be published) Renin release from the isolated juxtaglomerular apparatus depends on macula densa chloride transport. Am J Physiol
18. Churchill PC, Churchill MC, McDonald FD (1978) Renin secretion and distal tubule Na+ in rats. Am J Physiol 235:F611-F616
19. Schnermann J, Schubert G, Briggs JP (1982) In situ studies of the distal convoluted tubule in the rat. I. Evidence for NaCl secetion. Am J Physiol 243:F160-F166
20. Baines AD, Basmadjian D, Wang BC (1979) Computer simulation of flow-dependent absorption in microperfused short Henle's loop of rats. Biophys J 27:21-38
21. Churchill PC, Churchill MC, McDonald FD (1979) Effects of saline and mannitol on renin and distal tubule Na in rats. Circ Res 45:786-792
22. Di Bona GF (1971) Effect of mannitol diuresis and uretal occlusion on distal tubular reabsorption. Am J Physiol 221:511-514
23. Vander AJ (1968) Renin secretion during mannitol diuresis and ureteral occlusion. Proc Soc Exp Biol Med 128:518-520
24. Skøtt O (1988) Do osmotic forces play a role in renin secretion? Am J Physiol 255:F1-F10
25. Frederiksen O, Leyssac PP, Skinner SL (1975) Sensitive osmometer function of juxtaglomerular cells in vitro. J Physiol 252:669-679
26. Vander AJ, Miller R (1964) Control of renin secretion in the anaesthetized dog. Am J Physiol 207:537-546
27. Itoh S Carretero OA (1985) Role of the macula densa in renin release. Hypertension 7 (Suppl. 1):49-54
28. Gonzales E, Salomonsson M, Müller-Suur C, Persson AEG (1988) Measurements of macula densa cell volume changes in isolated and perfused rabbit cortical thick ascending limb. I. Isosmotic and anisosmotic cell volume changes. Acta Physiol Scand 133: 149-157
29. Kirchner KA, Kotchen TA, Galla JH, Luke RG (1978) Importance of chloride for acute inhibition of renin by sodium chloride. Am J Physiol 235:F444-F450
30. Kotchen TA, Welch WJ, Ott CE (1984) The renal tubular signal for renin release. J Hypertension 2(suppl 1):35-42
31. Abboud HE, Luke RG, Galla JH, Kotchen TA (1979) Stimulation of renin by acute selective chloride depletion in the rat. Circ Res 44:815-821
32. Rostand SG, Work J, Luke RG (1985) Effect of reduced chloride reabsorption on renin release in the isolated rat kidney. Pflugers Arch 405:46-51
33. Greger R (1985) Ion transport mechanisms in thick ascending limb of Henle's loop of mammalian nephron. Physiol Rev 65:760-797
34. Arend LJ, Haramati A, Thompson CL, Spielman WS (1984) Adenosine-induced decreases in renin release: dissociation from hemodynamic effects. Am J Physiol 247:F447-F452
35. Osswald H, Schmitz H-J, Heidenreich O (1975) Adenosine response of the rat kidney after saline loading, sodium restriction and hemorrhagia. Pflugers Arch 357:323-333
36. Tagawa A, Vander AJ (1970) Effects of adenosine compounds on renal function and renin secretion in dogs. Circ Res 26:327-338
37. Johns EJ, Singer B (1973) Effect of propranolol and theophylline on renin release caused by furosemide in the cat. Eur J Pharmacol 23:67-73
38. Oliw E, Anggard E, Fredholm BB (1977) Effect of indomethacin on the renal actions of theophylline. Eur J Pharmacol 43:9-16

39. Spielman WS (1984) Antagonistic effect of theophylline on the adenosine-induced decrease in renin release. Am J Physiol 247:F246–F251
40. Churchill PC, Bidani AK (1990) Adenosine and Renal Function. In: Adenosine and Adenosine Receptors, Williams M (ed), Humana, Clifton, pp 335–380
41. Cook CB, Churchill PC (1984) Effects of renal denervation on the renal responses of anesthetized rats to cyclohexyladenosine. Can J Physiol Pharmacol 62:934–938
42. Churchill PC, Churchill MC (1985) A_1 and A_2 adenosine receptor activation inhibits and stimulates renin secretion of rat renal cortical slices. J Pharmacol Exp Ther 232:589–594
43. Weihprecht H, Lorenz JN, Schnermann J, Skøtt O, Briggs JP (1990) Effect of adenosine$_1$-receptor blockade on renin release from rabbit isolated perfused juxtaglomerular apparatus. J Clin Invest apparatus. J Clin Invest 85:1622–1628
44. Itoh S, Carretero OA, Murray RD (1985) Possible role of adenosine in the macula densa mechanism of renin release in rabbits. J Clin Invest 76:1412–1417
45. Meyer DK, Benzing A (1979) Studies on the inhibitory effect of indomethacin and meclofenamate on the adrenalectomy-induced increase in plasma renin concentration. Naunyn Schmiedebergs Arch Pharmacol 309:25–27
46. Bailie MD, Crosslan K, Hook JB (1976) Natriuretic effect of furosemide after inhibition of prostaglandin synthetase. J Pharmacol Exp Ther 199:459–476
47. Olson RD, Skoglund ML, Nies AS, Gerber JG (1980) Prostaglandins mediate the macula densa stimulated renin release. Adv Prostaglandin Thromboxane Res 7:1135–1137
48. Smith WL, Bell YG (1978) Immunohistochemical localization of the prostaglandin-forming cyclooxygenase in renal cortex. Am J Physiol 235:F451–F457
49. Schlöndorff D, Ardaillou R (1986) Prostaglandins and other arachidonic acid metabolites in the kidney. Kidney Int 29:108–119
50. Mene P, Simonson MS, Dunn, MJ (1989) Physiology of the mesangial cell. Physiol Rev 69:1347–1424
51. Okuda T, Kojima I, Ogata E, Kurokawa K (1989) Ambient Cl^- ions modify rat mesangial cell contraction by modulating cell inositol trisphosphate and Ca^{2+} via enhanced prostaglandin E_2. J Clin Invest 84:1866–1872
52. Schnermann J, Briggs JP (to be published) Restoration of tubuloglomerular feedback in volume expanded rats by angiotensin II. Am J Physiol
53. Mitchell K, Navar LG (1988) Enhanced tubuloglomerular feedback during peritubular perfusions of angiotensins I and II. Am J Physiol 255:F383–F390

Macula Densa Control of Renin Secretion and Proximal Tubular Pressure

PAUL P. LEYSSAC[1]

SUMMARY. Early studies suggested that the proximal tubular pressure was regulated by a negative feedback mechanism operating via the juxtaglomerular (JG) apparatus, involving changes in renin secretion. Subsequent and recent studies have confirmed this hypothesis. The tubuloglomerular feedback (TGF) response oscillates with a frequency of about 30 mHz, and is sensitive to changes in late proximal flow of less than 3 nl.min^{-1}. It is specifically abolished by loop diuretics. Micropuncture studies have shown that single nephron renin release is increased when Henle loop flow is decreased and conversely, that single nephron renin release is decreased when Henle loop flow is increased. Studies on isolated JG-apparatuses have shown that this is due to the flow-dependent changes in luminal sodium chloride concentration at the level of the macula densa (M.D.). Thus, both the TGF-mediated afferent vasoconstriction and the M.D.-mediated renin secretion share the same luminal signal. The intracellular (i.c.) signal is probably also the same, since an increase in i.c. calcium causes vasoconstriction and inhibition of renin release from the JG cells. Both responses may therefore be considered as part of the TGF-mechanism.

Introduction

Present knowledge of glomerular and tubular pressures and flow rates through the different nephron segments indicates that the flow resistance across the glomerular membrane is 30–40 times less than the total resistance downstream from the proximal tubule. One could therefore predict that a primary change in the filtration pressure (P_{UF}) initially results in a nearly parallel increase in proximal tubular pressure (P_{prox}), thus leaving glomerular filtration rate (GFR) largely unchanged. However, the proximal hydrostatic pressure is very well regulated by tubuloglomerular feed-

---

[1]Institute of Experimental Medicine, University of Copenhagen, DK-2200 Copenhagen, Denmark

back mechanisms, and therefore rapidly returns to its control value [1]. In the steady state after such a change, at least after a moderate change of a few (e.g., 5) mm Hg, proximal intratubular pressure is always equal to its control value.

We have tested the concept that an increase in filtration pressure does in fact result in a parallel increase in proximal pressure, and that this pressure is regulated back to its stable steady state level by the TGF mechanism. We have also tested the postulate that the renin-angiotensin system (RAS) is involved in this regulation, and we conclude that it does participate, mainly by its effect on the efferent arteriolar resistance (R_e).

Results and Discussion

My first attempt dates back to 1969 [2], when tubular pressures were measured by the old-fashioned Landis technique, which only gives point-measurements. This is shown in Fig. 1, where pressure is followed as a function of time after an intravenous infusion of 2.5 ml of Ringer solution (equal to 1% of body weight), as shown by closed squares, or of rat plasma (circles), which gave the same plasma volume expan-

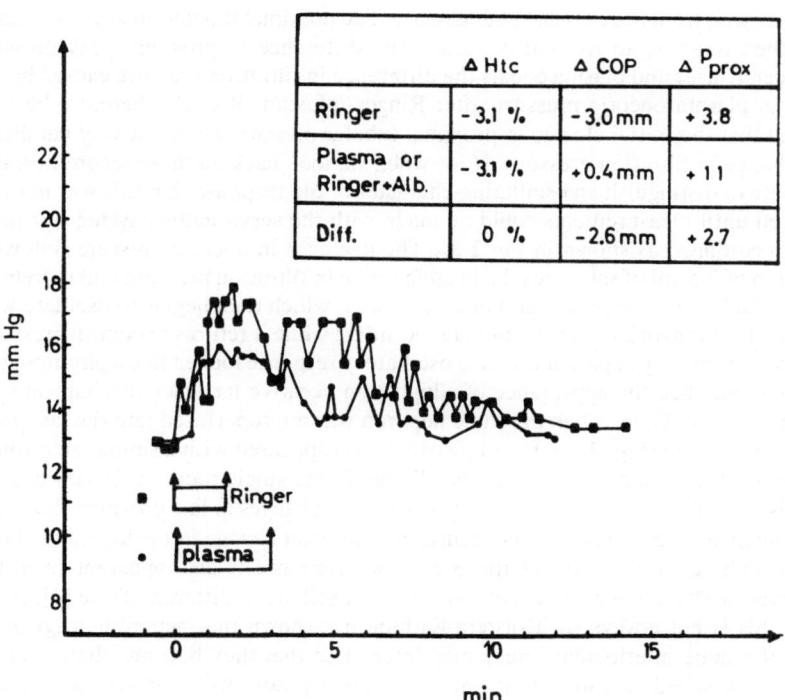

	Δ Htc	Δ COP	Δ P_{prox}
Ringer	- 3.1 %	- 3.0 mm	+ 3.8
Plasma or Ringer+Alb.	- 3.1 %	+0.4 mm	+ 11
Diff.	0 %	-2.6 mm	+ 2.7

Fig. 1. Changes in proximal intratubular pressure following extracellular volume expansion with 2.5 ml of Ringers and of rat plasma, respectively. Htc, hematocrit; COP, oncotic pressure (mm Hg); P_{prox}, proximal intratubular pressure (mm Hg)

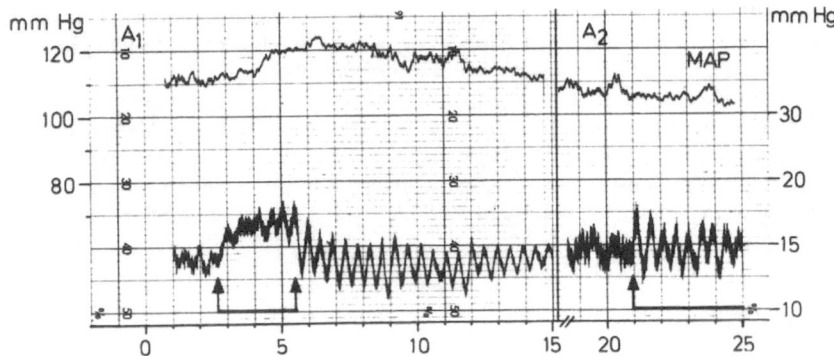

Fig. 2. Mean arterial pressure (*MAP*) and proximal tubular pressure recordings. **a₁** 2.5 ml of isotonic saline was given *between the arrows*. **a₂** After stabilization of the proximal pressure a microperfusion pipette was impaled into the last proximal convolution of the same nephron while leaving the pressure pipette in situ. The pump was started at 5 nl·min⁻¹ *at the arrow*. (From [3] with permission)

sion, as seen from the change in hematocrit. The proximal tubular pressure increased and then returned to its control value. The difference in proximal peak pressure between Ringer and plasma equals the difference in filtration pressure caused by the drop in plasma oncotic pressure after Ringer infusion. It could therefore be concluded that the initial change in proximal tubular pressure quantitatively paralleled the change in filtration pressure. Now, when we look back on these recordings, it is possible to distinguish an oscillating character of the response, but this was not recognized until measurements could be made with the servo-nulling system for pressure recordings, as shown in Fig 2 a₁. The decrease in oncotic pressure following infusion of 2.5 ml of saline results in an increase in filtration pressure and thereby in the initial increase in proximal tubular pressure, which then begins to oscillate with a regular rhythm of 2 cycles per minute (30 mHz) while it returns to control pressure.

It was intuitively apparent that this oscillatory response looked like a physiological response and had the appearance of a high-gain negative feedback mechanism with a certain delay. Then, when the same nephron was microperfused into the last proximal convolution (Fig. 2 a₂), the same oscillation appeared with a similar amplitude, indicating that this response could be elicited in the single individual nephron.

This rhythmic response is extremely sensitive to changes in late proximal flow rate. A difference of less than 3 nl/min causes a significant change in the amplitude [4].

The individual character of the oscillatory response is also apparent from the observation that neighboring nephrons usually oscillate in different phase [4]. However, this is not always so. Holstein-Rathlou has shown that nephrons originating from the same interlobular artery may interact so that they become phase-locked, i.e., synchronized, and so that a change in Henle loop flow in one nephron also results in a response in its neighbor [5].

Further evidence that these oscillations represent a TGF-mediated response transmitted by the macula densa were obtained from experiments with loop diuretics. Figure 3 shows the effect of late proximal microperfusion with furosemide on the

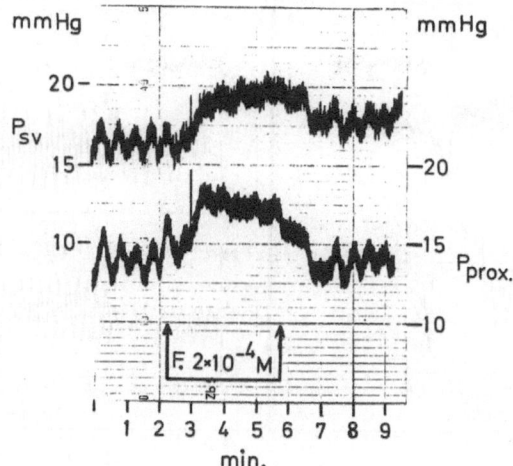

Fig. 3. Simultaneous recordings of pressures in the proximal tubule (P_{prox}) and in the star vessel of the same nephron (P_{SV}). Furosemide (F) was microperfused into the last proximal convolution at 7.1 nl·min^{-1} *between the arrows*. (From [4] with permission)

proximal tubular and star vessel pressures. The oscillations disappear, and the increase in pressure indicates that the nephron is no longer able to regulate its pressure, probably due to the afferent arteriolar vasodilation, as suggested also by the increase in efferent arteriolar pressure. This effect is specific for loop diuretics, since it is not seen after microperfusion with acetazolamide or amiloride [6].

Thus, it seems safe to conclude that the pressure oscillations reflect a TGF response transmitted by the reabsorptive function of the macula densa.

If this oscillatory phenomenon was simply the result of the operation of the TGF system, it should be possible to design a dynamic mathematical model by combining previous steady state models of all the individual steps. Holstein-Rathlou elegantly solved this task, and with this first dynamic model of the nephron we could now follow the changes in all parameter values with time, in response to a change in one of them, e.g., in the Henle loop flow rate [7].

The first version of the model consisted of a glomerular model, a tubular model, and a model of the afferent arteriolar feedback. Figure 4 shows various model simulations of effects after changes in Henle loop flow compared with direct experimental recordings of the same changes. It is seen how well the model simulates the in vivo responses, both regarding frequency and amplitude, and that the mean proximal free flow pressure is stabilized by the feedback.

However, there are significant differences, which indicate that the model is incomplete in this version. Firstly, increasing Henle loop flow, e.g., by i.v. isotonic saline infusion causes renal blood flow (RBF) to increase, whereas the model predicts that RBF is depressed. Secondly, the proximal tubular pressure is more accurately regulated in vivo than in the model simulations, as seen in Fig. 4. Thus, something is missing in the model. This could be the renin-angiotensin system.

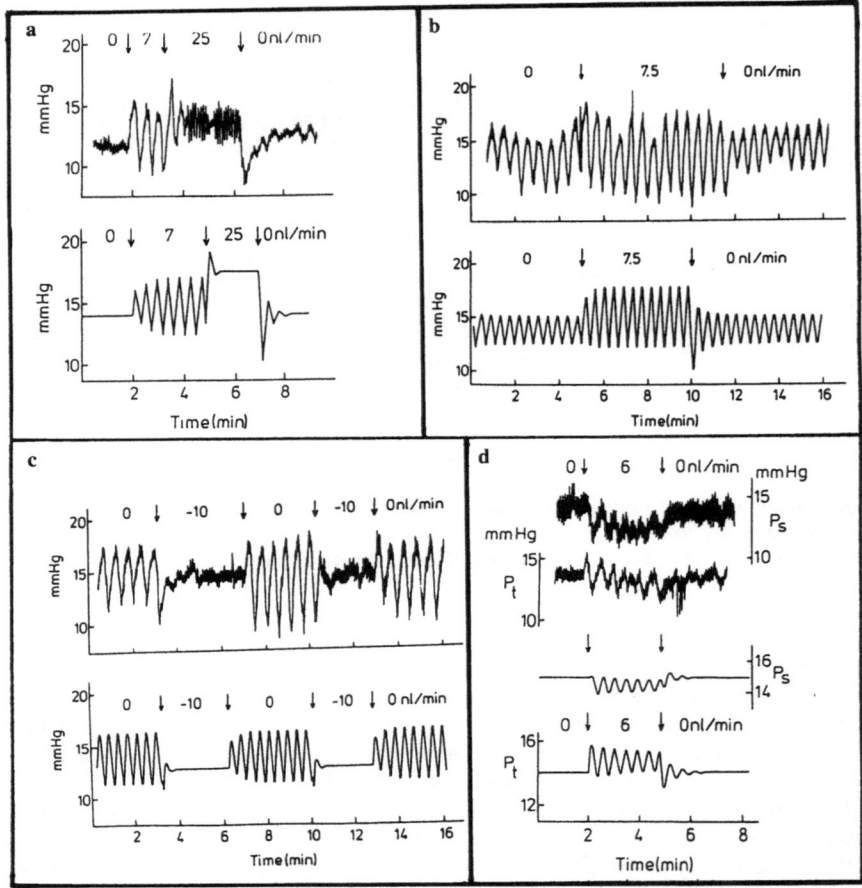

Fig. 4a-d. Effects of changing late proximal flow rate by microperfusion/suction. *Upper traces* experimental recordings of proximal intratubular pressures (**a,b,c**) and star vessel pressure (*P,*) (**d**). *Lower traces* corresponding model simulations P_t. (From [7] with permission)

Since 1964 I have hypothesized that the renin-angiotensin system is directly involved in the control of tubular pressure and flow by the effects of angiotensin-II on the efferent arteriole and on proximal tubular reabsorption [8]. For this regulation it was postulated that macula densa-mediated renin release is depressed by an increase in proximal pressure and Henle loop flow.

When a sufficiently sensitive radio-immunoassay (RIA) had been developed, we tested this hypothesis directly in vivo in two series of microperfusion experiments.

In one series, early proximal tubular fluid was collected before and after changing late proximal microperfusion rate. Tubular fluid renin concentration was measured by RIA, corrected for water reabsorption, and normalized with respect to the systemic plasma renin concentration. Increasing the late proximal flow rate from 12 to

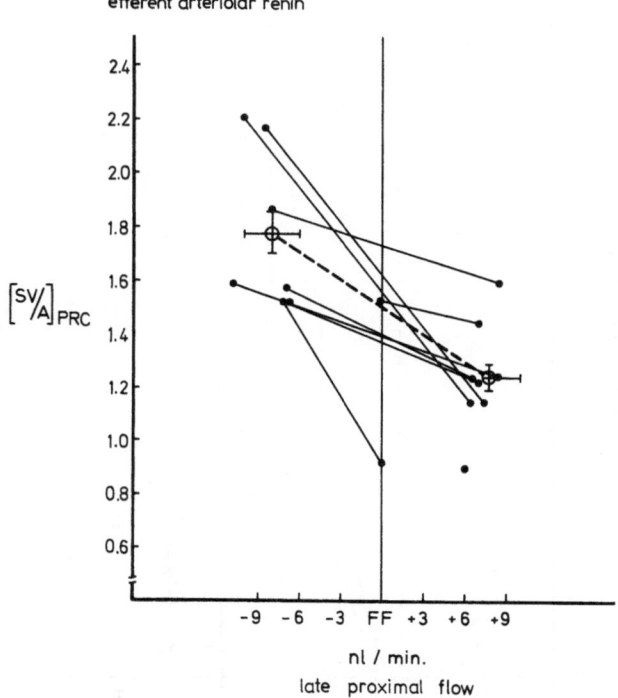

Fig. 5. Efferent arteriolar (*SV*) plasma renin concentration (*PRC*) versus changes in late proximal fluid flow. (From [9] with permission)

18 nl/min reduced tubular fluid renin concentration, while reducing the flow from 12 to 6 nl/min caused an increase in concentration [9]. In the other series, in order to ascertain that these changes in ultrafiltrate renin concentration represented changes in renin release rather than changes in glomerular membrane permeability to renin, blood was also collected at the end of the efferent arteriole, from the so-called star vessel [9].

The results are shown in Fig. 5, in which star vessel plasma renin concentration is normalized with respect to the systemic plasma renin concentration (PRC). Again, a reduction in late proximal flow caused an increase, while an increase in flow caused a decrease, in efferent arteriolar PRC. We conclude that an increase in Henle loop flow depresses macula densa-mediated renin release, and, conversely, that a decrease in Henle loop flow stimulates macula densa-mediated renin release. These results are in perfect agreement with those subsequently obtained by Skøtt and Briggs in their elegant in vitro studies with isolated, microperfused, and superfused juxtaglomerular apparatuses [10].

Thus, within recent years it has been firmly established that not only afferent arteriolar TGF, but also single nephron renin release responds to flow-dependent changes in sodium chloride concentration at the level of the macula densa.

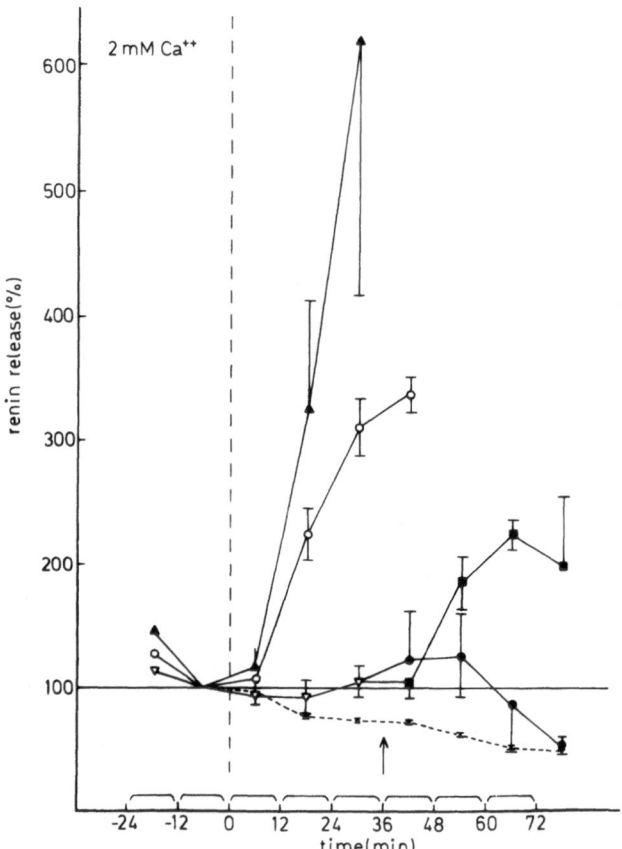

Fig. 6. Changes in renin release from isolated superfused glomeruli. Effect of changing super-fusate calcium in the presence or absence of the calcium ionophore A$_{23187}$. In the control period superfusate was bicarbonate-Ringer containing 2 mM calcium. At time zero superfusate composition was changed: to Ca-free Ringer with A$_{23187}$ (*open triangles*) and subsequently back to Ca-free Ringer without A$_{23187}$ (*closed squares*) or back to control Ringer (*closed circles*); or to Ca-free Ringer containing 0.5 mM EGTA without A$_{23187}$ (*open circles*) to be compared with Ca-free Ringer with A$_{23187}$ (*closed triangles*). The *dashed line* indicates basal renin release with time in control Ringer. Means ± SEM

These two responses from the afferent arteriole therefore share the same luminal signal. As for the intracellular signal in the afferent arteriole there is also an intriguing parallelism between the signal leading to vasoconstriction and the inhibition of renin release. The arterioles constrict when intracellular calcium increases. But much to our surprise we found 13 years ago that renin release was inhibited when calcium was increased [11]. Figure 6 shows these old data from isolated, superfused rat glomeruli. The data indicate that lowering intracellular calcium concentration stimulates renin release. This finding has been confirmed and extended by my collaborators Lars Baumbach and Ole Skøtt and by many others, and suggests that intracellular calcium may serve as a common trigger for the afferent vasoconstriction and the inhibition of renin release. The demonstration by Kurtz and Penner [12] that intracellular calcium concentration in the JG cells also oscillates with a frequency similar to that of the pressure, and the observation by Skøtt [13] that renin is released in pulses, fits together, and opens the possibility that a stimulus to renin release from the individual nephron may vary as a function of the amplitude of the pressure oscillation, in spite of a stable mean pressure and flow to the macula densa.

Viewed together, I think that it would be reasonable to consider both responses as part of the TGF mechanism. Both responses cooperate in changing glomerular capillary pressure and in counteracting any acute primary change in the filtration pressure and/or in the Henle loop flow rate, since an increase in Henle loop flow causes afferent vasoconstriction, and the accompanying decrease in renin release and local angiotensin concentration will cause relaxation mainly of the efferent arteriole, both of which will reduce glomerular capillary pressure.

References

1. Leyssac PP, Holstein-Rathlou N-H (1988) Dynamics of TGF mediated regulation of proximal tubular pressure. Role of the renin system. In: Persson AEG, Boberg U (eds) The juxtaglomerular apparatus, Fernström Foundation Series vol 11. Elsevier Scientific, Amsterdam, pp 237–247
2. Leyssac PP (1969) New aspects of the mechanisms of renal sodium excretion. Proc R Soc Med 62:1111–1116
3. Leyssac PP, Baumbach L (1983) An oscillating intratubular pressure response to alterations in Henle loop flow in the rat kidney. Acta Physiol Scand 117:415–419
4. Leyssac PP (1986) Further studies on oscillating tubulo-glomerular feedback responses in the rat kidney. Acta Physiol Scand 126:271–277
5. Holstein-Rathlou N-H (1987) Synchronization of proximal intratubular pressure oscillations: evidence for interaction between nephrons. Pflugers Arch 408:438–443
6. Leyssac PP, Holstein-Rathlou N-H (1986) Effects of various transport inhibitors on oscillating TGF pressure responses in the rat. Pflugers Arch 407:285–291
7. Holstein-Rathlou N-H, Leyssac PP (1987) Oscillations in the proximal intratubular pressure: a mathematical model. Am J Physiol 252:F560–F572
8. Leyssac PP (1964) The effect of partial clamping of the renal artery on pressures in the proximal and distal tubules and peritubular capillaries of the rat kidney. Acta Physiol Scand 62:449–456
9. Leyssac PP (1986) Changes in single nephron renin release are mediated by tubular fluid flow rate. Kidney Int 30:332–339
10. Skøtt O, Briggs JP (1987) Direct demonstration of macula densa-mediated renin secretion. Science 237:1618–1620
11. Baumbach L, Leyssac PP (1977) Studies on the mechanism of renin release from isolated superfused rat glomeruli: effects of calcium, calcium ionophore and lanthanum. J Physiol 273:745–764
12. Kurtz A, Penner R (1989) Angiotensin II induces oscillations of intracellular calcium and blocks anomalous inward rectifying potassium current in mouse renal juxtaglomerular cells. Proc Natl Acad Sci USA 86:3423–3427
13. Skøtt O (1986) Episodic release of renin from single isolated superfused rat afferent arterioles. Pflügers Arch 407:41–45

The Afferent Arteriole in Tubuloglomerular Feedback and Autoregulation

Leon C. Moore[1] and Daniel Casellas[2]

Introduction

The preglomerular vasculature of the kidney has long been known to be the principal site of autoregulatory adjustments in vascular resistance and the major effector site of the tubuloglomerular feedback (TGF) mechanism [1]. This paper will review some recent studies from our laboratories that have provided new evidence about the function of the renal preglomerular microvasculature and, in particular, the role of the afferent arteriole in autoregulation and TGF [2,3]. These results have helped to resolve several important issues regarding the regulation of renal hemodynamics.

Role of the Afferent Arteriole in Autoregulation

Although the afferent arteriole (AA), as a whole, is known to be an important site of nephron blood flow and filtration regulation [1,4–6], it has been proposed that the terminal, juxtaglomerular segment of the AA (jAA) is incapable of active vasoconstriction, owing to the low myosin content of the renin-positive granulated cells in this segment [7] and the lack of significant autoregulatory vasoconstriction in the terminal AA found in rat hydronephrotic kidneys [6]. Further, the descending myogenic hypothesis forwarded by Øien and Aukland [8] suggests that the autoregulatory responses of the terminal AA should only be manifested near the limits of the autoregulatory pressure range, after saturation of the autoregulatory responses of all upstream vascular segments.

We have recently succeeded in obtaining high resolution video images of the entire afferent arteriole and juxtaglomerular apparatus of blood-perfused juxtamedullary

[1]Department of Physiology and Biophysics, State University of New York, Stony Brook, NY 11794, USA
[2]Groupe Rein et Hypertension, St. Charles Hospital, Montpellier, France

(JM) nephrons in vitro. This has provided us with the ability to specifically examine the hemodynamic function of the juxtaglomerular and mid-afferent (mAA) segments of the afferent arteriole. The studies were conducted in vitro in the blood-perfused, JM nephron preparation [9]. This preparation is unique in that all preglomerular vascular segments and the macula densa (MD) are visible. The nephrons in this preparation retain basic vascular, glomerular, and tubular function [2–5,9,10]. Detailed descriptions of the in vitro perfused JM nephron preparation are available elsewhere [2,9,10]. Briefly, a rat kidney is removed and extensively dissected to expose an area of juxtamedullary cortex that lies under the pelvic mucosa. The major arteries supplying the rest of the kidney are ligated. During dissection, the kidney is perfused with a gassed Krebs-bicarbonate-Ringer (KBR) solution containing 4% albumin. During measurements, the kidney is perfused with a blood solution prepared from fresh rat blood. The red cells are separated, washed, and resuspended in KBR-6%-albumin solution (pH 7.4) to a hematocrit of 30%. The preparation is superfused with a warm (37°C) KBR solution with 1% albumin. In this region, AA length varies from around 200 to 1400 µm. Where possible, responses were measured at two sites in each AA, the terminal, juxtaglomerular segment (jAA) consisting of the final approximately 50 µm of the AA, and a mid-afferent site (mAA) located around 130–150 µm upstream from the vascular pole. In most JM nephrons, the jAA lumen also narrows by about 33% and the vessel wall thickens as it approaches the vascular pole. These jAA segments have been shown to contain renin [11].

Autoregulatory Responses of the AA

Figure 1 illustrates a typical autoregulatory response in the jAA segment of a JM AA, while Fig. 2 summarizes the results obtained for the mAA and the jAA. Significant perfusion-pressure-dependent vasoconstriction was found in both segments. In response to increasing perfusion pressure from 60 to 140 mmHg, mAA luminal diameter decreased by 23% ± 4%, while jAA diameter decreased by 40% ± 4%. In contrast, the diameter of the efferent arteriole was unaffected by perfusion pressure. The autoregulatory responses were calcium-dependent, as superperfusion with 1 µM nimodipine resulted in pressure-dependent dilation rather than constriction. These results are consistent with earlier measurements by others in mid afferent segments and with the results of micropressure measurements in JM vessels [4–6]. However, they extend previous findings by clearly demonstrating that the terminal, renin-containing segment of the AA is also capable of strong autoregulatory adjustments in resistance. These results also contrast sharply with studies of isolated rabbit AA in vitro, where only weak autoregulatory vasoconstriction was found in the distal region [12].

Another noteworthy feature of the autoregulatory responses of the distal AA and jAA is that they were distributed approximately uniformly over the pressure range of 60–140 mmHg, which exceeds the autoregulatory range in rat JM nephrons [13]. The monotonic, almost linear responses are basically inconsistent with the descending myogenic hypothesis (DMH) of renal blood flow autoregulation [8]. The DMH predicts little or no autoregulatory compensation by the distal AA at arterial pressures around the normotensive level, where all autoregulatory compensation is predicted to occur in the proximal preglomerular vascular segments. In contrast, our results show

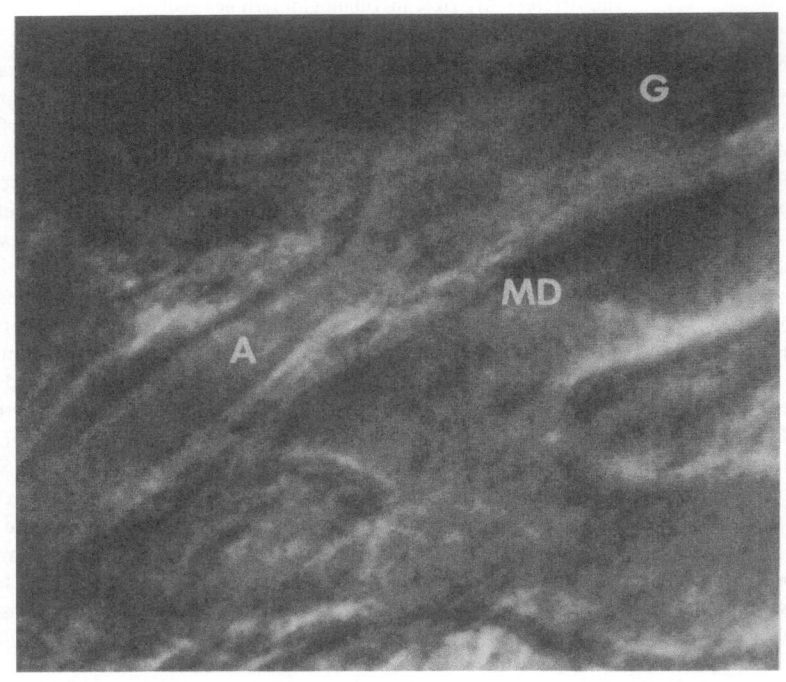

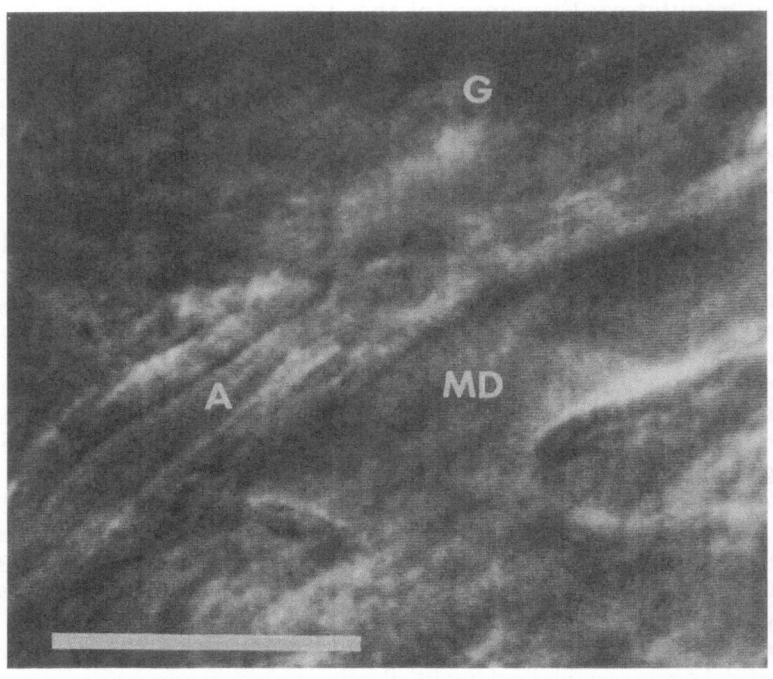

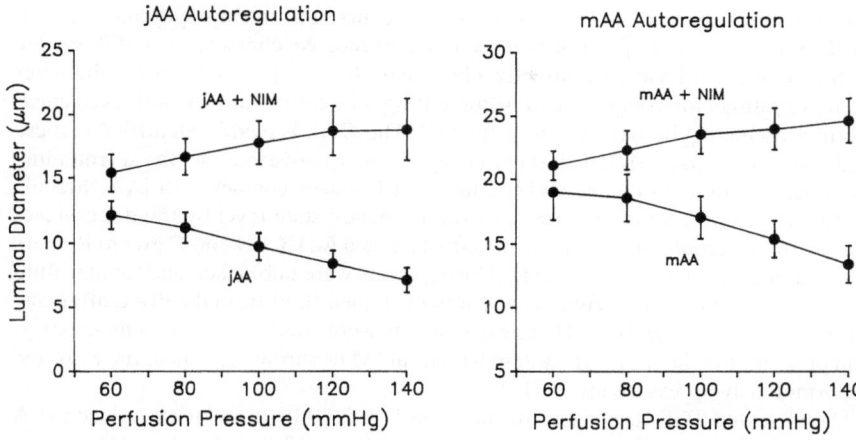

Fig. 2. Autoregulatory responses of the juxtoglomerular afferent arteriole (*jAA*), (*left*) and the mid-afferent arteriole (*mAA*), (*right*). Mean±SE, $n=8$ for jAA, $n=7$ for mAA. Responses are shown before and after calcium channel blockade with 1 µM nimodipine (*NIM*). The mAA and jAA responses and the inhibition by nimodipine were statistically significant in all cases. (Data from [2])

that the autoregulatory responses of the mid- and jAA are at least as strong in the region around 100 mmHg as they are at 60 and 140 mmHg. Hence, our results in JM vessels are inconsistent with the pattern of strong, sequential, descending responses predicted by the DMH. A similar conclusion was reached by Carmines et al. [4] on the basis of measurements of intravascular pressure in JM vessels. However, the DMH may be much more important in superficial cortical nephrons, where the cortical radial arteries are longer and show substantial autoregulatory ability [14].

TGF Responses in the Terminal Segment of the AA

It has long been known that the effector site of the TGF system was in the preglomerular vasculature, as TGF stimulation reduces glomerular capillary pressure and nephron glomerular filtration rate (GFR) in parallel [1]. However, the exact

---

◁

Fig. 1. Micrograph illustrating typical autoregulatory vasoconstriction in a juxtaglomerular afferent arteriole (*jAA*). *Upper* Control measurement of jAA lumen diameter at 60 mmHg perfusion pressure. *Lower* The same vessel at a perfusion pressure of 120 mmHg. The *bar* is 50 µm. A, jAA lumen; G, glomerular tuft; MD, macula densa. Vessels were visualized through a compound microscope (Leitz 12-FS) with a 25X long-working distance objective (Leitz Fluorotar). Illumination was provided by low-angle incident light from a fiber optic guide. Video images were obtained with a CCD camera, edge-enhanced on-line, and recorded. Vessel dimensions were measured with a video-caliper system

site at which TGF-mediated vasoconstriction occurs, and the strength and speed of the TGF response have never been directly measured. We characterized TGF system in JM nephrons in vitro by directly observing changes in jAA luminal diameter elicited by direct microinjection of isotonic Ringers solution into an unblocked cortical thick ascending limb (cTAL) near the MD. The cTAL is readily identified in these nephrons, owing to marked differences in appearance between it and the surrounding proximal convoluted tubules, and the fact that it makes contact with jAA. Macula densa NaCl concentration was raised from its steady state level by the direct injection, with a micropipette, of 30–80 nl/min of stained (0.1% FD and C green) Ringers solution into the cTAL near the MD. The nephrons were unblocked and tubular fluid flow was verified by observing the washout of stained fluid from the cTAL after cessation of the microinjection. These experiments were conducted at 60 mmHg perfusion pressure to relax the TGF system which, in JM nephrons, is almost fully excited at normotensive pressure levels [15].

The observed TGF responses are shown in Fig. 3. TGF stimulation reduced jAA diameter by 34% $\pm$ 4% ($n=8$) from a control value of 12.0 $\pm$ 1.0 μm. These measurements were made at sites averaging 22 $\pm$ 3 μm from the end of the AA. We also demonstrated that the response is rapid, requiring around 5 s to develop fully [2]. In the same nephrons, the addition of 0.1 mM furosemide to the injected fluid completely inhibited the TGF response, as observed in many earlier studies [1].

These are the first direct observations of TGF-mediated vasoconstriction, and the results demonstrate that the terminal portion of the AA is a major effector site of the TGF mechanism. Further, the magnitude and location of the TGF responses are similar to earlier conclusions reached by Schnermann and Kriz [16], who measured afferent arteriolar dimensions in sections of flash-frozen kidneys and found smaller diameters in nephrons subjected to maximal TGF stimulation.

Physiological Significance of AA Responses

An interesting feature of these results is the magnitude of TGF-mediated and autoregulatory jAA vasoconstriction. To explore the functional significance of the observed responses, we estimated the relative increments in segmental structural resistance elicited by TGF stimulation, and increased perfusion pressure. These values were calculated from the measured changes in vessel caliber, assuming an inverse 4th power relationship between vessel radius and resistance. The results of this analysis are shown in Fig. 4. For maximal TGF stimulation, the 34% $\pm$ 4% reduction in lumen diameter corresponds to an increase of about 5-fold in segmental vascular resistance. In response to a doubling of perfusion pressure, jAA segmental resistance increased approximately 4-fold, while mAA segmental resistance increased in proportion to perfusion pressure. At first glance, the degree of jAA autoregulatory and TGF-mediated vasoconstriction appears to be excessive. Similar large TGF-mediated increments in structural resistance were observed by Schnermann and Kriz in superficial rat nephrons [16]. However, in vessels of this size, the increment in the structural component of vessel resistance may substantially overestimate the true hemodynamic resistance, owing to the fact that the hematocrit and the apparent viscosity of blood in small vessels is an inverse function of vessel diameter [17]. The observations that glomerular capillary pressure is well autoregulated in JM nephrons

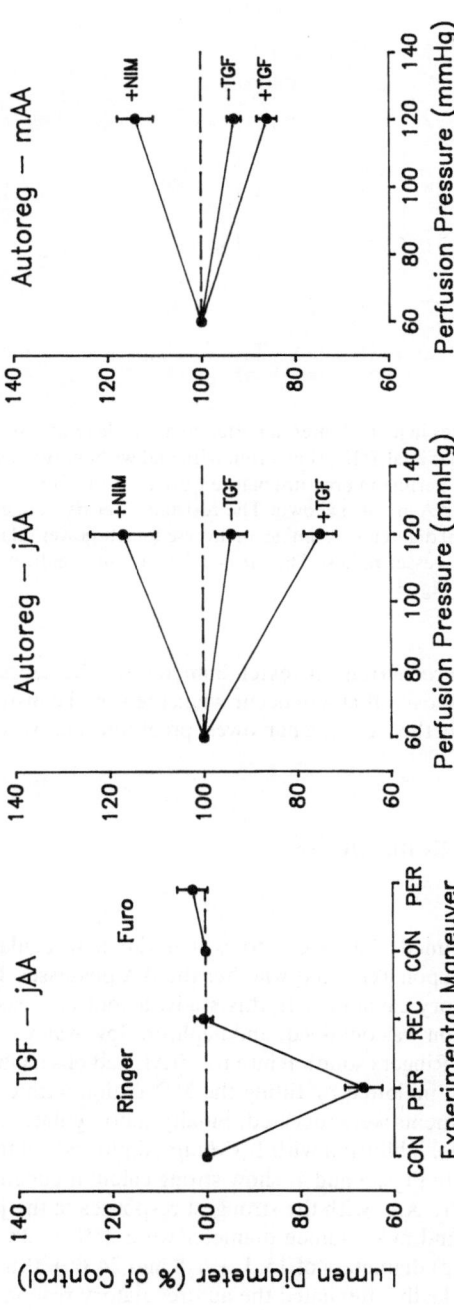

Fig. 3. TGF responses (*left*) (*n*=8) are shown before (*CON*), during (*PER*) and after (*REC*) the injection of Ringer solution into the macula densa region. Also shown are TGF responses in the juxtaglomerular afferent arteriole (*jAA*) (*n*=7) before (*Con*) and during microinjection of Ringer with 0.1 mM furosemide (*Furo*). The TGF response and the inhibition by furosemide were both statistically significant (*P*<0.05, paired t-test). Autoregulatory responses of the jAA (*middle*) and the mid-afferent arteri- ole (*mAA*) (*right*). Mean (±SE, *n*=8) responses are shown before (+*TGF*) and after TGF inhibition (−*TGF*), and after calcium channel blockade with 1 μM nimodipine (*NIM*). The inhibition of mAA and jAA responses by TGF inhibition and nimodipine were statistically significant in all cases, and the responses after TGF inhibition remained significant for both seg- ments (*P*<0.05, paired t-test). The jAA and mAA measuring sites were 19 ± 3 and 130 ± 9 μm from the vascular pole. (Data from [3])

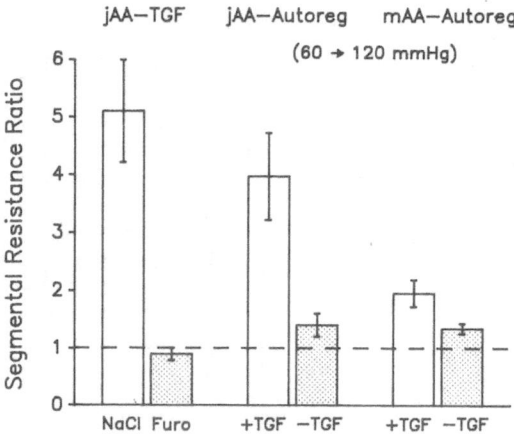

Fig. 4. Comparison of calculated increases in juxtaglomerular afferent arteriole (*jAA*) segmental structural resistance in response to maximal TGF stimulation with and without furosemide (*Furo*), and in response to a doubling of perfusion pressure before (*+TGF*) and after (*−TGF*) TGF inhibition. The responses of the mAA are also shown. The resistance ratios were calculated from measured decreases in luminal diameter assuming an inverse fourth-power relationship between segmental resistance and vessel radius. The *dashed line* at unity indicates no change in resistance. Data are given in Fig. 3

in vitro [4,5] suggest that such large reductions in vessel diameter may be necessary to counteract the decline in blood viscosity that will occur when the vessel constricts. This effect should be most apparent in the jAA, the narrowest preglomerular vascular segment.

Myogenic and TGF Components of AA Autoregulatory Responses

In a third investigation, we examined the extent to which the autoregulatory responses of the AA are dependent upon TGF, and whether the AA possesses TGF-independent, myogenic autoregulatory capability. In this study, a control measurement of jAA and mAA autoregulation was obtained, and nephron flow was verified by injecting a small bolus of stained Ringers solution into the cTAL and observing its washout. The TGF system was then inhibited by filling the MD region with castor oil, and the autoregulatory measurements were repeated. Finally, autoregulation was measured again after calcium-channel inhibition with 1 µM nimodipine added to the superfusate. The results, illustrated in Figs. 3 and 4, show strong calcium-dependent autoregulatory responses in the entire AA, with the strongest responses in the jAA. Mean fractional decreases in jAA and mAA lumen diameter were 25% ± 3% and 15% ± 2% from baseline (60 mmHg) diameters of 15.3 ± 1.8 and 24.0 ± 0.8 µm, respectively. Inhibition of TGF markedly attenuated the autoregulatory response of the jAA segment, reducing the mean fractional diameter decrease from 25% ± 3%

to 6% ± 3%. In the mAA, as in the jAA, the autoregulatory responses were also significantly attenuated by TGF inhibition, with the mean fractional reduction in mAA diameter reduced to 7% ± 2%. In both segments, however, there was also a significant degree of TGF-independent myogenic autoregulation that was most prominent in the mAA.

The dependence of afferent arteriolar autoregulation on TGF is consistent with micropuncture studies of single nephron GFR (SNGFR) autoregulation and with studies of isolated JM nephrons [1,5,16,18]. The results also explain the absence of substantial autoregulatory responses in late AA in hydronephrotic kidneys [6] and in AA segments in vitro [12], where the renal tubular system and, hence, TGF are absent. The results also clearly show a substantial TGF-independent myogenic autoregulatory component in both mAA and jAA segments, again in agreement with micropuncture and isolated nephron studies [1,4,18–20]. However, there is substantial evidence that relative contributions of the myogenic and TGF autoregulatory mechanisms may differ between species and may be altered by changes in physiological state. For example, autoregulation in the dog appears to be more dependent upon TGF than is autoregulation in the rat [21]. Further, two micropuncture studies have shown significantly enhanced myogenic autoregulation under conditions where the normal ability of TGF to participate in the autoregulatory process is inhibited by maintaining TGF under constant, maximal stimulation [19,20]. Although the mechanisms that underlie these intriguing observations of TGF-independent autoregulation are as yet unclear, they do suggest that renal autoregulation is a robust process, in that both TGF and myogenic mechanisms appear to be able to, at least partially, compensate when the other mechanism is impaired.

Communication Between Preglomerular Vascular Segments

Several recent studies have suggested that TGF responses that originate in the jAA can influence vascular reactivity in upstream AA segments and in neighboring nephrons. In our studies, we found substantial TGF-depencency of mAA autoregulation, where TGF inhibition attenuated the mAA autoregulatory increment in mAA segmental resistance by around 60%. This observation suggests that the effect of TGF stimulation can be seen over 100 μm upstream from the jAA segment. Further, the early studies by Schnermann and Kriz [16] in superficial cortical AA found that TGF stimulation resulted in a variable degree of vasoconstriction in the mid and early AA, with some vessels constricting along their entire length. Perhaps the most dramatic evidence that TGF has significant effects on upstream vessels is provided by a recent study by Källskog and Marsh [22]. They demonstrated that nephron stop-flow pressure, a variable that changes in parallel with glomerular capillary pressure, is reduced significantly when TGF in an adjacent nephron is subjected to maximal stimulation. As this response was seen only when both nephrons arose from a common feed vessel, the clear implication is that there is some communication pathway between afferent arterioles branching from the same cortical radial artery. The underlying mechanism has yet to be clearly identified. One possibility is electrotonic conduction of the local TGF signal for vasoconstriction along the arteriole. Although there are numerous gap junctions between endothelial cells in the AA, they are less prevalent between smooth muscle cells [23]. One investigation has failed to show extensive electrotonic conduction in the late AA in hydronephrotic kidneys [24], but it is unclear at present if results from this pathophysiological model can be extrapolated to normal renal vessels. A second possible mechanism is that a strong TGF response, localized in the jAA, enhances the degree of mAA myogenic vasoconstriction indirectly by increasing upstream intravascular pressure. Such a mechanism was first proposed by Johnson [25], and would operate in parallel with any electrotonic coupling mechanism that might operate along the arteriole. As yet, no direct evidence has been obtained concerning intravascular-pressure-mediated spread of the TGF response, although two mathematical models suggest that it might have a significant impact on renal autoregulation [20,26]. Much of our current understanding of the regulation of renal hemodynamics is based on single nephron and single vessel studies, yet overall kidney function is determined by the ensemble action of all individual nephrons. Hence, elucidating how TGF and autoregulatory responses are propagated along the afferent arteriole and, perhaps, to the large renal arterial vessels, is likely to be of critical importance in understanding renal autoregulation and how it is altered in disease.

Acknowledgments. These studies were supported by grants from INSERM (CRE 875003) and NIK (DK 26341). During these studies, L.C. Moore was the recipient of a Poste Orange Fellowship from INSERM. Expert technical assistance was provided by Aija Birzgalis and Annie Artuso.

References

1. Schnermann J, Briggs J (1985) Function of the juxtaglomerular apparatus: local control of glomerular hemodynamics. In: Seldin DW, Giebisch G (eds) The kidney: physiology and pathophysiology. Raven, New York, Ch 28
2. Casellas D, Moore LC (1990) Autoregulation and tubuloglomerular feedback in juxtamedullary glomerular arterioles. Am J Physiol 258:F660–F669
3. Moore LC, Casellas D (1990) Tubuloglomerular feedback dependency of autoregulation in rat juxtamedullary afferent arterioles. Kidney Int 37:1402–1408
4. Carmines PK, Inscho EW, Gensure RC (1990) Arterial pressure effects on preglomerular microvasculature of juxtamedullary nephrons. Am J Physiol 258:F94–F102
5. Sanchez-Ferrer CF, Roman RJ, Harder DR (1989) Pressure-dependent contraction of rat juxtamedullary afferent arterioles. Circ Res 64:790–798
6. Steinhausen M, Blum B, Fleming JT, Holz FG, Parekh N, Wiegman DL, Dussel R (1989) Visualization of renal autoregulation in the split hydronephrotic kidney of rats. Kidney Int 35:1151–1160
7. Taugner R, Rosivall L, Bührle CP, Gorschel-Steward U (1987) Myosin content and vasoconstrictive ability of the proximal juxtaglomerular (renin-positive) segments of the afferent arteriole. Cell Tissue Res 248:579–588
8. Øien AH, Aukland K (1983) A mathematical analysis of the myogenic hypothesis with special reference to autoregulation of renal blood flow. Circ Res 52:241–252
9. Casellas D, Navar LG (1984) In vitro perfusion of juxtamedullary nephrons in rats. Am J Physiol 246:F349–F358
10. Casellas D, Carmines PK, Navar LG (1985) Microvascular reactivity of in vitro blood perfused juxtamedullary nephrons from rats. Kidney Int 28:752–759

11. Casellas D, Taugner R (1987) Renin status of the afferent arteriole and ultrastructure of the juxtaglomerular apparatus in superficial juxtamedullary nephrons from rats. Renal Physiol 9:348–356
12. Edwards RM (1983) Segmental effects of norepinephrine and angiotensin II on isolated renal microvessels. Am J Physiol 244:F526–F534
13. Cohen HJ, Marsh DJ, Kayser B (1983) Autoregulation in the vasa recta of the rat kidney. Am J Physiol 245:F32–F40
14. Källskog O, Lindbom LO, Ulfendahl HR, Wolgast M (1976) Hydrostatic pressures within the vascular structures of the rat kidney. Pflugers Arch 363:205–210
15. Müller-Suur R, Ulfendahl HR, Persson AEG (1982) Evidence for tubuloglomerular feedback in juxtamedullary nephrons of young rats. Am J Physiol 244:F425–F431
16. Schnermann J, Briggs J, Kriz W, Moore LC, Wright FS (1980) Control of glomerular vascular resistance by the tubuloglomerular feedback mechanism. In: Leaf A, Giebisch G (eds) Renal pathophysiology. Raven, New York, pp 165–182
17. Fung YC (1984) Biodynamics Circulation. Springer, New York, pp 238–249
18. Moore LC (1984) Tubuloglomerular feedback and SNGFR autoregulation in the rat. Am J Physiol 247:F267–F276
19. Schnermann J, Briggs JP (1989) Interaction between loop of Henle flow and arterial pressure as determinants of glomerular pressure. Am J Physiol 256:F421–F429
20. Davis JM, Kawata T, Häberle D (1988) The influence of renal autoregulation on TGF control of glomerular filtration rate. In: Persson AEG, Boberg U (eds) The juxtaglomerular apparatus. Elsevier, Amsterdam, ch 34
21. Navar LG, Bell PD, Burke TJ (1982) Role of a macula densa feedback mechanism as a mediator of renal autoregulation. Kidney Int 22(Suppl 12):S157–S164
22. Kallskog O, Marsh DJ (to be published) TGF-initiated vascular interactions between adjacent nephrons in the rat kidney. Am J Physiol
23. Taugner R, Hackenthal E (1989) The Juxtaglomerular Apparatus. Springer, Berlin, pp 33–40
24. Nobiling R, Bührle CP (1989) Cell to cell coupling at the afferent arteriole: A combined electrophysiological and morphological study (abstract). Kidney Int 36:307
25. Johnson PC (1986) Autoregulation of blood flow. Circ Res 59:483–495
26. Moore LC, Rich A (1988) Mathematical model of ascending myogenic responses to tubuloglomerular feedback induced changes in afferent vascular resistance (abstract). Kidney Int 33:412

Systemic Dysfunctions in Renal Failure and Their Management

Chair: August Heidland (FRG)
Tsan-Shin Yen (Taipei, China)

Neutrophil Function in Uremia: Inhibition by Endogenous Plasma Inhibitor(s)

Walter H. Hörl[1]

Introduction

Infectious complications in patients with end-stage renal disease result in significant morbidity and mortality. Uremia is an immunocompromised state which is due to the direct effects of uremic toxins and to indirect factors, e.g., malnutrition, dialysis membranes with their effects on complement system and white blood cells, or vascular access for dialysis providing a portal of entry for microorganisms [1]. Dysfunction of polymorphonuclear cells (PMN) in uremia includes adherence, the first step in neutrophil migration, chemotaxis, phagocytotic capacity, generation of reactive oxygen intermediates, or intracellular killing of bacteria [2].

Chemotaxis and Phagocytotic Activity of PMN

A reduction in generation of chemotactic activity in experimentally induced acute renal failure has been reported by Clark et al. [3]. This reduction was proportional to the degree of azotemia. Baum et al. [4] demonstrated that chemotaxis of PMN was impaired in the presence of undialyzed uremic sera, but that hemodialysis seemed to correct the defect. A chemotactic inhibitor found in sera of uremic patients acted directly on leukotactic factors (C_3 and C_5 chemotactic fragment and bacterial factor) to render them irreversibly inactive [5]. Pedersen et al. [6] studied the ability of serum to attract PMN in uremic patients before and after hemodialysis. The chemotactic response toward serum from uremic patients were significantly decreased prior to hemodialysis and were normalized thereafter.

Phagocytosis in uremic patients is either normal or slightly diminished. Hirabayashi et al. [7] observed decreased phagocytic uptake of IgG-coated particles in

[1]Department of Medicine, Division of Nephrology, University of Saarland, D-6650 Homburg, Federal Republic of Germany

patients before hemodialysis therapy, which was restored by hemodialysis. The phagocytotic responsiveness of PMN increased after exposure to cuprophane filter, although exposure to polyacrylonitrile and polysulfone hemodialyzers did not affect phagocytotic activity [8]. A dramatic fall was observed in phagocytotic activity after 15 minutes of hemodialysis with cuprophane membranes. Reused cuprophane caused a minor decrease in phagocytotic activity, whereas hemodialysis with polyacrylonitrile and polysulfone produced no significant change in phagocyte populations at this time [8].

Kinetic measurements of the serum-independent uptake of IgG-coated polyvinyl toluene latex particles by isolated PMN cells have been performed in patients undergoing hemodialysis or peritoneal dialysis [9]. The mean phagocytic rate for the patient group was significantly reduced when compared to the reference group of apparently healthy individuals. After 4 months of adequate dialysis, the phagocytic uptake was significantly higher than the uptake shortly after the beginning of dialysis. It was suggested that elevated serum phosphate levels may, in part, be responsible for the impaired phagocytic activity of uremic patients [9].

Oxidative Metabolism and Glucose Metabolism

Ritchey et al. [10] studied superoxide anion production and luminol-amplified chemiluminescence in PMN from chronic hemodialysis patients and in age-matched controls in the resting state; he also studied response to phorbol myristate acetate (PMA). Studies in autologous serum showed higher chemiluminescence resting values in PMN from hemodialysis patients, with a significant reduction after dialysis. Cross-incubation studies indicated that this was a result of factor(s) in the patients' serum. In response to PMA, neutrophils from chronic hemodialysis patients in autologous serum had a significantly smaller increase in chemiluminescence compared with controls, suggesting that there was a defect intrinsic to the patient PMN [10]. Hirabayashi et al. [7] also found that impaired hydrogen peroxide production by PMA-stimulated PMN before dialysis was restored to the control level by hemodialysis.

Different changes in oxidative metabolism have been observed in PMN when exposed to a cuprophane filter, but not with a polyacrylonitrile filter membrane [11]. Reduced PMN activity of both chemiluminescence and H_2O_2 occurred as a consequence of hemodialysis when a cuprophane dialyzer was employed; however, the diminished activity was no longer detectable after the filter had been hemophane modified [12].

Markert et al. [13] found an increase, compared to the control cells, of lucigenin-amplified chemiluminescence, stimulated by phorbol myristate, acetate in PMN isolated after 5 and 60 minutes during hemodialysis with cuprophane, cellulose acetate, and polyacrylonitrile during the first and/or second use. Luminol increased chemiluminescence during the initial use of three filters: cuprophane, polycarbonate, and polysulfone.

Although numerous studies have affirmed changes of PMN metabolism and function in uremia, most of the evidence has come from data obtained before and during hemodialysis. However, information comparing PMN function after hemodialysis treatment with that prior to treatment is lacking. Studies on glucose metabolism have revealed that glucose intolerance and impaired utilization of glucose are improved

Table 1. Biological activity of granulocyte inhibiting protein (GIP)

Test condition	GIP concentration which inhibits 50% of maximal stimulation (IC_{50})
^{3}H d-glucose uptake[a]	5.2 ± 1.2 µg/ml ($n=5$)
Chemotaxis[a]	7.2 ± 1.7 µg/ml ($n=6$)
Oxidative metabolism[a]	8.1 ± 1.4 µg/ml ($n=5$)
Intracellular killing[b]	7.9 ± 1.7 µg/ml ($n=6$)

[a]stimulation with FMLP
[b]stimulation with *S. aureus* 502

significantly after uremic patients have undergone hemodialysis treatment. This suggests that a circulating plasma factor is responsible for inducing insulin resistance [14–16]. A variety of normal tissues obtained from animals have inhibited basal uptake of glucose following incubation with whole or partially purified sera obtained from uremic patients [17–19]. The insulin stimulation of glucose uptake and the metabolism of rat adipocytes were also reduced following preincubation with serum from uremic patients [20]. This irregularity occurred without affecting either insulin binding or the antilipolytic action of insulin [15].

Cellular activation of PMN by microbial antigens and certain toxins is achieved by the stimulation of phosphoinositol (PI) turnover and activation of protein kinase C. For example, the stimulus-response coupling in PMN is induced by a chemotactic peptide. Concanavalin A, immune complexes, and PMA showed an increase of calcium uptake preceding the onset of degranulation and of O_2-generation [21]. The stimulation of hexose transport by PMNs is associated with the activation of protein kinase C [22]. Furthermore, pertussis toxin, which is known to involve the activation of G proteins, effectively stimulates PI turnover with regard to increased formation of IP_3 and an increased elevation of intracellular calcium [23].

We have observed that PMN from uremic patients have diminished responsiveness to chemotactic peptide FMLP-induced hexose uptake, enzyme release, and chemotaxis [24]. This lack of responsiveness is improved after the patients have undergone hemodialysis. Moreover, when normal PMN were exposed to various concentrations of ultrafiltrates from uremic patients, there was an increased loss of responsiveness of these cells with regard to hexose uptake [25] and enzyme release. In addition, washing the PMN with buffered saline restored their function to normal, which suggests that a plasma-derived constituent is responsible for these effects. There is further evidence for the existence of such a putative entity, from initial experiments that have employed one species with a molecular weight (MW) of 8-30 Kda that was partly purified by column chromatography (Sephadex G-100) from the ultrafiltrate of uremic patients. The factor greater than 10 Kda MW appears to be heat labile, which suggests that it can be further purified, characterized, and its biochemical and immunochemical properties further elucidated.

Physiochemical Characterization of a Novel Polypeptide

Recently, a novel protein (molecular weight 28 Kda) was isolated and characterized from uremic serum of patients undergoing regular hemodialysis therapy. This polypeptide inhibits chemotaxis, oxidative metabolism, the uptake of glucose, and intracellular bacterial killing by polymorphonuclear leukocytes [26]. The IC_{50} of the granulocyte inhibiting protein required to inhibit both the biochemical and the functional changes is in the nanomolar range. Therefore, the efficacy of the protein is well within the range of physiological effector substances (Table 1). A specific rabbit polyclonal antibody raised against the protein nullified these inhibitory changes [26]. In summary, a granulocyte inhibitory protein was isolated from ultrafiltrates of patients on regular hemodialysis treatment. A polysulfone membrane (Fresenius, Oberursel, FRG) was used. The protein is capable of inhibiting four fundamental PMN cell functions. Its exact role remains to be elucidated.

References

1. Tolkoff NE, Rubin RH (1990) Uremia and host defenses. N Engl J Med 322:770–772
2. Haag-Weber M, Hable M, Schollmeyer P, Hörl WH (1989) Metabolic response of neutrophils to uremia and dialysis. Kidney Int 36(Suppl 27):S293–S298
3. Clark RA, Hamony BH, Ford G, Kimball HR (1972) Chemotaxis in acute renal failure. J Infect Dis 126:460–463
4. Baum J, Cestero RVM, Freeman RB (1975) Chemotaxis of polymorphonuclear leukocytes and delayed hypersensitivity in uremia. Kidney Int 7(Suppl 2):S147–S153
5. Siriwatratananonta P, Sinsakul V, Stern K, Slavin RG (1978) Defective chemotaxis in uremia. J Lab Clin Med 92:402–407
6. Pedersen JO, Knudsen F, Nielsen AH, Grunnet N (1987) The ability of uremic serum to induce neutrophil chemotaxis in relation to hemodialysis Blood Purif 5:24–28
7. Hirabayashi Y, Kobayashi T, Nishikawa A, Aoki T, Takaya J, Kobayashi Y (1988) Oxidative metabolism and phagocytosis of polymorphonuclear leukocytes in patients with chronic renal failure. Nephron 49:305–312
8. Vanholder RC, Dhondt A, Ringoir SMG (1988) Challenge of phagocyte metabolism by extracorporeal test. Trans Am Soc Artif Intern Organs 34:214–218
9. Hällgren R, Fjellström KE, Venge P (1979) Kinetic studies of phagocytosis. II. The serum-independent uptake of IgG-coated particles by polymorphonuclear leukocytes from uremic patients on regular dialysis treatment. J Lab Clin Med 94:277–284
10. Ritchey EE, Wallin JD, Shah SV (1981) Chemiluminescence and superoxide anion production by leukocytes from chronic hemodialysis patients. Kidney Int 19:349–358
11. Nguyen AT, Lethias C, Zingraff J, Herbelin A, Naret C, Descamps-Latscha B (1985) Hemodialysis membrane-induced activation of phagocyte oxidative metabolism detected in vivo and in vitro within microamounts of whole blood. Kidney Int 28:158–167
12. Kolb G, Schönemann H, Fischer W, Bittner K, Lange H, Höffken H, Damann V, Joseph K, Havemann K (1988) Hemodialysis with cuprophane membranes leads to alteration of granulocyte oxidative metabolism and leukocyte sequestion in the lung. In: Hörl WH, Heidland A (eds) Proteases: Potential role in health and disease II. Plenum, New York, pp 377–384
13. Markert M, Heierli C, Kuwahara T, Frei J, Wauters JP (1988) Dialyzed polymorphonuclear neutrophil oxidative metabolism during dialysis: a comparative study with 5 new and reused membranes. Clin Nephrol 29:129–136
14. McCaleb ML, Izzo MS, Lockwood DH (1985) Characterization and partial purification of a factor from uremic human serum that induces insulin resistance. J Clin Invest 75:391–396
15. DeFronzo RA, Tobin JD, Rowe JW, Andres R (1978) Glucose intolerance in uremia. J Clin Invest 62:425–435

16. Hampers CL, Soeldner JS, Doak PB, Merrill JP (1966) Effect of chronic renal failure and hemodialysis on carbohydrate metabolism. J Clin Invest 45:1719–1731
17. Balesteri P, Rindi P, Biagini M, Giovaneti S (1972) Effects of uremic serum, urea, creatinine and methylguanidine on glucose metabolism. Clin Sci 42:395–404
18. Morgan JM, Morgan RE (1964) Study of the effect of uremic metabolites on erythrocyte glycosis. Metabolism 13:629–635
19. Dzurik R (1980) Metabolic alterations caused by uremia. Proc Eur Dial Transplant Assoc 17:577–586
20. McCaleb ML, Mevorach R, Freeman RB, Izzo MS, Lockwood DH (1984) Induction of insulin resistance in normal adipose tissue by uremic human serum. Kidney Int 25:416–421
21. Korchak HM, Rutherford LE, Weissman G (1984) Stimulus response coupling in the human neutrophiles. I. Kinetic analysis of changes in calcium permeability. J Biol Chem 259:4070
22. McCall C, Schmitt J, Cousart S, O'Flaherty J, Bass D, Wykle R (1985) Stimulation of hexose transport by human polymorphonuclear leucocytes: a possible role of protein kinase C. Biochem Biophys Res Commun 126:450–456
23. Krause KH, Schlegel W, Wollheim CB, Andersson T, Waldvogel FA, Lew PD (1985) Chemotactic peptide activation of human neutrophils and HL-60 cells. Pertussis toxin reveals correlation between inositol triophate generation, calcium ion transients, and cellular activation. J Clin Invest 76:1348–1354
24. Haag-Weber M, Hable M, Schollmeyer P, Hörl WH (1989) Hemodialysis improves carbohydrate metabolism in polymorphonuclear neutrophils (PMN) (abstract). Kidney Int 35:248
25. Haag-Weber M, Schollmeyer P, Hörl WH (1989) Neutrophil activation during hemodialysis. In: Hörl WH, Schollmeyer P (eds) New perspectives in hemodialysis, peritoneal dialysis, arteriovenous hemofiltration, and plasmapheresis. Plenum, New York, pp 27–37
26. Hörl WH, Haag-Weber M, Georgopoulos A, Block LH (1990) The physicochemical characterization of a polypeptide present in uremic serum that inhibits the biological activity of polymorphonuclear cells. Proc Natl Acad Sci USA 87:6353–6357

The Impact of Anemia in the Pathogenesis of Endocrine Abnormalities in Chronic Renal Failure

Franciszek Kokot, Andrzej Więcek, Mariusz Klin[1],
and Jolanta Klepacka[2]

SUMMARY. Endocrine abnormalities are well characterized in uremic patients. On the other hand it is known that erythropoietin (EPO) treatment in patients with chronic uremia is accompanied by several beneficial, as well as by adverse effects, which suggest the participation of endocrine organs in the pathogenesis of this disease. In this paper we report the effects of three months EPO treatment on the function of several endocrine organs in hemodialyzed patients. Endocrine parameters were assessed before and after 3 months on EPO treatment, as well as 3 months after EPO administration was discontinued. Results obtained in these patients were compared with those established in appropriately selected healthy subjects, as well as with those found in hemodialyzed uremic patients (not receiving EPO) with a hematocrit value of the same magnitude as that determined in patients after EPO treatment. Treatment with EPO was followed by suppression of basal plasma levels of somatotropin, prolactin, follitropin, lutropin, adrenocorticotropic hormone (ACTH), cortisol, and aldosterone and by a moderate increase of plasma parathyroid hormone (PTH) and testosterone. Treatment with EPO did not significantly influence plasma calcitonin and 25-OH-D levels or the function of the pituitary-thyroid feedback. After 3 months of EPO treatment we found a suppression of plasma renin activity, but an increase of plasma atrial natriuretic peptide level. Treatment with EPO increased insulin, but suppressed plasma levels of glucagon, gastrin, and to a lesser degree, those of the pancreatic polypeptide. Some EPO-induced endocrine alterations were still present three months after the discontinuation of EPO therapy. From data presented in this study, it follows that EPO treatment is accompanied by profound endocrine alterations and that these alterations do not seem to be related only to the improvement of anemia.

[1]Department of Nephrology, Silesian School of Medicine, ul. Francuska 20, Katowice, Poland
[2]Institute of Transplantology, Medical Academy, Warsaw, Poland

Introduction

Erythropoietin (EPO) is a factor which undoubedly participates in the pathogenesis of anemia in patients with chronic renal failure. Several lines of evidence suggest that additional factors are also involved in the pathogenesis and maintenance of such anemia. Among these factors we refer to endocrine abnormalities [1]. On the other hand, some hormones (corticoids, thyroid, and gonadal hormones) are proven modulators of erythropoiesis, even under physiological conditions. Finally, from data obtained in the last 3–4 years, it seems that some clinical signs and symptoms, such as increased well-being, increased libido and potency, increased appetite, exacerbation of preexisting elevated blood pressure, and improvement of physical and mental activity, as well as some side effects of EPO treatment (hyperkalemia, hypocalcemia, periarticular inflammation due to calcified deposits) are not related only to the amelioration of anemia (for review see references in [1]).

In this paper we summarize our extensive studies on the influence of EPO treatment on the function of endocrine organs in hemodialyzed patients. Results of some of these studies are already published [2–5] while others are to be published [7–9]. In these studies we aimed to answer the following questions:

1) Does EPO treatment influence the function of endocrine organs in hemodialyzed patients with chronic renal failure? and
2) What is the impact of anemia in the pathogenesis of endocrine abnormalities in chronic renal failure?

Material and Methods

Three groups of patients were examined. The first one consisted of hemodialyzed patients treated with EPO (EPO group). The second one comprised hemodialyzed patients not treated with EPO (no EPO group), but who showed hematocrit values similar to those of patients in the first group after those patients had completed EPO therapy. The third group consisted of healthy control subjects. In the EPO group, baseline plasma levels of hormones were assessed before EPO treatment, after three months on EPO treatment, and three months after the discontinuation of EPO therapy, while in the other two groups baseline plasma concentrations of the individual hormonal parameters were estimated only once. The number of subjects examined is listed in Table 1. The mean age of the three groups was of similar magnitude. In hemodialyzed patients, blood samples for the assessment of the individual hormones were withdrawn from fasting subjects immediately before the dialysis session. EPO (EPREX from Cilag) was administered intravenously as a bolus injection at the end of the dialysis session three times per week. The mean dose of EPO was 75 U/kg b.w. In all blood samples, in addition to assessing parameters, hemoglobin concentration (Hb), hematocrit value (Hct), and plasma levels of calcium, phosphorus (inorganic), sodium, potassium, and creatinine were also assessed. All hormones were assessed by radioimmunoassay (for reference see [2]). Statistical evaluation of results was performed using Student's "t" test for paired and unpaired variables, respectively.

Table 1. Baseline plasma levels of hormones in patients of the NO-EPO group (*D*), in healthy subjects (*controls*) and in hemodialyzed patients before (*B*) and after (*A*) three months of EPO therapy, and 3 months after discontinuation of EPO therapy (*C*). Means ± SEM. The number of patients examined is shown in parentheses. The degree of statistical significance in EPO-treated patients concerns the difference B-A and B-C respectively, while in patients of the NO-EPO group the difference concerns D-A. CRF, chronic renal failure
$^xP < 0.05$ $^yP < 0.01$ $^zP < 0.001$

| | Patients with CRF on EPO | | | | |
| | Before EPO | After EPO | 3 Months after discontinued EPO | NO-EPO group | |
	B	A	C	D	Controls
Somatotropin (STH) ng/ml	9.5±1.1 (11)	4.8 ±0.7^z (11)	4.6±1.1^z (7)	7.0±1.7	3.5±0.5
ACTH pg/ml	58.8±4.4 (5)	13.2 ±2.2^z (5)	65.6±9.5 (5)	82.9±21.2^y (7)	23.6±1.9 (15)
Prolactin ng/ml	36.8±4.7 (11)	12.9 ±2.6^z (11)	48.2±14.2 (11	11.6±2.9 (7)	12.1±1.6 (12)
Follitropin (FSH) mU/ml	46.8±11.7 (5)	13.6 ±5.3^y (5)	16.4±9.0^x (5)	28.4±3.3^x (7)	5.7±0.4 (15)
Lutropin (LH) mU/ml	17.5±1.5 (5)	7.9 ±1.1^z (5)	5.4±1.7^z (5)	18.0±1.0^z (7)	8.2±0.5 (15)
Thyrotropin (TSH) mU/ml	2.2±0.3 (5)	2.2 ±0.4 (5)	2.1±0.3 (5)	2.0±0.2 (7)	2.6±0.3 (12)
Thyroxin (T$_4$) µmol/l	80.0±11.4 (5)	86.3 ±4.2 (5)	103.0±10.9 (5)	103.1±9.3 (7)	120.0±5.6 (12)
Triiodothyronine (T$_3$) mmol/l	1.2±0.2 (5)	1.3 ±0.2 (5)	1.7±0.1 (5)	2.0±0.2 (7)	2.1±0.2 (12)
Parathyroid hormone (PTH) ng/ml	1.6±0.3 (5)	2.08±0.31 (5)	1.7±0.3 (5)	1.3±0.4 (7)	0.6±0.05 (12)
Calcitonin (CT) pg/ml	109±20 (5)	149±11 (5)	133±9 (5)	194±31 (7)	23±14 (12)
25-OH-D ng/ml	17.4±2.4 (5)	19.7 ±1.6 (5)	12.5±0.8 (5)	14.0±0.8^y (7)	16.2±0.8 (12)
Plasma renin activity (PRA) ng/ml per h	5.4±0.8 (11)	3.3 ±0.6^y (11)	3.9±1.4 (11)	2.9±0.9 (7)	2.8±0.2 (10)
Aldosterone (Ald) ng/dl	14.8±1.4 (5)	11.3 ±1.3^x (5)	16.3±2.9 (5)	15.3±1.4^x (7)	9.8±0.7 (10)
Cortisol µg/dl	13.2±2.1 (5)	7.9 ±1.2^y (5)	18.7±4.7 (5)	19.2±1.3^z (7)	12.4±1.8 (12)
Atrial natriuretic peptide (ANP) pg/ml	159±13 (5)	255±38^x (5)	117±14 (5)	149±7^y (7)	74±1 (10)
Vasopressin pg/ml	6.4±1.7 (5)	6.2 ±1.3 (5)	9.8±1.6 (5)	9.3±1.5 (7)	2.1±0.2 (10)
Glucagon pg/ml	256±61 (5)	114±42^y (5)	275±28 (5)	174±43 (7)	115±17 (15)
Gastrin pg/ml	125±19 (5)	53±9^y (5)	120±9 (5)	265±16^z (7)	38±6 (15)
Pancreatic polypeptide (PP) pg/ml	735±92 (5)	526±93^x (5)	250±34^z (5)	682±32 (7)	80±12 (15)
Insulin µU/ml	19.8±3.6 (11)	29.2 ±3.4^x (11)	40.8±7.3^y (11)	27.9±6.2 (7)	8.6±1.2 (15)
Testosterone ng/ml	1.9±0.8 (5)	3.0 ±0.7^x (5)	1.9±0.3 (5)	4.2±0.5 (7)	8.2±0.3 (15)

Results

Influence of EPO Therapy on Blood Hemoglobin Concentration, Hematocrit Value, and Plasma Levels of Creatinine and Electrolytes

Treatment with EPO did not significantly influence plasma levels of creatinine (1208 $\pm$ 47 µmol/l before EPO vs 1236 $\pm$ 62 µmol/l after EPO treatment).

Treatment with EPO was accompanied by a significant increase of hemoglobin, from 4.47 $\pm$ 0.14 to 6.67 $\pm$ 0.15 mmol/l, and by a significant increase of the Hct value, from 23 $\pm$ 0.89 to 34.8 $\pm$ 0.75% ($P < 0.001$). Three months after EPO therapy was discontinued both Hb (=5.3 $\pm$ 0.15 mmol/l) and Hct (=27.6 $\pm$ 0.97%) values were found to have declined, although these values were still significantly ($P < 0.05$) higher than pre-EPO values.

Treatment with EPO did not influence plasma sodium levels, but was accompanied by a slight increase of plasma potassium (from 5.06 $\pm$ 0.09 to 5.38 $\pm$ 0.06 mmol/l) and inorganic phosphorus (from 1.68 $\pm$ 0.18 to 1.94 $\pm$ 0.2 mmol/l), and by a significant ($P < 0.05$) decline of plasma total calcium (from 2.44 $\pm$ 0.07 to 2.25 $\pm$ 0.08). Three months after EPO therapy was discontinued the respective plasma levels of K, Ca, and P did not differ from pretreatment values.

Endocrine Alterations Induced by EPO Therapy

As can be seen in Table 1, pretreatment baseline plasma levels of most hormones (cortisol, thyrotropin, T_3, T_4, 25-OH-D, and testosterone excepted) were significantly higher than the respective values in the control group. After three months of EPO therapy a significant decline or even normalization, of plasma levels of somatotropin (STH), ACTH, follitropin (FSH), lutropin (LH), prolactin, glucagon, gastrin, cortisol, and of plasma renin activity was noticed. In contrast EPO did not significantly influence plasma concentrations of thyrotropin (TSH), triiodothyronine (T_3), thyroxine (T_4), arginine vasopressin (AVP), parathyroid hormone (PTH), calcitonin (CT), and 25-OH-D, while a marked increase of atrial natriuretic peptide (ANP), insulin, and testosterone was observed. Three months after EPO therapy was discontinued, baseline plasma renin activity (PRA) and plasma levels of ACTH, prolactin, PTH, CT, aldosterone, vasopressin, cortisol, glucagon, gastrin and testosterone were similar to pretreatment values, while plasma levels of STH, FSH, LH and pancreatic polypeptide (PP) were still significantly lower than pretreatment values; in contrast, the plasma level of insulin was significantly higher, while ANP levels were significantly lower than their respective pretreatment concentrations.

Discussion

From the data presented in these studies it follows that EPO treatment markedly influences the function of many endocrine organs. Although the pathophysiology of most of these hormonal alterations has not been clarified, it seems that at least some of these alterations are of clinical relevance. For example, it seems likely that the observed suppression by EPO treatment of PRA and aldosterone, as well as the increase of plasma ANP levels, are purposeful compensatory mechanisms which counteract hypervolemia (induced by increased erythropoiesis), as recently suggested by Kühn et al. [10]. As is well known, hypervolemia suppresses the activity of the renin-angiotensin-aldosterone system, but stimulates ANP release. Based on this reasoning, a reduction of plasma AVP level should also be expected. As this was not the case (EPO did not change plasma AVP level), it seems that factors other than hypervolemia are involved in the pathogenesis of reduced PRA and aldosterone, and of increased ANP levels in EPO treated patients, and/or that EPO therapy does not normalize the normal volumetric regulation of AVP secretion in uremic patients.

As shown in Table 1, EPO treatment was followed by a significant decrease in the plasma levels of STH, ACTH, cortisol, prolactin, PP, glucagon, and gastrin. It remains to be clarified whether these endocrine alterations are caused by direct effects of EPO on the respective endocrine organs, or whether these alterations are a consequence of the improvement of anemia.

As recently reported by Schäfer et al. [4,5] EPO treatment significantly suppresses plasma prolactin levels in uremic patients. This EPO effect could be involved in the causation of the improved sexual activity of these patients. As already reported by Bommer et al. [11], suppression of prolactin secretion by α-bromcriptin is accompanied by improvement of sexual activity in patients with endstage renal failure. As EPO treatment was also followed by a significant increase in plasma testosterone levels, it seems likely that improved function of the Leydig's cells may be involved in the causation of improved sexual activity in these patients. Very recently, an increase of plasma testosterone level in EPO treated patients was also reported by other authors [12].

The importance of the observed increase of immunoreactive insulin (IRI) and decrease of plasma levels of STH, ACTH, cortisol, and glucagon in EPO treated patients has been insufficiently elucidated. It seems likely that these EPO induced alterations may be involved in the pathogenesis of improved carbohydrate tolerance in uremic patients [8].

As already mentioned, EPO treatment was accompanied by a mild increase of PTH plasma levels, probably induced by an enhanced ingestion of food (as a consequence of increased appetite). Short term EPO treatment did not significantly influence thyroid function in uremic patients.

As shown in Table 1, in patients of the No-EPO group (with a Hct values similar to the posttreatment values in the EPO group) plasma levels of several hormones differed significantly from the respective posttreatment values of the EPO group. This fact suggests the participation of factors other than anemia in the pathogenesis of endocrine alterations induced by EPO therapy.

The results presented in this paper suggest that, in patients with endstage renal failure, elevated levels of some hormones are not caused only by the reduced degradation or excretion of these hormones by the failing kidneys. Thus, reconsideration of the pathogenesis of endocrine abnormalities in patients with endstage renal failure seems to be mandatory. It remains to be clarified as to what extent endocrine alterations in EPO-treated patients are due to improvement of erythropoiesis and oxygen supply to different organs or whether they are specific EPO effects.

References

1. Kokot F, Więcek A (1989) Endocrine changes in chronic dialysis patients. In: Maher JF (ed) Replacement of renal function by dialysis. Kluwer, Dordrecht, pp 953–971
2. Kokot F, Więcek A, Grzeszczak W, Klepacka J, Klin M (1989) Influence of erythropoietin treatment on endocrine abnormalities in haemodialyzed patients. In: Baldamus CA, Scigalla P, Wieczorek L, Koch KM (eds) Erythropoietin: from molecular structure to clinical application. Contrib Nephrol, Karger, Basel, pp 257–272
3. Kokot F, Więcek A, Grzeszczak K, Klin M (1990) Influence of erythropoietin treatment on function of the pituitary adrenal axis and somatotropin secretion in hemodialyzed patients. Clin Nephrol 33:241–246
4. Schaefer RM, Kokot F, Heidland A (1989) Impact of recombinant erythropoietin on sexual function in hemodialysis patients. In: Baldamus CA, Scigalla P, Wieczorek al, Koch KM (eds) Erythropoietin: from molecular structure to clinical application. Contrib Nephrol, Karger, Basel, pp 273–282
5. Schaefer RM, Kokot F, Kürner B, Zech M, Heidland A (1988) Normalization of elevated prolactin levels in hemodialysis patients on erythropoietin. Nephron 50:400–401
6. Kokot F, Więcek A, Grzeszczak W, Klin M (1990) Influence of erythropoietin treatment on plasma renin activity, aldosterone, vasopressin and atrial natriuretic peptide in haemodialyzed patients. Min Electrol Metab 16:25–29
7. Kokot F, Więcek A, Grzeszczak W, Klin M (to be published) Influence of erythropoietin treatment on follitropin and lutropin response to luliberin and plasma testosterone levels in haemodialyzed patients. Nephron
8. Kokot F, Więcek A, Grzeszczak W, Klin M, Żukowska-Szczechowska E (to be published) Influence of erythropoietin treatment on glucose tolerance, insulin, glucagon, gastrin and pancreatic polypeptide secretion in haemodialyzed patients with endstage renal failure. Contrib Nephrol, Karger, Basel
9. Kokot F, Więcek A, Grzeszczak W, Klin M (to be published) Der Einfluss von Erythropoietin auf die Funktion der Schilddrüse und Nebenschildrüsen bei dialysierten Patienten mit chronischer Niereninsuffizienz. Z Klin Med
10. Kühn K, Talarschik H, Koch KM, Eisenhauer T, Nonast-Daniel B, Scheler F, Brunkhorst R, Reimers E (1988) Plasma atrial natriuretic peptide after partial correction of renal anaemia by recombinant human erythropoietin. Nephrol Dial Transplant 3:497–498
11. Bommer J, DelPozo E, Ritz E, Bommer G (1979) Improved sexual function in male haemodialysis patients on bromocriptin. Lancet II:496–497
12. Haley NR, Matsumoto AM, Eschbach JW, Adamson JW (1988) Low testosterone levels increase in male hemodialysis patients treated with recombinant human erythropoietin (abstract). 21st annual meeting of the American Society of Nephrology, December 11–12, 1988. San Antonio, USA

Growth Hormone Treatment for Patients with Renal Failure

Joel D. Kopple, Giuliano Brunori, Marc Leiserowitz, Crystal Mattimore, and Raimund Hirschberg[1]

Growth Hormone (GH), so called for its ability to induce an increase in linear growth, is secreted by the somatotrophes of the anterior pituitary gland. It is a single-chain polypeptide with a molecular weight of 22000 and contains 191 amino acid residues. Its configuration is determined by two intrachain disulfide bridges. The factors controlling the secretion and plasma levels of GH have been reviewed elsewhere [1].

GH exerts many metabolic and anabolic effects on skeletal and soft tissues. Some of these actions appear to be mediated directly by GH. Others GH effects are dependent on the synthesis and release of two polypeptide growth factors. These compounds are called, for their structural homology to proinsulin and similar activity to insulin, IGF-I and IGF-II [2]. Growth hormone stimulates IGF-I production in many cells including those in liver, kidney, cartilage, and the pituitary gland. Nutritional status also plays an important role in IGF-I production. During conditions associated with negative calorie balance or negative nitrogen balance, the circulating levels of IGF-I are reduced [3], even though plasma GH levels are elevated. IGF-II production is less GH-dependent; like IGF-I, it is produced in many tissues.

The most important metabolic effects of GH include increased cellular DNA, RNA, protein synthesis, and sulfate incorporation, positive nitrogen balance, enhanced lipolysis and release of free fatty acids. Growth hormone decreases urinary excretion of phosphorus, sodium, potassium and chloride. Acutely, GH may exert an insulin-like effect on carbohydrates; later it may cause insulin antagonism, carbohydrate intolerance and diabetes mellitus [1]. Thus, GH can be considered an anabolic hormone that stimulates postnatal growth and positive protein balance, antagonizes the glucose-lowering action of insulin, and possesses lipolytic activity.

The kidneys play an important role in the turnover of circulating GH. Johnson and Maack reported that in rats about 70% of the total turnover of GH occurs in the kid-

[1]Division of Nephrology and Hypertension, Harbor UCLA Medical Center and Schools of Medicine and Public Health, UCLA Torrance, CA 90509, USA

neys [4]. This may account for the increased plasma levels and decreased plasma turnover of GH in anephric animals and in humans with chronic renal failure.

Almost all studies of the nutritional status of patients with advanced chronic renal failure, including patients undergoing maintenance hemodialysis or peritoneal dialysis, indicate that they often demonstrate wasting or protein calorie malnutrition [5,6]. In many individuals, malnutrition is mild or moderate. There are a number of causes for wasting and malnutrition in renal failure. Probably the most important cause is poor dietary intake. Other causes include intercurrent illnesses, blood loss, the hemodialysis procedure itself, which may both stimulate protein breakdown and also engender losses of amino acids and proteins, and the altered metabolic and hormonal environment of renal failure. Malnutrition has been shown to be an important risk factor for high morbidity and mortality in patients with chronic renal failure [7,8]. It is not established whether low protein and calorie intake and malnutrition cause the adverse effects or whether underlying illnesses are responsible for both the inadequate intake and the increased morbidity and mortality. There is the sense among many nephrologists that poor nutritional intake negatively affects the course of patients with chronic renal failure.

Many studies have suggested that the uremic environment itself is antianabolic or catabolic. Indeed, inhibitors to protein synthesis, glucose uptake by muscle, and the effects of insulin-like growth factor-I (IGF-I, somatomedin C) have been described in uremic sera [9–11]. In both children and adults with chronic renal failure, serum GH levels are generally increased [4,12] and serum somatomedin C concentrations are normal or slightly elevated [11,13]. However, in children [14] and adults [11] with kidney failure, the biological activity of somatomedin C is reported to be reduced. Bioactivity of serum somatomedin C increases after a hemodialysis treatment [11].

Several investigators have attempted to use anabolic steroids to promote anabolism in acutely or chronically uremic patients [15,16]. These agents, which usually are similar in structure to androgens, could induce anabolic effects; but the results appear to be transient [15]. Because of the evidence for an inhibiting effect of uremia on IGF-1 activity [11] and the fact that GH has been shown to both increase IGF-1 levels and to promote anabolism, several researchers have began to investigate whether GH injections may improve the nutritional status and body composition of patients with chronic renal failure.

At present, most research on the effects of GH in renal failure has focused on children. Growth retardation is a prominent manifestation in children with advanced chronic renal failure. The heights and weights of children undergoing maintenance dialysis are frequently in the lower 3 percentile as compared to normal children of the same sex and chronological age [17]. With conventional treatment, children with advanced renal failure may grow normally, but catch-up growth is rare. Fortunately, bone epiphyses often close late and, hence, uremic children may continue to grow at a chronological age where height gain usually has ceased in normal individuals [17]. Nonetheless, children with advanced renal failure usually have short stature when they become adults. Children who have a renal transplant often continue to demonstrate low growth rates and short stature. Glucocorticoid therapy and the persistence of some degree of renal insufficiency in the transplanted kidney may contribute to this phenomenon. It should be emphasized that in children with end stage renal disease, body weight and most other anthropometric parameters, when adjusted for height age rather than chronological age, tend to be normal; on the other hand, their serum albumin is often low [18].

The pathogenesis of impaired growth in renal failure probably involves many factors including inadequate calorie and protein intake, the uremic environment, renal osteodystrophy, aluminum toxicity, 1,25-dihydroxycholecalciferol deficiency, acidemia, glucocorticoid therapy and superimposed illnesses [5,17]. As in adults, serum IGF-1 measured by bioassay is low, suggesting an inhibitory effect of the uremic environment on IGF-1 and, hence, GH activity.

Since the early 1960s GH, initially obtained by extraction from human pituitary glands, has been used to treat humans with catabolic stress [19]. The data suggested that GH promoted anabolism in these patients. As a result of the relative scarcity, cost and, more recently, the recognized potential hazards of human GH, its use was largely limited to growth retarded patients with GH deficiency [20]. With the development of recombinant human GH (rhGH), the potential for synthesizing large amounts of GH was now at hand, and its greater purity reduced the hazards of treatment. Several investigators have begun to explore the use of rhGH to promote growth and anabolism in patients with chronic renal failure. Initially, chronically azotemic rats were studied. Growth hormone extracted from human pituitary glands and injected intraperitoneally, 0.5 IU/day, was stated to be unsuccessful at increasing growth in azotemic or normal rats [21]. However, rhGH was successful at promoting growth and anabolism in these animals [21]. Subsequently, the growth promoting and anabolic effects of this hormone were tested, first in children and then in adults with chronic renal failure. The following paragraphs briefly review these studies.

Mehls et al. examined the effects of rhGH on the growth rate, the food conversion ratio and the rate of longitudinal growth at the proximal tibia level in female rats with subtotal nephrectomy or sham operation [21]. The rats received rhGH or vehicle either by continuous subcutaneous infusion using osmotic minipumps or by intraperitoneal injection for 14 days. Azotemic rats infused with GH, as compared to the pairfed azotemic rats given the vehicle, demonstrated significantly improved gain in body length (P < 0.01), and weight (P < 0.01) and an increased food utilization ratio (P < 0.01). The sham operated control rats infused with GH, as compared to pairfed sham animals given vehicle, also displayed a greater increase in growth and food utilization ratios. The growth velocity and weight gain in the azotemic rats given GH tended to be lower than the normal values of the sham-operated control rats treated with GH. These observations are consistent with the thesis that there is resistance to the actions of GH in chronic renal failure. The findings are also consistent with a lower ^{3}H-thymidine incorporation in cartilage chondrocytes in GH retarded chronically azotemic vs GH treated controls [22]. Curiously, serum IGF-1 levels did not rise in the GH treated rats.

Nakano and colleagues studied the effects of daily subcutaneous injections of rat GH in rats with mild to moderate renal insufficiency that were fed a low 8% protein diet [23]. The low protein diet was selected in order to reduce the potential hazards of higher protein diets on the survival of the remnant kidneys. Rats underwent 75% nephrectomy or sham surgery. The azotemic rats were randomly assigned to receive rat GH or vehicle; sham rats received only vehicle. Animals were studied for 20 days while they ate ad libitum. The azotemic rats treated with GH, as compared to azotemic animals given vehicle, demonstrated significantly greater body weight, length, head size, food efficiency ratios, and serum albumin. There were no apparent differences in these parameters between the azotemic GH treated rats and vehicle treated sham controls. In this experimental model of mild to moderate renal failure, GH was growth-enhancing, despite the low 8% protein diet.

Koch, Lippe, and associates studied the effects of rhGH in five children with chronic renal failure who were not receiving dialysis treatment and who had growth retardation [13]. All five patients were treated for one year with 0.125 mg/kg of rhGH (methionyl human GH [Protropin],Genentech Inc.) three times per week. Before treatment, the children had a mean annual growth velocity of 4.9 ± 1.4 (SD) cm/year, with a mean standard deviation score for height (height SDS) of less than -2.0. After one year of rhGH treatment, the mean growth rate increased to 8.9 ± 1.2 cm/year, and the mean height SDS rose from -2.98 ± 0.73 to -2.36 ± 0.83 (P < 0.02). In one patient, the rhGH dosage was increased after 6 months to 0.250 mg/kg three times per week, because the height gain with rhGH was only 20% greater than his baseline growth rate; there was no further increase in his growth velocity with the higher rhGH dose. For the five patients, the mean weight gain during the year before the therapy was 1.5 ± 0.5 kg/year; this increased to 2.8 ± 0.8 kg/year by the end of the rhGH treatment. The creatinine clearances remained stable during the period of the study in all five patients. This was an issue of some concern because of the possibility that the hyperfiltration induced by GH might accelerate the rate of progression of the renal failure [24]. The glucose tolerance test was not significantly different in the pre- vs the post-treatment period. Antibodies to GH did not develop in any patient. The mean acid-chromatographed serum IGF-1 levels were normal in all the children at the start of the study and increased during rhGH treatment.

Tonshoff and coworkers gave rhGH to nine prepubertal children, eight of whom were undergoing continuous ambulatory peritoneal dialysis (CAPD, $n=7$), or maintenance hemodialysis (HD, $n=1$) and one of whom had advanced chronic renal failure not treated with dialysis [25]. Patients received growth hormone, $4U/m^2$ (Genotropin, KabiVitrum), in daily subcutaneous injections for six months. During the six months of treatment, the mean annualized height velocity increased from -2.77 ± 1.69 (SD) to $+2.5 \pm 2.43$ (i.e., from 4.5 ± 2.47 cm to 8.3 ± 1.77 cm) (P < 0.01). Serum IGF-1 and IGF-II, measured by radioimmunoassay and expressed as percent of normal mean values, increased from 91 ± 60 to 308 ± 215 (P < 0.01), and from 155 ± 26 to 202 ± 23 (P < 0.01), respectively. Serum IGF-1 bioactivity, expressed as percent of normal, also rose from 40 ± 7 to 119 ± 35 (P < 0.01). Bone age increased by an average of only 0.4 years during the six months of treatment, suggesting that rhGH treatment will not accelerate bone aging and closure of the epiphyses. There was no change in glucose tolerance or in serum insulin levels.

Two studies with rhGH have been carried out in adult patients undergoing maintenance hemodialysis. Ziegler and colleagues performed six studies in four men and one woman undergoing maintenance hemodialysis as outpatients [26]. Patients received rhGH, 5 or 10 mg, subcutaneously, postdialysis, three times weekly for two weeks. Net urea generation fell from 6.2 ± 0.7 g/day during the week prior to treatment to 4.8 ± 0.6 and 4.5 ± 0.6 during the first and second weeks after therapy. Net protein catabolic rate also fell from 1.1 ± 0.1 g/kg per day before treatment to 0.9 ± 0.1 and 0.8 ± 0.1 (P < 0.05) during the first two weeks of treatment. Similarly, the mean weekly serum urea nitrogen (SUN) and the time averaged SUN fell during the two weeks of rhGH therapy. The authors reported that the dietary protein and energy intake did not change during treatment.

Table 1. Response of serum urea nitrogen (*SUN*) to daily growth hormone injections in a malnourished maintenance hemodialysis patient

Day of study	SUN (mg/dl) pre/post	Day of study	SUN (mg/dl) pre/post
5	90/32	21	93/35
7	91/37	22	Start GH, 0.05 mg/kg per day
12	97/43	23	82/33
14	92/40	26	75/33
19	96/44	28	56/26

GH, growth hormone

We have commenced a series of studies to evaluate the role of rhGH in malnourished maintenance hemodialysis patients. Criteria for acceptance into the study included evidence for protein-calorie malnutrition, as indicated by a body weight of 90% or less of desirable, determined from the Metropolitan Life Insurance Tables [27], or a serum albumin of 3.4 g/dl or less. Patients were studied for five weeks in the Clinical Research Center at Harbor UCLA Medical Center, where they ingested a constant diet that provided, each day, the patients' usual protein and energy intake. All diets were supplemented with calcium, at least 800 mg/day, and multivitamins, including folic acid. After the first 14 days of baseline study, rhGH (Somotrem [Genentech Inc.]) was administered at 0.05 mg/kg per day for 21 days. The key outcome measures included SUN, nitrogen balance, serum albumin and anthropometry.

At present two men and one women have been studied. All showed substantial evidence for malnutrition or protein calorie wasting. Edema-free relative body weights at the onset of study in the three patients were 70%, 74%, and 71%, respectively. The prestudy bone-free upper arm muscle areas in the three patients were in the <5, 7, and <5 percentiles, respectively, for normal adults of similar sex, height, and frame sizes and roughly similar age range. Patient 1 developed an unrelated illness and was removed from the study after 8 days of rhGH injections. Patients 2 and 3 left the study after 19 and 21 days of rhGH treatment.

After commencing the rhGH therapy, the predialysis SUN levels fell, even though the daily protein and energy intake and the hemodialysis regimen did not change. In Patient 1, the decrease in predialysis SUN appeared to begin within 24 hours of starting GH therapy (Table 1). Predialysis SUN also fell in Patients 2 and 3 within one day after starting daily growth hormone injections. However, the fall in SUN in Patient 3 was substantially less and transient, possibly because she developed pancreatitis during the course of the study. Analyses of the nitrogen balance data to date have been completed only in Patient 1. The results indicate that this patient went into markedly positive nitrogen balance.

These initial data suggest that rhGH may markedly improve protein balance in at least some malnourished maintenance hemodialysis patients. It must be emphasized that these GH studies are both very preliminary and of short duration. It has not yet been demonstrated that the chronic use of GH will improve body composition, clinical status, and quality of life, or that its chronic use will reduce symptoms, or reduce morbidity or mortality. Longterm studies of GH treatment in more maintenance hemodialysis patients will be necessary to examine these questions.

Another potential use of GH is for the treatment of patients with renal disease or acute or chronic renal failure who have a superimposed catabolic illness. It has been suggested that GH may reduce the degree of catabolism in these patients, and that this might improve host resistance, reduce morbidity and mortality, and facilitate recovery and convalescence. If these hypotheses can be proven, it could be particularly beneficial for the severely ill patient with acute renal failure. The mortality rate for acute renal failure patients remains very high. This is especially true for those acute renal failure patients who have surgical problems, have multiple complications, or require hemodialysis. Patients who have shock or sepsis as the cause of acute renal failure, and are not able to be nourished enterally because of a poorly functioning gastrointestinal tract, also have a marked morbidity and mortality rate; their overall mortality is about 85% [28–30].

These individuals may be severely catabolic, with a net rate of protein degradation that may rise to 150 g per day or greater [29,30]. Provision of intravenous nutrition to these individuals often has little effect on their degree of negative nitrogen balance. This is due to their metabolic status, which is programmed toward degrading fuel substrates, including protein and amino acids. It has been speculated that administration of anabolic agents, including growth factors, may alter the metabolic status of these patients and facilitate their ability to utilize both exogenous and endogenous nutrients more effectively. An hypothesis that underpins this approach is that if hypercatabolic individuals can be induced to improve their utilization of nutrients and to reduce their marked degree of wasting, they will demonstrate improved morbidity and mortality.

At present, growth hormone treatment has not been specifically studied in catabolic patients with renal failure. However, such studies have been performed in acutely catabolic or malnourished surgical patients who usually did not have renal failure. The results of these studies will be briefly reviewed, since the results may be pertinent to the use of GH for stressed patients with renal failure.

Okamura and associates studied the effects of rhGH on protein metabolism in rats with sepsis induced by cecal ligation [31]. Ten rats underwent sham-operation. All rats were nourished with total parenteral nutrition. Cumulative nitrogen balance was significantly more positive in the septic rats given TPN and 200 mU/day of rhGH as compared with the septic animals given TPN without rhGH. In the former rats, as compared to the sham-operated controls, cumulative nitrogen balance was not statistically different, although it tended to be less positive; serum albumin was slightly lower ($P < 0.05$), and urinary N^T-methylhistidine (3-methylhistidine), a marker of myofibrillar protein breakdown, was slightly greater ($P < 0.01$).

Several studies indicate that in postoperative patients, GH in pharmacological doses may promote an anabolic response [32–34]. Zhu-Ming et al. investigated the effects of hypocaloric feedings with or without injections of rhGH in 18 patients who underwent gastrointestinal surgery [32]. This was a placebo-controlled double blind randomized trial. Starting on the third day before surgery and continuing throughout the postoperative period of study, patients were given intravenous infusions of nutrient solutions providing 20 kcal/kg body weight per day and 1 g amino acids/kg per day. Commencing with the first day after the day of surgery, nine patients received daily subcutaneous injections of placebo (control group) and nine patients received intramuscular injections of 0.15 IU rhGH/kg per day. This rhGH regimen was continued for seven postoperative days. In the control group, the subjects were consistently in negative nitrogen balance (-32.6 ± 4.2 g/8 days). The urinary excretion of N^T-methylhistidine rose from preoperative values of 4.4 ± 0.7 to

7.26±1.01 umol/kg per day. In the GH treated group, the nitrogen balance was less negative, −7.1±3.12 g/8 days (P<0.001 vs controls), and the N^T-methylhistidine excretion was 3.6±0.3 and 4.4±0.3 umol/kg per day, respectively, before surgery and on postoperative day 7 (postoperative N^T-methylhistidine excretion in GH treated vs controls, P<0.05). The patients receiving rhGH lost, on average, 1.7% of their body weight, whereas the control group lost a mean of 6% of their body weight. Analysis of body composition revealed that the patients receiving GH maintained their lean body mass. The authors concluded that the postoperative catabolic response in patients receiving hypocaloric nutrients can be significantly ameliorated with the use of GH.

Ziegler et al. studied the metabolic effects of rhGH in nine clinically stable malnourished patients receiving hypocaloric parenteral nutrition [33]. Patients were studied for two consecutive 7-day periods while they received a hypocaloric intake that provided approximately 1100 kcal/day and 1.3 g amino acids/kg per day. During the 7 day control period, patients received a daily subcutaneous injection of saline; during the treatment period, the rhGH was given subcutaneously at a dose of 10 mg/day. In seven studies rhGH was given in the second week and in two studies it was given during the first week. Nitrogen balance was +0.5±0.9 (SEM) g/day during the control period and +3.4±0.5 g/day during the treatment period (P<0.001). Phosphorus balance was 0±29 mg/day during the control period and +218±32 mg/day during the GH period (P<0.001).

Six patients of Ziegler et al. received rhGH for 13–25 days [33]. Significantly positive nitrogen balance was observed for the entire period of rhGH administration. No side effects were observed. Serum IGF-1 increased markedly during rhGH treatment.

Manson and coworkers studied four healthy men who underwent eight paired studies in which they were given a constant amount of parenteral nutrition for two 7-day periods separated by at least two weeks [34]. The energy intake in the paired studies was calculated to provide 100% (2 studies), 50% (4 studies), or 30% (2 studies) of the subjects' calculated energy needs. During the first 7-day period, the individuals received GH, 10 mg/day, subcutaneously. In the second 7-day period, they received a daily injection of saline. With the GH as compared to the saline injections, the subjects demonstrated significantly more positive nitrogen balance and protein synthesis and increased serum insulin and plasma IGF-1 concentrations. After an oral glucose load, the GH-treated individuals appeared to show higher blood glucose values and attenuated muscle uptake of glucose and release of amino acids.

In contrast to these studies, Dahn et al. gave rhGH (methionyl human GH) 1 mg intramuscularly every six hours for 48 hours to acutely ill septic patients [35]. During the 48-hour period, the septic patients displayed no increase in plasma IGF-1 or in urinary urea nitrogen, and manifested a fall in splanchnic amino acid uptake. The normal control subjects, who were similarly treated with GH, showed a rise in plasma IGF-1, a fall in urinary urea nitrogen and no change in the splanchnic amino acid uptake. These findings suggest that GH may not be effective at promoting anabolism in acutely and severely stressed patients, at least when given over short periods of time. Since plasma IGF-1 also did not rise in response to the GH injections in these patients, it is possible that an injection of IGF-1 might be more effective at promoting anabolism in acutely and severely ill patients. It is pertinent in this regard that Mehls et al. found no increase in ^3H-thymidine incorporation into growing cartilage chondrocytes in rats with acute uremia that were given GH vs those given the solvent [22].

In summary, rhGH shows great promise for promoting longterm (i.e., at least one year) increased growth in children with chronic renal failure. In malnourished adults with chronic renal failure, preliminary studies indicate that rhGH increases nitrogen balance. Whether increased protein balance will enhance nutritional or clinical status or improve morbidity and mortality in these patients is not yet known. In nonuremic catabolic patients, GH may improve protein balance. However, in severely ill septic patients, GH may not exert these effects, at least during the first two days of treatment. It is possible that most, or all, of these effects of GH are mediated by IGF-1; whether giving IGF-1 will improve nutritional status in these patients is not known. The role of GH for growth enhancement in nondialyzed children with renal disease needs to be clarified; whether this therapy will accelerate the rate of progression of renal failure must be examined. Further studies are necessary to define more precisely the role for GH in the treatment of growth retarded, malnourished, or catabolic patients with acute or chronic renal disease and renal failure.

References

1. Felig P, Baxter JD, Broadus AE, Frohman LA (eds) (1987) Endocrinology and metabolism. McGraw-Hill, pp 264–269, 1584–1589
2. Daughday WH, Hall K, Salmon WD (1987) On the nomenclature of the somatomedins and insulin like growth factors. Endocrinology 121:1911–1912
3. Ronge H, Blum J (1989) Insulin-like growth factor I responses to recombinant bovine growth hormone during feed restriction in heifers. Acta Endocrinol (Copenh) 120:735–744
4. Johnson V and Maack T (1977) Renal extraction, filtration, absorption and catabolism of growth hormone. Am J Physiol 233 (3):F185–F196
5. Kopple JD (1978) Abnormal amino acid and protein metabolism in uremia. Kidney Int 14:340–348
6. Blumenkrantz MJ, Kopple JD, Gutman RA, Chan YK et al (1980) Methods for assessing nutritional status of patients with renal failure. Am J Clin Nutr 33:1567–1585
7. Acchiardo SR, Moore LW, Latour PA (1983) Malnutrition as the main factor in morbidity and mortality of hemodialysis patients. Kidney Int 24 (Suppl 16):S199–S203
8. Lowrie EG, Lew NC (1990) Death risk in hemodialysis patients: the predictive value of commonly measured variables and an evaluation of death rate differences between facilities. Am J Kidney Dis 15:458–482
9. Delaporte C, Gros F, Anagnostopoulos T (1980) Inhibitory effects of plasma dialysate on protein synthesis in vitro: influence of dialysis and transplantation. Am J Clin Nutr 33:1407–1410
10. Dzurik R, Hupkova V, Cernaceck P, Valovicova E, Niederland TR (1973) The isolation of an inhibitor of glucose utilization from the serum of uremic subjects. Clin Chim Acta 46:77–83
11. Phillips LS, Kopple JD (1981) Circulating somatomedin activity and sulfate levels in adults with normal and impaired kidney function. Metabolism 30:1091–1095
12. El-Bishti M, Counahan R, Bloom S (1978) Hormonal and metabolic responses to intravenous glucose in children on regular hemodialysis. Am J Clin Nutr 31:1865–1869
13. Koch VH, Lippe BM, Nelson PA, Boechat MI, Sherman BM, Fine RN (1989) Accelerated growth after recombinant human growth hormone treatment of children with chronic renal failure. J Pediatr 115:365–371

14. Mehls O, Fine RN (1989) The use of human recombinant growth hormone for treatment of growth failure in uremia. Semin Nephrol 9:43–48
15. Linder A, Tenckhoff H (1972) Influence of anabolic steroids on nitrogen balance in chronic peritoneal dialysis. Nephron 9:77–83
16. Gjorup S, Thaysen JH (1960) The effect of anabolic steroid (Durabolin [R]) in the conservative management of acute renal failure. Acta Med Scand 167:227
17. Fine RN (1984) Growth in children with renal insufficiency. In: Nissensen AR, Fine RN, Gentile DE (eds) Clinical Dialysis. Appleton-Century-Crofts, Norwalk, pp 661–669
18. Salusky IB, Fine RN, Nelson P, Blumenkrantz MJ, Kopple JD (1983) Nutritional status of children undergoing continuous ambulatory peritoneal dialysis. Am J Clin Nutr 38:595–611
19. Wilmore DW, Moylan JA, Bristow BF, Masom AD, Pruitt BA (1974) Anabolic effects of human growth hormone and high caloric feedings following thermal injury. Surg Gynecol Obstet 138:875–884
20. Brown P, Gajdusek DC, Gibbs CJ, Asher DM (1985) Potential epidemic of Creutzfeldt-Jakobs disease from human growth hormone therapy. N Engl J Med 313:728–731
21. Mehls O, Ritz E, Hunziker E-B, Eggli P, Heinrich U, Zapf J (1988) Improvement of growth and food utilization by human recombinant growth hormone in uremia. Kidney Int 33:45–52
22. Mehls O, Ritz E, Hunziker E-B, Tonshoff B, Heinrich U (1988) Role of growth hormone in growth failure of uremia. Perspective for application of recombinant growth hormone. Acta Paediatr Scand [Suppl] 343:118–126
23. Nakano M, Kainer G, Foreman JW, Ko D, Chan JCM (1989) The effects of exogenous rat growth hormone therapy on growth of uremic rats fed an 8% protein diet. Pediatr Res 26:204–207
24. Doi T, Striker LJ, Quaife C, Conti FG, Palmiter R, Behringer R, Brinster R, Striker GE (1988) Progressive glomerulosclerosis develops in transgenic mice chronically expressing growth hormone releasing factor but not in those expressing insulin like growth factor-1. Am J Pathol 131:398–403
25. Tonshoff B, Mehls O, Schauer A, Henrich U, Blum W, Ranke M (1989) Improvement of uremic growth failure by recombinant human growth hormone. Kidney Int 36 (Suppl 27):S201–S204
26. Ziegler TR, Lazarus JM, Young LS, Hakim R, Wilmore DW (1990) Growth hormone administration decreases urea generation in patients undergoing chronic hemodialysis. Clin Res 38:355A
27. Metropolitan Life Insurance Co (1983) Metropolitan height and weight tables. Stat Bull Metrop Life Found 64:1
28. Kopple JD (1988) Dietary considerations in patients with advanced chronic renal failure, acute renal failure and transplantation. In: Schrier RW, Gottschalk CW (eds) Diseases of the kidney. Little Brown, Boston, pp 3387–3436
29. Feinstein EI, Blumenkrantz MJ, Healy M, Koffler A, Silberman H, Massry SG, Kopple JD (1981) Clinical and metabolic responses to parenteral nutrition in acute renal failure. Medicine (Baltimore) 60:124–137
30. Feinstein EI, Kopple JD, Silberman H, Massry SG (1983) Total parenteral nutrition with high or low nitrogen intakes in patients with acute renal failure. Kidney Int 26 (Suppl. 16):S319–S323
31. Okamura K, Toshitada O, Tabira Y, Miyauchi Y (1989) Effect of administered human growth hormone on protein metabolism in septic rats. Journal Parenteral and Enteral Nutrition (Baltimore) 13:450–454
32. Zhu-Ming J, Gui-Zhen H, Si-Yuan Z, Xiu-Rong W, Nai-Fai Y, Yu Z, Wilmore DW (1989) Low-dose growth hormone and hypocaloric nutrition attenuate the protein catabolic response after major operation. Ann Surg 210:513–524

33. Ziegler TR, Lorraine SY, Manson JM, Wilmore DW (1988) Metabolic effects of recombinant human growth hormone in patients receiving parenteral nutrition. Ann Surg 208:6–16
34. Manson JM, Smith RJ, Wilmore DW (1988) Growth hormone stimulates protein synthesis during hypocaloric parenteral nutrition. Ann Surg 208:136–142
35. Dahn MS, Lange P, Jacobs LA (1988) Insulin like growth factor 1 production is inhibited in human sepsis. Arch Surg 123:1409–1414

Myocardial Function in Hemodialysis Patients

D.C. Schohn, P.A. Petitjean, and H.A. Jahn[1]

Summary. Myocardial impairment in hemodialysis patients is mainly due to the alterations induced by the predialytic uremic stage. Hemodialysis treatment may improve some of these disturbances: by maintaining a normal salt and fluid balance, by clearing uremic toxins, and by ameliorating nutritional status. But hemodialysis treatment may also have deleterious effects: due to A.V. fistula, to hypotension related to ultrafiltration or acetate dialysate, or due to bioincompatibility and β^2 accumulation with amyloid deposition.

Treatment of hypertension, anemia and hyperparathyroidism needs particular attention and care.

Introduction

Cardiovascular complications take a prominent place in the statistical evaluation of morbidity and mortality in hemodialysis patients and promoting the prevention of these complications remains a constant endeavor. Awareness of the fundamental alterations of the myocardium needs efficient diagnostic investigations of the cardiovascular status. These are most often based on pressure measurements, on ejection fraction and circumferential fiber shortening determinations, and on morphologic evaluations of ventricular wall thickening.

The tremendous work accomplished to elucidate the role of pathogenetic factors, such as ventricular pre and afterload modifications, metabolic, endocrine, toxic and nutritional disturbances may provide helpful hints for management strategies. In recent years great progress, which appears very promising, has been made in the control of hypertension, nutritional prevention of uremic toxemia and in the correction of anemia both in predialytic uremics and in hemodialysis patients.

[1]Nephrology Department, Louis Pasteur University, 67092 Strasbourg Cedex, France

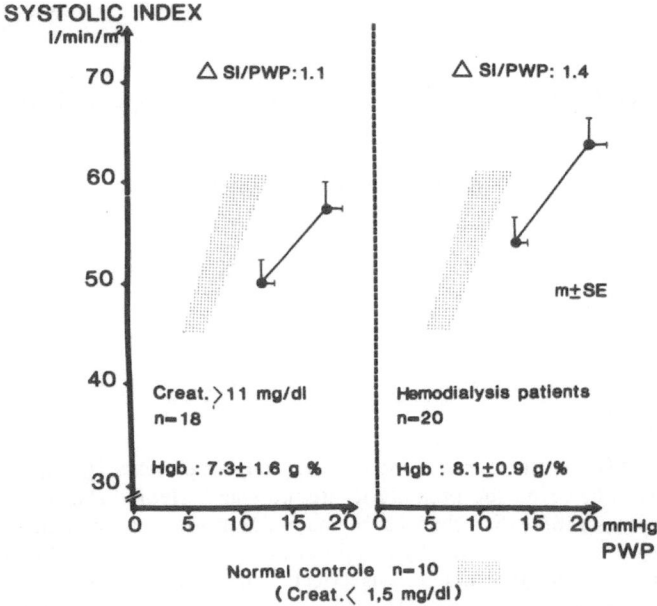

Fig. 1. Cardiac function curves (according to Frank and Starling) in chronic renal failure patients (creatinine > 11 mg/dl) and in hemodialysis patients compared with the area of normal function curves. PWP, pulmonary wedge pressure; SI, systolic index

The place of myocardial dysfunction in cardiovascular mortality statistics is difficult to evaluate. The European Dialysis and Transplant Association (EDTA) report of 1983 [1] mentions that cardiovascular disease represents 52.6% of all causes of death in hemodialysis patients, with the following origins: 14.1% cardiac failure, 12.9% cardiac arrest, 12.3% coronary disease, and 10.9% cerebrovascular lesions. Echocardiographic studies show that a high percentage of hemodialysis patients present with myocardial disturbances. Ejection fraction of left ventricle is reduced [2,3]. Left ventricular hypertrophy has been found in up to 66% of patients [4]. Invasive investigations have shown that cardiac function curves display reduced ventricular performance (Fig. 1).

Pressure Measurements and Myocardial Performance

Intracardiac pressures determine the cardiac output and reflect the adequacy of myocardial performance. In renal failure with disturbed volume homeostasis, pressure elevations are correlated to increased blood volume due to fluid overload. Pressure measurements are therefore an important clue for correction of volume disturbances. They represent the earliest sign of increased preload related to fluid overload and high fistula blood flows [5].

Table 1. Hemodynamic parameters in hemodialysis patients versus normal subjects and end stage renal failure patients

	AP (mm Hg)	HR (bpm)	$\overline{RAP}$ (mm Hg)	$\overline{PWP}$ (mm Hg)	CI (l/min per m²)	SI (ml/b per m²)	SVR (dyn/sec per cm⁻⁵)
* Normal subjects	103 ± 17	72 ± 8	0 ± 2	9 ± 3	3.08 ± 0.06	43.82 ± 6.11	1420 ± 210
$n=29$	(88 → 121)	(60 → 82)	(−3 → 3)	(5 → 13)	(2.91 → 3.36)	(36.12 → 53.11)	(799 → 1715)
* End stage renal failure	117 ± 15[a]	84 ± 13	4 ± 3[a]	12 ± 4[a]	4.11 ± 0.22[b]	50.17 ± 9.15[a]	1546 ± 329
$n=51$	(92 → 141)	(68 → 106)	(0 → 8)	(7 → 16)	(3.53 → 4.66)	(40.76 → 64.13)	(1022 → 2113)
* Hemodialysis patients	115 ± 14[a]	76 ± 8	5 ± 2[a]	13 ± 3[a]	3.97 ± 0.41[a]	54.25 ± 7.28[b]	1609 ± 281[a]
$n=113$	(88 → 136)	(64 → 91)	(1 → 10)	(8 → 18)	(3.01 → 4.42)	(37.16 → 71.81)	(713 → 2088)

m±sd

[a]$P<0.05$

[b]$P<0.01$ versus normal subject extreme values in brackets ( )

AP, arterial pressure; HR, heart rate; RAP, right atrial pressure; PWP, pulmonary wedge pressure; CI, cardiac index; SI, saturation index; SVR, systemic vascular resistance

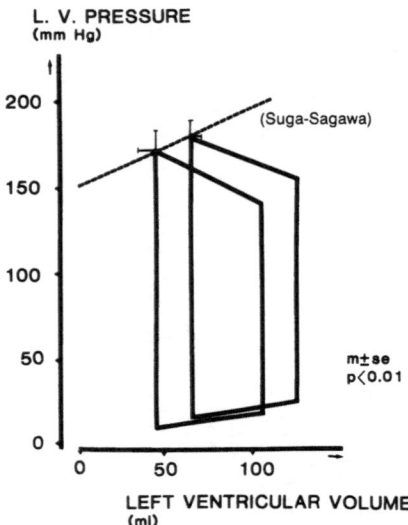

Fig. 2. Left ventricular pressure/volume relation before and after 0.9% saline infusion in dialysis patients ($n=7$) (plasma creat.: 10.6 ± 3.1 mg/dl). Suga-Sagawa line less steep than normal indicates reduced inotropic state

Usually, right atrial pressure and pulmonary wedge pressure are slightly higher in chronic hemodialysis patients than in normal subjects (Table 1). It is not clearly established whether these values indicate inadequacy of myocardial performance or a slight increase of volume. When distinctly elevated they usually indicate myocardial failure with more or less fluid overload [5].

In Table 1 we show the hemodynamic parameters obtained in normal subjects in chronic renal failure and in hemodialysis patients. The cardiac output and systolic index are increased and are related to the degree of anemia [5,6]. The cardiac function curves, following Frank Starling, obtained by volume expansion with saline [7] are shifted to the right and are less steep in comparison to normal curves. These curves display a diminished contractile state and impaired myocardial performance and may also imply a diminished myocardial compliance (Fig. 1).

The left ventricular systolo-diastolic pressure/volume loop permits a load independent evaluation of left ventricular performance. In hemodialyzed patients it is shifted to the right and the Suga-Sagawa curve is less steep, indicating reduced inotropy [5,7,8] (Fig. 2).

The echocardiographic established ejection fraction and circumferential fiber shortening of the left ventricle produce similar results when confirmed myocardial impairment exists; they are less efficient in early states characterized only by abnormal pressures.

Ventricular function seems, therefore, to be impaired in hemodialysis patients. The degree of impairment is different from patient to patient, extending from near normal to profound disturbance. Hyperdynamic circulatory states were observed due

Table 2. Echocardiographic studies

	51 CHD patients[a]		14 out of 51 CHD patients with L.V. hypertrophy	
Age (years)	50.14 ±	17.35	52.5 ±	19.1
Duration of dialysis (months)	34.96 ±	47.49	48.6 ±	70.49
Systolic AP (mmHg)	145.55 ±	32.6	155 ±	29.2
Diastolic AP (mmHg)	85.39 ±	13.78	87.76 ±	16.8
AP (mm Hg)	105.33 ±	17.31	104.9 ±	23
IST (mm)				
Systolic	13.87 ±	2.97	16.61 ±	2.47
Diastolic	10.46 ±	2.72	13.85 ±	1.75
LVPW (mm)				
Systolic	11.6 ±	2.55	13.33 ±	2.26
Diastolic	8.5 ±	2.0	9.9 ±	1.85
LVD (mm)				
Systolic	37.3 ±	8.8	40.1 ±	9.2
Diastolic	52.2 ±	7.6	54.1 ±	7.6
L.V. mass (gr)	243.7 ±	108	342.6 ±	140.8
EF (%)	63.4 ±	11.7	59 ±	14.5
Vcf (%)	29.3 ±	8.3	27.9 ±	9.8

CHD, chronic hemodialysis; AP, arterial pressure; IST, interventricular septum thickness; LVPW, left ventricular posterior wall; LVD, left ventricular dimension; EF, left ventricular ejection fraction; Vcf, circumferential fiber shortening of left ventricle
[a]mean values ± standard deviation

to anemia and to inotropic stimulation of parathyroidhormone. Associated heart disease contributes, in many situations, to the alterations of cardiac performance [9].

Immediate dialysate and ultrafiltration effects have been studied extensively: acetate dialysate enhances the peripheral contractile state due to vasodilatation and has a direct inotropic effect on the myocardium. During ultrafiltration, acetate vasodilatation mainly imprints the cardiovascular function and may induce severe hypotension [10,11]. Bicarbonate dialysate, per se, has no direct effect on myocardial performance; during ultrafiltration, peripheral vasoconstriction occurs and cardiac output diminishes.

Echomorphologic Changes of the Myocardium

Echocardiographic studies provide reliable information on the morphologic status of the myocardium; these studies comprise analysis of the interventricular septum, the left ventricular posterior wall, and the left ventricular mass and diameter.

The occurrence of the changes is diversely evaluated from 30% (Table 2)–66% [3,4]. The modifications consist of:

1) an increase in the diameter of the left and right atrium and left ventricle,
2) an increase in ventricular posterior wall thickness,
3) an asymmetric increase of interventricular septum,
4) an augmentation of left ventricular mass.

These modifications may all be found in the predialytic state.

Table 3. Risk involved in the genesis of arrhythmias in chronic hemodialysis patients

Myocardiopathy
Hypertrophy and/or dilatation
Pericardial disease
Electrolyte disturbances:
K^+, Ca^{2+}, Mg, Acidosis
Hypoxemia
Hypocapnia
Autonomous nervous system disturbances
Renin angiotensin system activation
Dialysis technique
rapid ultrafiltration
inadequate dialysate
Drugs: cardiac glycosides

A few observations provide some evidence of the role of hemodialysis in patients with uncontrollable weight gain. It is common to observe that fluid removal by ultrafiltration modifies the X ray silhouette and the echocardiographic images of the heart. In two observations we observed hypokinetic wall motion. In one patient it was located mainly in the right ventricle and was due to amyloid infiltration, perhaps related to bioincompatibility.

Severe morphologic abnormalities aggravate functional performance, conceivably both by impairment of myocardial compliance and contractility, but moderate modifications do not correlate with the results of functional investigations.

Clinical Manifestations

Slight impairments of myocardial performance remain asymptomatic or induce various intensities of exercise intolerance which are involved with the effects of anemia on oxygen supply.

In hemodialysis patients the degree of weight gain inducing dyspnea, may be a hint of the degree of myocardial impairment. Such weight gains are accompanied by elevations of pulmonary wedge pressure. Conversely, fluid removal by ultrafiltration may also be the expression of myocardial impairment: in such cases hypotension occurs as a consequence of inadaptation of cardiac output to removal of even a small volume of fluid.

Overt heart failure is rarely due to an impaired myocardial performance alone, usually other causes are added, such as salt and fluid overload; high A.V. fistula flows; hypertension; valvulopathy; coronary heart disease; and arrhythmias.

Myocardial intolerance may be expressed by dysrhythmias, tachycardia, and arrhythmia, which usually occur during dialysis treatment. Their pathogenesis is not yet clear (Table 3).

Factors Influencing Myocardial Function

Related to Renal Failure

Most of the disturbances of myocardial function and morphology may be present in the uremic state before dialysis treatment. Uremic myocardiopathy results from the

Table 4. Factors influencing myocardial function in chronic hemodialysis patients

---

Preload and/or afterload
  Weight gain and fluid overload
  Hypertension
  Hypotension
Pericardial involvements
Myocardial cell function
  K^+, Ca^{2+}, acidosis
  Oxygen supply:
    anemia
    coronary atherosclerosis
  Nutritional supply:
    amino acids, fatty acids, carnitine, insulin sensitivity
  Toxic influences:
    biocompatibility
    uremic toxins
Disturbed control systems
  Autonomic nervous system
  Catecholamines, receptors
  Hyperparathyroidism
  Hypocalcitriolemia
  Renin angiotensin

---

consequences of renal failure and the associated organic metabolic and endocrine disorder. (enumerated in Table 4).

Hypertension, with its increase of afterload, has the most deleterious effects on the heart. It is one of the main factors of left ventricular hypertrophy. Its effects on coronary arteries enhance development of atherosclerosis [12].

Anemia reduces oxygen supply. It is one of the factors which induces increased cardiac output and acceleration of heart rate [5].

Hyperparathyroidism may enhance cardiac contractility [13] but its ionophore effects determine myocytic calcinosis [14]. Its effects on mitochondrial energy production make excess parathyroid hormone a dangerous uremic toxin [15]. It has been shown to be responsible for myocardial hypertrophy [16].

Hypocalcitriolemia has been experimentally shown to be responsible for hypertrophy of myocardial interstitium at the expense of myofibrills [17]. Angiotensin may also contribute to the hypertrophy of myofibrills.

Autonomic nervous system disturbances comprise high levels of catecholamines and alteration of receptor activity. They therefore diminish the capacity of the myocardium to adapt to the necessity of the organism and to induce regulation which interferes with load problems. The sensitivity of the beta-adrenergic receptors is decreased in renal failure and is reduced much more in hemodialysis patients, as shown by the response of the heart rate to injection of increasing doses of isoproterenol. The dose response curve (injected dose of isoproterenol versus delta heart rate increase) is shifted to the right, compared with the curve obtained in normal subjects. The chronotropic dose 25 is significantly increased [18].

The negativity of nitrogen balance in uremia denotes profound effects on striated muscle cells. These problems with disturbed aminograms of uremia and altered carnitine metabolism have been implicated in the genesis of uremic myocardio-pathy [19].

Dialysis Related Effects

Fistula flow has been compared to the effects of arterio-venous aneurysm on heart function. High blood flow may induce modifications of preload. Heart failure has been reported. Shunt effects may also produce blood steeling effects on coronary flow.

Dialysis hypotension has deleterious effects on coronary circulation and must be avoided. The causes of hypotension are related to ultrafiltration rate, acetate dialysis, and bioincompatibility. These factors need therefore to be strictly monitored. Other factors which have to be taken into account are: antihypertensive drugs, autonomic neuropathy, and myocardiopathy itself.

Electrolyte disturbances and acidosis interfere with myocardial function and need to be monitored.

Beta 2 microglobulin which is retained in renal failure and is elevated in hemodialysis patients may be a factor in the genesis of amyloidosis.

Prevention of Myocardial Dysfunction

Prevention of myocardial dysfunction has to begin during the predialytic uremic state. Four main fields of progress seem to be promising:

1) The nutritional management of uremia, with drastic protein restriction and reduced accumulation of uremic toxins [20], usually supplemented with essential amino acids or keto acids of essential amino acids which ameliorate calcium phosphate metabolism and diminish hyperparathyroidism.
2) Administration of calcitriol may have protective effects per se on the myocardium [17] and may diminish hyperparathyroidism [21].
3) Administration of erythropoietin for correction of anemia maintains normal oxygen supply and avoids increased cardiac work. Data on beneficial effects have been reported [22,23].
4) The improved treatment of hypertension. Direct influences of medications on the myocardium have been suggested and need confirmation. Beta-blockers seem to prevent hypertrophy. Ca-channel blockers have been reported to influence coronary atherosclerosis. Converting enzyme inhibition prevents the hypertrophic effects of angiotensin II on myocardial cells.

Several improvements of hemodialysis techniques may reduce the influence of hemodialysis on the myocardial function.

It is most important to maintain the patient near his/her dry weight with normal pulmonary wedge pressure, to avoid the effects of increased preload.

Bicarbonate dialysate seems to ease fluid removal. Both hemofiltration and hemodiafiltration have, in this respect, advantages over conventional hemodialysis. More biocompatible membranes and better extractions of β^2 microglobulin will perhaps bring further ameliorations.

References

1. Geerling W, Tufveson G, Broyer M, Brunner FP, Brynger H, Fassbinder W (1983) Combined report on regular dialysis and transplantation in Europe. Proc Eur Dial Transplant Assoc 17:52–54
2. MacDonald IL, Uldall R, Buda AJ (1981) The effect of hemodialysis on cardiac rhythm and performance. Clin Nephrol 6:321–327
3. Lai KN, Whitford J, Buttfield I, Fasset RG, Mathew TH (1985) Left ventricular function in uremia: echocardiographic and radionuclide assessment in patients on maintenance hemodialysis. Clin Nephrol 23:125–133
4. London GM, Marchais SJ, Guérin AP, Fabiani F, Métivier F (1990) Fonction cardiovasculaire du sujet Hémodialysé. In: Hamburger J (ed) Actualités Néphrologiques. Flammarion, Paris, pp 283–302
5. Jahn HA, Schohn DC, Schmitt RL (1986) The heart in renal disease. In: Cheng Tsung O (ed) The international textbook of cardiology. Perga, New York, 988–1009
6. Jahn HA (1988) The cardiovascular system in uremia. Report of the Xth International Congress of Nephrology, London, pp 1026–1037
7. Jahn H, Schmitt R, Schohn D, Olier P (1984) Aspects of myocardial function in chronic renal failure. Contrib Nephrol 41:240–250
8. Kramer W, Wizemann V, Lämmlein G, Thormann J, Kindler M, Schlepper M, Schütter G (1986) Cardiac dysfunction in patients on maintenance hemodialysis. Contrib Nephrol 52:110–124
9. Kramer W, Wizemann V, Thormann J, Kindler M, Mueller K, Schlepper M (1986) Cardiac dysfunction in patients on maintenance hemodialysis. I) The importance of associated heat diseases in determining alterations of cardiac performance. Contrib Nephrol 52:97–109
10. Schohn D, Schmitt R, Jahn H (1986) Myocardial impairment in chronic hemodialysis patients. Effect of acetate hemodialysis. Contrib Nephrol 52:69–85
11. Jahn H, Schohn D, Schmitt R (1983) Hemodynamic modifications induced by fluid removal and treatment modalities in chronic hemodialysis patients. Blood Purif (1)80: 80–89
12. Rostand SG, Kirk KA, Rutsky EA (1982) Relationship of coronary risk factors to dialysis-associated ischemic heart disease. Kidney Int 22:304–308
13. Jahn H, Schohn D, Schmitt R Plasma parathormone levels (PTH) and heart function in end stage renal failure patients (abstract). IXth International Congress of Nephrology, June 11–16 1984. Los Angeles, USA, 51A
14. Massry SG (1987) Cardiovascular complications in chronic renal failure. Contrib Nephrol 54:177–189
15. Bogin E, Massry SG, Harray I (1981) Effects of parathyroid hormone on rat heart cells. J Clin Invest 67:1215–1227
16. London GM, Vernejoul De MC, Fabiani F, Marchais SJ, Guérin AP, Métivier F, London AM, Llach F (1987) Secondary hyperparathyroidism and cardiac hypertrophy in hemodialysis patients. Kidney Int 32:900–907
17. Weishaar RE, Sang-Nam K, Dwit ES, Robert US (1990) Involvement of vitamin D3 with cardiovascular function. III. Effects of physical and morphological properties. Am J Physiol 258:E134–E142
18. Schohn DC, Weidmann P, Jahn HA, Beretta-Piccoli C (1985) Norepinephrine-related mechanism in hypertension accompanying renal failure. Kidney Int 28:814–822
19. Drüeke T, Le Pailleur C (1981) Cardiomyopathy in uremia: hemodynamic and metabolic aspects. Nephrologie 2:63
20. Kopple JD (1988) Dietary considerations in patients with advanced chronic renal failure, acute renal failure and transplantation. In: Schrier RW, Gottschaltk CW (eds) Diseases of the kidney, vol 3, 4th edn. Little, Brown, New York pp 3387–3436

21. Mc Gonigle C, Fowler MB, Timmis AB, Weston MJ, Parsons Y (1984) Uremic cardiomyopathy: potential role of vitamin D and parathyroid hormone. Nephron 36:94-100
22. Tsutsui M, Suzuki M, Hirasawa Y (1989) Renewed cardiovascular dynamics induced by recombinant erythropoietin administration. Nephrol Dial Transplant 4:146-150
23. London GM, Zins B, Pannier B, Naret C, Berthelot JM, Jacquot C, Safar M, Drüeke TB (1989) Vascular changes in hemodialysis patients in response to recombinant human erythropoietin. Kidney Int 36:878-882

Electrophysiological and Biofunctional Abnormalities in Uremic Neuropathy

ALBERTO ALBERTAZZI, MARIO BONOMINI, and BRUNO DI PAOLO[1]

SUMMARY. The pathophysiology of central and peripheral nervous system dysfunctions in uremia has been extensively evaluated by neurophysiological studies and biofunctional techniques during the last few years. In order to investigate uremia-related nervous alterations in our cohort of patients clinical research was supported by electrophysiology and experimental work in synaptosomes drawn from uremic rats.

During a thirteen-year period, a cohort of 408 patients, subdivided into eight groups, was examined: 100 controls; 88 patients on a conventional low nitrogen diet (CLND); 25 on a very low nitrogen diet supplemented with a mixture of essential aminoacids and ketoanalogues (SD); 105 on Regular dialysis treatment (RDT); 10 on high-efficiency dialysis strategies with different membranes and techniques, 25 on continuous ambulatory peritoneal dialysis (CAPD); 23 treated with erythropoietin; the final group of 32 were transplanted. Data on electrogenesis of Evoked Potentials were drawn by: Electroencephalogram (EEG) with Berg's analysis, Visual (VEP), Brainstem (BAER), Somatosensory Evoked Potentials (SEP), electromyogram (EMG), and motor and sensory nerve conduction velocities (MNCV-SNCV). The synaptosomes were isolated from the cortices of normal and uremic rats (Blood urea nitrogen (BUN) $\simeq$ 250 mg%).

A good correlation was found between EEG activity, VEP, BAER, SEP wave modification and the decline of renal function and/or the quantitative estimates of dialysis treatments (RDT + CAPD). The nerve conduction velocity was lowered earlier in peroneal than in median nerve and the sensory conduction was implicated to a greater extent than the motor one. In the uremic synaptosomes, normal and stimulated Na^+ uptake was significantly increased when compared to the controls; the same behavior was seen for Ca^{++} uptake. Spontaneous evoked potentials and biochemical research appear to be promising methods for investigating uremic neuropathy. It is to be hoped that bio-functional abnormalities in the modifications

[1]Institute of Nephrology and Dialysis, S. Camillo De Lellis Hospital, Via C. Forlanini, 66100 Chieti, Italy

of energy reserves will yield an explanation for the intrinsic and functional defects of nervous structures.

Introduction

Neurologic abnormalities specifically related to uremia occur constantly in chronic renal failure, although they do not become clinically well defined until late in the course of the uremic syndrome [1]. The presence of clinical features of uremic encephalopathy and neuropathy seems to correlate with the severity of the renal failure [2]. The symptomatology, the electrophysiology, and the biochemistry of uremic encephalopathy are incompletely relieved by dialysis and are generally ameliorated after successful renal transplantation [3-5]. It has not been established whether uremic encephalopathy is due to "uremic intoxication" per se, to the unphysiological nature of different dialysis treatments, or whether it is due to more strictly technical factors such as the type of membrane employed, the dialysis schedule, the composition of the dialysate or trace elements in it, or to concomitant therapy [6]. The pathogenesis of neurologic abnormalities is still speculative and is the subject of continuing investigation. It is desirable to utilize noninvasive methods for the early detection of neurological impairments. The reproducibility of modern electrophysiological tests, which we have utilized for many years, has allowed even early alterations of the nervous system to be revealed while clinical symptomatology was completely silent.

In order to exemplify a very complicated issue — in one word, the pathophysiology of uremic encephalopathy — clinical research has attempted to evaluate the effects of uremia on the central and peripheral nervous systems by using the sophisticated techniques of electrophysiology and of subcellular analysis. Many studies are now beginning to appear; they utilize additional techniques for assessing the relationships between electrocortical activity and uremia [7]. The present study deals with the evaluation of the effects of chronic renal failure, of uremia and of metabolic derangements related to the central and peripheral nervous systems. In order to determine the possible causes of electrophysiological abnormalities we designed functional and biochemical assessments of pathways and of nervous cells whose alterations are associated with the uremic state.

Material and Methods

During a thirteen-year period, 408 subjects, subdivided into various groups, were examined: 100 were healthy subjects; 88 were patients with chronic renal failure (creatinine clearance 15.5 ± 8.20 ml/min), treated with a conventionally low nitrogen diet (0.6 g/kg bw/daily of proteins, CLND); 25 patients (creatinine clearance 6.83 ± 3.31 ml/min) whose very low nitrogen diet (0.3 g/kg bw/daily of unselected proteins) was supplemented with a mixture of essential aminoacids and ketoanalogues (SD); 105 patients who underwent regular dialysis treatment (RDT) for 12 to 15 hours/weekly for 70.5 ± 13.4 months, and 10 patients who were on high-efficiency dialysis strategies with different membranes (polysulphon, polymethylmethacrylate, polyacrylonitrile) and different techniques (hemofiltration, hemodiafiltration, biofiltration) using such replacement only fluids as lactate and bicarbonate. Twenty-five patients were on CAPD from 34.5 ± 10.7 months, essentially with commercially available 2000 ml bags which were changed four times a day. The CAPD was performed in accordance with internationally recommended guidelines [8]. Twenty-three dialysis patients were treated with r-HuEPO given as an i.v. bolus 50-100 UI/kg thrice weekly, for at least 6 months. Thirty-two patients underwent cadaver-donor renal transplantation (T) from 13.4 ± 7.5 months, and were treated with methyl-prednisolone plus cyclosporine A, azathioprine or both. Patients with diabetes mellitus and/or systemic diseases which can involve the nervous system were excluded. Medications, antihypertensives in particular, that influence the nervous system, were not given to any of the patients, or were stopped two weeks before the examination.

The following electrophysiological parameters were studied: Electroencephalogram with Berg's analysis (EEG), Visual Evoked Potentials (VEP), Brainstem Auditory Evoked Potentials (BAER), Somatosensory Evoked Potentials (SEP), Electromyogram with Motor and Sensitive Nerve Conduction Velocities (EMG, MNCV, SNCV). All the tests were recorded in accordance with our previous papers [9] and checked at least once per year in the same patient during the span of the study period. Particular attention was paid to the modifications induced by conservative dietary treatment, by different dialysis techniques at various degrees of efficiency, and after renal transplantation.

Since numerous attempts have been made to elucidate the mechanisms by which uremia interferes with brain electrocortical activity, we performed biochemical and functional studies to ascertain the biochemical basis of dysfunctions of the central nervous system. These were done in vitro models such as the vesicles of synaptic junctions, called synaptosomes. Basically, the synaptosomes showed abnormalities both in enzyme activity and in certain transport phenomena. When brain tissue is homogenized in isoosmotic solution, the bulblike presynaptic nerve endings are sheared off and resealed to form intact vesicles. The synaptosomes function morphologically and biochemically as intact nerve endings [10]. Similarly to nerve terminals, the synaptosomes contain synaptic vesicles, mitochondria, and cytoplasmic volume and are metabolically active. Synaptosomes have been used for the investigation of the synthesis, storage and release of neurotransmitters; because of their unique properties, they appear to be appropriate models for the investigation of the effects of uremia on the central nervous system.

The synaptosomes were isolated from 200 g male Sprague-Dawley rats; the isolation was carried out in paired groups of normal and uremic rats. The rats were made acutely uremic (blood urea nitrogen ≃ 250 mg%) by performing bilateral ureteral ligation under intramuscularly administered general anesthesia. At 45 h the rats were killed by decapitation; their forebrains were removed and immediately placed in 10 ml of ice-cold isolation medium at 0-4°C. The normal and uremic brains were processed simultaneously, but kept separately in distinctly marked containers.

In the synaptosomes we carried out protein determination; we calculated the total intern synaptosomal volume, ATP, Na^+-uptake, K^+-uptake, ATP-stimulated Na^+-uptake, oxygen consumption, and investigated enzymes. We measured Na^+ uptake using $^{22}Na^+$ under controlled conditions and under treatment with veratridine or tetrodotoxin. These studies were carried out in pH- and temperature-controlled conditions. Furthermore, our study was designed to investigate the role that the calcium transport may play in the abnormalities of synaptosomes taken from uremic rat brain cerebral cortex.

Results

The neurological manifestations of uremia are quite numerous. EEG changes include disorganization, slowing down and loss of alpha frequency, slow background activity together with an excess of theta and delta waves, linked with a decreased metabolic rate typical of all metabolic encephalopathies. There is a good correlation between the percentage of EEG frequencies and power below 7 Hz and the decline of renal function as estimated by serum creatinine [11]. The measurement of Central Nervous System function might yield quantitative estimates of relevant impairment in uremic patients, as well as their responses to treatment. That is why we employed some electrophysiological and biochemical dynamic measures which reflect the activity of central and peripheral neurons.

The VEPs represent a useful method of studying and following the cerebral alterations of the uremic cerebral cortex. In our experience P_{100} wave latency increased in the uremic population (115.7 ± 8.4 msec vs 106.4 ± 7.7 msec, $P < .01$) and correlated directly with serum creatinine concentration ($P < .01$). The uremic patients exhibited an increase in latency of BAER waves I, III, and V and an increase in interpeaks I-III, I-V, and III-V compared to normal subjects. The BAER were abnormal in 32/88 patients (36.3%) on CLND, in 44/105 (41.9%) on RDT, and in 13/25 (52%) on CAPD. The peak latencies for spinal and cortex SEP from median and peroneal nerves are summarized in Figs. 1 and 2. During median nerve stimulation the peaks were delayed in 43 out of 88 (48.8%) CLND patients and in 43/130 (33.0%) dialyzed patients (RDT + CAPD). During peroneal nerve stimulation the lumbar compound action potential was polyphasic in 17 out of 88 (19.3%) CLND patients and in 20 out of 130 dialyzed (RDT + CAPD) patients (15.3%). Latencies and morphologies of peroneal SEP were quite different in CLND and RDT patients.

Even though the whole EMG is extremely useful in the evaluation of uremic myopathy, the Fast Fourier Transform is fundamental in analyzing the sinusoidal components of a given waveform. In the uremic patients we found different populations of motor unit potentials. A normal one with a spectral distribution around 150–200 Hz was found in 25% of CLND patients, in 19% of RDT patients, and in all the transplanted patients; a high frequency-low voltage wave group around 500 Hz was found in 44% of CLND patients and in 35% of the RDT group, and a polymorphic pattern with a multiple spectral distribution at low and high frequencies was found in 24% of CLND and in 43% of RDT patients. Figs. 3 and 4 compare MNCV and SNCV in the control, CLND, RDT, and T groups. Decreased MNCV was found in 37% from the lower limb and in 32% from the upper limb of CLND patients, while RDT patients had slowed MNCV in 45% and 40% respectively. The SNCV was compromised more frequently than the MNCV in 44% and 35%, respectively, of CLND patients and in 52% and 45%, respectively, of RDT patients. In the first 6 months after transplantation the conduction velocity and the distal latency in median and peroneal nerves improved somewhat in all patients; a few achieved normal values. By 12 months most values were normal; the others were only slightly prolonged.

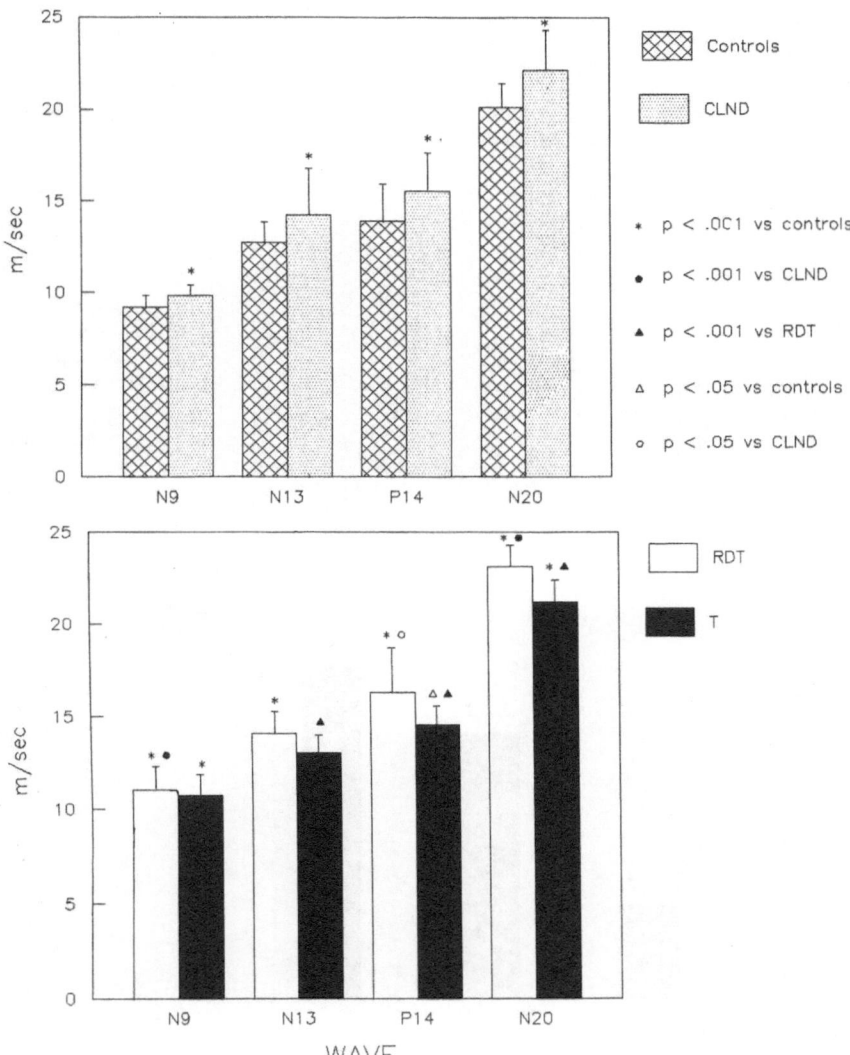

Fig. 1. Somatosensory evoked potentials (*SEP*) from median nerve in controls, diet (*CLND*), dialysis (*RDT*), and transplanted (*T*) patients. Latencies of main waves registered in posterior roots ganglia (*N9*), cervical medulla (*N13*), and pre-rolandic area (*P14* and *N20*)

Paradoxically, during the first year after transplantation, the improvement was greater in those patients affected most severely prior to transplantation. The synaptosomes function morphologically, biochemically, and from an electrophysiological point of view, as intact nerve endings do. To assess the ability of uremic synaptosomes to transport sodium, we first evaluated Na⁺ uptake in normal synaptosomes.

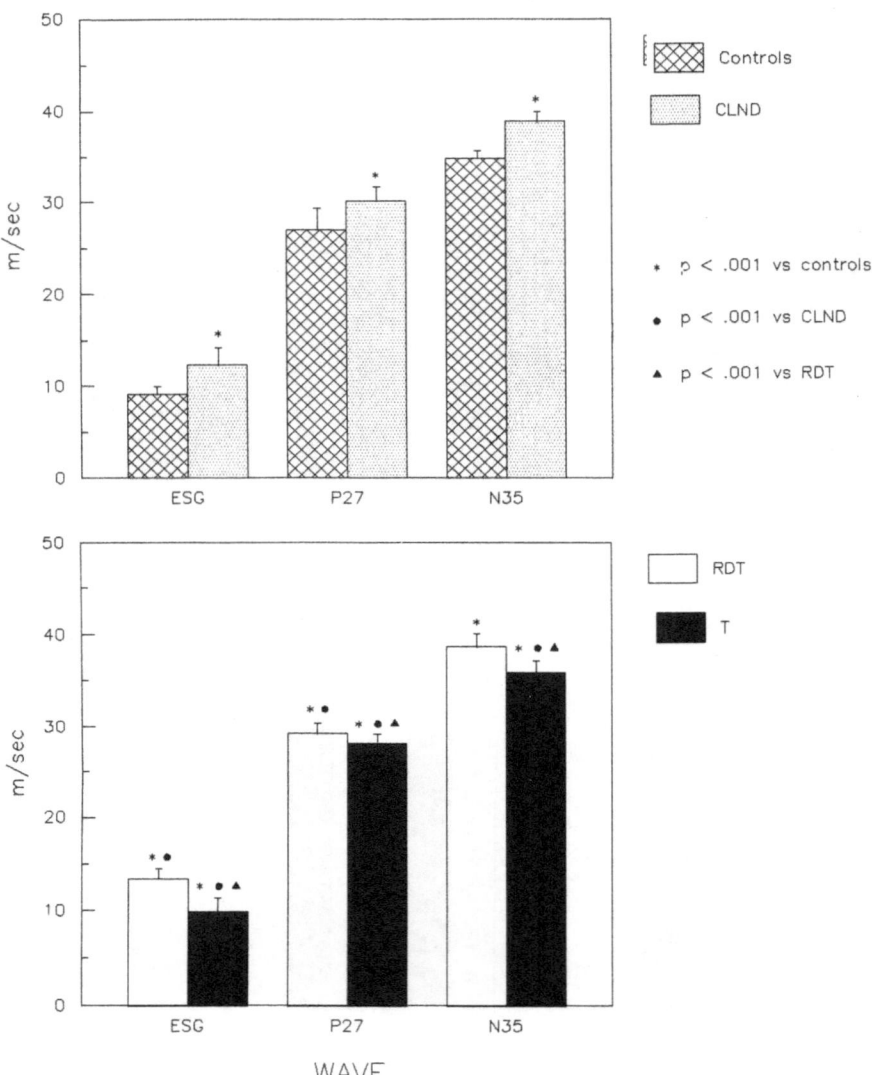

Fig. 2. Somatosensory evoked potentials (*SEP*) from peroneal nerve in controls, diet (*CLND*), dialysis (*RDT*), and transplanted (*T*) patients. Latencies of main waves registered from third lumbar vertebra (*ESG*) and cortical post-rolandic area (*P27* and *N35*)

Using synaptosomes from uremic rats, stimulated Na^+ uptake was increased significantly when compared with normal (4.12 nmol/mg vs 5.53 nmol/mg of protein, P < .001 respectively). Potassium uptake in uremic synaptosomes was only 78% of normal (6.0 nmol/mg vs 7.7 nmol/mg of protein) and was significantly less than normal (P < .005).

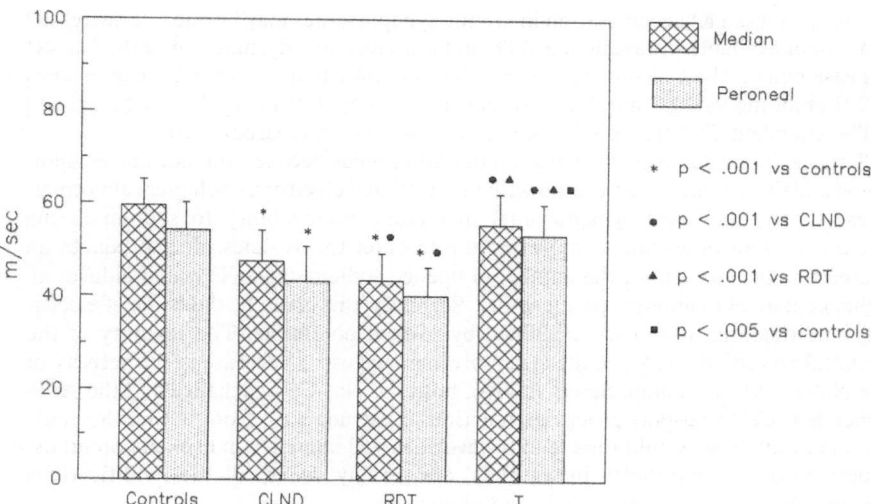

Fig. 3. Motor nerve conduction velocities (*MNCV*) from median and peroneal nerves comparing controls, diet (*CLND*), dialysis (*RDT*), and transplanted (*T*) patients

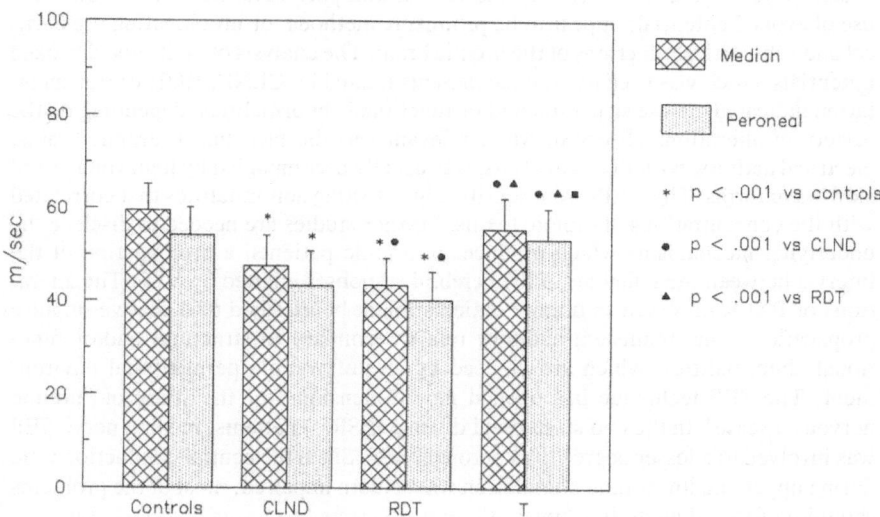

Fig. 4. Sensory nerve conduction velocities (*SNCV*) from median and peroneal nerves comparing controls, diet (*CLND*), dialysis (*RDT*), and transplanted (*T*) patients

The decreased K^+ accumulation in uremic synaptosomes may be due to a decreased amount of available intravesicular ATP and therefore to a dysfunction of the Na^+-K^+ ATPase pump. The Ca^{2+}-uptake was greater in uremic than in normal synaptosomes (13.0 nmol/mg vs 10.3 nmol/mg protein, $P < .005$). Both Na^+-Ca^{2+} exchange and ATP-dependent Ca^{2+} transport processes appear to be increased in uremia.

Two likely mechanisms may explain the differences between the normal synaptosome and the uremic synaptosome with its correlated electrophysiological abnormalities: firstly, increased synaptosomal membrane permeability to sodium in the uremic synaptosomes allows more sodium to enter the vesicles. This produces an increase in the size and/or the number of opened sodium channels which induces an enhancement of membrane permeability. Secondly, this could be the cause of electrical modifications which we examined by evoked potentials. The inability of the accumulated sodium to leave the synaptosomes suggests a decrease in the activity of the Na^+-K^+ ATPase pump. Since, in vivo, both the Na^+-Ca^{2+} exchange and the ATP-dependent Ca^{2+} transport processes function to extrude Ca^{2+} from within the cells, both abnormalities would thus tend to favor delayed latencies in evoked potentials, modification of amplitudes in wavelets, and in any event, all the modifications documented by electrophysiological examinations.

Discussion

Electrophysiological evaluation of the central and peripheral nervous systems and use of evoked potentials appear to be promising methods for investigating the cortical and sub-cortical functions of the uremic brain. The analysis of multimodal evoked potentials which was used to evaluate patients treated by CLND, RDT, or transplantation indicated diffuse structural and/or functional abnormalities, depending on the variety of alterations observed. More relevant was the fact that in uremic brains, electrical activity, with Berg's analysis, was usually accompanied by high voltage and slow wave forms. The VEPs were sensitive in detecting abnormalities that correlated with the concentrations of uremic toxins. Further studies are needed to disclose the underlying mechanisms which produce, in uremic patients, a prolongation of the interval between the latencies of the cerebral responses elicited by VEP. The alterations of BAER observed in uremic patients might be ascribed to defective impulse propagation along brainstem auditory relays secondary to structural and/or functional abnormalities, which are induced by an unfavorable perineuronal environment. The SEP technique has opened new dimensions for the study of "uremic nervous disease". In the end stage renal disease (ESRD) patients, median nerve SEP was involved to a lesser degree than peroneal SEP. Since the central conduction time during upper and lower limb stimulation was seldom impaired, most of the problems should be focused along the spinal afferents connected to lower limb receptors.

It was therefore suggested that most of the latency delay of the scalp SEP to peroneal nerve stimulation was secondary to defective propagation in the most distal axons. This is the mechanism proposed to explain uremic neuropathy; it implies that circulating agents might primarily affect the large diameter bipolar dorsal root ganglion cells, decreasing the axoplasmic flow in the most distal areas of their central and peripheral prolongations, which have the longest trajectories. A slowed lumbar-to-vertex central velocity could be due partly to a synaptic malfunction. However, this does not satisfactorily explain why, within the same anatomical structures, synapses interrupting ascending pathways from lower limbs should be more affected than those interposed between long sensory fibers from upper limbs. Slowing of the velocities of SEP, BAER, and VEP could be due partially to a synaptic malfunction, even though within the same anatomical loci, some synapses would be more affected than others.

Thus, it appears that the effects of uremia on both central and peripheral nervous systems are generated by intrinsic functional defects in various membranes. This could be the general meaning of uremic neuropathy and that is why we decided to study, in the synaptosomes, the biofunctional abnormalities induced by uremia. Our findings of increased Na^+ concentration and of decreased Na^+-K^+ ATPase pump activity may be significant factors in the observed central nervous system manifestations of uremia. The calcium transport in uremic synaptosomes is altered and this alteration results in increased Ca^{2+} uptake by both Na^+-Ca^{2+} exchange mechanisms and by the ATP-dependent calcium transport system [12]. The demonstrated in vitro abnormalities of intracellular Na^+ and Ca^{2+} flux in the uremic central nervous system may in fact lead to alterations in vivo in any of these electrophysiological processes mentioned. All these defects do not appear to be due to "uremic toxins" per se, but rather to an effect of uremia that alters synaptosomial function. In uremia, central nervous system function is impaired and is only partially corrected by dialysis, which corrects the abnormalities found in the uremic milieu (elevated BUN, creatinine, metabolic acidosis, etc.).

Further research into the role of brain energy metabolism in uremia should probably be addressed toward metabolic rates and electrophysiological implications rather than toward static levels of uremic metabolites. It is quite possible that the demonstration of a more than strict correlation between the electrophysiology of the nervous system and energy-using-producing reactions may not be a useful concept for investigating the pathophysiology of uremic encephalopathy. From a clinical point of view, the "neutralization" of uremic neurotoxicity, as achieved by a functioning transplant seems to be quite important [13]. Modern guidelines in the treatment of uremic neuropathy are leading towards the control of hypertension, towards counteracting anemia and aluminum intoxication, towards the employment of more biocompatible membranes in dialysis, and towards taking all those measures that modern research can foster.

References

1. Albertazzi A, Di Paolo B (1989) Neurologic abnormalities of uremia. In: Bonomini V, Scolari MP, Stefoni S, Vangelista A (eds) Biotechnology in renal replacement therapy. Contrib Nephrol, Karger, Basel, pp 188–193
2. Albertazzi A, Di Paolo B, Cappelli P, Spisni C, Del Rosso G (1985) Evoked potentials in uremia. In: D'Amico G, Colasanti G (eds) Advances in nephrology and dialysis. Contrib Nephrol, Karger, Basel, pp 60–68
3. Raskin NH, Fishman RA (1976) Neurologic disorders in renal failure. N Engl J Med 294:143–148, 204–210
4. Teschan PE, Arieff Al (1985) Uremic and dialysis encephalopathies. In: McCandless DW (ed) Cerebral energy metabolism and metabolic encephalopathy. Plenum, New York, pp 263–286

5. Arieff Al (1985) Effects of water, electrolyte and acid base disorders on the central nervous system. In: Arieff Al, DeFronzo RA (eds) Fluid, electrolyte and acid base disorders. Churchill Livingstone, New York, pp 969-1040

6. Savazzi GM (1988) Pathogenesis of cerebral atrophy in uremia. Nephron 49: 94-103

7. Di Paolo B, Arieff Al, Del Rosso G, Di Mizio GF, Campanella M, Muscianese P, Colacelli R, Bonomini M, Albertazzi A (1989) Alterazioni del trasporto di Na^+ e Ca^{2+} in sinaptosomi de encefalo di ratto uremico: vi è correlazione con la trasmissione sinaptica? In: Saporiti E, Bazzato G (eds) Atti del XXX Congresso Nazionale della Società Italiana di Nefrologia. Acta Medica Roma 835-836

8. Clayton S, Quinton C, Oreopoulos D (1981) Training technique for continuous ambulatory peritoneal dialysis (with discussion). Perit Dial Bull 1: S23-S28

9. Di Paolo B, Di Marco T, Cappelli P, Spisni C, Del Rosso G, Palmieri PF, Evangelista M, Albertazzi A (1988) Electrophysiological aspects of nervous conduction in uremia. Clin Nephrol 29: 253-260

10. Booth RFG and Clark JB (1978) A rapid method for the preparation of relatively pure metabolically competent synaptosomes from rat brain. Biochem J 176: 365-370

11. Albertazzi A, Di Paolo B, Del Rosso G, Gambi D, Rossini PM (1981) Neurophysiological abnormalities in uraemic encephalopathy. In: Robinson BHB, Hawkins JB, Davison AM (eds) Proc XVIII EDTA. Pitman, London, pp 652-656

12. Rasmussen H, Goodman DBP (1977) Relationships between calcium and cyclic nucleotides in cell activation: cellular calcium metabolism and calcium-mediated cellular processes. Physiol Rev 57: 428-441

13. Albertazzi A, Di Paolo B, Cappelli P, Evangelista M, Di Marco T, Varanese L (1985) Uremic polyneuropathy: electrophysiologic findings after renal transplantation. In: Najarian JF, Bach FH, Sutherland DER (eds) Transplantation proceedings, Grune and Stratton, New York, p 127

ATPases of the Kidney

Chair: Peter Leth Jørgensen (Denmark)
Stephen L. Gluck (USA)

Localization of Transport ATPases in the Mammalian Nephron

Adrian I. Katz[1]

SUMMARY. Tubule microdissection and enzymatic microassays have allowed measurement of transport adenosine triphosphatases (ATPases) in individual nephron segments. Such studies have mapped the distribution of ATPases involved in the active transport of Na^+, K^+, Ca^{2+}, and H^+ along the nephron of several mammalian species, and have enabled investigators to correlate the activity of these enzymes with transport events mediated by them in the same tubule segment. This brief survey summarizes current knowledge of the nephron localization and function of Na-K-ATPase, the most abundant and best studied transport ATPase in the kidney, as well as of low- and high affinity Ca-ATPases, proton translocating ATPases, and K-activated ATPase—which have been examined in isolated tubules only in the last decade. In view of the remarkable functional heterogeneity of the nephron, information obtained about transport ATPases in its component units has contributed to an improved understanding of kidney function.

Introduction

In the preceding two decades, studies utilizing tubule microdissection and microperfusion techniques have revealed the remarkable biochemical diversity of the nephron and the heterogeneity of transport processes along its longitudinal axis [1-4]. By examining metabolic and transport functions in discrete tubule segments, such studies have greatly expanded previous knowledge obtained with classical biochemical methods in tissue slices or homogenates, or with clearance measurements which provided information about the kidney as a whole rather than about its component units. Given the functional specialization of different regions of the nephron, it is easy to appreciate why understanding kidney function requires its examination in the

[1]Department of Medicine, The University of Chicago Pritzker School of Medicine, Chicago, IL 60637, USA

individual segment(s) of interest. This is particularly true for epithelial transport and the various ATPases which are responsible for the active translocation of electrolytes across the renal tubule, as physiologic alterations, hormones, and dietary manipulations that affect transport do so in certain regions of the nephron and not in others. Equally important, determination of ATPase in specific nephron segments allows quantitative correlations between its activity and transport events measured in the corresponding segment with micropuncture or isolated tubule microperfusion techniques.

Localization of ATPases in the nephron has been attempted principally with two techniques: immunohistochemistry, lately utilizing monoclonal antibodies to the purified enzyme or its subunits [5–7] and, more often, tubule microdissection and enzymatic microassay (see below). The latter offers the advantage of quantitative measurements in nephron segments of unequivocal origin which, in addition, have preserved their linear architecture and cell orientation. Despite the technical difficulty and low tissue yield of this technique, its use has generated a large body of information on the location and function of transport ATPases in the nephron [8–10].

Na-K-ATPase

Na-K-ATPase, the biochemical equivalent of the Na:K pump, mediates the active reabsorption of Na from lumen to blood and secretion of potassium in the opposite direction by effecting the coupled countertransport of these ions at the basolateral membrane of renal tubule cells. In addition, Na-K-ATPase participates indirectly in the translocation of numerous other solutes ("secondary-active transport") via the sodium gradient that it generates. Because of its central role in epithelial transport in general, and kidney function in particular, this enzyme was the first and most extensively studied of renal transport ATPases.

Na-K-ATPase is not distributed evenly in the kidney, its activity being highest in the outer medulla, intermediate in the cortex, and lowest in the inner medulla-papilla. Because the concentration of Na:K pumps varies along the nephron, these differences reflect the relative abundance of the different nephron segments in each of the 3 zones of the kidney. For example, the renal outer medulla is rich in Na-K-ATPase because it contains chiefly thick ascending limbs of Henle's loops, one of the segments with the highest density of Na:K pumps in the nephron.

The first measurements of Na-K-ATPase in discrete nephron segments were reported by Schmidt and Dubach, who examined lyophilized tubules and used an enzymatic cycling method based on the fluorometric measurement of generated NADPH [11,12]. Because the use of freeze-dried tissue has certain limitations and because the method in general was too cumbersome for routine application, my colleagues and I developed an alternative technique that utilizes freshly microdissected tubules and measures directly radiolabeled P, liberated from the hydrolysis of [γ-^{32}P]ATP [13,14]. This method is simple enough to allow simultaneous measurement of Na-K-ATPase in large numbers of tubules, and sufficiently sensitive to determine the enzyme activity in tubule segments 100–200 μm in length. Alternative techniques that combine certain features of those listed above have been introduced more recently [15,16].

Na-K-ATPase activity has been determined in individual nephron segments of several species, including the rabbit, rat, and mouse (see Table 1). Not surprisingly,

Table 1. Distribution of Transport ATPases in the Mammalian Nephron

ATPase	Species	Segment with highest activity	pmol·mm⁻¹·h⁻¹	PCT	PST	tDL	tAL	MAL	CAL	DCT	CNT	CCT	OMCT	IMCT	Ref.
								(% of segment with highest activity)							
Na⁺-K⁺-ATPase	Rabbit	MAL	3080^a	33^b / 75^c	–^{d}	–	–	100	41	–	–	37	29	–	17
	Rabbit	DCT	3091	75	21	(3.5)^e	–	80	32	100	–	27	17	–	14
	Mouse	DCT	5171	34	9	5	–	71	71	100	–	21	5	–	14
	Rat	DCT	6679	36	8	4	(2)	68	74	100	–	12	11	–	14
	Rabbit	DCT	9120	69	15	(3)	(2)	82	20	100	83	15	13	–	15
Ca²⁺-ATPase (low-affinity)	Rabbit	DCT	1200	36	32	11	–	92	23	100	–	79	65	–	19
Ca²⁺-Mg²⁺-ATPase (high-affinity)	Rabbit	DCT	243	58	40	–	–	56	21	100	–	86	21	–	20
H⁺-ATPase (NEM-sensitive)	Rat	PCT	550	100	64	–	–	66	78	–	–	64	45	–	21
	Rat	DCT	1980	–	–	–	–	44	49	100	–	39	38	32	23
	Rabbit^f	CNT	1810	–	–	–	–	–	28	76	100	29	30	25	22
	Rat	PCT	450	100	9	0	0	51	80	82	–	61	48	72/17^g	24
HCO₃⁻-ATPase	Rabbit	PST	330	64	100	–	–	(7)	(2)	55	91^h	50	39	–	26
K⁺-ATPase	Rabbit	CNT^h	328	0	0	–	–	0	0	(3)	100^h	55	20	–	27
	Rabbit	CNT	1000	(11)	(9)	–	–	(3)	(2)	(20)	100	40	54	–	28

^{a}calculated from authors' data; ^{b}cortical nephron; ^{c}juxtamedullary nephron; ^{d}not measured; ^{e}values in parentheses are not significantly different from zero; ^{f}adrenalectomized rabbits receiving aldosterone replacement (1.5 μg/100g per day × 7); ^{g}before/after entry into the ducts of Bellini; ^{h}granular (terminal) portion of DCT PCT, proximal convoluted tubule; PST, proximal straight tubule; tDL,tAL, thin descending and ascending limb of Henle's loop; MAL,CAL, medullary and cortical thick ascending limb of Henle's loop; DCT, distal convoluted tubule; CNT, connecting tubule; CCT, cortical collecting tubule; OMCT, IMCT, outer and inner medullary (papillary) collecting tubule

the absolute levels of enzyme activity measured by different investigators using diverse methods corresponded only for some segments and differed for others. In contrast, however, the enzyme distribution profile along the nephron was remarkably similar regardless of species studied or methods used, the greatest activity being always measured in the distal convoluted tubule (DCT) and thick ascending limb. Considerable activity is also found in proximal convoluted tubules (PCT), but the enzyme is present in lesser amounts in the collecting tubule and pars recta (PST), and is barely detectable in the thin limbs of Henle's loops [14,15,17]. When measured with the same technique, Na-K-ATPase activity was, in general, comparable in the three species studied, being greater in the rat, lesser in the rabbit, and intermediate in the mouse [14]. It should be noted, however, that even in the same nephron segment the enzyme is not distributed homogeneously. In the collecting tubule of the rat, for example, it is found in principal, but not in intercalated cells [5]. Finally, examination of Table 1 reveals that Na-K-ATPase is by far the most abundant transport ATPase in the nephron.

The nonuniform distribution of Na-K-ATPase activity along the nephron poses the question whether the enzyme has the same characteristics in all its subdivisions. Earlier studies which showed that cortical and outer medullary Na-K-ATPase have the same affinity (K_m) for ATP and sodium appear to support this view, as did observations that pump density ([³H] ouabain binding) varies along the nephron exactly in parallel with Na-K-ATPase hydrolytic activity, so that the turnover rate of the pump is the same in all nephron segments. In contrast, a more recent report describing increased sensitivity to ouabain of the cortical collecting tubule (CCT) compared with the thick ascending limb and PCT [18] raised speculations that Na-K-ATPase may vary in different nephron segments, for example because it may contain different isoforms of its catalytic (α) subunit. As of the time of this writing, however, there is no convincing evidence for the presence of other isoforms of the enzyme besides α_1 in the kidney, and therefore its different affinity for ouabain probably reflects the local influence of factors extrinsic to the pump itself, as originally suggested by the authors.

Ca-ATPases

The bulk of filtered Ca is reabsorbed in the proximal convoluted tubule, but substantial reabsorption also occurs in the pars recta, thick ascending limb, distal convoluted tubule, and early cortical collecting tubule; indeed, the final regulation of Ca excretion takes place in the distal segments of the nephron.

The mechanisms responsible for tubular Ca reabsorption are incompletely understood, as both active and passive modes of transport have been proposed, sometimes for the same nephron segment. Cytoplasmic free Ca concentrations are several orders of magnitude lower than in plasma, and this gradient is maintained both by ATP-dependent Ca pumps and Ca:Na and Ca:H exchange mechanisms located in the plasma membrane as well as in cell organelles. When located in the membrane of transporting epithelia these systems participate in the vectorial transport of Ca, besides maintaining cell Ca homeostasis.

Ca-activated ATPases have been demonstrated in kidney cortex homogenates, suspensions of cortical tubules, and microsomes or membrane vesicles from several species. Supporting a physiologic role of these enzymes is their location in the basolateral membrane, across which the large Ca concentration gradient is maintained, and observations that they operate optimally in the presence of ATP concentrations found in kidney cells' cytosol.

Low-Affinity Ca-ATPase

A calcium-stimulated ATPase that could be activated by either Ca *or* Mg in millimolar amounts has been described in basolateral membranes of kidney cortex. We determined the distribution of this enzyme along the rabbit nephron with the microassay previously used for measuring Na-K-ATPase in individual nephron segments [13]. The enzyme was found along the entire nephron, and was activated by millimolar concentrations of Ca or Mg, neither of which was necessary for activation by the other cation [19]. This Ca-ATPase originated both in the mitochondria and in the plasma membrane, as it was inhibited to a substantial extent by oligomycin and azide; its activity in the combined presence of these inhibitors ranged between 200 and 400 pmols Pi.mm^{-1}·h^{-1} in most segments examined, being lower in the cortical thick ascending limb.

The physiologic role of this enzyme in transmembrane Ca transport (i.e., whether it behaves like a Ca pump) is not clear, because it is activated by Ca in millimolar concentrations, whereas cytosolic free Ca in kidney cells is orders of magnitude lower. Although its function remains obscure, it is of interest that such an enzyme was also found in red blood cell ghosts, brain synaptosomes, and eel gills. Perhaps its high capacity compensates for its low affinity, or it may act at the outer surface of the membrane.

High-Affinity Ca-Mg-ATPase

A more attractive hypothesis is that calcium extrusion from renal tubule cells is mediated, in part, by a high-affinity calcium-stimulated ATPase, activated by Ca in concentrations normally present in the cytosol. Supporting this view is the identification of such an enzyme exclusively in basolateral membrane vesicles, and the correspondence between the K_m for calcium of this Ca-Mg-ATPase and that of the ATP-dependent Ca uptake in this preparation. It is also recalled that cytosolic free Ca in kidney cells averages 0.1–0.45 μM. For these reasons we sought to determine whether a high-affinity calcium-ATPase could be detected in isolated rabbit tubules and to measure its activity in individual nephron segments [20].

A Mg-dependent ATPase, maximally activated by Ca concentrations between 1.1 and 2.3 μM and with an apparent K_m of 0.3 to 0.4 μM (hence Ca-Mg ATPase), was found in all the nephron segments examined: Its activity was greatest ($\geq$ 200 pmols.mm^{-1}.h^{-1}) in distal convoluted and cortical collecting tubules, intermediate in the proximal convoluted tubule and medullary thick ascending limb, and least in the pars recta, cortical thick ascending limb, and medullary collecting tubule [20]. Because we measured Ca-Mg-ATPase in intact tubules, the cellular component where it originates is uncertain. However, sodium azide, an inhibitor of mitochondrial ATPase, did not affect the enzyme, so that enzyme location in the plasma membrane (or in the endoplasmic reticulum) seems likely. This enzyme differed from the

Ca-ATPase described above in its absolute requirement for magnesium, high affinity for calcium, and lack of inhibition by azide.

To our knowledge Ca-Mg-ATPase has not been determined in microdissected nephron segments by other investigators. Borke et al. [6] have demonstrated this enzyme in basolateral membranes of the human DCT with an immunohistochemical method, using monoclonal antibodies against Ca-Mg-ATPase purified from red cell ghosts.

H-ATPase

ATPases in general are classified into two broad categories: Those of the F_0-F_1 type, characterized by a complex structure with several subunits, lack of a phosphorylated intermediate, and resistance to vanadate; and those of the E_1-E_2 type, which have a simpler subunit structure, undergo phosphorylation in the catalytic cycle, and are inhibited by vanadate. In recent years much attention has been devoted to a proton-translocating ATPase (H-ATPase) not strictly belonging to either type. This enzyme is associated with cell organelles such as clathrin-coated vesicles and lysosomes, and is not affected by ouabain, vanadate, oligomycin or azide, but is inhibited by dicyclo-hexylcarbodiimide (DCCD) and N-ethylmaleimide (NEM), which helps define it operationally. This vacuolar H-ATPase, thought to be the biochemical expression of proton pumps involved in ATP-dependent H secretion, has been characterized in the turtle urinary bladder and purified from bovine renal medulla, where it is found in the intercalated cells of collecting ducts. Its activity is regulated by insertion of vesicles into the membrane, e.g., in response to respiratory acidosis or increased ambient CO_2 in vitro.

Active H secretion in the kidney occurs primarily in the proximal tubule, where it brings about the reclamation of filtered bicarbonate, and in the collecting tubule, where it regenerates bicarbonate consumed in metabolism. Proton secretion in the proximal tubule is largely sodium-dependent and electroneutral, whereas in the collecting tubule it has the opposite characteristics. Proximal acidification is thus accomplished mainly via luminal Na:H exchange, but recent studies also suggest a role for a proton pump in the proximal tubule, as well as in the other segments besides the collecting tubule (reviewed in [7]). Distal acidification, on the other hand, is mediated by the electrogenic proton pump found in the intercalated cells of the collecting tubule, especially in its medullary portion.

Several studies have attempted to localize the vacuolar proton pump in the nephron, taking advantage of its inhibition by N-ethylmaleimide. Ait-Mohamed et al. [21] were the first to describe the distribution of a NEM-sensitive ATPase along the nephron. Interestingly, the highest activity was found in proximal convoluted tubules, whereas the activity in medullary collecting tubules, although substantial, was lowest among the segments tested. More recently, Garg and Narang have measured NEM-sensitive ATPase in the distal segments of the rat and rabbit nephron [22,23], where it was highest in the DCT and connecting tubule (CNT), respectively; the activity of this enzyme in outer and inner medullary collecting tubules was about one third that in the DCT and CNT (see Table 1). Finally, in a study that included the proximal nephron, Sabatini et al. [24] found a distribution of NEM-sensitive ATPase in the rat nephron similar to that originally reported in this species [21].

The distribution of vacuolar H-ATPase in the kidney has also been examined by immunocytochemistry, using affinity-purified antibodies to several subunits of the proton pump from bovine kidney medulla [7]. This study also revealed a widespread occurrence of the enzyme, which was found in most nephron segments. In the PCT it was present in the apical plasma membrane, where it would be expected to reside if it contributed to H transport. In the collecting duct only intercalated cells showed staining, which was located to the apical membrane in cells of the medullary portion, but to either side of the cell membrane in cells of the cortical collecting duct. The latter observation reflects the presence of different populations of intercalated cells (α and β subtypes) involved in proton − or bicarbonate secretion, respectively.

Besides being stimulated by respiratory acidosis, NEM-sensitive ATPase in distal segments is also stimulated by aldosterone [22], metabolic acidosis [24,25], and K-depletion [23,25]. Although abundant in PCT, the enzyme therein (to the extent that it has been tested) is not increased by these stimuli, and its precise role in urine acidification remains unclear.

HCO_3-ATPase

Another enzyme putatively involved in H secretion is an ATPase stimulated by intracellular HCO_3 (HCO_3-ATPase). However, the nature of this enzyme, and specifically whether it is of mitochondrial or extramitochondrial origin, has been the subject of intense controversy that continues to the present. Advocates of a plasma membrane location of HCO_3-ATPase postulate that by stimulating H secretion via this mechanism, reabsorbed HCO_3 may act as a positive promoter of additional HCO_3 reabsorption from the tubular lumen, but the role of this enzyme is far from being settled.

Perhaps because of the controversy surrounding its cellular location and physiologic function, HCO_3-ATPase in isolated tubules has been studied less extensively than other transport ATPases. In a thorough study describing an extramitochondrial HCO_3-ATPase in discrete rabbit nephron segments [26], the highest activity was found in proximal straight tubules and in the late ("granular") DCT, although substantial activity was also found in all other segments examined except in the thick ascending limb of Henle's loop (see Table 1). In distal portions of the nephron the enzyme was stimulated by chronic desoxycorticosterone acetate (DOCA) treatment [26].

K-ATPase

An enzyme stimulated by potassium and inhibited by vanadate (but not by ouabain) has been recently reported by two groups of investigators [27,28]. Unlike all the other ATPases described in this review, this enzyme is present only in distal portions of the nephron, where its activity is highest in the late ("granular") DCT [27] or connecting tubule [28], and decreases in the cortical and medullary collecting duct. Distribution of the enzyme is proportional to the number of intercalated cells in these segments, and its activity is stimulated by K depletion. For these reasons it has been postulated that K-ATPase is located in intercalated cells where it participates in active K reabsorption, although it should be mentioned that enzyme activity is highest at nephron sites proximal to the outer medullary collecting duct where most of the K reabsorption is thought to occur.

Because of certain shared characteristics with the gastric H-K-ATPase, including inhibition by vanadate, omeprazole, and Sch 28080, it has also been proposed that the K-ATPase found in distal nephron segments might be similar to or identical with the gastric enzyme. This intriguing hypothesis depends, first, on the demonstration that H-K-ATPase is present in the kidney. While this has not yet been established with certainty, preliminary studies suggest that the rat kidney expresses a mRNA encoding for a molecule closely related to (albeit not identical with) gastric H-K-ATPase [29]. Madin-Darby canine kidney (MDCK) cells, derived from a distal tubular epithelium, may have a H-K-pump, but this appears to be immunologically distinct from the gastric pump [30].

Acknowledgment. This paper was supported by National Institutes of Health Grant DK 13601 and by the American Heart Association.

References

1. Jacobson HR (1981) Functional segmentation of the mammalian nephron. Am J Physiol 241:F203–F218
2. Ross BD, Guder WG (1982) Heterogeneity and compartmentation in the kidney. In: Sies H (ed) Metabolic Compartmentation. Academic, New York, pp 363–409
3. Berry CA (1982) Heterogeneity of tubular transport processes in the nephron. Annu Rev Physiol 44:181–201
4. Schlondorff D (1986) Isolation and use of specific nephron segments and their cells in biochemical studies. Kidney Int 30:201–207
5. Kashgarian M, Biemesderfer D, Caplan M, Forbush B (1985) Monoclonal antibody to Na, K-ATPase: immunocytochemical localization along nephron segments. Kidney Int 28: 899–913
6. Borke JL, Minami J, Verma A, Penniston JT, Kumar R (1987) Monoclonal antibodies to human erythrocyte membrane $Ca^{2+}Mg^{2+}$ adenosine triphosphatase pump recognize an epitope in the basolateral membrane of human kidney distal tubule cells. J Clin Invest 80: 1225–1231
7. Brown D, Hirsh S, Gluck S (1988) Localization of a proton-pumping ATPase in rat kidney. J Clin Invest 82:2114–2126
8. Katz AI (1986) Distribution and function of classes of ATPases along the nephron. Kidney Int 29:21–31
9. Doucet A (1988) Function and control of Na-K-ATPase in single nephron segments of the mammalian kidney. Kidney Int 34:749–760
10. Katz AI (1988) Role of Na-K-ATPase in kidney function. In: Skou JC, Norby JG, Maunsbach AB, Esmann M (eds) The Na^+,K^+-Pump, Part B: Cellular Aspects. Alan R Liss, New York, pp 207–232
11. Schmidt U, Dubach U (1969) Activity of (Na^+K^+)-stimulated adenosintriphosphatase in the rat nephron. Pflugers Arch 306:219–226
12. Schmidt U, Dubach U (1974) Induction of Na K ATPase in the proximal and distal convolution of the rat nephron after uninephrectomy. Pflugers Arch 346:39–48
13. Doucet A, Katz AI, Morel F (1979) Determination of Na,K-ATPase activity in single segments of the mammalian nephron. Am J Physiol 237:F105–F113
14. Katz AI, Doucet A, Morel F (1979) Na,K-ATPase activity along the rabbit, rat and mouse nephron. Am J Physiol 237:F114–F120

15. Garg LC, Knepper MA, Burg MB (1981) Mineralocorticoid effects on Na,K-ATPase in individual nephron segments. Am J Physiol 240:F536–F544
16. O'Neil RG, Dubinsky WP (1984) Micromethodology for measuring ATPase activity in renal tubules: Mineralocorticoid influence. Am J Physiol 247:C314–C320
17. Schmidt U, Horster M (1977) Na-K-activated ATPase: activity maturation in rabbit nephron segments dissected in vitro. Am J Physiol 233:F55–F60
18. Doucet A, Barlet C (1986) Evidence for differences in the sensitivity to ouabain of Na-K-ATPase along the nephron of rabbit kidney. J Biol Chem 261:993–995
19. Katz AI, Doucet A (1980) Calcium-activated adenosine triphosphatase along the rabbit nephron. Int J Biochem 12:125–129
20. Doucet A, Katz AI (1982) High-affinity Ca-Mg-ATPase along the rabbit nephron. Am J Physiol 242:F346–F352
21. Ait-Mohamed AK, Marsy S, Barlet C, Khadouri C, Doucet A (1986) Characterization of N-ethylmaleimide-sensitive proton pump in the rat kidney. Localization along the nephron. J Biol Chem 261:12526–12533
22. Garg LC, Narang N (1988) Effects of aldosterone on NEM-sensitive ATPase in rabbit nephron segments. Kidney Int 34:13–17
23. Garg LC, Narang N (1990) Effects of low-potassium diet on N-ethylmaleimide-sensitive ATPase in the distal nephron segments. Renal Physiol Biochem 13:129–136
24. Sabatini S, Laski ME, Kurtzman NA (1990) NEM-sensitive ATPase activity in rat nephron: effect of metabolic acidosis and alkalosis. Am J Physiol 258:F297–F304
25. Hayashi M, Chekal MA, Katz AI (1986) Proton ATPase in isolated rat medullary collecting tubules: effects of systemic acidosis, K depletion and aldosterone. Kidney Int 29:368
26. Ben Abdelkhalek M, Barlet C, Doucet A (1986) Presence of an extramitochondrial anion-stimulated ATPase in the rabbit kidney: localization along the nephron and effect of corticosteroids. J Membr Biol 89:225–240
27. Doucet A, Marsy S (1987) Characterization of K-ATPase activity in distal nephron: stimulation by potassium depletion. Am J Physiol 253:F418–F423
28. Garg LC, Narang N (1988) Ouabain-insensitive K-adenosine triphosphatase in distal nephron segments of the rabbit. J Clin Invest 81:1204–1208
29. Okusa MD, Unwin R, Wright FS, Giebisch G, Caplan MJ (1990) H^+,K^+-ATPase mRNA expression in rat kidney. Kidney Int 37:568
30. Eisen TD, Caplan MJ, Boron WF (1990) Intracellular pH regulation in MDCK cells. Kidney Int 37:535

Regulation of Tubular Na-K-ATPase

C. Barlet-Bas, L. Cheval, E. Feraille, S. Marsy, and A. Doucet[1]

Summary. This review summarizes some studies from our laboratory which illustrate the wide variety of mechanisms through which renal Na-K-ATPase activity is controlled by hormones. A special emphasis is given to those regulation processes which alter Na-K-ATPase activity and renal Na handling with similar time-courses. Analysis of Na-K-ATPase was carried out at the level of single nephron segments obtained by microdissection of collagenase-treated kidneys.

Introduction

The functional polarization of renal epithelial cells results from the presence of segregated permeability and transport properties in apical and basolateral membranes (Fig. 1). In fact most uphill transepithelial transport processes in tubular cells are coupled to cell metabolism through Na-K-ATPase, either directly or undirectly. This enzyme, which is located in basolateral cell membranes [1,2], converts the energy-rich P_i bond of ATP into electrochemical gradients of Na and K. The low intracellular Na concentration generated thereby can drive Na entry across the luminal cell membrane, and thus creates a net transepithelial, transcellular Na reabsorption flux. Despite the marked axial heterogeneity of the nephron, this general scheme applies to the successive nephron segments, which differ from one another mainly by the nature of transport systems which allow luminal sodium entry.

In renal cells, transcellular Na flux is intense, since it accounts for 1–10 times the intracellular Na content per minute, according to the cell type. Furthermore, in a given nephron segment this flux may vary within a wide range according to the metabolic and/or hormonal status of the organism. Confronted which such large variations of the transcellular sodium flux, maintaining cellular homeostasia requires the

---

[1]Laboratoire de Physiologie Cellulaire, URA 219 CNRS, Collège de France, 11 Place M. Berthelot, 75231 Paris Cedex 05, France

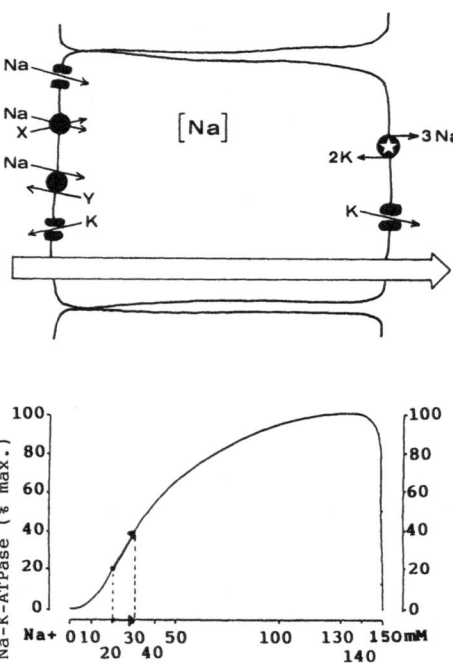

Fig. 1. *Top*, schematic representation of the segregation of Na transport systems in apical and basolateral membrane which leads to Na-K-ATPase generated transcellular Na transport. *Bottom*, activation of Na-K-ATPase activity by increasing Na concentration. Na-K-ATPase, expressed as percent of its V_{max}, was determined in the presence of varying Na concentrations, the sum of Na and K concentrations being maintained equal to 150mM. The *left part of the curve* corresponds to what occurs at the intracellular site (low Na, high K). It indicates that increasing Na concentration activates Na-K-ATPase which will extrude more Na out of the cell and, thereby, decrease Na concentration

existence of a tight coupling between the Na-transporting systems which operate at both cell borders. Thus, Na flux through Na-K-ATPase must exactly balance luminal Na entry, whatever the changes of the latter might be.

It has long been admitted that the adaptation of Na-K-ATPase pumping rate to alterations of luminal Na entry was accounted for by changes in intracellular Na concentration. Indeed, since intracellular Na is rate limiting for Na-K-ATPase, any increase in luminal Na entry will increase intracellular Na concentration, and thereby activate Na-K-ATPase. In turn, the pump will extrude more Na out of the cell, thus contributing to restore basal conditions (Fig. 1). Conversely, decreased luminal Na entry will inhibit basolateral Na exit through the pump. Although efficient, this automatic control process does require transient changes in Na (and K) concentration, which may be prejudicial to cell survival, even in the short term. The purpose of this work is to present evidence that, besides its control by intracellular Na concentration, the activity of renal Na-K-ATPase can be controlled by metabolic and/or hormonal parameters through other mechanisms, although within short latency.

As long as the cellular heterogeneity of the nephron can be overcome, the renal tubule reveals itself as a highly suitable model for the study of Na-K-ATPase regulation because: 1) it is the target for a great number of hormones, 2) some of these hormones induce very large changes in the Na transport capacity of target cells, and 3) within the same organ, some cells are sensitive to a given hormone whereas others are not, which proves useful for assuming the specificity of the responses. Our approach to circumvent the renal heterogeneity has consisted in measuring Na-K-ATPase in single nephron segments obtained by microdissection of collagenase-treated kidney [3]. This allowed us to obtain large numbers of well-characterized nephron segments which, although not suitable for in vitro microperfusion, could be used for biochemical studies since they displayed a cellular polarity, they responded to hormones, and they could be maintained in vitro for several hours while keeping their transport and regulatory properties.

On such samples, the hydrolytic activity of Na-K-ATPase can be measured by the rate of ouabain-sensitive production of $^{32}P_i$ from $[\gamma^{-32}P]ATP$ [4]. Although it has been fruitful, this methodological approach suffers several limitations. First, it permits the measurement of Na-K-ATPase activity mainly under V_{max} conditions, which may mask regulatory phenomena which do not alter V_{max}. Secondly, it requires the previous permeabilization of cell membranes to allow the entrance of exogenous ATP, and this leads to the loss of transmembrane gradients, and possibly of intracellular regulatory components. To palliate these limitations we recently developed another microassay which permits the quantitation of Na-K-ATPase-mediated ionic flux in intact tubular cells, i.e., transport generated through the cellular metabolism and against the transmembrane gradients prevailing under physiological conditions. This assay is based on the determination of the initial rate of ouabain-sensitive ^{86}Rb influx in single nephron segments [5].

To elucidate the molecular mechanisms underlying changes in Na-K-ATPase activity, in particular to determine whether such changes are due to activation of preexisting pump units or to induction of new ones, it has been necessary to quantitate the number of active Na-K-ATPase units. This is feasible by measuring specific ^{3}H-ouabain binding under saturating conditions in intact tubules [6]. Unfortunately, this method is hardly applicable to the rat nephron, because of the very low affinity for ouabain of this species. Therefore, we are presently developing a substitutive method, utilizable in all species, which consists in quantifying the phosphointermediate of the Na-K-ATPase cycle. The simultaneous application of these methods, which are not further discussed in this article, allowed the characterization of some regulatory processes of tubular Na-K-ATPase which are summarized below. A special emphasis will be given to those processes which do not involve long term, secondary adaptations of tubular cells.

Activation of Na-K-ATPase Activity by Intracellular Na

As discussed above, intracellular Na is the main rate limiting factor of Na-K-ATPase activity. Thus, changes in its concentration modify the pump activity in a way which tends to restore basal Na level. In addition, it should also be noted that Na-K-ATPase sensitivity to Na is modulated by intracellular K, since the two cations compete for the occupancy of intracellular Na sites [7,8]. Thus the apparent $K_{0.5}$ for Na deter-

Table 1. Kinetic properties of Na-K-ATPase along the rabbit nephron

	App $K_{0.5}$ for Na (mM)		App K_i for ouabain (μM)	App K_D for ouabain (μM)
	[K]=5mM	[Na]+[K]=150mM		
Proximal tubule	9.5	65.0	1.8	4.0
Thick ascending limb	10.2	48.0	0.5	0.6
Collecting tubule	3.1	25.0	0.06	0.1

Apparent $K_{0.5}$ for Na was measured either at low K concentration ([K]=5mM) or at high K concentration, under conditions in which the sum of the Na and K concentrations remained constant and equal to 150mM([Na]+[K]=150mM). The apparent $K_{0.5}$ for K was 0.4 mM for all nephron segments. (Data from [9] and [10])

mined at low K concentration ([K] = 5mM) is five–eightfold lower than that measured at high K concentration ([Na] + [K] = 150mM) (Table 1). In other words, at a constant Na concentration, Na-K-ATPase activity increases when intracellular K concentration decreases, and this is particularly marked when the latter varies within the 120–100mM range [9], i.e., within the physiological range of variation of cell K concentration. If one assumes that the sum of Na and K concentrations within the cell remains constant under all conditions, this property enhances the self regulatory ability of Na-K-ATPase. Indeed, in response to increased intracellular Na concentration, Na-K-ATPase will be stimulated through: 1) the enhancement of the concentration of its rate limiting substrate, i.e., Na, and 2) the enhancement of its affinity for Na (due to decreased K concentration).

A specific feature of kidney cells is that the sensitivity of Na-K-ATPase for Na varies along the nephron: The collecting tubule is two-threefold more sensitive to Na than more proximal segments, whether this sensitivity is determined at low or high K concentration (Table 1). Therefore, the collecting tubule is more sensitive to physiological changes of intracellular Na concentration, a property likely related to the role of this nephron segment in the ultimate control of Na/K excretion.

Again it should be emphasized that these auto-regulation processes of Na-K-ATPase activity require changes in intracellular Na concentration, which often are not observed, and which may be unsuitable for the maintenance of cellular homeostasia.

Can Endogenous Ouabain-Like Factor Control Renal Na-K-ATPase?

It is beyond the scope of this review to analyze the pieces of evidence which suggest that the specific ouabain-binding site present on the catalytic subunit (α) of Na-K-ATPase may be the receptor for a circulating modulator (hormone?) of this enzyme. If one admits that such a modulator(s) exists, which is most likely, even though it proves difficult to purify, the problem in question here is whether the kidney may or may not be a target for its action. Indeed, there was a paradox in the findings that kidney has a low affinity for ouabain on the one hand [10], and that ouabain-like factors are natriuretic on the other [11].

However, analysis of renal ouabain-sensitivity at the level of single nephron segments instead of whole kidney homogenates or membrane fractions thereof revealed that, conversely to most nephron segments, the collecting tubule is highly sensitive to ouabain [12]. Indeed, apparent K_i as well as apparent K_D for ouabain are 10–30-fold lower in the rabbit collecting tubule (either in its cortical or medullary portions) than in more proximal nephron segments (Table 1). A posteriori, it appears obvious that such a property could not be observed on whole kidney preparations because Na-K-ATPase activity originating in the collecting tubule represents only a minute fraction of the whole kidney enzyme's activity since: 1) this nephron segment represents a small fraction ($<5\%$) of total kidney mass, and 2) the collecting tubule has among the lowest Na-K-ATPase activities, when expressed per millimeter of tubule length (or per unit of mass). These results suggest that ouabain-like factors may act on the kidney, and that the collecting tubule likely represents their target site.

Together with the higher affinity for Na described above (Table 1), the higher affinity of the collecting tubule for ouabain may suggest that this nephron segment expresses the α_3 isoform of the catalytic subunit of Na-K-ATPase rather than the α_1 isoform, which is admittedly found in kidney [13]. However, confirmation of this hypothesis will require different experimental approaches at the level of isolated segments of collecting tubule. In any case, whether α_3 is present in the collecting tubule or not, this does not change the conclusion that this nephron segment is the major renal target of ouabain-like factors. In contrast, this has functional implications regarding the regulation of the synthesis of Na-K-ATPase, since the genes encoding for the α_1 and α_3 subunits are likely not controlled by the same parameters.

Control of Na-K-ATPase Synthesis by Aldosterone in the Collecting Tubule

Among the numerous hormones which control renal Na-K-ATPase, mineralocorticoids play a central role because the kidney is their major target. The antinatriuretic action of mineralocorticoids results from the induction of specific genes encoding for aldosterone-induced proteins (AIP) which are responsible for the hormonal action. Since adrenalectomy decreases Na-K-ATPase activity in the collecting tubule [14,15] and since in vivo administration of aldosterone to adrenalectomized rats [14] or rabbits [15] restores it within 3 h, the question arises, whether or not Na-K-ATPase is an AIP.

In vitro experiments [16] demonstrated that incubation, for 2.5 h at 37° C, of cortical collecting tubules of 7-day-adrenalectomized rats resulted in a marked stimulation of Na-K-ATPase activity and specific binding of ^{3}H-ouabain (Fig. 2). This stimulation was totally abolished in the presence of actinomycin D or of cycloheximide (Fig. 2), suggesting that aldosterone induced the synthesis of Na-K-ATPase. Alternatively, however, these results could suggest that aldosterone induces the synthesis of a protein which, in turn, would activate preexisting units of Na-K-ATPase. The demonstration that aldosterone indeed induces Na-K-ATPase synthesis was provided by the work of Verrey et al. who showed that in A_6 cells, aldosterone enhances the number of mRNAs encoding for the α and β subunits of the enzyme [17].

Although it is usually admitted that Na-K-ATPase has a long half-life (7–15 h), it is noteworthy that the time-course of aldosterone action on the pump synthesis is fast (30 min latency, maximal stimulation within 2.5–3 h) and coincides with the

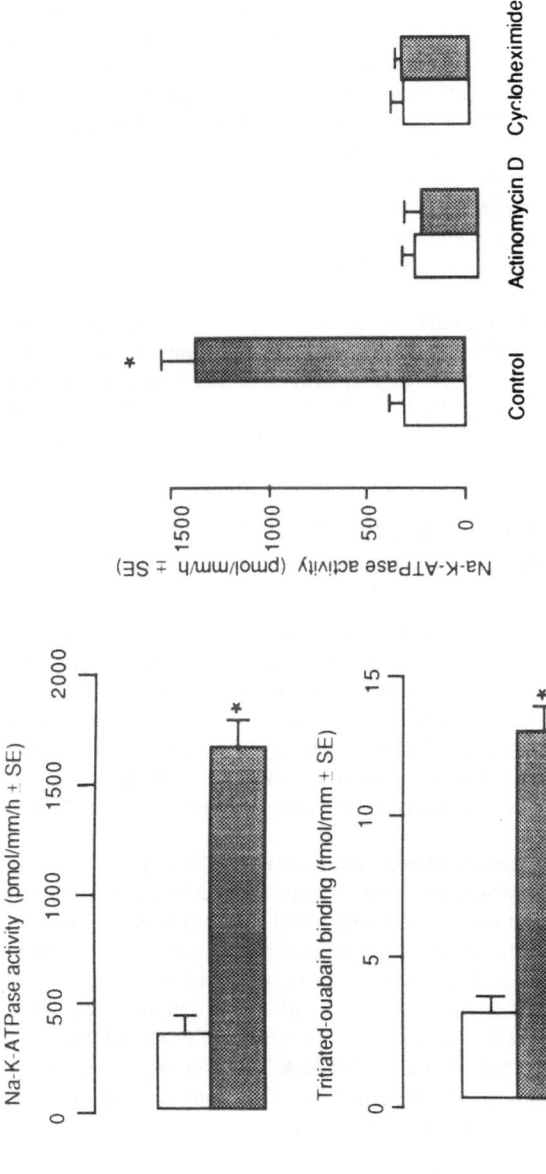

Fig. 2. Effect of aldosterone on Na-K-ATPase in the cortical collecting tubule (*CCT*) of 7-day-adrenalectomized rats. *Left*, Na-K-ATPase activity and specific binding of ³H-ouabain were measured in CCT incubated for 2.5h at 37°C in the absence (*open bars*) or in the presence of 10⁻⁸M aldosterone (*dark bars*). *Right*, CCT were incubated without (*open bars*) or with aldosterone (*dark bars*) in same conditions as above, and in the presence of 5µM actinomycin D, 20µM cycloheximide or in the absence of drug (control). Statistical significance according to Student's t-test:*P<0.005. (Redrawn from [16])

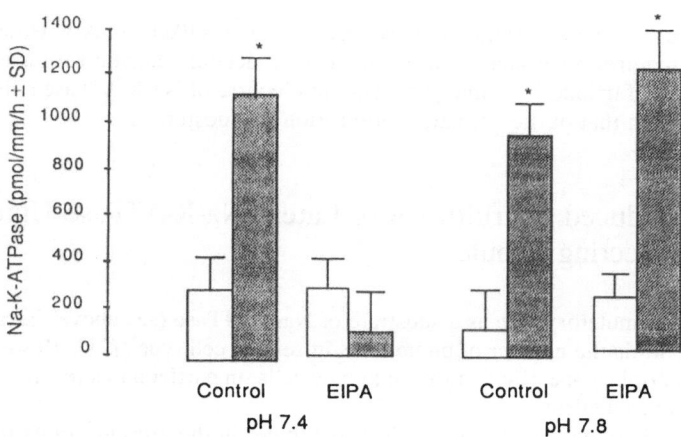

Fig. 3. Effect of ethylisopropyl amiloride (*EIPA*) and pH on aldosterone action in the cortical collecting tubule (*CCT*) of adrenalectomized rats. Na-K-ATPase activity was measured in CCT incubated for 2.5h at 37°C in the absence (*open bars*) or in the presence of 10^{-8}M aldosterone (*dark bars*), under normal conditions (control) or in the presence of 25µM EIPA. The pH of the medium was adjusted to either 7.4 or 7.8, which corresponds to intracellular pH of 7.3 and 7.6, respectively. Statistical significance according to Student's t-test:*,P < 0.001

antinatriuretic response to aldosterone [14]. Despite this synchronization between the actions of aldosterone on Na-K-ATPase activity and on urinary Na excretion, it has been postulated that induction of Na-K-ATPase synthesis could be a secondary action of aldosterone due to enhanced intracellular Na concentration, itself brought about by the primary stimulation by aldosterone of luminal Na channels. This hypothesis was based on the finding that in vivo administration of the Na channel blocker amiloride prior to aldosterone abolished the stimulation of collecting tubule Na-K-ATPase [18]. However, such inhibitory action of amiloride could result from unspecific effects of this drug which, depending on its concentration, can also inhibit the Na/H exchanger [19], Na-K-ATPase [20], and even protein synthesis [21]. And indeed, low concentrations of amiloride sufficient to inhibit Na channels, but with no action on other systems had no effect on the in vitro induction of Na-K-ATPase by aldosterone, whereas higher concentrations known to inhibit the Na/H exchanger totally abolished Na-K-ATPase stimulation [16]. That induction of Na-K-ATPase synthesis by aldosterone requires the integrity of the Na/H exchanger is confirmed by experiments showing that ethylisopropylamiloride (EIPA), a specific inhibitor of the Na/H exchanger [19], totally abolished aldosterone action (Fig. 3). Thus, induction of ATPase synthesis by aldosterone may require the preliminary stimulation of the Na/H exchanger which has previously been observed by Oberleithner et al. [22]. In fact, it seems to require an intracellular alkalinization, brought about by stimulation of Na/H exchanger, since the inhibitory action of EIPA can be curtailed when artificial intracellular alkalinization is produced by incubating the samples at pH 7.8 (which corresponds to a pH$_i$ of 7.6) instead of 7.4 (which corresponds to a pH$_i$ of 7.3) (Fig. 3).

In conclusion, Na-K-ATPase of the collecting tubule is likely an AIP. However, its induction requires other factors, which include intracellular alkalinization as well as the presence of triiodothyronine [16]. The time-course of Na-K-ATPase stimulation correlates with that of the antinatriuretic action of aldosterone.

Sodium-Induced Recruitment of Latent Na-K-ATPase Units in the Collecting Tubule

Besides its stimulatory role as a substrate of Na-K-ATPase (see above) intracellular Na also controls the number of pump units in several cell types [23]. However, this regulation displays specific features in kidney cells, in particular as regards its time-course and mechanism.

Thus, incubation of rat cortical collecting tubules in the presence of extracellular Na and of Na ionophores such as nystatin or amphotericin B results, within 2–3 h, in a marked stimulation of Na-K-ATPase activity, and, to a similar extent, of the specific ^{3}H-ouabain binding (Fig. 4). However, this induction of new pump units by increased intracellular Na concentration does not involve de novo synthesis of the enzyme, since it is not altered by either actinomycin D or cycloheximide (Fig. 4). Rather, these observations suggest the existence of a pool of latent Na-K-ATPase units which can be recruited in response to a transient increment of intracellular Na concentration [24]. The localization of this pool and its mode of recruitment are not, as yet, known.

Another feature of this regulatory process is that the latent pool of Na-K-ATPase does not exist (or is not recruitable) in collecting tubules of adrenalectomized rats [24], suggesting that its synthesis is controlled by corticosteroids. In fact, during the first 24 h following adrenalectomy, the pool of latent Na-K-ATPase is progressively recruited so as to maintain constant the pool of active Na-K-ATPase; this latter decreasing because of the decline in its rate of synthesis (see above). Thus, following adrenalectomy, a decreased rate of Na-K-ATPase synthesis may generate an increase in intracellular Na concentration, which triggers the recruitment of the latent pool of ATPase, until its total disappearance.

Besides the nature and the intracellular localization of this latent pool of Na-K-ATPase, several other questions have to be solved. Among them, it will be important to know whether or not this reserve of Na-K-ATPase is a special feature of the collecting tubule.

Control of Na-K-ATPase Activity by Locally Generated Mediators

Another mechanism of rapid regulation of Na-K-ATPase involves metabolites of arachidonic acid which can be produced in the medullary thick ascending limb (MTAL) in response to vasopressin (AVP).

Thus, we observed [25] that incubation of MTAL, microdissected from normal rats, in the presence of AVP 10^{-7} M for 15 min induced a marked inhibition of Na-K-ATPase

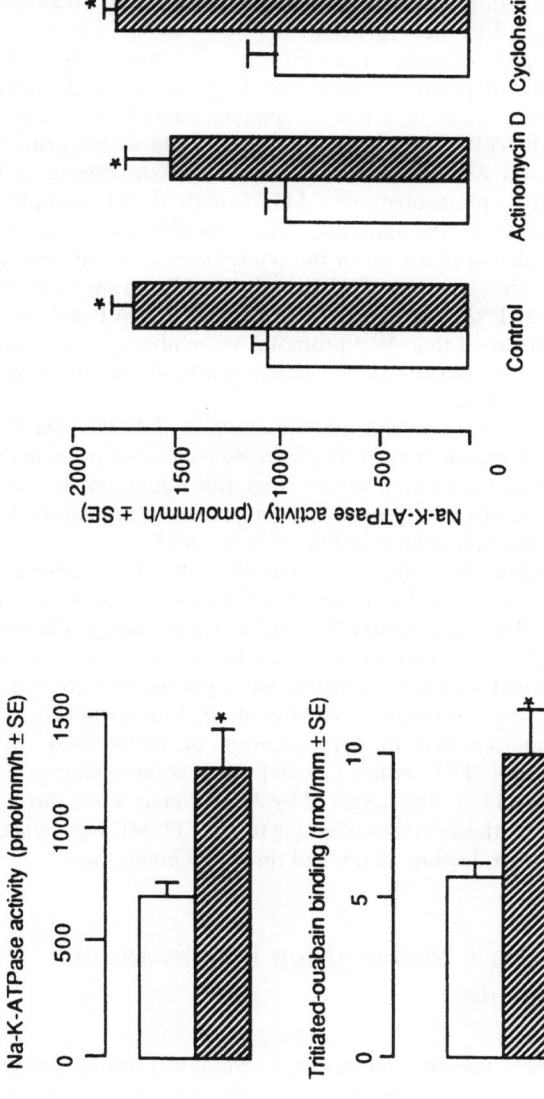

Fig. 4. Effect of increasing intracellular Na concentration on Na-K-ATPase in rat cortical collecting tubule (*CCT*). *Left,* Na-K-ATPase activity and specific binding of ^{3}H ouabain were measured in CCT incubated for 2.5h at 37°C in the absence (*open bars*) or in the presence of 0.1U/μl of the sodium ionophore nystatin (*hatched bars*). *Right,* Before incubation without (*open bars*) or with nystatin (*hatched bars*) for 2h in same conditions as above, CCT were preincubated for 1 h with 5μM actinomycin D, 20μM cyclohexi-mide, or in the absence of drug (control). Statistical significance according to Student's t-test:*P < 0.001. (Redrawn from [24])

activity (control: 3740 ± 210 pmol/mm per h $\pm$SE; AVP: 2280 ± 110 pmol/mm per h $\pm$ SE; n=5, P<0.001 by Student's t-test). This inhibition was dose-dependent (app $K_{0.5} \sim 2.10^{-8}$M) and reached its maximum within 5 min. Inhibition of Na-K-ATPase activity by AVP was accompanied by a similar inhibition of ouabain-sensitive ^{86}Rb uptake (Control: 42.8 ± 2.8 pEq/mm per min $\pm$SE; AVP: 29.9 ± 1.9 pEq/mm min $\pm$SE, n=6, P<0.005). Inhibition of ATPase activity and Rb uptake was mediated by cyclic AMP since it was mimicked by cAMP generating hormones (calcitonin and glucagon), by forskolin, and by dibutyryl cAMP.

Earlier, Schwartzman and colleagues reported that cells from rabbit MTAL displayed a cytochrome P450-dependent monoxygenase pathway which metabolized arachidonic acid into two biologically active compounds, one of which was a potent inhibitor of purified Na-K-ATPase [26]. Thus, we investigated whether this metabolite could be responsible for AVP-induced inhibition of Na-K-ATPase in rat MTAL.

Results indicated that: 1 – preincubation of MTAL with 10^{-4}M arachidonic acid mimicked the action of AVP; 2 – the inhibitory actions of AVP and arachidonic acid were not additive; 3 – addition of 10^{-5}M of the phospholipase A_2 inhibitor, quinacrine, abolished the inhibitory action of AVP, and 4 – addition of 5.10^{-5}M of the monoxygenase inhibitor SKF525A curtailed the actions of both AVP and arachidonic acid. These findings confirmed that AVP promotes its inhibitory action on Na-K-ATPase by inducing the monoxygenase-dependent synthesis of an arachidonate-derived inhibitor of Na-K-ATPase.

From a physiological point of view, this inhibitory action of AVP on Na-K-ATPase is paradoxical, since this hormone is known to increase Na reabsorption in the thick ascending limb [27]. It is possible, however, that the inhibitory action, which requires higher concentrations of hormone, may represent a regulatory feedback mechanism preventing excessive dilution of the tubular fluid.

Other local mediators have been shown to control Na-K-ATPase activity. Thus, prostaglandins, which were reported to inhibit Na-K-ATPase in the gastric mucosa [28], liver [29], and brain [30], also inhibit the renal enzyme. Indeed, Cordova et al. have shown that Na-K-ATPase activity was increased in the cortical collecting tubule of rabbits chronically treated with the prostaglandin synthesis inhibitor indomethacin [31]. Similar results were observed by Wald et al. [32] on rat MTAL. Furthermore, these authors reported that in vitro addition of 10^{-4}M PGE_2 inhibited Na-K-ATPase activity in rat MTAL within 15 min [32]. It is interesting to note that this regulatory pathway could also be triggered by AVP in vivo, since this hormone stimulates prostaglandin synthesis in the collecting tubule [33,34], from where it can be expected to act on both collecting tubule and thick ascending limb.

Control of Na-K-ATPase Mediated Ion Flux by Insulin in the Collecting Tubule

Besides its metabolic effects, insulin controls urinary sodium excretion directly at the tubular level. Thus, insulin reduces natriuresis in isolated kidneys perfused at constant GFR [35]. Since, in several tissues, insulin was shown to stimulate Na-K-ATPase activity [36–38], we investigated whether the antinatriuretic action of insulin could be mediated by stimulation of the pump activity. A likely target for this

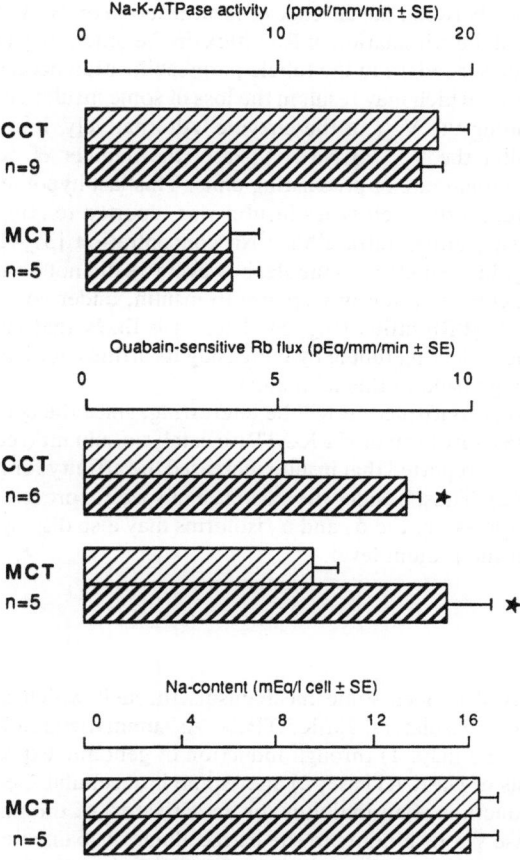

Fig. 5. Effect of insulin on Na-K-ATPase and Na concentration in rat cortical (*CCT*) and medullary collecting tubule (*MCT*). Na-K-ATPase activity, ouabain sensitive Rb uptake and intracellular Na concentration were measured in CCT and MCT incubated for 15–120 min at 37°C in the *absence* (▨) or in the *presence* of 10^{-8}M insulin (▨). Statistical significance according to Student's t-test:*,P < 0.05

action is the collecting tubule, since it has been reported previously that insulin increased active transepithelial Na transport in amphibian bladder and in cultured A_6 cells [39,40].

In vitro preincubation of rat collecting tubules at 37°C for 15–120 min in the presence of 10^{-8}M insulin did not modify the V_{max} of the ATP hydrolytic activity of Na-K-ATPase (Fig. 5). However, under the same conditions, insulin markedly increased (+60%) the ouabain-sensitive influx of Rb (Fig. 5). This stimulation was dose-dependent (app $K_{05} \sim 10^{-9}$M) and reached its maximum within the first 5 min of incubation with insulin (E. Feraille et al., unpublished work).

Such a discrepancy between the absence of insulin action on Na-K-ATPase activity on the one hand, and the stimulation of Rb influx on the other, may have several origins. First, it may be secondary to the tubule permeabilization necessary to measure Na-K-ATPase activity, which may result in the loss of some insulin-sensitive intracellular factor controlling the V_{max} of the enzyme. Alternatively, it may indicate that insulin does not alter the V_{max} of Na-K-ATPase (the number of pump units), but rather alters the pumping rate of preexisting units. This last hypothesis seems more likely, since in several other cell types insulin was reported to stimulate the pump activity by increasing either intracellular Na concentration [37,41] or the pump affinity for Na [42]. In the collecting tubule, however, we did not observe any change in intracellular Na concentration in response to insulin, under conditions in which this hormone increased Rb influx (Fig. 5). Thus, it is likely that insulin stimulates Na-K-ATPase in the collecting tubule by increasing its affinity for Na. This hypothesis is presently being tested in this laboratory.

If this hypothesis is confirmed, it will be interesting, since the collecting tubule is likely to contain the α_3 isoform of Na-K-ATPase catalytic subunit (see above) and, in adipocytes, Lytton has reported that insulin increased the affinity for Na of the α_3 isoform exclusively [42]. Thus, besides the existence of specific processes of regulation of their genomic expression, the α_1 and α_3 isoforms may also display different regulation properties at the protein level.

Conclusions

This review briefly describes some mechanisms through which a hormone may control the activity of basolateral Na-K-ATPase. As summarized in Fig. 6 (from top to bottom), a hormone may: 1) through induction of genomic expression, increase the rate of synthesis of Na-K-ATPase; 2) alter some intracellular metabolic pathway leading to the production of an inhibitor (or an activator) of the pump; 3) directly inhibit Na-K-ATPase via its binding to the extracellular ouabain site; or 4) increase intracellular Na concentration through activation of luminal Na entry, and thereby either activate preexisting pump units (substrate effect) or induce the recruitment of latent pump units (possibly through exocytosis). Other possible mechanisms which have been described in the literature include alterations of the basolateral membrane potential (which might alter the pump activity because of its electrogenicity) or alterations of the basolateral K conductance associated with the recycling of K [43,44]. Finally, it has also been proposed that, in the proximal tubule, Na-K-ATPase could be controlled through a G protein [45].

The two main conclusions which can be drawn are the following: Firstly, in many circumstances, control of Na-K-ATPase activity in kidney cells is fast and is concomitant with the hormone action on Na transport. Thus, changes in Na-K-ATPase primarily participate in the hormonal response, rather than being, as considered hitherto, secondary adaptations to this response. Secondly, there is a wide heterogeneity of hormone actions on Na-K-ATPase along the nephron (even though the collecting tubule appears as a major site of control). This heterogeneity may be due either to the distinct nature of regulatory proteins present in each cell type (hormone receptors, transduction mechanisms, intracellular metabolic pathways, . . .) or to the very nature of Na-K-ATPase itself, i.e., the presence of α_1 versus α_3 isoforms of the pump.

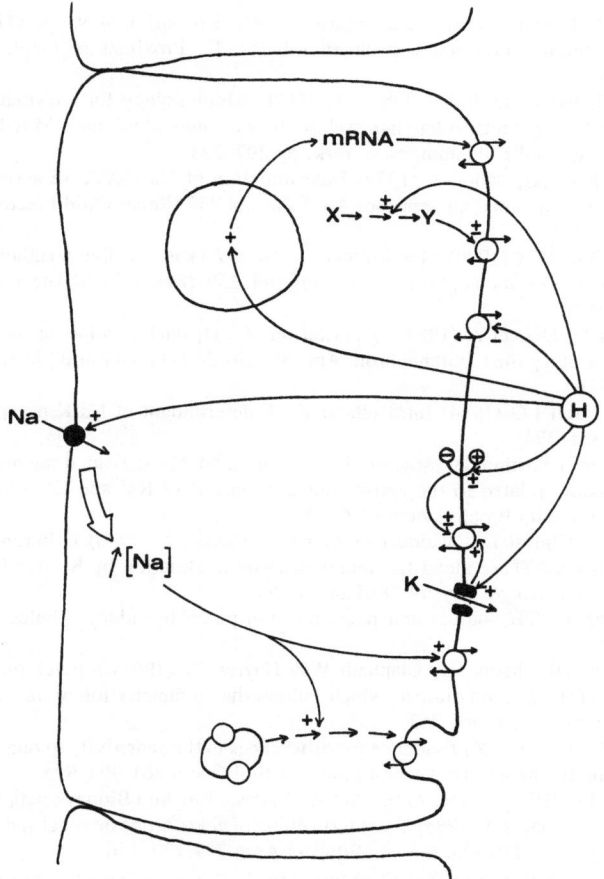

Fig. 6. Schematic summary of the different modes of control of Na-K-ATPase by a hormone (*H*)

Acknowledgments. The authors are grateful to L. Bonnet-Lericque for her secretarial assistance during the preparation of this manuscript. Work from our laboratory was supported in part by grants from the Centre National de la Recherche Scientifique to the Unité de Recherche Associée 219. L. Cheval and E. Feraille were assisted by grants from the Ministère de la Recherche et de la Technologie and from the Fondation pour la Recherche Médicale, respectively.

References

1. Kyte J (1976) Immunoferritin determination of the distribution of Na, K-ATPase over the plasma membranes of renal convoluted tubules. I. Distal segment. J Cell Biol 68:287–303

2. Kyte J (1976) Immunoferritin determination of the distribution of Na, K-ATPase over the plasma membranes of renal convoluted tubules. II. Proximal segment. J Cell Biol 68:304–318

3. Morel F, Chabardes D, Imbert-Teboul M (1978) Methodology for enzymatic studies of isolated tubular segments: Adenylate cyclase. In: Martinez-Maldonado M (ed) Methods in Pharmacology, vol 4B. Plenum, New York, pp 297–323

4. Doucet A, Katz AI, Morel F (1979) Determination of Na-K-ATPase activity in single segments of the mammalian nephron. Am J Physiol 237 (Renal Fluid Electrolyte Physiol 6):F105–F113

5. Cheval L, Doucet A (1990) Measurement of Na-K-ATPase-mediated rubidium influx in single segments of rat nephron. Am J Physiol 259 (Renal Fluid Electrolyte Physiol 28):F111–F121

6. El Mernissi G, Doucet A (1984) Quantitation of [^{3}H] ouabain binding and turnover of Na-K-ATPase along the rabbit nephron. Am J Physiol 247 (Renal Fluid Electrolyte Physiol 16):F158–F167

7. Knight AB, Welt LG (1974) Intracellular K. A determinant of Na:K pump rate. J Gen Physiol 63:351–373

8. Skou JC (1960) Further investigations of a Mg^{2+} and Na^+-activated adenosine triphosphatase possibly related to the active, linked transport of Na^+ and K^+ across the nerve membrane. Biochim Biophys Acta 42:6–23

9. Barlet-Bas C, Cheval L, Khadouri C, Marsy S, Doucet A (1990) Difference in the Na affinity of Na-K-ATPase along the rabbit nephron:modulation by K. Am J Physiol 259 (Renal Fluid Electrolyte Physiol 28):F246–F250

10. Jorgensen PL (1980) Sodium and potassium ion pump in kidney tubules. Physiol Rev 60:864–917

11. De Wardener HE, Mills IH, Clapham WF, Hayter CJ (1961) Studies on the efferent mechanism of the sodium diuresis which follows the administration of intravenous saline in the dog. Clin Sci 21:249–263

12. Doucet A, Barlet C (1986) Evidence for differences in the sensitivity to ouabain of Na-K-ATPase along the nephrons of rabbit kidney. J Biol Chem 261:993–995

13. Sweadner KJ (1989) Isozymes of the Na^+/K^+-ATPase. Biochim Biophys Acta 988:185–220

14. El Mernissi G, Doucet A (1983) Short-term effect of aldosterone on renal sodium transport and tubular Na-K-ATPase in the rat. Pflugers Arch 399:139–146

15. El Mernissi G, Doucet A (1983) Short term effects of aldosterone and dexamethasone on Na-K-ATPase along the rabbit nephron. Pflugers Arch 399:147–151

16. Barlet-Bas C, Khadouri C, Marsy S, Doucet A (1988) Sodium-independent in vitro induction of Na-K-ATPase by aldosterone in renal target cells: permissive effect of triiodothyronine. Proc Natl Acad Sci USA 85:1707–1711

17. Verrey F, Schaerer E, Zoerkler P, Paccolat MP, Geering K, Kraehenbuhl JP, Rossier BC (1987) Regulation by aldosterone of Na^+, K^+-ATPase mRNAs, protein synthesis, and sodium transport in cultured kidney cells. J Cell Biol 104:1231–1237

18. Petty KJ, Kokko JP, Marver D (1981) Secondary effect of aldosterone on Na-K-ATPase activity in the rabbit cortical collecting tubule. J Clin Invest 68:1514–1521

19. Frelin C, Vigne P, Barbry P, Lazdunski M (1987) Molecular properties of amiloride action and of its Na^+ transporting targets. Kidney Int 32:785–793

20. Soltoff SP, Mandel LJ (1983) Amiloride directly inhibits the Na, K-ATPase activity of rabbit kidney proximal tubules. Science 20:957–959

21. Leffert HL, Koch KS, Fehlmann M, Heiser W, Lad PJ, Skelly H (1982) Amiloride blocks cell-free protein synthesis at levels attained inside cultured rat hepatocytes. Biochem Biophys Res Commun 108:738–745

22. Oberleithner H, Weigt M, Westphale HJ, Wang W (1987) Aldosterone activates Na^+/H^+ exchange and raises cytoplasmic pH in target cells of the amphibian kidney. Proc Natl Acad Sci USA 84:1464–1468

23. Fambrough DM, Wolitzky BA, Tamkun MM, Takeyasu K (1987) Regulation of the sodium pump in excitable cells. Kidney Int 32:S97–S112

24. Barlet-Bas C, Khadouri C, Marsy S, Doucet A (1990) Enhanced intracellular sodium concentration in kidney cells recruits a latent pool of Na-K-ATPase whose size is modulated by corticosteroids. J Biol Chem 265:7799–7803

25. Doucet A (1988) Multiple hormonal control of the Na/K-ATPase activity in the thick ascending limb. In: Davison AM (ed) Nephrology, vol 1. Baillière Tindall, London, pp 247–254

26. Schwartzman M, Ferreri NR, Carroll MA, Songu-Mize E, McGiff JC (1985) Renal cyto-chrome P450-related arachidonate metabolite inhibits $(Na^+ + K^+)$ ATPase. Nature 314: 620–622

27. Greger R (1985) Ion transport mechanisms in thick ascending limb of Henle's loop of mammalian nephron. Physiol Rev 65:760–797

28. Mazsik G, Kutas J, Nagy L, Nameth G (1974) Inhibition of Mg^{2+}, Na^+-K^+-dependent ATPase system in human gastric mucosa by prostaglandin E_1 and E_2. Eur J Pharmacol 29:133–137

29. Verna R (1984) Effects of prostaglandins on rat liver plasma membrane-bound Na^+-K^+-ATPase. In: Braquet P, et al (eds) Prostaglandins and membrane ion transport. Raven, New York, pp 227–233

30. Yasuko S, Hideramro O, Masarori S, Yasahiko S, Hisashi T (1982) Inhibitory effect of PGA_2 on Na-K-ATPase in synoptic plasma membrane of rat brain in vitro. Int J Biochem 14:347–350

31. Cordova HR, Kokko JP, Marver D (1989) Chronic indomethacin increases rabbit cortical collecting tubule Na^+-K^+-ATPase activity. Am J Physiol 256 (Renal Fluid Electrolyte Physiol 25)F570–F576

32. Wald H, Scherzer P, Rubinger D, Popovtzer MM (1990) Effect of indomethacin in vivo and PGE_2 in vitro on MTAL Na-K-ATPase of the rat kidney. Pflugers Arch 415:648–650

33. Kirschenbaum MA, Lowe AG, Trizna W, Fine LG (1982) Regulation of vasopressin action by prostaglandins. Evidence for prostaglandin synthesis in the rabbit cortical collecting tubule. J Clin Invest 70:1193–1204

34. Schlondorff D, Satriano JA, Schwartz GJ (1985) Synthesis of prostaglandin E_2 in different segments of isolated collecting tubules from adult and neonatal rabbits. Am J Physiol 248 (Renal Fluid Electrolyte Physiol 17):F134–F144

35. Nizet A, Lefèbvre P, Crabbé J (1971) Control by insulin of sodium potassium and water excretion by the isolated dog kidney. Pflugers Arch 323:11–20

36. Clausen T, Flatman JA (1987) Effects of insulin and epinephrine on Na^+-K^+ and glucose transport in soleus muscle. Am J Physiol 252 (Endocrinol Metab 15)E492–E499

37. Gelehrter TD, Shreve PD, Dilworth VM (1984) Insulin regulation of Na/K pump activity in rat hepatoma cells. Diabetes 33:428–434

38. Rosic NK, Standaert ML, Pollet RJ (1985) The mechanism of insulin stimulation of $(Na^+$-$K^+)$-ATPase transport activity in muscle. J Biol Chem 260:6206–6212

39. Cobb MH, Yang CPH, Brown JA, Scott WN (1986) Insulin stimulated sodium transport in toad urinary bladder. Biochim Biophys Acta 856:123–129

40. Fidelman ML, May JM, Biber TVL, Watlington CO (1982) Insulin stimulation of Na^+ transport and glucose metabolism in cultured kidney cells. Am J Physiol 242 (Cell Physiol 11):C121–C123

41. Resh MD, Nemenoff RA, Guidotti G (1980) Insulin stimulation of (Na^+,K^+)-adenosine triphosphatase dependent $^{86}Rb^+$ uptake in rat adipocytes. J Biol Chem 255:10938–10945

42. Lytton J (1985) Insulin affects the sodium affinity of the rat adipocyte (Na^+,K^+)-ATPase. J Biol Chem 260:10075–10080

43. Capasso G, Lin JT, DeSanto NG, Kinne R (1985) Short term effect of low doses of tri-
    iodothyronine on proximal tubular membrane Na-K-ATPase and potassium permeability in
    thyroidectomized rats. Pflugers Arch 403:90–96
44. Schultz SG (1981) Homocellular regulatory mechanisms in sodium-transporting epithelia:
    Avoidance of extinction by "flush-through." Am J Physiol 241 (Renal Fluid Electrolyte
    Physiol 10):F579–F590
45. Bertorello A, Aperia A (1989) Regulation of Na^+-K^+-ATPase activity in kidney proximal
    tubules: involvement of GTP binding proteins. Am J Physiol 256 (Renal Fluid Electrolyte
    Physiol 25):F57–F62

Properties and Function of the Kidney Vacuolar H+ ATPase: a Versatile Proton Pump Responsible for Urinary Acidification

STEPHEN GLUCK, BAHAR BASTANI, RAOUL NELSON, HENRY PURCELL, ZHI-QIANG WANG, KUN ZHANG, MICHAEL MARUSHACK, BETH LEE, XIAO-LI GUO, KHALID MASOOD, and PHILIP HEMKEN[1]

Introduction

Approximately 30%–40% of hydrogen ion transport in the proximal tubule, and most or all of proton transport in the distal nephron, is generated by proton pumps belonging to the vacuolar class of H+ATPases. This ubiquitous type of proton pump is found in all eukaryotic cells, where it serves to acidify intracellular compartments, such as endosomes, lysosomes, and secretory vesicles, in the endocytic and secretory pathways. Certain renal tubular epithelial cells have amplified the expression of the enzyme, and are able to direct it in a polarized manner to specific domains of the plasma membrane, where it carries out transepithelial proton secretion. How amplified expression and polarized localization are achieved, how the enzyme is regulated, and the abnormalities in these processes that underlie disease processes, remain among the most important unanswered questions in this field.

Structure of the Vacuolar H+ ATPases

Progress in understanding the structure and function of the vacuolar class of H+ATPases has come from studies in several systems, including the fungal and plant enzymes, and the kidney, coated vesicle, and chromaffin granule enzymes from mammalian sources. The vacuolar H+ATPases were first identified as electrogenic proton pumps that were resistant to azide and oligomycin, inhibitors of the mitochondrial proton pump, and resistant to vanadate, an inhibitor of the gastric electroneutral H+/K ATPase. The plant, fungal, and mammalian enzymes were all purified independently from different sources, but showed remarkably similar structures. The vacuolar H+ATPases are all 500–600000 molecular weight (Mr) proteins with, generally, at

---

[1]Depts. of Medicine and Cell Biology and Physiology, Washington University School of Medicine, and The Renal Division, Jewish Hospital, St. Louis, MO 63178, USA

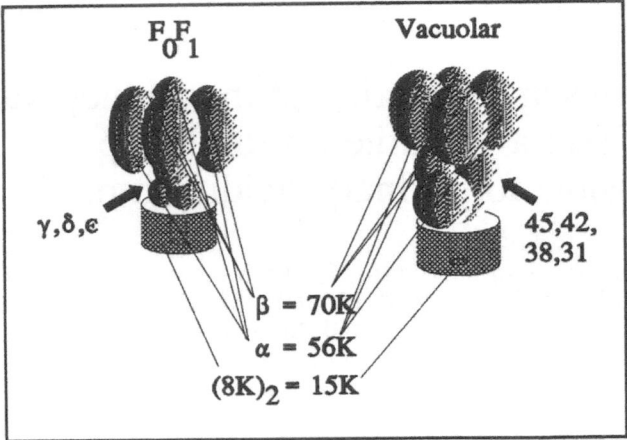

Fig. 1

least 8 different component subunits. All have subunits of approximately 70 kD, 56 kD, several subunits between 30 and 50 kD, and at least one low molecular weight subunit of 17 kD. In all of the enzymes, most of the large molecular weight proteins are peripheral membrane proteins that do not have any membrane spanning portions, and the small molecular weight proteins are intrinsic membrane proteins that span the lipid bilayer. Purification of the bovine kidney H^+ATPase by two different methods yielded an identical pattern of composite polypeptides with relative molecular weights of 70, 56 (a cluster), 45, 42, 38, 33, 31, 15, 14, and 12 kD.

Advance in understanding the basic structure of the enzyme and the function of the subunits has been relatively rapid because of the remarkable similarity of these enzymes to the F0F1 class of H^+ATPases, whose structure and function have been investigated extensively. The known structure of the F0F1 H^+ATPases has provided a conceptual framework for most of the experiments probing the structure of the vacuolar enzymes (Fig. 1). The α and β subunits which form the major structural part of the catalytic domain of the F0F1 ATPases share significant sequence homology with the 56 kD and 70 kD subunits of the vacuolar enzymes. Recent sequence analysis shows that the sequences of the 70 kD and 56 kD subunits are also highly similar to the two largest subunits of the archaebacterial H^+ATPases. Thus, it is likely that the vacuolar and F0F1 classes of H^+ATPases share a common ancestral proton pump, from which both diverged, dating back to the earliest life forms.

The vacuolar H^+ATPases have two major domains, the cytoplasmic domain and the transmembrane domain, each of which is composed of a multitude of subunits. The cytoplasmic domain is the locus of the catalytic and probably regulatory sites of the enzyme, and is composed of peripheral membrane proteins. The transmembrane domain forms the channel through which protons cross the lipid bilayer, and is composed of intrinsic membrane proteins which span the cytoplasmic domain and anchor it on the membrane (Fig. 2).

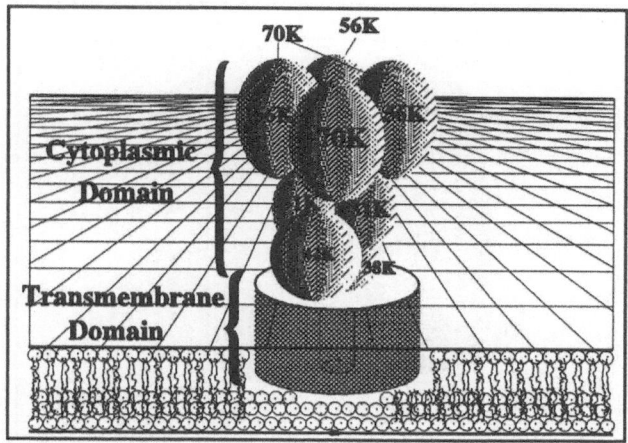

Fig. 2

The Cytoplasmic Domain

The 70 kD molecular weight of the vacuolar H⁺ATPases appears to be the site where ATP is hydrolyzed during proton transport. Thee are three duplicates of the subunit in each complete proton pump. The evidence available at present suggests that there is only one gene for the 70 kD subunit. The sequences of the 70 kD subunit and its homolog have a highly conserved domain in the mid coding region, which probably comprises the nucleotide binding and catalytic site. The sequence of the bovine kidney subunit, compared with the subunits of plant and fungal enzymes, shows wide divergence at the amino-terminal and carboxyl-terminal domains, with no sequence conservation. It is possible that these regions have a regulatory or non-catalytic role.

There are three duplicates of this subunit per H⁺ATPase as well. The function of the 56 kD subunit is uncertain. The subunit is homologous to the α subunit of the F0F1 H⁺ATPases. The α subunit does not have a catalytic ATP binding site, but is required for catalytic activity. It has a high affinity nucleotide binding site, which is though to be involved either in regulation of the enzyme, or as a non-hydrolytic part of the reaction mechanism. The function of the 56 kD subunit of the vacuolar H⁺ATPases is unknown, although evidence from the plant enzyme suggests that it may have an ATP binding site. In kidney H⁺ATPase, isolated by affinity chromatography on a monoclonal antibody column, several 56 kD subunits were observed which differed slightly in M_r. cDNA cloning of the subunit has revealed that there are at least two different isoforms of the 56 kD subunit in the kidney, and that these are encoded by different genes. The isoforms have 93% sequence identity in the mid coding region, but are completely different at the amino and carboxyl terminal domains. H⁺ATPase affinity purified from a bovine kidney cortex microsomal fraction had different enzymatic properties from H⁺ATPase isolated from bovine kidney brush border. The microsomal enzyme also exhibited a pattern of 56 kD polypeptides that differed from

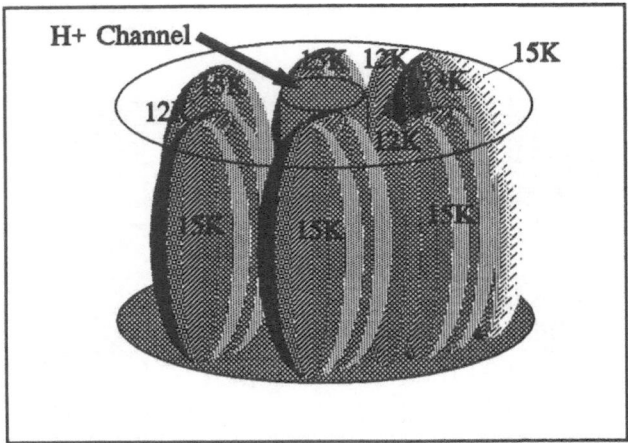

Fig. 3

the 56 kD subunit pattern in the H⁺ATPase isolated from brush border. The 56 kD subunit may therefore have an important role in determining the enzymatic properties or compartmentation of the vacuolar H⁺ATPase.

There are from one to three duplicates of the 31 kD subunit per H⁺ATPase; the exact composition is unresolved. Results to date indicate only one gene for this subunit in mammalian cells. The amino acid sequence of the subunit is 98% identical in different mammalian species, far higher than for the 70 and 56 kD subunits. The function of the 31 kD subunit is unknown. Experiments on the biosynthesis of the enzyme suggest a possible role in nucleating its extramembranous catalytic head. Free 70 and 56 kD subunits could be immunoprecipitated from the cytosol of 35-S methionine-labeled cultured renal cells, but free 31 kD subunit could not, although this subunit could be immunoprecipitated associated with the other two subunits.

The function of the other subunits of the cytosolic domain is not established, but they may constitute a "stalk" domain connecting the catalytic portion to the intrinsic membrane domain, a construction similar to that of the F0F1 enzymes.

The Transmembrane Domain

The transmembrane domain forms a proton conducting channel that spans the lipid bilayer. Although the entire composition of this portion of the enzyme remains in dispute, all of the vacuolar H⁺ATPases have an approximately 17 kD (or 15 kD in the kidney) polypeptide that reacts readily with the hydrophobic carboxyl reagent DCCD. The F0F1 H⁺ATPases all have a DCCD binding protein which is approximately 8 kD, and is present in 9 or more duplicates per enzyme. The 17 kD subunit of the mammalian and fungal H⁺ATPases has been cloned, and the vacuolar subunit appears to have arisen from a duplication and fusion of the F0F1 gene.

This suggests that this subunit forms at least part of the proton conducting channel spanning the membrane. The function of the other subunits is unclear. Evidence from other vacuolar H⁺ATPases suggests that the 33 kD subunit may be part of the transmembrane domain. By functional analogy with the F0F1 H⁺ATPases, it may serve as a binding and regulatory subunit for anchoring the cytosolic domain on the membrane.

Specialized Use of the Vacuolar H⁺ATPase in Renal Hydrogen Ion Excretion

As indicated above, most eukaryotic cells have the vacuolar H⁺ATPase primarily, or exclusively, on the plasma membrane. This is true even in cultured renal epithelial cells such as the LLC-PK1 and MDCK lines. However, some specialized cells, such as certain proton-transporting renal epithelial cells, are able to direct the enzyme to the plasma membrane and employ it to engender hydrogen ion or bicarbonate secretion. To do so, proton transporting renal epithelial cells impart four specialized functions to the vacuolar H⁺ATPase, functions not observed in other cells: 1) Amplified expression of the H⁺ATPase, 2) appearance of the enzyme in abundance on the plasma membrane, 3) polarization to different plasma membrane or cellular domains, and 4) physiologic regulation geared to maintain extracellular fluid homeostasis. How the kidney uses the enzyme to accomplish these tasks, while still employing vacuolar H⁺ATPases to acidify and energize transport in intracellular compartments, remains a central question.

Several lines of evidence indicate that the vacuolar H⁺ATPase in mammalian kidney is actually composed of a mixture of several different enzymes with subtle differences in structure. We postulate that these structural variations impart different physiologic properties to the enzyme, enabling renal cells to establish the differentiated functions outlined above. The first evidence for different forms of the H⁺ATPase was obtained from the SDS gels of fractions from a high performance liquid chromatography (HPLC) ion exchange column originally used to purify the bovine kidney enzyme (Fig. 4). Two partially resolved peaks of ATPase activity were observed eluting off the column. Gels of these revealed the complicated polypeptide composition described above. However, the first peak of ATPase activity had a polypeptide at Mr 58 kD, whereas the second peak of activity had a peak at 56 kD. This suggested that different forms of the ATPase might exist, which differed in the composition of the 56 kD subunit. Recent experiments have continued to provide support for this view. As discussed above, at least two different genes for the 56 kD subunit are expressed in mammalian kidney, and these differ in composition prominently at the amino and carboxyl termini, while the central portion, which contains the domain thought to participate in catalysis, is highly conserved.

A second approach to this question has been to compare the properties of vacuolar H⁺ATPase isolated from different kidney membrane compartments, such as microsomes (which likely includes plasma membrane from intercalated cells), and brush border microvilli. H⁺ATPase, purified from kidney microsomes and brush border on a monoclonal antibody affinity column and analyzed on 2D gels, revealed a different composition of polypeptides in the 56 kD Mr range. H⁺ATPase purified from brush

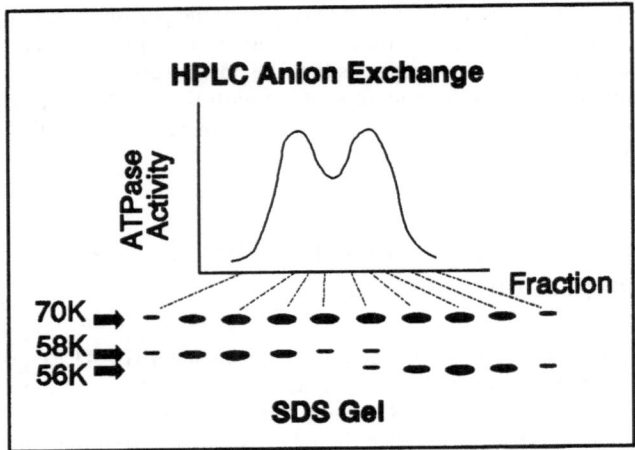

Fig. 4

border had different enzymatic properties from H⁺ATPase purified from renal microsomes, with different pH optima, ATP:GTP substrate preference, and response to the addition of various divalent cations. We have subsequently isolated H⁺ATPase from bovine kidney cortex lysosomes, and found that its properties differ from both the microsomal and brush border enzymes.

The 31 kD subunit may also be a site for variations in structure between different forms of the H⁺ATPase (Fig. 5). Two monoclonal antibodies, E11 and H8, were

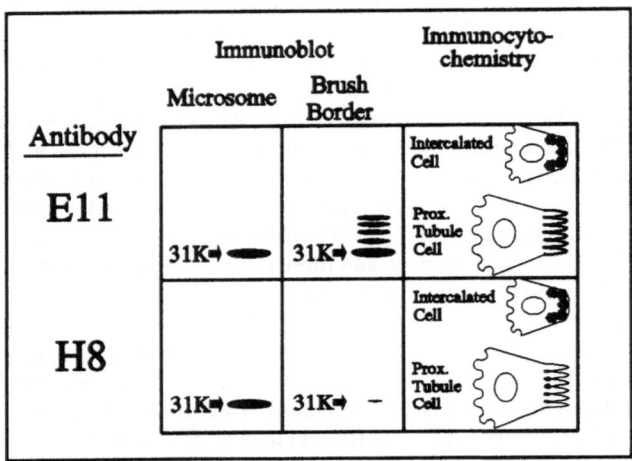

Fig. 5

generated to the 31 kD subunit. The patterns of reactivity of the two antibodies on immunoblots of the isolated brush border and microsomal H+ATPase, and the distribution of immunocytochemical staining with the two antibodies differed greatly. E11 reacted strongly with both the microsomal and brush border enzymes, but the brush border immunoblot showed several additional immunoreactive bands at apparent molecular weights slightly higher than 31 kD. H8 reacted strongly with the microsomal H+ATPase, but showed only faint immunoreactivity against the brush border enzyme. On immunocytochemistry, both E11 and H8 stained the intercalated cells strongly. E11 also stained both the brush border and the invaginations at the base of the brush border in the proximal tubule. H8 stained only the invaginations, and did not stain the brush border. These observations suggest that structural differences in the 31 kD subunit exist between the brush border and microsomal H+ATPase, and that the differences may have a role in directing the enzyme to the brush border. The higher molecular weight forms of the 31 kD subunit were visible on two dimensional silver stained gels of the purified brush border H+ATPase, but were not seen in the microsomal H+ATPase.

These observations show that enzymatic differences exist between vacuolar H+ATPase isolated from different kidney membrane fractions, and that structural differences can be detected in at least two of the subunits of the enzyme. It remains to be determined whether these differences in structure underlie the specialized functions of the vacuolar H+ATPase in epithelial cells, discussed above.

Mechanisms for Regulating Renal Hydrogen Ion Secretion

Hydrogen ion transport could be regulated, in principle, by three different mechanisms, illustrated in Fig. 6. Regulation could involve a redistribution of the enzyme,

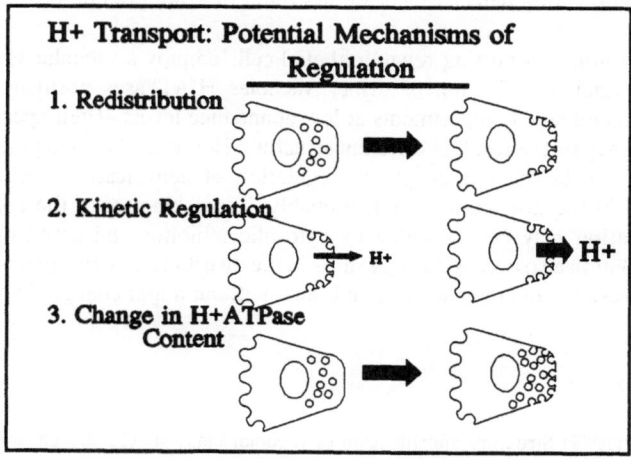

Fig. 6

kinetic regulation of the enzyme, or a change in the quantity of enzyme. Acute redistribution of the enzyme is known to occur in the kidney in response to a change in pCO_2. Increases in the pCO_2 stimulate the recruitment of $H^+ATPase$ from intracellular membrane vesicles, and its insertion in the plasma membrane. This response is prevented by the microtubule destabilizing agent, colchicine. Recent micropuncture studies have shown that in the outer stripe of the outer medulla, only half of the increase in hydrogen ion secretion in response to CO_2 is inhibited by colchicine, suggesting that mechanisms other than insertion operate to regulate hydrogen ion transport.

Our laboratory recently discovered that kidney cytosol contains proteins that both inhibit and stimulate the purified $H^+ATPase$, and that these proteins appear to do so by binding to the enzyme. The binding of the activator is enhanced at low pH, implying that the protein could activate the $H^+ATPase$, were cytosolic pH to fall. The binding of the inhibitor protein is prevented at low pH. The partially purified inhibitor suppresses both purified $H^+ATPase$ and proton transport in vesicles by up to 80%, but has no activity against Na-K, Ca^{2+}, or F0F1 ATPases. Though additional studies are needed to establish the cellular distribution and physiologic role of these proteins, they appear to be candidates as kinetic regulators.

Renal hydrogen ion excretion increases in response to acid loading, which has prompted the speculation that the response is, in part, due to an increase in the $H^+ATPase$ content of the intercalated cells. We examined this directly by using monoclonal antibodies and a cDNA clone probe for the 31 kD subunit to measure quantities of $H^+ATPase$ protein, 31 kD subunit transcript, and the distribution of the $H^+ATPase$ by immunocytochemistry in rats subjected to acid and alkali loading over a 14-day period. No change in 31 kD subunit protein or in mRNA levels was detected during the 2-week period, either in the cortex or in the medulla. In contrast, there was a striking change in the distribution of the enzyme. In both the inner and outer stripe of the outer medulla, acid loading produced a progressive shift of $H^+ATPase$ from intracellular vesicles to the plasma membrane. Similar changes were seen in a major subpopulation of intercalated cells in the cortex. Changes in the distribution of the $H^+ATPase$ also appear to have a role in the adaptive response of the remnant kidney, and in the acidification defect which follows relief of acute ureteral obstruction.

SUMMARY. Proton transporting renal epithelial cells employ a vacuolar $H^+ATPase$ to produce the final acidification of urine. Vacuolar $H^+ATPases$ normally reside in intracellular membrane compartments at low abundance levels. Their specialized use in renal cells may be the result of different structural isoforms of the enzyme that serve unique functions in the kidney. Acute regulation of acidification occurs through changes both in the distribution, and, probably, in the kinetics of the enzyme, and kinetic regulation may be controlled by cytosolic inhibitor and activator proteins. Chronic regulation also occurs through shifts in the distribution of the enzyme between intracellular vesicles and the plasma membrane, without major changes in abundance.

References

1. Forgac M (1989) Structure and function of vacuolar class of ATP-driven proton pumps. Physiol Rev 69:765–796
2. Steinmetz PR (1974) Cellular mechanisms of urinary acidification. Physiol Rev 54:890

3. Gluck S, Caldwell J (1988) Proton-translocating ATPase from bovine kidney medulla: partial purification and reconstitution. Am J Physiol (Renal Fluid Electrolyte Physiol 23)254:F71–F79
4. Gluck S, Caldwell J (1987) Immunoaffinity purification and characterization of vacuolar H⁺ATPase from bovine kidney. J Biol Chem 262:15 780–15 789
5. Yurko M, Gluck S (1987) Production and characterization of a monoclonal antibody to vacuolar H⁺ATPase of renal epithelia. J Biol Chem 262:15 770–15 779
6. Brown D, Gluck S, Hartwig J (1987) Structure of the novel membrane-coating material in proton-secreting cells and identification as an H⁺ATPase. J Cell Biol 105:1637–1648
7. Brown D, Hirsch S, Gluck S (1988) An H⁺ATPase in opposite plasma membrane domains in kidney epithelial cell subpopulations. Nature 331:622–624
8. Brown D, Hirsch S, Gluck S (1988) Localization of a proton-pumping ATPase in rat kidney. J Clin Invest 82:2114–2126
9. Madsen KM, Tisher CC (1984) Response of intercalated cells of rat outer medullary collecting duct to chronic metabolic acidosis. Lab Invest 51:268–276
10. Hirsch S, Strauss A, Masood K, Lee S, Sukhatme V, Gluck S (1988) Isolation and sequence of a cDNA clone encoding the 31-kDa subunit of bovine kidney vacuolar H⁺ATPase. Proc Natl Acad Sci USA 85:3004–3008
11. Alper S, Natale J, Gluck S, Lodish H, Brown D (1989) Intercalated cell subtypes in rat kidney collecting duct defined using antibodies against erythrocyte band 3 and renal vacuolar H⁺ATPase. Proc Natl Acad Sci USA 86:5429–5433
12. Gluck S, Cannon C, Al-Awqati Q (1982) Exocytosis regulates urinary acidification in turtle bladder by rapid insertion of H⁺ pumps into the luminal membrane. Proc Natl Acad Sci USA 79:4327–4331
13. Wang Z-Q, Gluck S (to be published) Isolation and properties of bovine kidney brush border vacuolar H⁺ATPase. A proton pump with enzymatic and structural differences from kidney microsomal H⁺ATPase. J Biol Chem
14. Wang Z-Q, Hemken P, Gluck S (1989) Role of the vacuolar H⁺ATPase 31K subunit in targeting to renal brush border. J Cell Biol 109:297a
15. Hemken P, Wang Z-Q, Gluck S (1990) Role of 31k subunit in targeting renal H⁺ATPase to brush border. Kidney Int 37:225a
16. Schwartz GJ, Al-Awqati Q (1985) Carbon dioxide causes exocytosis of vesicles containing H⁺ pumps in isolated perfused proximal and collecting tubules. J Clin Invest 75:1638–1644

Role of Ca^{2+} ATPase and Plasma Membrane Ca^{2+} Pump in Ca^{2+} Transport by the Mammalian Kidney

John T. Penniston[1]

SUMMARY. Current evidence suggests that Ca^{2+} transport in the distal nephron involves transit of Ca^{2+} through the epithelial cells and movement out of these cells on the basolateral side via the ATP-powered plasma membrane Ca^{2+} pump.

Introduction

In its role of reclaiming the Ca^{2+} from the filtrate, the kidney faces very different problems in the proximal and distal portions of the nephron. In the proximal nephron the freshly formed ultrafiltrate has nearly the same Ca^{2+} concentration as does the blood, so that the Ca^{2+} needs to be moved up only a very shallow concentration gradient as it moves into the blood. In the distal nephron, the Ca^{2+} concentration in the ultrafiltrate is very low and the remaining Ca^{2+} must be moved up a steep concentration gradient in order to reclaim it. Since plasma membrane Ca^{2+} pumps are ubiquitous in mammalian cells [1], it is natural to suppose that an asymmetrical distribution of the Ca^{2+} pumps in the epithelial cells of the nephron might be responsible for Ca^{2+} transport. In order for this to work, Ca^{2+} would have to enter the epithelial cells from the villous side and then be extruded by Ca^{2+} pumps located only on the basolateral side. This supposition has been supported by studies on plasma membranes isolated from whole kidney homogenates; when basolateral kidney membranes were isolated, they contained Ca^{2+} pump, consistent with the suggestion that Ca^{2+} pumps were present in these membranes, but not ruling out their presence in the villous membranes on the other side of the epithelium [2,3]. The studies on isolated plasma membranes also did not address the question of whether the amount and location of Ca^{2+} pump differed in the proximal and distal nephrons.

---

[1]Department of Biochemistry and Molecular Biology, Mayo Clinic, Rochester, MN 55905, USA

Table 1. Ca^{2+} pump and Na^+/Ca^{2+} exchange in Ca^{2+} efflux

	V_{max} nmol/(mg,min)	
	Ca^{2+} pump	Na^+/Ca^{2+} exchange
Kidney	80	10
Heart	90	1200

Additional information on localization was provided by the use of monoclonal antibody 5F10, raised against the human erythrocyte Ca^{2+} pump. This antibody cross-reacted with tissues other than erythrocyte and with species other than human. When applied to the kidney, this antibody stained specifically the basolateral side of epithelial cells only in the distal nephron (not in the proximal). This was observed in both human and rat kidneys [4,5]. This results suggests that the proximal and distal portions of the nephron employ different strategies to move Ca^{2+} across the epithelium. The lack of an obvious asymmetric staining in the proximal nephron may mean that transcellular Ca^{2+} transport is not highly important here, but that paracellular Ca^{2+} transport mechanisms are in operation. In paracellular transport, the Ca^{2+} does not pass into an epithelial cell, but rather passes through a channel between epithelial cells. This Ca^{2+} transport may be driven by the potential difference across the epithelial layer. On the other hand, the distal nephron must put more energy into the Ca^{2+} transport process in order to move Ca^{2+} up the steep concentration gradient between the filtrate and the blood. This can be done by allowing Ca^{2+} to diffuse passively into the cell. Although the Ca^{2+} concentration in the ultrafiltrate is much lower than that in the blood, it is high compared with that inside the cell, so that no energy input is needed for this phase of the Ca^{2+} movement. By allowing Ca^{2+} to enter the cell, the epithelium can employ the cell's highly developed mechanisms for controlling Ca^{2+}. In other types of cells, these same mechanisms are used to manage the intracellular Ca^{2+} signal, which controls contraction, secretion, etc. Once the Ca^{2+} has entered the cell, it must be exported through the basolateral membrane, up a 10000-fold concentration gradient. The necessity of moving Ca^{2+} up such a steep gradient is not unique to epithelial cells; in mammals all types of cells must extrude Ca^{2+} against such a gradient. The plasma membrane Ca^{2+} pump exists in all kinds of mammalian cells and is specialized for moving Ca^{2+} up this gradient. Thus, it appears likely that the specific staining for Ca^{2+} pump in the distal nephron reflects a special role for this pump in Ca^{2+} transport by the epithelial cells of the distal nephron.

In considering the ejection of Ca^{2+} from cells, the Na^+/Ca^{2+} exchanger must also be taken into account. This exchanger performs a specific exchange of Na^+ for Ca^{2+} in such a way that the gradient of Na^+ ions across the plasma membrane drives the ejection of Ca^{2+}. Table 1 is a brief summary of data accumulated by Van Os [6], showing the relative capacities of the Na^+/Ca^{2+} exchanger and the plasma membrane Ca^{2+} pump in kidney and in heart. As Table 1 shows, the Na^+/Ca^{2+} exchanger is extremely active in heart muscle (and also in nervous tissue and skeletal muscle). In these tissues, the exchanger probably moves most of the Ca^{2+} out of the cell. However, in kidney, the situation is very different; the Na^+/Ca^{2+} exchanger is present only in rather low concentrations and is probably not capable of moving very much Ca^{2+} out of the cell. This indicates that the Ca^{2+} pump is probably a primary mechanism of transepithelial Ca^{2+} transport.

We still do not know whether the packaging of Ca^{2+} into vesicles [7] is an important part of transcellular Ca^{2+} movements in any tissue. The formation of vesicles packed with Ca^{2+} at one side of the cell, followed by the movement of the vesicle through the cell and the dumping of this Ca^{2+} on the other side of the cell is still a possible mechanism for transcellular Ca^{2+} transport. However, no conclusive evidence in favor of the existence of such a mechanism has yet been introduced.

A feature of plasma membranes which complicates the study of the Ca^{2+} pump is the presence of non-pump Ca^{2+} ATPases. Plasma membranes in many kinds of cells have very active ATPases which are stimulated by the presence of Ca^{2+}. These ATPases are entirely separate from the Ca^{2+} pump and frequently are so high in activity as to mask the Ca^{2+} ATPase activity of the pump. Several different kinds of enzymes can give such ATPase activity, so that the use of ATPase to measure pump activity requires great care and definitive proof that the ATPase activity observed is due to the Ca^{2+} pump. In kidney plasma membranes, an ATPase activity stimulated by either Mg^{2+} or Ca^{2+} is present at an activity of about 700 nmol/(mg,min) [2,3,8]. This ATPase is not specific for ATP, but hydrolyzes other nucleotides equally well [2]. Compared to the ATPase activity of this enzyme, the ATPase due to the Ca^{2+} pump is relatively low in activity, being between 10 and 50 nmol/(mg,min). By taking special care, it is possible to demonstrate the presence of the Ca^{2+} ATPase due to the pump, but routine measurements of Ca^{2+} ATPase will measure primarily the other activity. Thus, in order to measure with certainty the activity of the Ca^{2+} pump in various parts of the kidney or along the nephron, it is necessary to measure Ca^{2+} uptake by inside-out plasma membrane vesicles or to measure Ca^{2+} ATPase with special precautions such as were used in the references cited above.

Four different genes which code for the plasma membrane Ca^{2+} pump in mammals are now known [9–12]. Northern blots performed on messenger RNA (mRNA) from rats shows that, of the first three isozymes, only the mRNA of isozyme 1 is present to a significant degree in rat kidney [11]. The mRNA for this isozyme was present in all tissues tested, so that kidney is not unusual in having it. The functions of the isozymes are not known, and much remains to be done in determining the details of the role of the plasma membrane Ca^{2+} pump in Ca^{2+} transport by the kidney.

References

1. Penniston JT (1983) Plasma membrane Ca^{2+}-ATPases as active Ca^{2+} pumps. In: Cheung WY (ed) Calcium and cell function, vol 4. Academic, New York, pp 99–149
2. Ghijsen W, Gmaj P, Murer H (1984) Ca^{2+}-stimulated Mg^{2+}-independent ATP hydrolysis and the high affinity Ca^{2+}-pumping ATPase. Two different activities in rat kidney basolateral membranes. Biochim Biophys Acta 778:481–488
3. van Heeswijk MPE, Geertsen JAM, van Os CH (1984) Kinetic properties of the ATP-dependent Ca^{2+} pump and the Na^+/Ca^{2+} exchange system in basolateral membranes from rat kidney cortex. J Membr Biol 79:19–31
4. Borke JL, Minami J, Verma A, Penniston JT, Kumar R (1987) Monoclonal antibodies to human erythrocyte membrane Ca^{2+}-Mg^{2+} adenosinetriphosphatase pump recognize an epitope in the basolateral membrane of human kidney distal tubule cells. J Clin Invest 80:1225–1231

5. Borke JL, Minami J, Verma AK, Penniston JT, Kumar R (1988) Co-localization of erythrocyte Ca^{2+}-Mg^{2+} ATPase and vitamin D-dependent 28-kilodalton calcium binding protein in the cells of human kidney distal tubules. Kidney Int 34:262–267
6. van Os CH (1987) Transcellular calcium transport in intestinal and renal epithelial cells. Biochim Biophys Acta 906:195–222
7. Terepka AR, Coleman JR, Armbrecht HJ, Gunter TE (1976) Transcellular transport of calcium. Symposia of the Society for Experimental Biology, No. XXX, Calcium in biological systems. Cambridge University Press, Cambridge, pp 117–140
8. Gmaj P, Murer H, Carafoli E (1982) Localization and properties of a high-affinity Ca^{2+} + Mg^{2+} ATPase in isolated kidney cortex plasma membranes. FEBS Lett 144:226–230
9. Verma AK, Filoteo AG, Stanford DR, Wieben ED, Penniston JT, Strehler EE, Fischer R, Heim R, Vogel G, Matthews S, Strehler-Page MA, James P, Vorherr T, Krebs J, Carafoli E (1988) Complete primary structure of a human plasma membrane Ca^{2+} pump. J Biol Chem 263:14152–14159
10. Strehler EE, James P, Fischer R, Heim R, Vorherr T, Filoteo AG, Penniston JT, Carafoli E (1990) Peptide sequence analysis and molecular cloning reveal two calcium pump isoforms in the human erythrocyte membrane. J Biol Chem 265:2835–2842
11. Greeb J, Shull GE (1989) Molecular cloning of a third isoform of the calmodulin-sensitive plasma membrane Ca^{2+}-transporting ATPase that is expressed predominantly in brain and skeletal muscle. J Biol Chem 264:18569–18576
12. Shull GE, Greeb J (1988) Molecular cloning of two isoforms of the plasma membrane Ca^{2+}-transporting ATPase from rat brain. Structural and functional domains exhibit similarity to Na^{+}, K^{+}- and other cation transport ATPases. J Biol Chem 263:8646–8657

Vitamin D and
Uremic Bone Disease

Chair: Francisco Llach (USA)
Shozo Koshikawa (Japan)

Vitamin D$_3$ and Uremic Bone Disease

HARMUT H. MALLUCHE and MARIE-CLAUDE FAUGERE[1]

SUMMARY. The failure of patients with renal insufficiency to produce vitamin D$_3$ plays a major role in the initiation and progression of uremic bone disease. The longevity that dialysis affords patients is accompanied by severe clinical symptoms which reduce the quality of life of chronically dialyzed patients.

Relative or absolute D$_3$ deficiency results in secondary hyperparathyroidism [1]. Research is under way to determine the mechanisms which link the diminished endocrine function of the kidneys and increased synthesis and secretion of parathyroid hormone (PTH) seen in patients with early renal failure [2–4].

The uremic bone disease seen in end-stage renal failure and in chronically dialyzed patients is caused by a variety of independent and interrelated factors. These factors include altered set point for calcium-regulated PTH secretion, phosphate retention, hypocalcemia, aluminum intoxication, metabolic acidosis, putative abnormalities in calcitonin secretion, primary kidney disease and dialytic therapies [5]. This explains the heterogeneity of the syndrome.

Histological Abnormalities of Uremic Bone Disease

Mild to Moderate Renal Failure

Uremic bone disease develops in the early stages of loss of kidney excretory function. Half of those patients with a glomerular filtration rate (GFR) equal to or less than 50% of normal exhibit abnormal bone histology. Bone biopsies indicate increased PTH activity, increased volume and surface of osteoid bone, and increased number of osteoclasts and osteoblasts. Mineralization status, as measured by tetracycline uptake, is usually normal until the GFR reaches 40 ml/min. Below 40 ml/min, woven

[1]Department of Medicine, Division of Nephrology, Bone and Mineral Metabolism, University of Kentucky Medical Center, Lexington, KY 40536-0084, USA

osteoid is present and some individuals exhibit impaired mineralization at the osteoid surface [6].

Advanced Renal Failure

When end-stage renal failure ensues, necessitating chronic dialysis, nearly all patients have abnormal bone histology and approximately 5% have stainable aluminum at the mineralization front [7].

Advanced renal bone disease can be divided into three primary histological groups: predominant hyperparathyroid bone disease, low turnover osteomalacia and adynamic bone disease, and mixed uremic osteodystrophy [8]. These groups do not represent fully separate entities and transformation from one form to another can occur. However, characterization is useful because therapy can be tailored according to the predominant histological finding.

Predominant Hyperparathyroid Bone Disease

This disease is seen in 5%–30% of dialyzed patients and is characterized by a marked increase in bone turnover due to longstanding, excessive PTH secretion. The morphological cellular abnormalities present are accompanied by profound perturbation of cell function. Excessive production of collagen fibers results in an increase in osteoid surface and volume. Osteoid is primarily of the woven, irregular type. Although mineralization sites and apposition rate are increased, as documented by tetracycline labelling, mineralization of woven osteoid is deficient and haphazard.

Cortical bone volume is reduced due to increased bone turnover, while cancellous bone volume depends upon calcium balance. However, bone mass cannot be equated with bone strength in predominant hyperparathyroid bone disease, because of the prevalence of mechanically deficient woven bone.

Low Turnover Osteomalacia and Adynamic Bone Disease

This disease is seen in 5%–35% of individuals on chronic maintenance dialysis and is characterized by a profound decrease in the number of active remodelling sites. In addition to aluminum overload, pathogenetic factors include parathyroidectomy, medications, and underlying disease.

The dramatic reduction in the number of bone forming and resorbing cells is associated with greatly diminished bone formation and mineralization. Osteoblasts in particular are reduced in number and/or activity.

Two subgroups may be characterized: adynamic bone disease, where few osteoid seams are present, and low turnover osteomalacia, where an accumulation of unmineralized matrix prevails.

Bone volume is usually reduced in adynamic uremic bone disease. Although total bone volume may vary in low turnover osteomalacia, mineralized bone volume is invariably low. This, in addition to increased osteoid, renders osteomalacic bone soft and subject to deformity and fractures.

Mixed Uremic Osteodystrophy

This disease is seen in 45%–80% of patients on chronic dialysis, and in most individuals in end-stage renal failure. Hyperparathyroidism and defective mineralization, with or without decreased bone formation, are pathogenetic factors in mixed uremic osteodystrophy.

Woven osteoid may be found adjacent to lamellar sites. Mineralization surfaces and apposition rates are increased in woven bone, whereas in lamellar bone the obverse is true.

Bone volume is variable within this group and is relative to the predominant pathogenetic factor.

Aluminum-Related Bone Disease

Aluminum-related bone disease may be found superimposed upon any of the three groups previously described.

Aluminum deposition at the bone-osteoid interface and within trabecules is seen in approximately 90% of patients with low turnover uremic bone disease, in 50% of patients with mixed uremic bone disease and in 10%–15% of those individuals with predominant hyperparathyroid osteodystrophy [7] for whom aluminum deposition should not be regarded as an epiphenomenon [9].

The influence of parathyroid hormone on aluminum-related bone disease is controversial. On the one hand, the occurrence of stainable aluminum in patients with predominent hyperparathyroid bone disease is less frequent than in the other types of uremic bone disease [7,10]. On the other hand, high serum PTH levels seem to augment aluminum uptake [11]. Indeed, clinicians point out that patients with severe hyperparathyroid bone disease may have higher total bone aluminum content than patients with aluminum-related osteomalacic.

Prophylaxis and Therapy of Uremic Bone Disease Using Vitamin D_3

Supplementation of the renal hormone vitamin D_3 has been in use since 1972 for the prevention of uremic bone disease. Reversal of secondary hyperparathyroidism and increased growth velocity in children have been observed.

Effects of Vitamin D_3 on Bone in Mild to Moderate Renal Failure

Widespread prophylactic use of the active vitamin D metabolite by $1,25D_3$ has been hampered by its cost, concern regarding a deleterious effect on renal function, and by the metabolite's tendency to suppress bone turnover. Recent trials using low dose therapy (not exceeding 0.50 µg/day) and careful monitoring of serum and urinary calcium failed to demonstrate impaired renal function [12]. Suppression of bone turnover can be avoided by intermittent therapy.

Effects of Vitamin D$_3$ on Bone in Advanced Uremic Bone Disease

Most studies indicate that vitamin D$_3$ has a beneficial effect on the biochemical and histological abnormalities seen in hyperparathyroid bone disease. The drug's effect on osteomalacic abnormalities must be re-evaluated in the light of aluminum's pathogenetic influence on uremic bone disease. Moreover, studies indicate that the presence or absence of aluminum may influence the efficacy of vitamin D$_3$ therapy.

Recently, 1,25(OH)$_2$D$_3$ became available for intravenous injection. Daily injections of vitamin D$_3$ may induce hypercalcemia, a situation further aggravated by use of calcium salts to bind aluminum. Alternative approaches such as "pulse therapy," with high doses of the metabolite given twice weekly at the end of dialysis, or modulation of calcium supplement, dialysate calcium, and oral vitamin D$_3$ dosage have been shown to decrease hyperparathyroidism while reducing the incidence of hypercalcemia [13–15].

The efficacy and safety of intravenous vitamin D$_3$ administration needs further study.

New Avenues for Research

Recent studies report the mechanisms involved in the effects of vitamin D$_3$ on bone histology [16].

Vitamin D$_3$ exerts an antiproliferative effect on bone cells and promotes their activity, whereas parathyroid hormone stimulates increased numbers of cells. This explains how vitamin D$_3$ suppresses the accelerated bone turnover characteristic of hyperparathyroid osteodystrophy (by decreasing parathyroid hormone secretion), but is able to promote normal lamellar bone growth. In contrast, vitamin D$_3$ is of little value in low turnover states characterized by a paucity of bone cells.

Parathyroid hormone had long been thought to be influenced solely by abnormalities in plasma calcium. Current studies in our laboratory indicate that during early renal failure serum phosphorus and calcium concentrations increase as 1,25 vitamin D$_3$ levels decline. This is followed by increased PTH levels, while calcium remains elevated and serum phosphorus decreases toward normal. After normalization of serum phosphorus, serum calcium remains high and serum 1,25 Vit D$_3$ rises. Consequently, we have advanced the hypothesis that PTH secretion (secondary hyperparathyroidism) functions as a compensatory mechanism used to correct low levels of circulating vitamin D$_3$ occurring during the earliest stages of loss of kidney function.

References

1. Oldham SB, Smith R, Hartenbower DL (1979) The acute effects of 1,25-dihydroxycholecalciferol on serum immunoreactive parathyroid hormone in the dog. Endocrinology 104:248–254
2. Silver J, Russell J, Serwood LM (1985) Regulation by vitamin D metabolites of messenger ribonucleic acid for preproparathyroid hormone in isolated bovine parathyroid cells. Proc Natl Acad Sci USA 82:4270–4273

3. Lopez-Hilker S, Galceran T, Chan U-L, Rapp N, Martin KJ, Slatopolsky E (1986) Hypocalcemia may not be essential for the development of secondary hyperparathyroidism in chronic renal failure. J Clin Invest 78:1097–1102
4. Faugere M-C, Friedler RM, Fanti P, Malluche HH (1988) Lack of histologic signs of Vit D deficiency in early development of renal osteodystrophy. J Bone Mineral Res 3(Suppl 1):S95
5. Malluche HH, Faugere M-C (1990) Renal bone disease 1990: An unmet challenge for the nephrologist. Kidney Int 38:193–211
6. Maluche HH, Ritz E, Lange HP, Lutschere K, Hodgson M, Seiffert U, Schoeppe W (1976) Bone histology in incipient and advanced renal failure. Kidney Int 9:355–362
7. Smith AJ, Faugere M-C, Abreo K, Fanti P, Julian B, Malluche HH (1986) Aluminum related bone disease in mild and advanced renal failure. Evidence for high prevalence and morbidity, and studies on etiology and diagnosis in 197 patients. Am J Nephrol 6:275–283
8. Malluche HH, Faugere M-C (1986) Atlas of Mineralized Bone Histology. S. Karger, New York
9. Malluche HH, Faugere M-C, Smith AJ, Friedler RM (1986) Aluminum intoxication of bone in renal failure: Fact or fiction? Kidney Int 29(Suppl 18):70–73
10. Ott SM, Maloney NA, Coburn JW, Alfrey AC, Sherrard DJ (1982) The prevalence of bone aluminum deposition in renal osteodystrophy and its relation to the response to calcitriol therapy. N Engl J Med 307:709–713
11. Alfrey AC, Sedman A, Chan Y-L (1985) The compartmentalization and metabolism of aluminum in uremic rats. J Lab Clin Med 105:227–233
12. Baker LRI, Abrams SML, Roe CJ, Faugere M-C, Fanti P, Subayti Y, Malluche HH (1989) 1,25(OH)₂D₃ administration in moderate renal failure: A prospective double-blind trial. Kidney Int 35:661–669
13. Slatopolsky E, Weerts C, Thielan J, Horst R, Harter H, Martin KJ (1984) Marked suppression of secondary hyperparathyroidism by intravenous administration of 1,25-dihydroxycholecalciferol in uremic patients. J Clin Invest 74:2136–2143
14. Salusky IB, Goodman WC, Norris KC, Horst R, Fine RN, Coburn JW (1988) Bioavailability of calcitriol: comparison of oral, intravenous and intraperitoneal routes of administration in CAPD patients (abstract). Kidney Int 33:250
15. Andress DL, Norris KC, Coburn JW, Slatopolsky EA, Sherrard DJ (1989) Intravenous calcitriol in refractory osteitis fibrosa of chronic renal failure. N Engl J Med 321:274–279
16. Malluche HH, Matthews CM, Faugere M-C, Fanti P, Friedler RM (1986) 1,25 dihydroxyvitamin D maintains bone cell activity and parathyroid hormone modulates bone cell number in dogs. Endocrinology 119:1298–1304

The Therapeutic Role of 24,25 Dihydroxycholecalciferol in Dialysis Patients with Secondary Hyperparathyroidism

MORDECAI M. POPOVTZER[1]

SUMMARY. In early renal insufficiency, secondary hyperparathyroidism can be controlled with calcium/vitamin D and low-phosphate intake. In advanced disease, secondary hyperparathyroidism becomes refractory, displaying variable suppression with high levels of $1,25(OH)_2D_3$. However, $1,25(OH)_2D_3$ directly blocks bone formation and induces resorption, the latter being undesirable.

As shown in experimental and clinical studies, $24,25(OH)_2D_3$ administration (1) lowers parathyroid hormone (PTH) mRNA, (2) directly blocks PTH action on the bone, (3) reduces osteoclast number, suppresses resorption, and normalizes mineralizing surface, when combined with 1 alpha$(OH)D_3$ analogues. These findings demonstrate that $24,25(OH)_2D_3$, combined with 1 alpha$(OH)D_3$, reverses the osseous abnormalities of secondary hyperparathyroidism and proves to be an effective therapy for uremic osteodystrophy in patients on chronic dialysis.

Introduction

Secondary hyperparathyroidism is evident in the majority of patients with chronic renal disease, even in those with minimal functional impairment [1–4]. The pathogenesis of this abnormality is still unknown. In the early phase of renal disease there is already a decrease in the urinary excretion and an increase in the fractional reabsorption of calcium and an increase in the fractional excretion of phosphate, both factors reflecting secondary hyperparathyroidism [3,4]. Serum levels of calcium and phosphate are not significantly altered, whereas $1,25(OH)_2D_3$ levels are variable, but still in the normal range [5,6]. At this early stage the parathyroid hyperactivity is amenable to suppression by intravenous calcium [1,4] and can be normalized with dietary phosphate restriction and oral physiological doses of $1,25(OH)_2D_3$ [7]. As

[1]Nephrology and Hypertension Services, Hadassah University Hospital, 91120 Jerusalem, Israel

renal failure progresses the parathyroid glands become less suppressible [1,4] and eventually become refractory to most medical treatments. The end-organ damage that is caused by secondary hyperparathyroidism consists of an incapacitating bone disease, osteitis fibrosa cystica [8], metastatic calcifications, and presumed damage to many other systems, including the central nervous system, the bone marrow, and the heart muscle.

The deleterious consequences of secondary hyperparathyroidism have led to clinical trials in which attempts have been made to optimize the management of this complication. Attempts to reduce PTH levels by calcium supplementation have met with variable success [9]. In patients with end-stage renal disease the parathyroid glands exhibit a reduced sensitivity to calcium suppression. This abnormality can be quantitated by the assessment of the "set point," which is defined as the calcium level that produces 50% of the maximum decrement in PTH level. In patients on dialysis there is a shift in that "set point," i.e., to achieve a 50% of maximum suppression of PTH, "supraphysiological" degrees of hypercalcemia are necessary [10]. Yamamoto et al. [11] have recently shown that in rats with normal kidney function, sustained moderate hypercalcemia can elicit a significant decrease in the steady state levels of PTH messenger RNA in the parathyroid tissue. This finding implied that hypercalcemia not only suppresses the secretion, but also inhibits the synthesis of PTH. The effect of sustained hypercalcemia on messenger RNA levels in rats with chronic renal failure has not been studied in detail. Hypercalcemia induced by the intravenous infusion of calcium in patients on dialysis fails to produce a substantial decrease in PTH level [10].

Vitamin D Treatment of Secondary Hyperparathyroidism

In vivo experiments have demonstrated that physiological or nearly physiological amounts of $1,25(OH)_2D_3$ inhibit the levels of messenger RNA, independent of serum calcium levels [12,13]. These findings, reported in rats with both normal and reduced renal effects of $1,25(OH)_2D_3$ on PTH-gene transcription, suggested that this active metabolite of vitamin D directly regulates PTH synthesis. Furthermore, it has been shown that the suppression of PTH mRNA by $1,25(OH)_2D_3$ is dose-dependent [12,13].

In patients undergoing chronic dialysis, the oral administration of 1 alpha-hydroxylated analogues of vitamin D, in many instances, failed to elicit a therapeutically effective suppression of PTH [15,16]. Two major disadvantages are inherent in the oral route of administration. First, the direct action on the gut absorption of minerals may result in prohibitively high concentrations of calcium and phosphate that limit continuation of therapy. Second, the enhanced intestinal break-down of orally administered $1,25(OH)_2D_3$ [17] precludes achievement of high serum levels of this metabolite, which are essential for a direct suppression of PTH synthesis in uremic patients.

In view of the above limitations of oral therapy with 1 alpha-hydroxylated analogues of vitamin D, the intravenous route of administration has emerged. In clinical studies, intravenous administration of $1,25(OH)_2D_3$ was associated with a striking increase in serum levels that led to a fall in PTH levels, an effect which could not be accomplished with equal oral doses of $1,25(OH)_2D_3$ [15]. The suppression of PTH levels in uremic patients receiving the intravenous $1,25(OH)_2D_3$ was apparent before measurable changes in serum calcium were evident [15]. Furthermore, the intravenous administration of $1,25(OH)_2D_3$ was associated with a shift toward normal in the set point for PTH suppression [10]. In a recent clinical trial it was shown that long term treatment with intravenous $1,25(OH)_2D_3$, in patients with secondary hyperparathyroidism undergoing chronic dialysis, was associated with significant changes in bone histology [16]. These changes consisted of a striking and significant decrease in bone formation without significant changes in the osteoclast number [16]. The authors commented that these changes in bone histology could not be fully explained by the suppression of PTH, and a possible direct effect of $1,25(OH)_2D_3$ on the bone was implied. High levels of $1,25(OH)_2D_3$ are known to exert a direct effect on the bone which is independent of the inhibitory effect on PTH secretion. This direct effect on the bone consists of: 1] An induction of osteoclast differentiation from proliferating and from post-mitotic precursors, 2] an enhanced formation of multinucleated cells bearing the characteristics of osteoclasts including an augmented osteoclastic resorption [18–22], 3] a decrease in the rate of bone matrix apposition and a decrease in the rate of osteoblast proliferation, 4] a suppression of collagen synthesis [18–25], and 5] an impairment of bone mineralization [22]. It is felt that the anabolic effects of $1,25(OH)_2D_3$ on bone growth are mediated by its intestinal actions through an increased supply of calcium and phosphate to the bone [22]. Popovtzer et al. [27] were the first to demonstrate a complete clinical and histological healing of vitamin D deficiency osteomalacia in man, without vitamin D therapy, solely with the intravenous administration of calcium and phosphate.

The net effect of high levels of $1,25(OH)_2D_3$ on bone metabolism will be determined by the balance of the two main processes triggered by this active metabolite:

1) Suppression of PTH secretion.
2) Direct action on the bone.

Suppression of PTH will remove the major stimulus for the increased bone turnover rate which is the main feature of secondary hyperparathyroidism. This will reduce equally both the bone formation and the bone resorption. In clinical studies, the intravenous administration of $1,25(OH)_2D_3$ was associated with a reduction in PTH [16]; however, even after a prolonged treatment the PTH level was still very high. Through its direct action $1,25(OH)_2D_3$ will reduce bone formation, yet will increase bone resorption. Thus, the interaction between declining PTH levels and high $1,25(OH)_2D_3$ will result in a synergism with respect to bone formation, but will result in an antagonism with respect to bone resorption (see Table 1). This interaction will invariably result in reduced bone formation, whereas the effect on resorption will vary.

In a recent report we described the effects of high doses of $1,25(OH)_2D_3$ in rats with 5/6 nephrectomy [28]. The elevated PTH in these animals declined to a normal level and bone formation decreased markedly; however, the osteoclast number did not change significantly. Similar results were recorded in a recent clinical study employing long-term intravenous therapy with $1,25(OH)_2D_3$ in uremic patients with secondary hyperparathyroidism [16]. There was a significant fall in PTH levels, normalization of bone formation rate, and a non-significant change in the osteoclast count.

The above clinical and experimental studies suggest that high circulating concentrations of $1,25(OH)_2D_3$ may suppress PTH hyperactivity, however, their direct resorptive actions on the bone may be therapeutically counterproductive (Table 1).

Table 1. Effects of the interaction of $1,25(OH)_2D_3$ with suppressed PTH on bone metabolism

	Bone formation	Bone resorption
1. Direct effect of $1,25(OH)_2D_3$ on the bone	↓	↑
2. Effect of suppressed PTH on the bone[a]	↓	↓
3. Net result of the combined effects of 1. and 2. on the bone	↓↓	0

[a]Suppressed by high levels of $1,25(OH)_2D_3$. ↓, Decreased; ↑, Increased

In this regard, the administration of $24,25(OH)_2D_3$ in combination with 1 alpha hydroxylated metabolites of vitamin D, as will be further elaborated, may be the optimal formulation of vitamin D therapy for uremic patients.

Treatment with $24,25(OH)_2D_3$ in Combination with 1 Alphahydroxylated Analogues of Vitamin D

Experimental Studies

The exact physiological function of $24,25(OH)_2D_3$ has not yet been fully elucidated. There is, however, an accumulation of experimental and clinical data suggesting a biological role for $24,25(OH)_2D_3$ in bone metabolism. Galus et al. [29] showed, in vitamin D deficient dogs, that the administration of $24,25(OH)_2D_3$ increased bone formation and mineralization, but decreased bone resorption, while 1 alpha(OH)D_3 increased both bone mineralization and bone resorption. Thus, the difference in the action of these two metabolites was with respect to bone resorption; $24,25(OH)_2D_3$ effected a decrease while 1 alpha(OH)D_3 caused an increase in this parameter.

In a dose-dependent manner, $24,25(OH)_2D_3$ blocked PTH-activated adenylate cyclase in rat calvaria and in osteoblastic cells [30,31], but enhanced calcitonin-stimulated adenylate cyclase. Long-term administration of $24,25(OH)_2D_3$ to vitamin D replete rats obliterated PTH-sensitive adenylate cyclase activity in crude calvarial membrane fractions [31]. Activation of adenylate cyclase is believed to be the mechanism of the skeletal action of PTH. Specific inhibition of this activity by $24,25(OH)_2D_3$ both in vivo and in in vitro experiments, suggests that $24,25(OH)_2D_3$ interferes directly with the skeletal action of PTH [30–32].

We have shown that $24,25(OH)_2D_3$ suppresses the hypercalcemic effect of $1,25(OH)_2D_3$ in rats with reduced renal mass (5/6 nephrectomy), a model of chronic renal failure with secondary hyperparathyroidism [33]. Furthermore, our histomorphometric bone studies demonstrated that the effect of $24,25(OH)_2D_3$ in blunting the hypercalcemic effect of $1,25(OH)_2D_3$ was associated with striking decrease in osteoclastic activity [34]. In this experimental model, even though $1,25(OH)_2D_3$ lowered the elevated PTH to normal levels, it reduced osteoclastic bone resorption only modestly [28]. The combined administration of $24,25(OH)_2D_3$ with $1,25(OH)_2D_3$ elicited the most profound suppression of osteoclastic resorption, even though it did not reduce the PTH to a level below that achieved with $1,25(OH)_2D_3$

alone. These findings implied that $24,25(OH)_2D_3$ acts to reverse osteoclastic bone resorption in rats with chronic renal failure, independent of PTH suppression. The synergism with $1,25(OH)_2D_3$, however, is probably related to calcitriol's inhibitory action on PTH secretion.

In rats with intact kidney function, $24,25(OH)_2D_3$ similarly to $1,25(OH)_2D_3$, suppresses the levels of prepro PTH mRNA. It is, however, less potent than $1,25(OH)_2D_3$ in this regard. At a dose of 100 pmol, $24,25(OH)_2D_3$ elicits a 52% decrease in prepro PTH mRNA in 24 hours, compared with an 82% reduction with an equimolar dose of $1,25(OH)_2D_3$ [12,13]. Fukagawa et al. [14] have recently shown, in rats 4 weeks after 5/6 nephrectomy, a steady state elevation of PTH mRNA. They were able to suppress the elevated PTH mRNA with either 100 pmol of $1,25(OH)_2D_3$ or 500 pmol of $24,25(OH)_2D_3$. Fukagawa et al. suggested that the diminished levels of these 2 metabolites of vitamin D in chronic renal failure may play a critical role in the pathogenesis of secondary hyperparathyroidism. These results suggest that $24,25(OH)_2D_3$ directly suppresses PTH synthesis. This effect, however, is by far smaller when compared with that of $1,25(OH)_2D_3$.

Clinical Studies

Brickman et al. [35] and Piraino et al. [36] demonstrated a calcium lowering effect of $24,25(OH)_2D_3$, both in normocalcemic and in hypercalcemic patients undergoing chronic hemodialysis. It has been pointed out that when $24,25(OH)_2D_3$ is added to 1 alpha-hydroxylated analogues of vitamin D it lowers the risk of hypercalcemia and increases the tolerance to these agents.

Long-term administration of $24,25(OH)_2D_3$, in combination with dehydrotachysterol, to children undergoing chronic hemodialysis brought about a 70% reduction in bone surface covered with osteoclasts [37].

Mortensen et al. [31,32] showed that serum levels of $24,25(OH)_2D_3$ in normals and in patients with chronic renal failure were inversely correlated with PTH-stimulated adenylate cyclase from iliac crest biopsies. The adenylate cyclase activity correlated directly with bone resorption. This finding was interpreted to indicate that $24,25(OH)_2D_3$ serves as an important physiological modulator of PTH-induced bone resorption. Mortensen et al. [32] extended their observations by investigating 3 groups of uremic patients: (1) Patients treated with $1,25(OH)_2D_3$ alone, (2) patients treated with a high dose of $24,25(OH)_2D_3$, and (3) patients treated with a combination of both $1,25(OH)_2D_3$ and $24,25(OH)_2D_3$. Net bone PTH-activated adenylate cyclase was completely abolished after 2 months of treatment with $24,25(OH)_2D_3$ or with the combination, while $1,25(OH)_2D_3$ alone yielded a minor decrease in the enzyme activity. The authors concluded that the effect of $24,25(OH)_2D_3$ might be to restore normal bone turnover in uremia in concert with $1,25(OH)_2D_3$.

We have conducted the first controlled trial evaluating the effect of $24,25(OH)_2D_3$ combined with 1 alpha$(OH)D_3$, as compared with the effect of 1 alpha$(OH)D_3$ alone on renal osteodystrophy in patients undergoing chronic hemodialysis [38].

Fifty eight patients were randomly divided into: (1) a control group receiving 1 alpha$(OH)_2D_3$ alone and (2) a combined treatment group receiving both $24,25(OH)_2D_3$ and 1 alpha$(OH)D_3$. In 41 patients two bone biopsies, the first pretrial and the second at the end of the trial, about 12 months apart, were suitable for histomorphometric analysis. Nineteen patients were in the control and 22 in the

Table 2. Effects of the interaction of $1,25(OH)_2D_3$ and $24,25(OH)_2D_3$ with suppressed PTH on bone metabolism

	Bone formation	Bone resorption
1. Direct effect of $1,25(OH)_2D_3$ on the bone	↓	↑
2. Direct effect of $24,25(OH)_2D_3$ on the bone	↑	↓↓
3. Effect of suppressed PTH on the bone[a]	↓	↓
4. Net result of the combined effects of 1., 2., and 3. on the bone	↓	↓↓

[a]Suppressed both by high levels of $1,25(OH)_2D_3$ and by $24,25(OH)_2D_3$.
↓, Decreased; ↑, Increased

combined treatment group. No differences between the control and the combined treatment group were recorded in $25(OH)D_3$ and $1,25(OH)_2D_3$ levels in the serum; $24,24(OH)_2D_3$ levels remained below normal in the control, but increased markedly in the combined treatment groups. Changes from the first to the second biopsy in the control were compared with those in the combined treatment group. A striking decrease (-10.5%) in the eroded surface was observed in the combined treatment, but not in the control group, leading to a significant difference in this change between the two groups ($P < 0.01$). A significant decrease ($-0.22mm^{-1}$) in the osteoclast number was observed in the combined treatment, but not in the control group, resulting in a significant difference in this change between the two groups ($P < 0.05$). Likewise, a significant decrease (-15.8%) in mineralizing surface was recorded in the combined treatment, but not in the control group, leading to a significant difference in this change between the 2 groups ($P < 0.01$). An increase ($+5.6\%$) in bone volume was recorded in the control, but not in the combined treatment group, resulting in a significant difference in this change between the 2 groups ($P < 0.01$).

The above results clearly demonstrated that the combined administration of $24,25(OH)_2D_3$ with 1 alpha(OH)D$_3$ produced a striking improvement in the hyperparathyroid bone disease [38]. This was highlighted by a substantial fall in osteoclast number and a reduction in mineralizing surface. As summarized in Table 2, the combined administration of $24,25(OH)_2D_3$ with 1 alphahydroxylated vitamin D$_3$ features an optimal integrated treatment with vitamin D. Not only does $24,25(OH)_2D_3$ attenuate the effects of bone-resorbing factors, including those of PTH, but it also facilitates the effects of 1 alphahydroxylated vitamin D analogues in suppressing PTH secretion. Furthermore, $24,25(OH)_2D_3$ has no significant side-effects. These unique attributes make $24,25(OH)_2D_3$ an important therapeutic agent in the treatment of uremic osteodystrophy when given in combination with 1 alphahydroxylated vitamin D analogues.

References

1. Reiss E, Canterbury JH, Canter A (1969) Circulating PTH in chronic renal failure. Arch Intern Med 124:417–420

2. Popovtzer MM, Massry SG, Coburn JW, Kleeman CR (1969) The interrelationship between sodium, calcium and magnesium excretion in advanced renal failure. J Lab Clin Med 73:763–771
3. Popovtzer MM, Schainuck Ll, Massry SG, Kleeman CR (1970) Divalent ion excretion in chronic kidney disease. Relation to degree of renal insufficiency. Clin Sci 38:297–307
4. Popovtzer MM, Massry SG, Coburn JW, Koppel M, Drinkard JH, Kleeman CR (1970) Calcium infusion test in chronic renal failure. Nephron 7:400–412
5. Llach F, Massry SG (1985) On the mechanism of secondary hyperparathyroidism in moderate renal insufficiency. J Clin Endocrinol Metab 61:601–606
6. Wilson L, Felsenfeld A, Drezner MK (1985) Altered divalent ion metabolism in early renal failure: role of 1,25(OH)$_2$D$_3$. Kidney Int 27:565–573
7. Portale AA, Booth BE, Halloran BP, Morris RC (1984) The effect of dietary phosphorus on circulating concentrations of 1,25(OH)$_2$D$_3$ and immunoreactive parathyroid hormone in children with moderate renal insufficiency. J Clin Invest 73:1580–1589
8. Huffer WE, Kuzela D, Popovtzer MM (1975) Metabolic bone disease in chronic renal failure. I. Dialyzed uremics. Am J Pathol 78:365–385
9. Popovtzer MM, Pinggera WF, Hutt MH, Robinette J, Halgrimson CG, Starzl TE (1972) The effect of sustained normocalcemia on serum levels of parathyroid hormone and renal handling of phosphorus in patients with chronic renal disease. J Clin Endocrinol Metab 35:213–218
10. Delmez JA, Tindira C, Grooms P, Dusso A, Windus DW, Slatopolsky E (1989) Parathyroid hormone suppression by intravenous 1,25-dihydroxyvitamin D. J Clin Invest 83:1349–1355
11. Yamamato M, Igarashi T, Muramatsu M, Fukagawa M, Motokra T, Ogata E (1989) Hypocalcemia increases and hypercalcemia decreases the steady-state level of parathyroid hormone messenger RNA in the rat. J Clin Invest 83:1053–1056
12. Silver J, Naveh-Many T, Mayer H, Schmelzer HJ, Popovtzer MM (1986) Regulation by vitamin D metabolites of parathyroid hormone gene transcription in vivo in the rat. J Clin Invest 78:1296–1301
13. Silver J, Naveh-Many T, Schmelzer H, Mayer H, Popovtzer MM (1987) Vitamin D metabolites regulate PTH gene transcription in vivo in the rat. In: DV Cohn, TJ Martin, PJ Meunier (eds) Calcium regulation and bone metabolism. Basic and clinical aspects, vol 9. Excerpta Medica, Amsterdam, pp 782–784
14. Fukagawa M, Kaname S, Igarashi T, Kurokawa K (1989) Regulation of PTH messenger RNA levels in parathyroid glands of chronic renal failure in rats. Kidney Int 35:392A.
15. Slatopolsky E, Weerts C, Thielan J, Horst R, Harter H, Martin KJ (1984) Marked suppression of secondary hyperparathyroidism by intravenous administration of 1,25-dihydroxycholecalciferol in uremic patients. J Clin Invest 74:2136–2143
16. Andress DL, Norris KC, Coburn JW, Slatopolsky E, Sherrard DJ (1989) Intravenous calcitriol in the treatment of refractory osteitis fibrosa of chronic renal failure. N Engl J Med 321:274–279
17. Napoli JL, Premanik BC, Royal PM, Reinhardt TA, Horst RL (1983) Intestinal synthesis of 24-keto 1,25-dihydroxyD$_3$. J Biol Chem 258:2100–2107
18. Raisz LG, Trummel CL, Holick MF, DeLuca HF (1972) 1Alpha,25-dihydroxycholecalciferol, a potent stimulator of bone resorption in tissue culture. Science 175:768–769
19. Bar-Shavit Z, Teitelbaum SL, Rietsma P, Hall A, Peg LE, Trail J, Kahn AJ (1983) Induction of monocytic differentiation and bone resorption by 1,25-dihydroxyvitamin D$_3$. Proc Natl Acad Sci USA 80:5907–5911
20. Pharaoh M, Heersche JNM (1985) 1,25-dihydroxyvitamin D$_3$ causes an increase in the number of osteoclast-like in cat bone marrow cultures. Calcif Tissue Int 37:276–281

21. McSeehy PMJ, Chambers TJ (1987) 1,25-Dihydroxyvitamin D_3 stimulates rat osteoblastic cells to release a soluble factor that increases osteoclastic bone resorption. J Clin Invest 80:425–428
22. Raisz LG (1990) Recent advances in bone cell biology: interactions of vitamin D with other local and systemic factors. Bone Min 9:191–197
23. Hock JM, Kream BE, Raisz LG (1982) Autoradiographic study of the effect of 1,25-dihydroxyvitamin D_3 on bone matrix synthesis in vitamin D replete rats. Calcif Tissue Int 34:347–351
24. Raisz LG, Kream BE, Smith MD, Simmons HA (1980) Comparison of the effects of vitamin D metabolites on collagen synthesis and resorption of fetal rat bone in organ culture. Calcif Tissue Int 32:135–138
25. Rowe DW, Kream BE (1982) Regulation of collagen synthesis in fetal rat calvaria by 1,25-dihydroxyvitamin D_3. J Biol Chem 257:8009–8015
26. Skjodt H, Gallagher JA, Beresford JN, Couch M, Poser JW, Russell RG (1985) Vitamin D metabolites regulate osteocalcin synthesis and proliferation of human bone cells in vitro. J Endocrinol 105:391–396
27. Popovtzer MM, Matthay R, Alfrey A, Block M, Beck P, Reeve EB (1973) Vitamin D deficiency osteomalacia: Healing of the bone disease in the absence of vitamin D with intravenous calcium and phosphorus infusion. In: Frame B, Parfitt AM, Duncan H (eds) Clinical aspects of metabolic bone disease. International Congress Series No. 270. Excerpta Medica, Amsterdam, pp 382–387
28. Rubinger D, Moscovitz A, Popovtzer MM, Bernheim J, Bab I, Gazit D (1990) $24,25(OH)_2D_3$ in combination with calcitriol reverses osteoclastic hyperactivity in chronic renal failure (CRF): evidence for a direct effect on the bone. Kidney Int 37:451A
29. Galus K (1980) Effects of 1alpha-hydroxyvitamin D_3 and 24,25-dihydroxyvitamin D_3 on bone remodeling. Calcif Tissue Int 31:209–213
30. Gordeladze JO, Gautvik KM (1986) Hydroxycholecalciferols modulate parathyroid hormone and calcitonin sensitive adenylyl cyclase in bone and kidney of rats. A possible physiological role for 24,25-dihydroxyvitamin D_3. Biochem Pharmacol 35:899–902
31. Mortensen B, Gordeladze JO, Aksnes L, Gautvik KM (1990) Long term administration of vitamin D_3 metabolites alters PTH-responsive osteoblastic adenylate cyclase in rats. Calcif Tissue Int 46:339–345
32. Mortensen B, Klem KH, Jablonski G, Haug E, Aarseth HP, Gautvik KM, Gordeladze JO (1990) The permissive role of $24,25(OH)_2D_3$ in treatment of renal osteodystrophy. Calcif Tissue Int 46:A56
33. Rubinger D, Cojocaru T, Popovtzer MM (1987) $24,25(OH)_2D_3$ attenuates the calcemic effect of $1,25(OH)_2D_3$ in rats with reduced renal mass. Proc Soc Exp Biol Med 186:64–69
34. Rubinger D, Moscovitz A, Popovtzer MM, Bab I, Gazit D (1989) $24,25(OH)_2D_3$ in combination with $1,25(OH)_2D_3$ ameliorates renal osteodystrophy in rats. Kidney Int 35:379(A)
35. Brickman AS, Llach FL, Coburn JW (1979) Preliminary report of biological actions of $24,25(OH)_2D_3$ in normal man and in patients with advanced renal failure. In: Norman, Schaefer, Herrath, Grigsleit, Coburn, DeLuca, Mawer, Suda (eds) Vitamin D, basic research and its clinical applications. Walter de Gruyter, Berlin, pp 1085–1090
36. Piraino BM, Rault R, Greenberg A, Dominguez JH, Wallia R, Houck P, Segre GV, Chent T, Foti FM, Puschett JB (1986) Spontaneous hypercalcemia in patients undergoing dialysis. Etiologic and therapeutic considerations. Am J Med 80:607–615
37. Van Diemen-Steenvoorde R, Donckerwolcke RA, Visser WJ, Raymakers JA, Duursma SA (1985) Treatment of renal osteodystrophy in children with dihydrotachysterol and 24,25-dihydroxyvitamin D_3. Clin Nephrol 24:292–299
38. Popovtzer MM (1989) $24,25(OH)_2D_3$ (OSTEO-D) combined with 1alpha(OH)D_3 is an effective therapy for uremic bone disease. Report of the Collaborative Israeli Multicenter trial. Calcif Tissue Int 44:S–86

The Future of New Vitamin D Analogs in Uremic Bone Disease

ALEX BROWN, JANE FINCH, SILVIA LOPEZ-HILKER, ADRIANA DUSSO,
JEREMIAH MORRISSEY, JUNKO ABE, TAKASHI MORI, YASUHO NISHII[2],
and EDUARDO SLATOPOLSKY[1]

SUMMARY. The spectrum of activities promoted by calcitriol has been found to extend far beyond a role in calcium homeostasis. Calcitriol has been shown to have important immunomodulating properties. The major limitation of calcitriol therapy is its accompanying calcemic activity. The recent development of analogs of vitamin D, that retain the properties of calcitriol with less calcemic activity, may offer a potential therapeutic tool in the treatment of uremic bone disease and other clinical conditions such as psoriasis and leukemia. Among these analogs 22-oxacalcitriol (OCT), $1,25\text{-}(OH)_2\text{-}24\text{-homo-}D_3$, $1,25\text{-}(OH)_2\text{-}22\text{-ene-}24\text{-homo-}D_3$, formerly MC 903 (now Calcipotriol), and $1,25\text{-}(OH)_2\text{-}16\text{-ene-}23\text{-yne-}D_3$ have been shown to have important biological effects.

In studies in rats and dogs OCT has a low calcemic activity both in vitro and in vivo. In primary culture of bovine parathyroid cells, OCT is as active as calcitriol in suppressing parathyroid hormone (PTH) release. In studies in normal and uremic rats, OCT produced a significant decrease in pre-pro PTH mRNA. In addition, OCT decreased PTH secretion in dogs with chronic renal failure. This analog may provide a unique therapeutic tool for the treatment of secondary hyperparathyroidism in patients with chronic renal failure.

Introduction

In the past 10 years the biological functions induced by $1,25\text{-}(OH)_2D_3$ (calcitriol) have been found to extend far beyond a role in calcium homeostasis. Calcitriol has been shown to have important cell differentiating activities and immunomodulating properties. Because hypercalcemia may preclude the administration of large

[1] The Renal Division, Department of Medicine, Washington University School of Medicine, St. Louis, MO 63110, USA
[2] Chugai Pharmaceutical Company Limited, 2-1-9 Kyobashi, Chuo-ku, Tokyo, 104 Japan

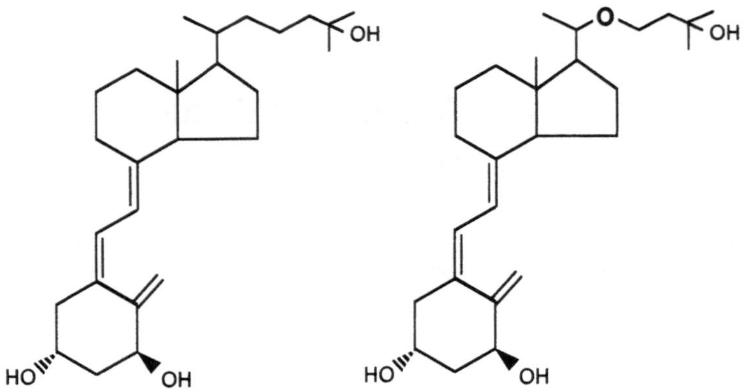

1α, 25(OH)$_2$D$_3$
calcitriol

22-oxa-1α, 25(OH)$_2$D$_3$
22-oxacalcitriol (OCT)

Fig. 1. Structure of 1,25-(OH)$_2$D$_3$ and 22-oxa-1,25-(OH)$_2$D$_3$[22-oxa-calcitriol (OCT). (Modified from [2])

doses of vitamin D in certain clinical disorders, the recent development of analogs of vitamin D that retain the properties of calcitriol with less calcemic activity may offer a potential therapeutic tool for the treatment of secondary hyperparathyroidism and renal osteodystrophy.

New Analogs of Vitamin D with Low Calcemic Activity

In 1986, Murayama et al. [1] studied the effects of a new analog with selective activity. This compound, 22-oxacalcitriol (OCT), developed by Chugai Pharmaceutical Co. in Japan, differs from 1,25-(OH)$_2$D$_3$ solely by the substitution of an oxygen atom for the methylene group at carbon 22 (Fig. 1). Abe et al. [2] demonstrated that OCT is more effective than 1,25-(OH)$_2$D$_3$ in suppressing cell growth and in inducing phagocytic activity in a mouse myelomonocytic leukemia cell line, WEHI-3. In addition, OCT is 10 times more effective than 1,25-(OH)$_2$D$_3$ in suppressing cell growth and in inducing phagocytic activity in a human leukemia cell line, HL-60. Despite this higher activity, OCT was found to bind 14 times less avidly to chicken intestinal receptor [1]. Calcemic activity was tested in vitro by measuring release of ^{45}Ca from prelabelled fetal mouse calvaria. OCT appeared to be 50–100 times less effective than 1,25-(OH)$_2$D$_3$ [2]. This low calcemic activity of OCT has been confirmed in vivo in both mice [2] and rats [3]. This analog is 100 times less effective than 1,25(OH)$_2$D$_3$ in mobilizing bone calcium and 1000 times less effective in stimulating intestinal calcium transport. Subsequently, Abe et al. [4] demonstrated that OCT markedly enhanced the immune response in mice. When mice were injected with a dose of antigen (10^7 sheep erythrocytes) that gave a submaximal antibody response, treatment with either OCT or 1,25-(OH)$_2$D$_3$ significantly increased the number of antibody-producing spleen cells. OCT was 50 times more potent than 1,25-(OH)$_2$D$_3$.

Fig. 2. Northern blot analysis of cytoplasmic RNA extracted from the parathyroid glands of normal, 1,25-$(OH)_2D_3$-treated and OCT-treated rats. The blot was hybridized with PTHm122cDNA. (Reproduced from the *Journal of Clinical Investigation* by copyright permission of the American Society for Clinical Investigation [3])

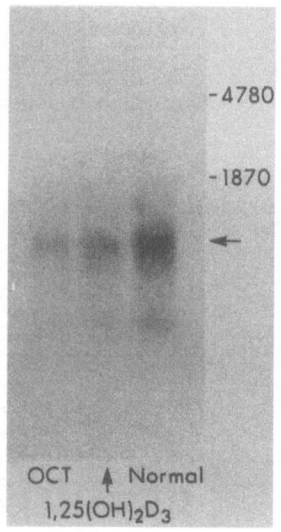

The doses of OCT that enhance the immune response are much lower than those capable of increasing serum calcium.

Further investigations of the activities of OCT by Brown et al. [3] have demonstrated that this analog can suppress the synthesis and secretion of PTH. The ability of OCT to suppress PTH secretion was assessed initially in primary cultures of parathyroid cells. Exposure of the cells to various doses of OCT and 1,25-$(OH)_2D_3$ for 48 hours revealed a similar dose-dependent inhibition of PTH secretion by these two compounds. The suppressive action of OCT in vivo was confirmed by measuring the pre-pro PTH mRNA levels in the parathyroid glands of normal rats 48 hours after a single 40 ng dose of 1,25-$(OH)_2D_3$ or OCT. Northern analysis and slot blot analysis showed that both 1,25-$(OH)_2D_3$ and OCT suppressed PTH mRNA levels by about 60%–80% (Fig. 2).

More recently in a preliminary study, we have confirmed that OCT effectively suppressed N-terminal PTH levels in dogs with chronic renal failure [5]. Administration of a single intravenous dose of 5 µg OCT decreased PTH by 80% toward normal levels in 24 hours. PTH levels were still suppressed at 69 hours. With this dose of OCT, no changes in serum calcium or phosphorus were observed (Fig. 3). Further studies indicate that even lower doses of OCT are capable of suppressing PTH to a similar degree. These data indicate that OCT may be effective for the treatment of secondary hyperparathyroidism.

In 1987, Ostrem et al. [6,7] demonstrated the effects of non-calcemic analogs that retained the ability of 1,25-$(OH)_2D_3$ to differentiate myeloid leukemia cells. Two of the analogs, 1,25-$(OH)_2$-24-homo-D_3 and 1,25-$(OH)_2$-22-ene-24-homo-D_3 had very low bone mobilizing activity. On the other hand, these analogs were about 10 times more potent than 1,25-$(OH)_2D_3$ in differentiating HL-60 cells, as assessed by the appearance of the macrophage-like activities, non-specific esterase and phagocytosis, after four days of exposure to the compounds. These analogs contain an extra carbon atom in the side chain; one also contains a double bond at the 22 position.

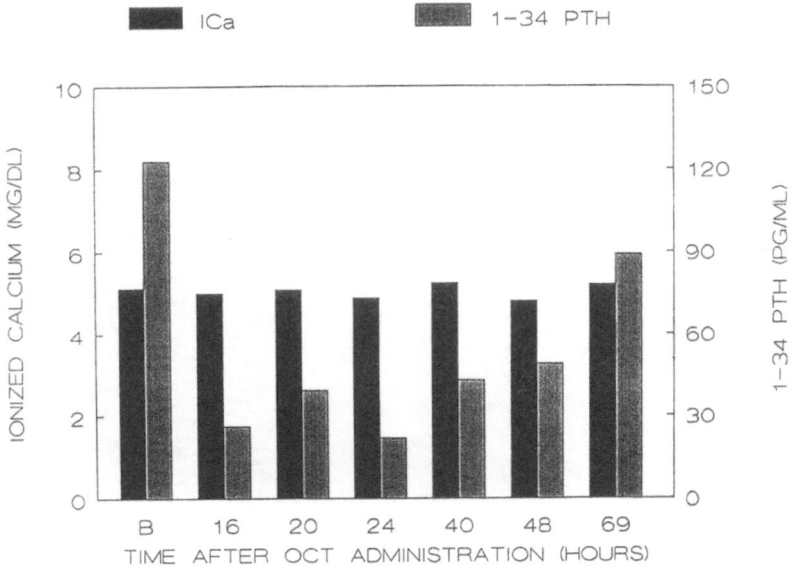

Fig. 3. The effects of a single dose of OCT (5 µg), given intravenously, on ionized calcium and amino-terminal PTH in a dog with chronic renal failure. (Reprinted from *Kidney International* with permission [5])

In 1988, Leo Pharmaceutical Products in Denmark [8] developed a new analog which was originally designated as MC 903 but is now referred to as calcipotriol. In this compound, the 26 and 27 carbons of the vitamin D side chain have been joined in a cyclopropyl ring, and the hydroxyl group is at the 24 position. Also, there is a double bond at the 22 position. This analog has twice the activity of $1,25\text{-}(OH)_2D_3$ in blocking the proliferation of the histiocytic lymphoma cell line, U937. The calcemic response of MC 903 was assessed in normal rats on 1% calcium diet following daily intraperitoneal administration for one week. This analog was more than 200 times less potent than $1,25(OH)_2D_3$ in its ability to increase urinary and serum calcium and decrease bone mass. Two clinical studies [9,10] have reported that topically-applied MC 903 is effective in the treatment of psoriasis, but has no effect on serum ionized calcium.

Recently Zhou et al. [11] tested eight analogs for their effects on hemopoietic cell growth and calcium metabolism. The most potent of these analogs in HL-60 cells is $1,25\text{-}(OH)_2\text{-}16\text{-ene-}23\text{-yne-}D_3$. This compound is four times more effective than $1,25\text{-}(OH)_2D_3$ in blocking HL-60 cell growth but is 33 times less active in stimulating intestinal calcium absorption and 50 times less active in bone calcium mobilization.

The general properties of these non-calcemic analogs can be summarized as follows: (1) All of these analogs are modified in the side chain, implicating this portion of the molecule in their selective action; (2) All of these analogs show selective activity on leukemia cells. They are more active than $1,25\text{-}(OH)_2D_3$ in the differentiation of these malignant cells, but have much lower calcemic activity. (3) One analog,

OCT, is active in vivo in suppressing PTH synthesis and secretion and in enhancing the immune response, indicating that the lack of calcemic activity, at least for this analog, is not due to rapid clearance or inactivation in vivo.

The reason for the selective action of these analogs is not clear. Every analog tested had a relatively low affinity for the vitamin D binding protein (DBP) ranging from 50–500 times less than that of $1,25\text{-}(OH)_2D_3$. The possible consequences of this low affinity for DBP are: (1) A higher proportion of the analog will be in the free, or active, form. This may explain why the analogs have a higher differentiating activity than expected based on the receptor-binding affinity. All leukemia cell cultures contained serum, usually 10%, during incubation with vitamin D compounds. Under these conditions, the greater proportion of the analogs will be unbound and more accessible to the cells. This hypothesis has not yet been tested. Bikle and Gee [12] indicate that in keratinocyte cell culture the free rather than the total $1,25\text{-}(OH)_2D_3$ is responsible for the regulation of $25(OH)D_3$ metabolism; (2) The analogs will be cleared more rapidly from the circulation which generally will decrease their effectiveness. Presumably, one of the important functions of DBP is to prolong the lifetime of $1,25\text{-}(OH)_2D_3$ in the circulation. Despite the more rapid clearance, however, OCT is still active in vivo on the parathyroid glands and the immune system; (3) The low affinity for DBP suggests that these analogs may be carried by other serum proteins. Okano et al. [13] demonstrated that OCT is associated primarily with lipoproteins. A number of other possibilities also exist for the selective action of these analogs. Rapid degradation in the non-responsive target tissues, bone and intestine, may prevent the action of the analogs. Currently, little is known about the metabolism of any of these vitamin D analogs. Recently, Tanaka et al. [14] demonstrated that during differentiation of HL-60 cells, OCT differs from $1,25\text{-}(OH)_2D_3$ in that it does not increase cytosolic calcium or prime the cells for oxidative burst. It is not known whether OCT is defective in stimulating cytosolic calcium in all target tissues or whether this phenomenon is related to its lack of calcemic activity. Although currently there is no clear explanation for the selective action of these analogs, their low calcemic activity may be useful for the treatment of a number of diseases that have been shown to respond to $1,25\text{-}(OH)_2D_3$.

Therapeutic Potential of Non-Calcemic Analogs of Vitamin D

Suda and his co-workers demonstrated that $1,25\text{-}(OH)_2D_3$ could differentiate myeloid leukemia cells from both mice and humans to non-proliferating monocyte/macrophage-like cells [15,16]. Smith et al. demonstrated an effect of $1,25\text{-}(OH)_2D_3$ in the normal maturation of skin cells [17]. These newly discovered functions of $1,25\text{-}(OH)_2D_3$ have also suggested new therapeutic uses of this hormone for the treatment of leukemia and psoriasis. The major limitation of $1,25\text{-}(OH)_2D_3$ therapy is its accompanying calcemic activity. Thus, several investigators are currently determining the potential clinical application of these new vitamin D analogs. M C903 has been shown to be effective in the treatment of psoriasis [9,10]. Morimoto et al. demonstrated that OCT inhibited the growth of psoriatic fibroblasts more effectively than $1,25\text{-}(OH)_2D_3$ [18]. We have found that OCT suppresses PTH synthesis and secretion. Studies in normal rats clearly demonstrated that OCT has a significant suppressive effect on pre-pro PTH mRNA. In addition, in preliminary studies on dogs with chronic renal failure, OCT greatly decreased the levels of circulating PTH, with no change in serum ionized calcium. This may be of utmost importance in the treatment of secondary hyperparathyroidism in patients with renal failure. The control of serum phosphorus is critical before calcitriol is administered to uremic patients. Since the long term administration of phosphate-binders containing aluminum is associated with a multitude of deleterious effects, calcium carbonate is currently the phosphate-binder of choice. However, the simultaneous administration of large doses of calcium carbonate, e.g., 6–10 gm daily, and calcitriol frequently induces severe hypercalcemia, precluding the administration of therapeutic doses of calcitriol. Thus, OCT, an analog of vitamin D which is without a calcemic effect, but which has properties similar to those of calcitriol in its action on PTH synthesis and release, may provide a unique therapeutic tool for the treatment of secondary hyperparathyroidism in patients with chronic renal failure.

References

1. Murayama E, Miyamoto K, Kubodera N, Mori T, Matsunaga I (1986) Synthetic studies of vitamin D_3 analogues. VIII. Synthesis of 22-oxavitamin D_3 analogues. Chem Pharm Bull (Tokyo) 34:4410–4413
2. Abe J, Morikawa M, Miyamoto K, Kaiho S-I, Fukushima M, Miyaura C, Abe E, Suda T, Nishii Y (1987) Synthetic analogues of vitamin D compounds with an oxygen atom in the side chain. FEBS Lett 226:58–62
3. Brown AJ, Ritter CS, Finch JL, Morrissey J, Martin KJ, Murayama E, Nishii Y, Slatopolsky E (1989) The noncalcemic analogue of vitamin D, 22-oxacalcitriol, suppresses parathyroid hormone synthesis and secretion. J Clin Invest 84:728–732
4. Abe J, Takita Y, Nakano T, Miyaura C, Suda T, Nishii Y (1989) A synthetic analogue of vitamin D_3, 22-oxa-1,25-dihydroxyvitamin D_3, is a potent modulator of in vivo immunoegulating activity without inducing hypercalcemia in mice. Endocrinology 124:2645–2647
5. Brown AJ, Finch JL, Lopez-Hilker S, Dusso A, Ritter C, Pernalete N, Morrissey J, Nishii Y, Slatopolsky E (1990) New active analogues of vitamin D with low calcemic activity. Kidney Int 38 S 29 22–27
6. Ostrem VK, Lau WF, Lee SH, Perlman K, Ikekawa N (1987) Induction of monocytic differentiation of HL-60 cells by 1,25-dihydroxyvitamin D analogues. J Biol Chem 262:14164–14171
7. Ostrem VK, Tanaka Y, Prahl J, DeLuca HF, Ikekawa N (1987) 24-and 26-homo-1,25-dihydroxyvitamin D_3: Preferential activity in inducing differentiation of human leukemia cells HL-60 in vitro. Proc Natl Acad Sci USA 84:2610–2614
8. Binderup L, Bramm E (1988) Effects of a novel vitamin D analogue MC903 on cell proliferation and differentiation in vitro and on calcium metabolism in vivo. Biochem Pharmacol 37:889–895
9. Staberg B, Roed-Petersen J, Menne T (1989) Efficacy of topical treatment in psoriasis with MC903, a new vitamin D analogue. Acta Derm Venereol (Stockh) 69:147–150
10. Kragballe K (1989) Treatment of psoriasis by the topical application of the novel cholecalciferol analogue calcipotriol (MC 903). Arch Dermatol 125:1647–1652
11. Zhou J-Y, Norman AW, Lubbert M, Collins ED, Uskokovic MR, Koeffler HP (1989) Novel vitamin D analogues that modulate leukemic cell growth and differentiation with little effect on either intestinal calcium absorption or bone calcium mobilization. Blood 74:82–93
12. Bikle DD, Gee E (1989) Free, and not total, 1,25-dihydroxyvitamin D regulates 25-hydroxyvitamin D metabolism by keratinocytes. Endocrinology 124:649–654

13. Okano T, Tsugawa N, Masuda S, Takeuchi A, Kobayashi T, Nishii Y (1989) Protein-binding properties of 22-Oxa-1α, 25-dihydroxyvitamin D₃, a synthetic analogue of 1α,25-dihydroxyvitamin D₃. J Nutr Sci Vitaminol (Tokyo) 35:529-533
14. Tanaka H, Hruska KA, Seino Y, Nishii Y, Teitelbaum SL (1989) Dissociation of the macrophage-maturational effects of vitamin D from respiratory burst priming. J Bone Mineral Res 4:S197
15. Abe E, Miyaura C, Sakagami H, Takeda M, Konno K, Yamazaki T, Yoshiki S, Suda T (1981) Differentiation of mouse myeloid leukemia cells induced by 1,25-dihydroxyvitamin D₃. Proc Natl Acad Sci USA 78:4990-4994
16. Tanaka H, Abe E, Miyaura C, Kuribayashi T, Konno K, Nishii Y, Suda T (1982) 1,25-Dihydroxycholecalciferol and a human myeloid leukemia cell line (HL-60). Biochem J 204:713-719
17. Smith EL, Walworth NC, Holick MF (1986) Effect of 1,25-dihydroxyvitamin D₃ on the morphologic and biochemical differentiation of cultured human epidermal keratinocytes grown in serum-free conditions. J Invest Dermatol 86:709-714
18. Morimoto S, Imanaka S, Koh E, Shiraishi T, Nabata T, Kitano S, Muyashita Y, Nishii Y, Ogihara T (1989) Comparison of the inhibitions of proliferation of normal and psoriatic fibroblasts by 1α,25-dihydroxyvitamin D₃ and synthetic analogues of vitamin D₃ with an oxygen atom in their side chain. Biochem Int 19:1143-1149